For Reference

The GALE
ENCYCLOPEDIA of
NEUROLOGICAL
DISORDERS

The GALE
ENCYCLOPEDIA *of*
NEUROLOGICAL
DISORDERS

VOLUME

2

M - Z

GLOSSARY

INDEX

STACEY L. CHAMBERLIN, BRIGHAM NARINS, EDITORS

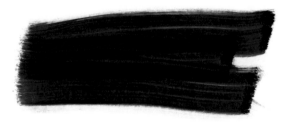

THOMSON

★ ™

GALE

Detroit • New York • San Francisco • San Diego • New Haven, Conn. • Waterville, Maine • London • Munich

The Gale Encyclopedia of Neurological Disorders

Project Editors
Stacey L. Chamberlin, Brigham Narins

Editorial
Erin Watts

Editorial Support Services
Andrea Lopeman

Indexing Services
Synapse

Rights Acquisitions Management
Margaret Chamberlain, Jackie Jones, Shalice Shah-Caldwell

Imaging and Multimedia
Randy Basset, Lezlie Light, Dan Newell, Robyn V. Young

Product Design
Michelle DiMercurio, Tracey Rowens, Kate Scheible

Composition and Electronic Prepress
Evi Seoud, Mary Beth Trimper

Manufacturing
Wendy Blurton, Dorothy Maki

LIBRARY OF CONGRESS CATALOGING-IN-PUBLICATION DATA

The Gale encyclopedia of neurological disorders / Stacey L. Chamberlin, Brigham Narins, editors.
        p.   ; cm.
    Includes bibliographical references and index.
    ISBN 0-7876-9150-X (set hardcover : alk. paper) — ISBN
0-7876-9151-8 (v. 1) — ISBN
0-7876-9152-6 (v. 2)
    1. Neurology—Encyclopedias.
    [DNLM: 1. Nervous System Diseases—Encyclopedias—English. 2. Nervous System Diseases—Popular Works. WL 13 G151 2005] I. Title: Encyclopedia of neurological disorders. II. Chamberlin, Stacey L. III. Narins, Brigham, 1962– IV. Gale Group.

RC334.G34 2005
616.8'003—dc22
                                                2004021644

CONTENTS

LIST OF ENTRIES

A

Abulia
Acetazolamide
Acupuncture
Acute disseminated encephalomyelitis
Adrenoleukodystrophy
Affective disorders
Agenesis of the corpus callosum
Agnosia
AIDS
Alcohol-related neurological disease
Alexander disease
Alpers' disease
Alternating hemiplegia
Alzheimer disease
Amantadine
Amnestic disorders
Amyotrophic lateral sclerosis
Anatomical nomenclature
Anencephaly
Aneurysms
Angelman syndrome
Angiography
Anosmia
Anticholinergics
Anticonvulsants
Antiepileptic drugs
Antimigraine medications
Antiparkinson drugs
Antiviral drugs
Anxiolytics
Aphasia
Apraxia
Arachnoid cysts
Arachnoiditis
Arnold-Chiari malformation
Arteriovenous malformations
Aspartame
Asperger's disorder
Assistive mobile devices
Ataxia-telangiectasia
Ataxia
Atomoxetine
Attention deficit hyperactivity disorder
Autism
Autonomic dysfunction

B

Back pain
Bassen-Kornzweig syndrome
Batten disease
Behçet disease
Bell's palsy
Benign positional vertigo
Benzodiazepines
Beriberi
Binswanger disease
Biopsy
Blepharospasm
Bodywork therapies
Botulinum toxin
Botulism
Brachial plexus injuries
Brain anatomy
Brain and spinal tumors
Brown-Séquard syndrome

C

Canavan disease
Carbamazepine
Carotid endarterectomy
Carotid stenosis
Carpal tunnel syndrome
Catechol-O-methyltransferase inhibitors
Central cord syndrome
Central nervous system
Central nervous system stimulants
Central pain syndrome
Cerebellum
Cerebral angiitis
Cerebral cavernous malformation
Cerebral circulation
Cerebral dominance
Cerebral hematoma
Cerebral palsy
Channelopathies
Charcot-Marie-Tooth disorder
Cholinergic stimulants
Cholinesterase inhibitors
Chorea

Chronic inflammatory demyelinating polyneuropathy
Clinical trials
Congenital myasthenia
Congenital myopathies
Corpus callosotomy
Corticobasal degeneration
Craniosynostosis
Craniotomy
Creutzfeldt-Jakob disease
CT scan
Cushing syndrome
Cytomegalic inclusion body disease

D

Dandy-Walker syndrome
Deep brain stimulation
Delirium
Dementia
Depression
Dermatomyositis
Devic syndrome
Diabetic neuropathy disease
Diadochokinetic rate
Diazepam
Dichloralphenazone
Dichloralphenazone, Isometheptene, and Acetaminophen
Diencephalon
Diet and nutrition
Disc herniation
Dizziness
Dopamine receptor agonists
Dysarthria
Dysesthesias
Dysgeusia
Dyskinesia
Dyslexia
Dyspraxia
Dystonia

E

Electric personal assistive mobility devices

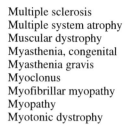

PLEASE READ—IMPORTANT INFORMATION

The Gale Encyclopedia of Neurological Disorders is a medical reference product designed to inform and educate readers about a wide variety of diseases, syndromes, drugs, treatments, therapies, and diagnostic equipment. Thomson Gale believes the product to be comprehensive, but not necessarily definitive. It is intended to supplement, not replace, consultation with a physician or other healthcare practitioner. While Thomson Gale has made substantial efforts to provide information that is accurate, comprehensive, and up-to-date, Thomson Gale makes no representations or warranties of any kind, including without limitation, warranties of merchantability or fitness for a particular purpose, nor does it guarantee the accuracy, comprehensiveness, or timeliness of the information contained in this product. Readers are advised to seek professional diagnosis and treatment for any medical condition, and to discuss information obtained from this book with their healthcare providers.

INTRODUCTION

The Gale Encyclopedia of Neurological Disorders (GEND) is a one-stop source for medical information that covers diseases, syndromes, drugs, treatments, therapies, and diagnostic equipment. It keeps medical jargon to a minimum, making it easier for the layperson to use. *The Gale Encyclopedia of Neurological Disorders* presents authoritative and balanced information and is more comprehensive than single-volume family medical guides.

SCOPE

Almost 400 full-length articles are included in *The Gale Encyclopedia of Neurological Disorders.* Articles follow a standardized format that provides information at a glance. Rubrics include:

Diseases

- Definition
- Description
- Demographics
- Causes and symptoms
- Diagnosis
- Treatment team
- Treatment
- Recovery and rehabilitation
- Clinical trials
- Prognosis
- Special concerns
- Resources
- Key terms

Drugs

- Definition
- Purpose
- Description
- Recommended dosage
- Precautions
- Side effects
- Interactions
- Resources
- Key terms

Treatments

- Definition
- Purpose
- Precautions
- Description
- Preparation
- Aftercare
- Risks
- Normal results
- Resources
- Key terms

INCLUSION CRITERIA

A preliminary topic list was compiled from a wide variety of sources, including professional medical guides, consumer guides, and textbooks and encyclopedias. The advisory board, made up of seven medical and healthcare experts, evaluated the topics and made suggestions for inclusion. Final selection of topics to include was made by the medical advisors in conjunction with Gale editors.

ABOUT THE CONTRIBUTORS

The essays were compiled by experienced medical writers, physicians, nurses, and pharmacists. GEND medical advisors reviewed most of the completed essays to insure that they are appropriate, up-to-date, and medically accurate.

HOW TO USE THIS BOOK

The *Gale Encyclopedia of Neurological Disorders* has been designed with ready reference in mind:

- Straight **alphabetical arrangement** allows users to locate information quickly.

- Bold faced terms function as print hyperlinks that point the reader to full-length entries in the encyclopedia.

- A list of **key terms** is provided where appropriate to define unfamiliar words or concepts used within the context of the essay.

- **Cross-references** placed throughout the encyclopedia direct readers to where information on subjects without their own entries can be found. Cross-references are also used to assist readers looking for information on diseases that are now known by other names; for example, there is a cross-reference for the rare childhood disease commonly known as Hallervorden-Spatz disease that points to the entry entitled Pantothenate kinase-associated neurodegeneration.

- A **Resources** section directs users to sources of further information, which include books, periodicals, websites, and organizations.

- A **glossary** is included to help readers understand unfamiliar terms.

- A comprehensive **general index** allows users to easily target detailed aspects of any topic.

GRAPHICS

The Gale Encyclopedia of Neurological Disorders is enhanced with over 100 images, including photos, tables, and customized line drawings.

ADVISORY BOARD

An advisory board made up of prominent individuals from the medical and healthcare communities provided invaluable assistance in the formulation of this encyclopedia. They defined the scope of coverage and reviewed individual entries for accuracy and accessibility; in some cases they contributed entries themselves. We would therefore like to express our great appreciation to them:

CONTRIBUTORS

Lisa Maria Andres, MS, CGC
Certified Genetic Counselor and Medical Writer
San Jose, CA

Paul Arthur
Science writer
London, England

Bruno Verbeno Azevedo
Espirito Santo University
Vitória, Brazil

Deepti Babu, MS, CGC
Genetic Counselor
Marshfield Clinic
Marshfield, WI

Laurie Barclay, MD
Neurologist and writer
Tampa, FL

Julia Barrett
Science Writer
Madison, WI

Danielle Barry, MS
Graduate Assisstant
Center of Alcohol Studies
Rutgers University
Piscataway, NJ

Maria Basile, PhD
Medical Writer
Roselle, NJ

Tanja Bekhuis, PhD
Science Writer and Psychologist
TCB Research
Boalsburg, PA

Juli M. Berwald, PhD
Geologist (Ocean Sciences)
Chicago, Illinois

Robert G. Best, PhD
Director
Division of Genetics
University of South Carolina School of Medicine
Columbia, SC

Michelle Lee Brandt
Medical Writer
San Francisco, CA

Dawn J. Cardeiro, MS, CGC
Genetic Counselor
Fairfield, PA

Francisco de Paula Careta
Espirito Santo University
Vitória, Brazil

Rosalyn Carson-DeWitt, MD
Physician and Medical Writer
Durham, NC

Stacey L. Chamberlin
Science Writer and Editor
Fairfax, VA

Bryan Richard Cobb, PhD
Institute for Molecular and Human Genetics
Georgetown University
Washington, D.C.

Adam J. Cohen, MD
Craniofacial Surgery, Eyelid and Facial Plastic Surgery, Neuro-Ophthalmology
Downers Grove, IL

Tish Davidson, AM
Medical Writer
Fremont, CA

James Paul Dworkin, PhD
Professor
Department of Otolaryngology, Voice/Speech Pathology Program and Laboratory
Wayne State University
Detroit, MI

L. Fleming Fallon, Jr., MD, DrPH
Professor
Department of Public Health
Bowling Green State University
Bowling Green, OH

Antonio Farina, MD, PhD
Department of Embryology, Obstetrics, and Gynecology
University of Bologna
Bologna, Italy

Kevin Fitzgerald
Science Writer and Journalist
South Windsor, CT

Paula Anne Ford-Martin
Medical Writer
Warwick, RI

Lisa A. Fratt
Medical Writer
Ashland, WI

Rebecca J. Frey, PhD
Freelance Medical Writer
New Haven, CT

Sandra L. Friedrich, MA
Science Writer
Clinical Psychology
Chicago, IL

Sandra Galeotti, MS
Science Writer
Sao Paulo, Brazil

Larry Gilman, PhD
Electrical Engineer and Science Writer
Sharon, VT

Laith Farid Gulli, MD
Consulting Psychotherapist
Lathrup Village, MI

Stephen John Hage, AAAS, RT(R), FAHRA
Medical Writer
Chatsworth, CA

Brook Ellen Hall, PhD
Science Writer
Loomis, CA

Dan Harvey
Medical Writer
Wilmington, DE

Hannah M. Hoag, MSc
Science and Medical Writer
Montreal, Canada

Brian Douglas Hoyle, PhD
Microbiologist
Nova Scotia, Canada

Cindy L. Hunter, CGC
Genetic Counselor
Medical Genetics Department
Indiana University School of Medicine
Indianapolis, IN

Alexander I. Ioffe, PhD
Senior Scientist
Geological Institute of the Russian Academy of Sciences
Moscow, Russia

Holly Ann Ishmael, MS, CGC
Genetic Counselor
The Children's Mercy Hospital
Kansas City, MO

Joel C. Kahane, PhD
Professor, Director of the Anatomical Sciences Laboratory
The School of Audiology and Speech-Language Pathology
The University of Memphis
Memphis, TN

Kelly Karpa, PhD, RPh
Assistant Professor
Department of Pharmacology
Pennsylvania State University College of Medicine
Hershey, PA

Karen M. Krajewski, MS, CGC
Genetic Counselor, Assistant Professor of Neurology
Wayne State University
Detroit, MI

Judy Leaver, MA
Behavioral Health Writer and Consultant
Washington, D.C.

Adrienne Wilmoth Lerner
University of Tennessee College of Law
Knoxville, TN

Brenda Wilmoth Lerner, RN
Nurse, Writer, and Editor
London, UK

K. Lee Lerner
Fellow (rt)
Science Policy Institute
London, UK

Agnieszka Maria Lichanska, PhD
Department of Microbiology and Parasitology
University of Queensland
Brisbane, Australia

Peter T. Lin, MD
Research Assistant
Member: American Academy of Neurology, American Association of Electrodiagnostic Medicine
Department of Biomagnetic Imaging
University of California, San Francisco
Foster City, CA

Iuri Drumond Louro, MD, PhD
Adjunct Professor
Human and Molecular Genetics
Espirito Santo University
Vitória, Brazil

Nicole Mallory, MS, PA-C
Medical Student
Wayne State University
Detroit, MI

Igor Medica, MD, PhD
Assistant Professor
School of Medicine
University of Rijeka
Pula, Croatia

Michael Mooney, MA, CAC
Consultant Psychotherapist
Warren, MI

Alfredo Mori, MD, FACEM, FFAEM
Emergency Physician
The Alfred Hospital
Victoria, Australia
Oxford's Program in Evidence-Based Health Care
University of Oxford
Oxford, England

Marcos do Carmo Oyama
Espirito Santo University
Vitória, Brazil

Greiciane Gaburro Paneto
Espirito Santo University
Vitória, Brazil

Borut Peterlin, MD, PhD
Neurologist; Consultant Clinical Geneticist; Director
Division of Medical Genetics
University Medical Center
Lubiana, Slovenia

Toni I. Pollin, MS, CGC
Research Analyst
Division of Endocrinology, Diabetes, and Nutrition
University of Maryland School of Medicine
Baltimore, MD

J. Ricker Polsdorfer, MD
Medical Writer
Phoenix, AZ

Scott J. Polzin, MS, CGC
Medical Writer
Buffalo Grove, IL

Jack Raber, PharmD
Principal
Clinipharm Services
Seal Beach, CA

Robert Ramirez, DO
Medical Student
University of Medicine and
    Dentistry of New Jersey
Stratford, NJ

Richard Robinson
Medical Writer
Tucson, AZ

**Jennifer Ann Roggenbuck, MS,
    CGC**
Genetic Counselor
Hennepin County Medical Center
Minneapolis, MN

Nancy Ross-Flanigan
Science Writer
Belleville, MI

Stephanie Dionne Sherk
Freelance Medical Writer
University of Michigan
Ann Arbor, MI

Lee Alan Shratter, MD
Consulting Radiologist
Kentfield, CA

Genevieve T. Slomski, PhD
Medical Writer
New Britain, CT

Amie Stanley, MS
Genetic Counselor
Medical Genetics
The Cleveland Clinic
Cleveland, OH

Constance K. Stein, PhD
*Director of Cytogenetics, Assistant
    Director of Molecular
    Diagnostics*
SUNY Upstate Medical University
Syracuse, NY

Roger E. Stevenson, MD
*Senior Clinical Geneticist, Senior
    Clinical Laboratory Geneticist*
Greenwood Genetic Center
Greenwood, SC

Roy Sucholeiki, MD
*Professor, Director of the
    Comprehensive Epilepsy
    Program*
Department of Neurology
Loyola University Health System
Chicago, IL

Kevin M. Sweet, MS, CGC
Cancer Genetic Counselor
James Cancer Hospital, Ohio State
    University
Columbus, OH

David Tulloch
Science Writer
Wellington, New Zealand

Carol A. Turkington
Medical Writer
Lancaster, PA

Samuel D. Uretsky, PharmD
Medical Writer
Wantagh, NY

**Chitra Venkatasubramanian,
    MBBS, MD (internal
    medicine)**
Resident in Neurology
Department of Neurology and
    Neurosciences
Stanford University
Stanford, CA.

Bruno Marcos Verbeno
Espirito Santo University
Vitória, Brazil

Beatriz Alves Vianna
Espirito Santo University
Vitória, Brazil

Machado-Joseph disease

Definition

Machado-Joseph disease (MJD), also known as **spinocerebellar ataxia** Type 3 (SCA 3), is a rare hereditary disorder affecting the **central nervous system**, especially the areas responsible for movement coordination of limbs, facial muscles, and eyes. The disease involves the slow and progressive degeneration of brain areas involved in motor coordination, such as the cerebellar, extrapyramidal, pyramidal, and motor areas. Ultimately, MJD leads to paralysis or a crippling condition, although intellectual functions usually remain normal. Other names of MJD are Portuguese-Azorean disease, Joseph disease, Azorean disease.

Description

Machado-Joseph disease was first described in 1972 among the descendants of Portuguese-Azorean immigrants to the United States, including the family of William Machado. In spite of differences in symptoms and degrees of neurological degeneration and movement impairment among the affected individuals, it was suggested by investigators that in at least four studied families the same gene mutation was present. In early 1976, investigators went to the Azores Archipelago to study an existing neurodegenerative disease in the islands of Flores and São Miguel. In a group of 15 families, they found 40 people with neurological disorders with a variety of different symptoms among the affected individuals.

Another research team in 1976 reported an inherited neurological disorder of the motor system in Portuguese families, which they named Joseph disease. During the same year, the two groups of scientists both published independent evidence suggesting that the same disease was the primary cause for the variety of symptoms observed. When additional reports from other countries and ethnic groups were associated with the same inherited disorder, it was initially thought that Portuguese-Azorean sailors had been the probable disseminators of MJD to other populations around the world during the sixteenth century period of Portuguese colonial explorations and commerce. Presently, MJD is found in Brazil, United States, Portugal, Macau, Finland, Canada, Mexico, Israel, Syria, Turkey, Angola, India, United Kingdom, Australia, Japan, and China. Because MJD continues to be diagnosed in a variety of countries and ethnic groups, there are current doubts about its exclusive Portuguese-Azorean origin.

Causes and symptoms

The gene responsible for MJD appears at chromosome 14, and the first symptoms usually appear in early adolescence. **Dystonia** (**spasticity** or involuntary and repetitive movements) or gait **ataxia** is usually the initial symptoms in children. Gait ataxia is characterized by unstable walk and standing, which slowly progresses with the appearance of some of the other symptoms, such as hand dysmetria, involuntary eye movements, loss of hand and superior limbs coordination, and facial dystonia (abnormal muscle tone). Another characteristic of MJD is clinical anticipation, which means that in most families the onset of the disease occurs progressively earlier from one generation to the next. Among members of the same family, some patients may show a predominance of muscle tone disorders, others may present loss of coordination, some may have bulging eyes, and yet another sibling may be free of symptoms during his/her entire life. In the late stages of MJD, some people may experience **delirium** or **dementia**.

According to the affected brain area, MJD is classified as Type I, with extrapyramidal insufficiency; Type II, with cerebellar, pyramidal, and extrapyramidal insufficiency; and Type III, with cerebellar insufficiency. Extrapyramidal tracts are networks of uncrossed motor nerve fibers that function as relays between the motor areas and corresponding areas of the brain. The pyramidal tract consists of groups of crossed nerves located in the white matter of the spinal cord that conduct motor impulses originated in

Key Terms

Autosomal   Relating to any chromosome besides the X and Y sex chromosomes. Human cells contain 22 pairs of autosomes and one pair of sex chromosomes.

Cerebellar   Involving the part of the brain (cerebellum) that controls walking, balance, and coordination.

Dysarthria   Slurred speech.

Dystonia   Painful involuntary muscle cramps or spasms.

Extrapyramidal   Refers to brain structures located outside the pyramidal tracts of the central nervous system.

Genotype   The genetic makeup of an organism or a set of organisms.

Mutation   A permanent change in the genetic material that may alter a trait or characteristic of an individual, or manifest as disease. This change can be transmitted to offspring.

Penetrance   The degree to which individuals possessing a particular genetic mutation express the trait that this mutation causes. One hundred percent penetrance is expected to be observed in truly dominant traits.

Phenotype   The physical expression of an individual's genes.

Spasticity   Increased mucle tone, or stiffness, which leads to uncontrolled, awkward movements.

Trinucleotide   A sequence of three nucleotides.

the opposite area of the brain to the arms and legs. Pyramidal tract nerves regulate both voluntary and reflex muscle movements. However, as the disease progresses, both motor systems tracks will eventually suffer degeneration.

Diagnosis

Diagnosis depends mainly on the clinical history of the family. Genetic screening for the specific mutation that causes MJD can be useful in cases of persons at risk or when the family history is not known or a person has symptoms that raise suspicion of MJD. Initial diagnosis may be difficult, as people present symptoms easily mistaken for other neurological disorders such as **Parkinson** and **Huntington diseases**, or even **multiple sclerosis**.

Treatment

Although there is no cure for Machado-Joseph disease, some symptoms can be relieved, The medication Levodopa or L-dopa often succeeds in lessening muscle rigidity and **tremors**, and is often given in conjunction with the drug Carbidopa. However, as the disease progresses and the number of neurons decreases, this palliative (given for comfort) treatment becomes less effective. Antispasmodic drugs such as baclofen are also prescribed to reduce spasticity. **Dysarthria**, or difficulty to speak, and dysphagia, difficulty to swallow, can be treated with proper medication and speech therapy. Physical therapy can help patients with unsteady gait, and walkers and wheelchairs may be needed as the disease progresses. Other symptoms also require palliative treatment, such as muscle cramps, urinary disorders, and sleep problems.

Clinical Trials

Further basic research is needed before **clinical trials** become a possibility for MJD. Ongoing genetic and molecular research on the mechanisms involved in the genetic mutations responsible for the disease will eventually yield enough data to provide for future development and design of experimental gene therapies and drugs specific to treat those with MJD.

Prognosis

The frequency with which such genetic mutations trigger the clinical onset of disease is known as penetrance. Machado-Joseph disease presents a 94.5% penetrance, which means that 94.5% of the mutation carriers will develop the symptoms during their lives, and less than 5% will remain free of symptoms. Because the intensity and range of symptoms are highly variable among the affected individuals, it is difficult to determine the prognosis for a given individual. As MJD progresses slowly, most patients survive until middle age or older.

Resources

BOOKS

Fenichel, Gerald M. *Clinical Pediatric Neurology: A Signs and Symptoms Approach,* 4th ed. Philadelphia: W. B. Saunders Company, 2001.

OTHER

National Institute of Neurological Disorders and Stroke. *Machado-Joseph Disease Fact Sheet.* May 5, 2003 (June 7, 2004). <http://www.ninds.nih.gov/health_and_medical/pubs/machado-joseph.htm>.

ORGANIZATIONS

Dystonia Medical Research Foundation. 1 East Wacker Drive, Suite 2430, Chicago, IL 60601-1905. (312) 755-0198; Fax: (312) 803-0138. dystonia@dystonia-foundation.org. <http://www.dystonia-foundation.org>.

International Machado-Joseph Disease Foundation, Inc. P.O. Box 994268, Redding, CA 96099-4268. (530) 246-4722. MJD@ijdf.net. <http://www.ijdf.net>.

National Ataxia Foundation (NAF). 2600 Fernbrook Lane, Suite 119, Minneapolis, MN 55447-4752. (763) 553-0020; Fax: (763) 553-0167. naf@ataxia.org. <http://www.ataxia.org>.

National Organization for Rare Disorders (NORD). P.O. Box 1968 (55 Kenosia Avenue), Danbury, CT 06813-1968. (203) 744-0100 or (800) 999-NORD (6673); Fax: (203) 798-2291. orphan@rarediseases.org. <http://www.rarediseases.org>.

Worldwide Education & Awareness for Movement Disorders (WE MOVE). 204 West 84th Street, New York, NY 10024. (212) 875-8312 or (800) 437-MOV2 (6682); Fax: (212) 875-8389. wemove@wemove.org. <http://www.wemove.org>.

Sandra Galeotti

Macrencephaly *see* **Megalencephaly**

Mad cow disease *see* **Creutzfeldt-Jakob disease**

▌Magnetic resonance imaging (MRI)

Definition

Magnetic resonance imaging (MRI) scanners rely on the principles of atomic nuclear-spin resonance. Using strong magnetic fields and radio waves, MRI collects and correlates deflections caused by atoms into images. MRIs (magnetic resonance imaging tests) offer relatively sharp pictures and allow physicians to see internal bodily structures with great detail. Using MRI technology, physicians are increasingly able to make diagnosis of serious pathology (e.g., tumors) earlier, and earlier diagnosis often translates to a more favorable outcome for the patient.

Description

A varying (gradient) magnetic field exists in tissues in the body that can be used to produce an image of the tissue. The development of MRI was one of several powerful diagnostic imaging techniques that revolutionized medicine by allowing physicians to explore bodily structures and functions with a minimum of invasion to the patient.

In the last half of the twentieth century, dramatic advances in computer technologies, especially the development of mathematical algorithms powerful enough to allow difficult equations to be solved quickly, allowed

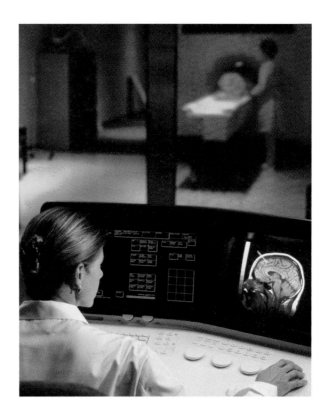

Technician conducting an MRI. (*Will & Deni McIntyre/Photo Researchers, Inc. Reproduced by permission.*)

MRI to develop into an important diagnostic clinical tool. In particular, the ability of computer programs to eliminate "noise" (unwanted data) from sensitive measurements enhanced the development of accurate, accessible and relatively inexpensive noninvasive technologies.

Nuclear medicine is based upon the physics of excited atomic nuclei. Nuclear magnetic resonance (NMR) was one such early form of nuclear spectroscopy that eventually found widespread use in clinical laboratory and medical imaging. Because a proton in a magnetic field has two quantized spin states, NMR allowed the determination of the complex structure of organic molecules and, ultimately, the generation of pictures representing the larger structures of molecules and compounds (such as neural tissue, muscles, organs, bones, etc.). These pictures were obtained as a result of measuring differences between the expected and actual numbers of photons absorbed by a target tissue.

Groups of nuclei brought into resonance, that is, nuclei-absorbing and -emitting photons of similar electromagnetic **radiation** (e.g., radio waves), make subtle yet distinguishable changes when the resonance is forced to change by altering the energy of impacting photons. The speed and extent of the resonance changes permit a nondestructive (because of the use of low energy photons) determination of anatomical structures. This form of NMR became the physical and chemical basis of the powerful diagnostic technique of MRI.

The resolution of MRI scanning is so high that they can be used to observe the individual plaques in **multiple sclerosis**. In a clinical setting, a patient is exposed to short bursts of powerful magnetic fields and radio waves from electromagnets. MRI images do not utilize potentially harmful ionizing radiation generated by three-dimensional x-ray computed tomography (CT) scans, and there are no known harmful side effects. The magnetic and radio wave bursts stimulate signals from hydrogen atoms in the patient's tissues that, when subjected to computer analysis, create a cross-sectional image of internal structures and organs.

Healthy and diseased tissues produce different signal patterns and thus allow physicians to identify diseases and disorders.

American chemist and physicist Paul Lauterbur and British physicist Sir Peter Mansfield shared the 2003 Nobel Prize in Physiology or Medicine for their discoveries concerning the use of magnetic resonance to visualize different structures.

MRI tests, brain scans, and potential security issues

Studies of the potential of new brain wave scanners explore the possibility that MRI tests could be part of a more accurate form of polygraph (lie detector). Current polygraphs are of debatable accuracy (usually they are not admissible in court as evidence) and measure observable fluctuations in heart rate, breathing, perspiration, etc.

In a 2001 University of Pennsylvania experiment using MRI, 18 subjects were given objects to hide in their pockets, then shown a series of pictures and asked to deny that the object depicted was in their pockets. Included was a picture of the object they had pocketed and so subjects were "lying" (making a deliberate false statement) if they claimed that the object was not in their pocket. An MRI recorded an increase of activity in the anterior cinglate, a portion of the brain associated with inhibition of responses and monitoring of errors, as well as the right superior frontal gyrus, which is involved in the process of paying attention to particular stimuli.

After the September 11, 2001, terrorist attacks, a number of government agencies in the United States began to take a new look at brain scanning technology as a potential means of security screening. Such activity, along with an increase of interest in potential brain-wave scanning by the Federal Bureau of Investigation (FBI), has raised concerns among civil-liberties groups, which view brain-wave scanning as a particularly objectionable invasion of privacy.

Key Terms

Magnetic resonance imaging MRI An imaging technique used in evaluation and diagnoses of the brain and other parts of the body.

Resonance A condition in which the applied force (e.g., forced vibrations, forced magnetic field, etc.) becomes the same as the natural frequency of the target (e.g., tissue, cell structure, etc.).

Resources

PERIODICALS
Young, Emma. "Brain Scans Can Reveal Liars." *New Scientist* (November 12, 2001).

WEBSITES
Hornak, J. P. *The Basics of MRI.* May 9, 2004 (June 2, 2004). <http://www.cis.rit.edu/htbooks/mri/>.
Johnson, K. A., and J. A. Becker. *The Whole Brain Atlas.* May 9, 2004 (June 2, 2004). <http://www.med.harvard.edu/AANLIB/home.html>.

Paul Arthur

Megalencephaly

Definition

Megalencephaly (also called macrencephaly) describes an enlarged brain whose weight exceeds the mean (the average weight for that age and sex) by at least 2.5 standard deviations (a statistical measure of variation). Megalencephaly may also be defined in terms of volume rather than weight. Hemimegalencephaly (or unilateral megalencephaly) is a related condition in which brain enlargement occurs in one hemisphere (half) of the brain.

Description

A person with megalencephaly has a large, heavy brain. In general, a brain that weighs more than 1600 grams (about 3.5 pounds) is considered megalencephalic. The heaviest brain on record weighed 2850 grams (about 6.3 pounds). Macrocephaly, a related condition, refers to an abnormally large head. Macrocephaly may be due to megalencephaly or other causes such as **hydrocephalus** (an excess accumulation of fluid in the brain), and brain edema. Megalencephaly may be an isolated finding in an otherwise normal individual or it can occur in association with neurological problems (such as **seizures** or **mental retardation**) and/or somatic abnormalities (physical

Key Terms

Autosomal dominant A pattern of inheritance in which only one of the two copies of an autosomal gene must be abnormal for a genetic condition or disease to occur. An autosomal gene is a gene that is located on one of the autosomes or non-sex chromosomes. A person with an autosomal dominant disorder has a 50% chance of passing it to each of their offspring.

Autosomal recessive A pattern of inheritance in which both copies of an autosomal gene must be abnormal for a genetic condition or disease to occur. An autosomal gene is a gene that is located on one of the autosomes or non-sex chromosomes. When both parents have one abnormal copy of the same gene, they have a 25% chance with each pregnancy that their offspring will have the disorder.

Chromosome A microscopic thread-like structure found within each cell of the human body and con-

sisting of a complex of proteins and DNA. Humans have 46 chromosomes arranged into 23 pairs. Chromosomes contain the genetic information necessary to direct the development and functioning of all cells and systems in the body. They pass on hereditary traits from parents to child (like eye color) and determine whether the child will be male or female.

Gene A building block of inheritance, which contains the instructions for the production of a particular protein, and is made up of a molecular sequence found on a section of DNA. Each gene is found on a precise location on a chromosome.

Inborn error of metabolism One of a group of rare conditions characterized by an inherited defect in an enzyme or other protein. Inborn errors of metabolism can cause brain damage and mental retardation if left untreated. Phenylketonuria, Tay-Sachs disease, and galactosemia are inborn errors of metabolism.

---

problems or birth defects of the body). Dysmorphic facial features (abnormal shape, position or size of facial features) may also be observed in an affected individual.

According to the National Institute of Neurological Disorders and Stroke (NINDS), megalencephaly is one of the cephalic disorders, congenital conditions due to damage to or abnormal development of the nervous system. There have been various attempts to classify megalencephaly into subcategories based on etiology (cause) and/or pathology (the condition of the brain tissue and cells). Dekaban and Sakurgawa (1977) proposed three main categories: primary megalencephaly, secondary megalencephaly, and hemimegalencephaly. DeMyer (1986) proposed two main categories: anatomic and metabolic. Gooskens and others (1988) modified these classifications and added a third category: dynamic megalencephaly. The existence of different classification systems highlights the inherent difficulty in categorizing a condition that has a wide range of causes and associated pathology.

Demographics

The incidence of megalencephaly is estimated at between 2% and 6%. There is a preponderance of affected males; megalencephaly affects males three to four times more often than it does females. Among individuals with macrocephaly, estimates of megalencephaly are between 10 and 30%. Hemimegalencephaly is a rare condition and occurs less frequently than megalencephaly.

Causes and symptoms

Both genetic and non-genetic factors may produce megalencephaly. Most often, megalencephaly is a familial trait that occurs without extraneural (outside the brain) findings. Familial megalencephaly may occur as an autosomal dominant (more common) or autosomal recessive condition. The autosomal recessive form is more likely than the autosomal dominant form to result in mental retardation. Other genetic causes for megalencephaly include single gene disorders such as **Sotos syndrome** (an overgrowth syndrome), **neurofibromatosis** (a neurocutaneous syndrome), and **Alexander disease** (a **leukodystrophy**); or a chromosome abnormality such as Klinefelter syndrome. Non-genetic factors such as a transient disorder of cerebral spinal fluid may also contribute to the development of megalencephaly. Finally, megalencephaly can be idiopathic (due to unknown causes).

The cells that make up the brain (neurons and other supporting cells) form during the second to fourth months of pregnancy. Though the precise mechanisms behind megalencephaly at the cellular level are not fully understood, it is thought that the condition results from an increased number of cells, an increased size of cells, or accumulation of a metabolic byproduct or abnormal substance due to an inborn error of metabolism. It is possible that more than one of these processes may explain megalencephaly in a given individual.

There is variability in age of onset, symptoms present, rate of progression, and severity of megalencephaly. The disorder typically presents as a large head circumference (distance around the head) either prenatally (before birth), at birth, or within the first few years of life. The head circumference may increase rapidly in the span of a few months or may progress slowly over a longer period of time. Head shape may be abnormal and skull abnormalities such as widened or split sutures (fibrous joints between the bones of the head) may occur. There may also be increased cranial pressure and bulging fontanels (the membrane covered spaces at the juncture of an infant's cranial bones which later harden).

From a neurological standpoint, the clinical picture of megalencephaly varies widely. Manifestations may range from normal intellect, as with case of benign familial megalencephaly, to severe mental retardation and seizures, as with Alexander disease, an inherited leukodystrophy (disease of the brain's white matter). Neurological symptoms that may be present or develop in a person with megalencephaly include:

• delay of motor milestones such as holding up head, rolling over, or sitting

• mental retardation

• speech delay

• poor muscle tone

• body asymmetry

• paralysis of one or both sides of the body

• poor coordination

• involuntary movements

• visual disturbances

Brain abnormalities that may be seen in individuals with megalencephaly include:

• gyral abnormalities

• neuronal heterotopias

• corpus callosum dysgenesis

• myelum dysplasia

• abnormal or an excess amount of neurons

• abnormal or an excess amount of glia cells

Diagnosis

A diagnosis of megalencephaly is based on clinical findings and results of brain imaging studies. Since megalencephaly can be a benign condition, there may well be many individuals who never come to medical attention. Though no longer used as a primary means of diagnosing megalencephaly, an autopsy may provide additional evidence to support this diagnosis. The evaluation of a patient with suspected megalencephaly will usually consist of questions about medical history and family history, a physical exam that includes head measurements, and a developmental and/or neurological exam. It may be necessary to obtain head circumference measurements for first-degree relatives (parents, siblings, children). Depending upon the history and clinical findings, a physician may recommend imaging studies such as CT (computed tomography) scan or **MRI (magnetic resonance imaging)**. Findings on **CT scan** or MRI consistent with a diagnosis of megalencephaly are an enlarged brain with normal-sized ventricles and subarachnoid spaces. The volume (size) of the brain may be calculated or estimated using measurements from the CT or MRI. A patient with megalencephaly may be referred to specialists in neurology or genetics for further evaluation. Laboratory testing for a genetic condition or chromosome abnormality may also be performed.

Treatment

There is no specific cure for megalencephaly. Management of this condition largely depends upon the presence and severity of associated neurological and physical problems. In cases of benign familial megalencephaly, additional management beyond routine health care maintenance may consist of periodic head measurements and patient education about the inheritance and benign nature of the condition. For patients with neurological and/or physical problems, management may include anti-epileptic drugs for seizures, treatment of medical complications related to the underlying syndrome, and rehabilitation for neurological problems such as speech delay, poor muscle tone, and poor coordination. Placement in a residential care facility may be necessary for those cases in which megalencephaly is accompanied by severe mental retardation or uncontrollable seizures.

Treatment team

The types of professionals involved in the care of patients is highly individualized because the severity of symptoms varies widely from patient to patient. For patients with associated neurological and/or physical problems, the treatment team may include specialists in neonatology, neurology, radiology, orthopedics, rehabilitation, and genetics. Genetic counseling may be helpful to the patient and family, especially at the time of diagnosis. Participation in a support group may also be beneficial to those families adversely affected by megalencephaly.

Recovery and rehabilitation

The optimal remedial strategies for individuals with megalencephaly depend upon the presence and severity of associated neurological and physical problems. Interventions such as speech, physical, and occupational therapy may be indicated for individuals with megalencephaly. Early intervention services for young children and special education or other means of educational support for school-aged children may be recommended if developmental delays, learning disabilities, or other barriers to learning are present. The goal of these therapies is to maximize the patient's success in school, work, and life in general. A child with megalencephaly may be eligible to have an Individual Education Plan (IEP). An IEP provides a framework from which administrators, teachers, and parents can meet the educational needs of a child with learning disabilities. Depending upon severity of symptoms and the degree of learning difficulties, some children with megalencephaly may be best served by special education classes or a private educational setting.

Clinical trials

As of 2004, there were no active **clinical trials** specifically designed to study megalencephaly. Patients with underlying syndromes that produce megalencephaly may be candidates for clinical trials that relate to that particular syndrome. For more information, interested individuals may search for that specific condition (for example, neurofibromatosis) at www.clinicaltrails.gov.

Prognosis

The prognosis for megalencephaly varies according to the presence and severity of associated problems such as intractable seizures, paralysis, and mental retardation. Hemimegalencephaly is often associated with severe seizures, hemiparesis (paralysis of one side of the body), and mental retardation and as such, it carries a poor prognosis. In the case of a fetus diagnosed with megalencephaly, prediction of outcome remains imprecise.

Resources

BOOKS

Greer, Melvin. "Structural Malformations," Chapter 78. In *Merritt's Textbook of Neurology*, 10th edition, edited by L. P. Rowland. Baltimore, MD: Williams and Wilkins, 2000.

Graham, D. I., and P. L. Lantos, eds. *Greenfield's Neuropathology*, volume I, 7th edition. London: Arnold, 2002.

Parker, James N., and Philip M. Parker, eds. *The Official Parent's Sourcebook on Alexander Disease: A Revised and Updated Directory for the Internet Age.* San Diego, CA: ICON Health Publications, 2003.

PERIODICALS

Bodensteiner, J. B. and E. O. Chung. "Macrocrania and megalencephaly in the neonate." *Seminars on Neurology* 13 (March 1993): 84–91.

Cutting, L. E., K. L. Cooper, C. W. Koth, S. H. Mostofsky, W.R. Kates, M. B. Denckla, and W. E. Kaufmann. "Megalencephaly in NF1: predominantly white matter

contribution and mitigation by ADHD." *Neurology* 59 (November 2002): 1388–94.

DeMyer, W. "Megalencephaly: types, clinical syndromes and management." *Pediatric Neurology* 2 (1986): 321–28.

Gooskens, R. H. J. M., J. Willemse, J. B. Bijlsma, and P. Hanlo. "Megalencephaly: Definition and classification." *Brain and Development* 10 (1988): 1–7.

Johnson, A. B., and M. Brenner. "Alexander's disease: clinical, pathologic, and genetic features." *Journal of Child Neurology* 18 (September 2003): 625–32.

Singhal, B. S., J. R. Gorospe, and S. Naidu. "Megalencephalic leukoencephalopathy with subcortical cysts." *Journal of Child Neurology* 18 (September 2003): 646–52.

WEBSITES

The National Institute of Neurological Disorders and Stroke (NINDS). *Megalencephaly Information Page.* <http://www.ninds.nih.gov/health_and_medical/ disorders/megalencephaly.htm>.

The National Institute of Neurological Disorders and Stroke (NINDS). *Cephalic Disorders Fact Sheet.* <http:// www.ninds.nih.gov/health_and_medical/pubs/ cephalic_disorders.htm>.

Online Mendelian Inheritance In Man (OMIM). *Megalencephaly.* <http://www.ncbi.nlm.nih.gov/ entrez/dispomim.cgi?id=155350>.

ORGANIZATIONS

National Institute of Child Health and Human Development (NICHD) Information Resource Center. P. O. Box 3006, Rockville, MD 20847. (301) 496-7101 or (800) 370-2943. NICHDInformationResourceCenter@mail.nih.gov. <http://www.nichd.nih.gov>.

National Institute of Neurological Disorders and Stroke (NINDS, Brain Resources and Information Network (BRAIN). P. O. Box 5801, Bethesda, MD. (800) 352-9424. <http://www.ninds.nih.gov>.

National Organization for Rare Disorders (NORD). PO Box 1968, 55 Kensonia Avenue, Danbury, CT 06813. (203) 744-0100 or 800-999-NORD (6673); Fax: (203) 798-2291. orphan@rarediseases.org. <http://www.rare diseases.org>.

Dawn J. Cardeiro, MS, CGC

Meige syndrome *see* **Hemifacial spasm**

Melodic intonation therapy

Definition

Melodic intonation therapy (MIT) uses melodic and rhythmic components to assist in speech recovery for patients with **aphasia**.

Purpose

Although MIT was first described in the 1970s, it is considered a relatively new and experimental therapy. Few research studies have been performed to analyze the effectiveness of treatment with large numbers of patients. Despite this, some speech therapists use the method for children and adults with aphasia as well as for children with developmental **apraxia** of speech.

The effectiveness of MIT derives from its use of the musical components melody and rhythm in the production of speech. A group of researchers from the University of Texas have discovered that music stimulates several different areas in the brain, rather than just one isolated area. They also found a strong correlation between the right side of the brain that comprehends music components and the left side of the brain that comprehends language components. Because music and language structures are similar, it is suspected that by stimulating the right side of the brain, the left side will begin to make connections as well. For this reason, patients are encouraged to sing words rather than speak them in conversational tones in the early phases of MIT. Studies using **positron emission tomography** (**PET**) scans have shown Broca's area (a region in the left frontal brain controlling speech and language comprehension) to be reactivated through repetition of sung words.

Precautions

Patients and caregivers should be aware that there is little research to support consistent success with MIT. Theoretically, this form of therapy has the potential to improve speech communication to a limited extent.

Description

Melodic intonation therapy was originally developed as a treatment method for speech improvements in adults with aphasia. The initial method has had several modifications, mostly adaptations for use by children with apraxia. The primary structure of this therapy remains relatively consistent however.

There are four steps, or levels, generally outlining the path of therapy.

- Level I: The speech therapist hums short phrases in a rhythmic, singsong tone. The patient attempts to follow the rhythm and stress patterns of phrases by tapping it out. With children, the therapist uses signing while humming and the child is not initially expected to participate. After a series of steps, the child gradually increases participation until they sign and hum with the therapist.
- Level II: The patient begins to repeat the hummed phrases with the assistance of the speech therapist. Children at this level are gradually weaned from therapist participation.

- Level III: For adults, this is the point where therapist participation is minimized and the patient begins to respond to questions still using rhythmic speech patterns. In children, this is the final level and the transition to normal speech begins. *Sprechgesang* is the technique used to transition the constant melodic pitch used up to this point with the variable pitch in normal conversational speech.
- Level IV: The adult method incorporates *sprechgesang* at this level. More complex phrases and longer sentences are attempted.

Preparation

Preparation for MIT involves some additional research into the therapy and discussions with a **neurologist** and a speech pathologist. It is important to have an understanding of the affected brain areas. MIT is most likely to be successful for patients who meet certain criteria such as non-bilateral brain damage, good auditory aptitude, non-fluent verbal communication, and poor word repetition. The speech pathologist should be familiar with the different MIT methodologies as they relate to either adults or children.

Aftercare

There is no required aftercare for MIT.

Risks

There are no physical risks associated with the use of melodic intonation therapy.

Normal results

The expected outcome after completion of the MIT sequence is increased communication through production of intelligible word groups. Patients are typically able to form short sentences of 3–5 words, but more complex communication may also be possible depending on the initial cause of speech impairment.

Resources
BOOKS

Aldridge, David. *Music Therapy in Dementia Care*. Jessica Kingsley Publishing, 2000.

PERIODICALS

Baker, Felicity A. "Modifying the Melodic Intonation Therapy Program for Adults with Severe Non-fluent Aphasia." *Music Therapy Perspectives* 18, no. 2 (2000): 110–14.

Belin, P., et al. "Recovery from Nonfluent Aphasia After Melodic Intonation Therapy: A PET Study." *Neurology* 47, no. 6 (December 1996): 1504–11.

Bonakdarpour, B., A. Eftekharzadeh, and H. Ashayeri. "Preliminary Report on the Effects of Melodic Intonation Therapy in the Rehabilitation of Persian Aphasic

Key Terms

Aphasia Loss of the ability to use or understand language, usually as a result of brain injury or disease.

Apraxia Loss of the ability to carry out a voluntary movement despite being able to demonstrate normal muscle function.

Pitch The property of sound that is determined by the frequency of sound wave vibrations reaching the ear.

Patients." *Iranian Journal of Medical Sciences* 25 (2000): 156–60.

Helfrich-Miller, Kathleen. "A Clinical Perspective: Melodic Intonation Therapy for Developmental Apraxia." *Clinics in Communication Disorders* 4, no. 3 (1994): 175–82.

Roper, Nicole. "Melodic Intonation Therapy with Young Children with Apraxia." *Bridges* 1, no. 8 (May 2003).

Sparks R, Holland A. "Method: melodic intonation therapy for aphasia." *Journal of Speech and Hearing Disorders.* 1976;41:287–297.

ORGANIZATIONS

American Speech-Language-Hearing Association. 10801 Rockville Pike, Rockville, MD 20852. (301) 897-5700 or (800) 638-8255; Fax: (301) 571-0457. action center@asha.org. <http://www.nsastutter.org>.

Music Therapy Association of British Columbia. 2055 Purcell Way, North Vancouver, British Columbia V7J 3H5, Canada. (604) 924-0046; Fax: (604) 983-7559. info@mtabc.com. <http://www.mtabc.com>.

The Center For Music Therapy. 404-A Baylor Street, Austin, TX 78703. (512) 472-5016; Fax: (512) 472-5017. info@centerformusictherapy.com. <http://www.centerfor musictherapy.com>.

Stacey L. Chamberlin

Méniere's disease

Definition

Méniere's disease is a disorder characterized by recurrent vertigo, sensory hearing loss, tinnitus, and a feeling of fullness in the ear. It is named for the French physician, Prosper Méniere, who first described the illness in 1861. Méniere's disease is also known as idiopathic endolymphatic hydrops; "idiopathic" refers to the unknown or spontaneous origin of the disorder, while "endolymphatic hydrops" refers to the increased fluid pressure in the inner ear that causes the symptoms of Méniere's disease.

Description

Patients with Méniere's disease have periodic attacks characterized by four major symptoms:

• Vertigo. This is a spinning or whirling sensation that affects the patient's sense of balance; it is sometimes violent. The vertigo is often accompanied by nausea and vomiting.

• Fluctuating loss of hearing.

• Tinnitus. This is a sensation of ringing, buzzing, or roaring noises in the ear. The most common type of tinnitus associated with Méniere's is a low-pitched roaring.

• A sensation of fullness, pressure, or discomfort in the ear.

Some patients also experience **headaches**, diarrhea, and **pain** in the abdomen during an attack.

Attacks usually come on suddenly and last from two or three to 24 hours, although some patients experience an aching sensation in the affected ear just before an attack. The attacks typically subside gradually. In most cases, only one ear is affected; however, 10–15% of patients with Méniere's disease are affected in both ears. After a severe attack, the patient often feels exhausted and sleeps for several hours.

The spacing and intensity of Méniere's attacks vary from patient to patient. Some people have several acute episodes relatively close together, while others may have one or two milder attacks per year or even several years apart. In some patients, attacks occur at regular intervals, while in others, the attacks are completely random. In some patients, acute attacks are triggered by psychological stress, menstrual cycles, or certain foods. Patients usually feel normal between episodes; however, they may find that their hearing and sense of balance get slightly worse after each attack.

Demographics

The National Institute on Deafness and Other Communication Disorders (NIDCD) estimates that, as of 2003, there are about 620,000 persons in the United States diagnosed with Méniere's disease. Another expert gives a figure of 1,000 cases per 100,000 people. About 46,000 new cases are diagnosed each year; some neurologists, however, think that the disorder is underdiagnosed.

Méniere's disease has been diagnosed in patients of all ages, although the average age at onset is 35–40 years of age. The age of patients in several controlled studies of the disorder ranged from 49 to 67 years.

Although Méniere's disease has not been linked to a specific gene or genes, it does appear to run in families. About 55% of patients diagnosed with Méniere's have significant family histories of the disorder. Women are slightly more likely than men to develop Ménière's; various studies report female-to-male ratios between 1.1:1 and 3:2.

There is no evidence as of 2003 that Ménière's disease occurs more frequently in some racial or ethnic groups than in others.

Causes and symptoms

The underlying causes of Ménière's disease are poorly understood as of late 2003. Some geneticists proposed in 2002 that Ménière's disease might be caused by a mutation in the COCH gene, which is the only human gene known to be associated with inherited hearing loss related to inner ear dysfunction. In 2003, however, two groups of researchers in Japan and the United Kingdom reported that mutations in the COCH gene are not responsible for Ménière's. Other theories about the underlying causes of Ménière's disease that are being investigated include virus infections and environmental noise pollution.

One area of research that shows promise is the possible relationship between Ménière's disease and migraine headache. Dr. Ménière himself suggested the possibility of a link, but early studies yielded conflicting results. A rigorous German study published in late 2002 reported that the lifetime prevalence of migraine was 56% in patients diagnosed with Ménière's disease as compared to 25% for controls. The researchers noted that further work is necessary to determine the exact nature of the relationship between the two disorders.

The immediate cause of acute attacks is fluctuating pressure in a fluid inside the inner ear known as endolymph. The endolymph is separated from another fluid called perilymph by thin membranes containing nerves that govern hearing and balance. When the endolymph pressure increases, there is a sudden change in the rate of nerve cells firing, which leads to vertigo and a sense of fullness or discomfort inside the ear. In addition, increased endolymph pressure irritates another structure in the inner ear known as the organ of Corti, which lies inside a shell-shaped structure called the cochlea. The organ of Corti detects pressure impulses, which it converts to electrical impulses that travel along the auditory nerve to the brain. The organ of Corti contains four rows of hair cells that govern a person's perception of the pitch and loudness of a sound. Increased pressure from the endolymph affects the hair cells, causing loss of hearing (particularly the ability to hear low-pitched sounds) and tinnitus.

Diagnosis

Diagnosis of Ménière's disease is a complex process requiring a number of different procedures:

• Patient history, including family history. A primary care physician will ask the patient to describe the symptoms experienced during the attacks, their severity, the dates of recent attacks, and possible triggers.

• Physical examination. Patients often come to the doctor's office with signs of recent vomiting; they may be pale and sweaty, with a fast pulse and higher than normal blood pressure. There may be no unusual findings during the physical examination, however, if the patient is between episodes. If the doctor suspects Ménière's disease on the basis of the patient's personal or family history, he or she will examine the patient's eyes for nystagmus, or rapid and involuntary movements of the eyeball. At this point, a primary care physician may refer the patient to an audiologist or other specialist for further testing.

• Hearing tests. There are several different types of hearing tests used to diagnose Ménière's. The Rinne and Weber tests use a tuning fork to detect hearing loss. In Rinne's test, the examiner holds the stem of a vibrating tuning fork first against the mastoid bone and then outside the ear canal. A person with normal hearing or Ménière's disease will hear the sound as louder when it is held near the outer ear; a person with conductive hearing loss will hear the tone as louder when the fork is touching the bone. In Weber's test, the vibrating tuning fork is held on the midline of the forehead and the patient is asked to indicate the ear in which the sound seems louder. A person with conductive hearing loss on one side will hear the sound louder in the affected ear, while a person with Ménière's disease will hear the sound louder in the unaffected ear. Other hearing tests measure the person's ability to hear sounds of different pitches and volumes. These may be repeated in order to detect periodic variations in the patient's hearing.

• Balance tests. The most common balance tests used to diagnose Ménière's disease are the Romberg test, in which the patient is asked to stand upright and steady with eyes closed; the Fukuda test, in which the patient is asked to march in place with eyes closed; and the Dix-Hallpike test, in which the doctor moves the patient from a sitting position to lying down while holding the patient's head tilted at a 45-degree angle. Patients with Ménière's disease tend to lose their balance or move from side to side during the first two tests. The Dix-Hallpike test is done to rule out benign paroxysmal positional vertigo (BPPV), a condition caused by small crystals of calcium carbonate that have collected within a part of the inner ear called the utricle. Some patients with Ménière's disease may have a positive score on the Dix-Hallpike test, indicating that they also have BPPV.

• Blood tests. These are ordered to rule out metabolic disorders, autoimmune disorders, anemia, leukemia, or infectious diseases (**Lyme disease** and neurosyphilis).

• Transtympanic electrocochleography (ECoG). This test involves the placement of a recording electrode close to

Key Terms

Audiologist A healthcare professional who specializes in diagnostic testing of hearing impairments and rehabilitation of patients with hearing problems.

Cochlea A spiral-shaped tubular structure resembling a snail's shell that forms part of the inner ear.

Conductive hearing loss A type of medically treatable hearing loss in which the inner ear is usually normal, but there are specific problems in the middle or outer ears that prevent sound from getting to the inner ear in a normal way.

Endolymph The fluid contained inside the membranous labyrinth of the inner ear.

Endolymphatic hydrops Another term for Ménière's disease. It defines the disorder in terms of increased fluid pressure in the inner ear.

Idiopathic Of unknown cause or spontaneous origin. Ménière's disease is considered an idiopathic disorder.

Labyrinth The inner ear. It consists of the membranous labyrinth, which is a system of sacs and ducts made of soft tissue; and the osseous or bony labyrinth, which surrounds and contains the membranous labyrinth.

Labyrinthectomy Surgical removal of the labyrinth of the ear. It is done to treat Ménière's disease only when the patient has already suffered severe hearing loss.

Mastoid bone The bony area behind and below the ear.

Nystagmus Rapid and involuntary movements of the eyeball. Measuring and recording episodes of nystagmus is part of the differential diagnosis of Ménière's disease.

Otolaryngology The branch of medicine that treats disorders of the ear, nose, and throat.

Otology The branch of medicine that specializes in medical or surgical treatment of ear disorders.

Perilymph The fluid that lies between the membranous labyrinth of the inner ear and the bony labyrinth.

Prophylaxis A measure taken to prevent disease or an acute attack of a chronic disorder.

Tinnitus A sensation of ringing, buzzing, roaring, or clicking noises in the ear.

Vertigo An illusory feeling that either one's self or the environment is revolving. It is usually caused either by diseases of the inner ear or disturbances of the central nervous system.

the cochlea of the patient's ear; it is done to detect distortion of the membranes in the inner ear. ECoG is most accurate when performed during an attack of Ménière's.

- Electronystagmography (ENG). This test is done to evaluate the functioning of the patient's vestibular and oculomotor (eye movement) systems. It takes about 60–90 minutes to complete and includes stimulating the inner ear with air or water of different temperatures as well as measuring and recording the patient's eye movements in response to lights and similar stimuli. ENG can cause **dizziness** and nausea; patients are told to discontinue all medications for two weeks before the test and to take the test on an empty stomach.

- Imaging studies. **MRIs** and **CT scans** are done to detect abnormalities in the shape or structure of the cochlea and other parts of the inner ear, to rule out tumors, and to detect signs of multiple sclerosis.

Treatment team

A family care practitioner may suspect the diagnosis of Ménière's disease on the basis of the patient's history and physical examination, but the tests required to rule out other diseases or disorders may require specialists in endocrinology, neurology, cardiology, otolaryngology, and internal medicine. Diagnostic hearing tests may be administered by an audiologist. Surgical treatment of Ménière's is usually performed by an otolaryngologist or otologist. A nutritionist or dietitian should be consulted to plan a low-salt diet for the patient.

Patients whose attacks are triggered by emotional stress may be helped by therapists who teach biofeedback, meditation, or other techniques of stress reduction.

Treatment

Medical treatment

Medical management of Ménière's disease involves prophylaxis (prevention of acute attacks) as well as direct treatment of symptoms. Prophylactic treatment begins with **diet and nutrition**. A low-salt diet is recommended for almost all patients with Ménière's, as reducing salt intake helps to lower the body's overall fluid volume. Lowered fluid volume in turn reduces the amount of fluid in the inner ear. Patients should avoid foods with high sodium content, including pizza, smoked or pickled fish, and other preserved foods. Other foods that commonly trigger acute attacks include chocolate; beverages containing caffeine or alcohol, particularly beer and red wine; and foods with high carbohydrate or high cholesterol content. Since nicotine also triggers Ménière's attacks, patients are advised to stop smoking. The doctor may also prescribe a diuretic, usually Dyazide or Diamox, to lower the fluid pressure in the inner ear. Diuretic medications help to prevent acute attacks but will not stop an attack once it has begun.

Medications that are given to treat the symptoms of an attack include drugs that help to control vertigo by numbing the brain's response to nerve impulses from the inner ear. These include such benzodiazepine tranquilizers as **diazepam** (Valium) or alprazolam (Xanax), and such antinausea drugs as prochlorperazine (Compazine). The doctor may also prescribe steroid medications to reduce inflammation in the inner ear.

Surgical treatment

Surgery is usually considered if the patient has not responded to 3–6 months of medical treatment and is healthy enough to undergo general anesthesia. There are four surgical procedures that are commonly done to treat Ménière's disease:

- Endolymphatic sac decompression or shunt. In this procedure, the surgeon inserts a small tube or valve to drain excess endolymph fluid into a space near the mastoid bone and/or removes some of the bone surrounding the endolymphatic sac in order to reduce pressure on it. The success rate is about 60–90% for controlling vertigo, but the procedure often improves the patient's hearing.

- Vestibular nerve sectioning. This procedure is typically done in patients who still have fairly good hearing in the affected ear. The surgeon enters the internal canal of the ear and separates the nerve bundles governing hearing from the nerve bundles that govern the sense of balance, in order to control the patient's vertigo without sacrificing hearing.

- Labyrinthectomy. Labyrinthectomies are performed only in patients whose hearing has already been damaged or destroyed by the disease. The surgeon removes the entire labyrinth of the inner ear. Both vestibular nerve sectioning and labyrinthectomy have a 95–98% success rate in controlling vertigo, but the patient's hearing may be impaired.

- Transtympanic medication perfusion. This procedure involves delivering medications into the middle ear through an incision in the eardrum. Once in the middle ear, the drugs are absorbed into the inner ear. Two types

of drugs are used—steroids and aminoglycoside antibiotics (most commonly gentamicin). Medication perfusion is reported to have a 90% success rate.

Complementary and alternative (CAM) treatments

Acupuncture is an alternative treatment that has been shown to help patients with Ménière's disease. The World Health Organization (WHO) lists Ménière's disease as one of 104 conditions that can be treated effectively with acupuncture. In addition, such stress management techniques as autogenic training, visualization, deep breathing, and muscle stretching are helpful to many patients in lowering the frequency of acute attacks.

Recovery and rehabilitation

Patients with Ménière's are referred to rehabilitation therapy if they have not benefited from dietary changes or medication. In vestibular rehabilitation therapy, the therapist first assesses the patient's general muscular strength and coordination, gait and balance, and the triggers as well as the severity and frequency of the vertigo. Rehabilitation itself involves both balance retraining exercises and habituation exercises, which are designed to weaken the brain's response to specific positions or movements that trigger vertigo.

Clinical trials

As of 2003, no **clinical trials** for Ménière's disease were listed in the National Institutes of Health (NIH) database.

Prognosis

Ménière's disease is not fatal; however, there is no cure for it. Medical treatment between attacks and/or surgery are intended to lower the patient's risk of further hearing loss. Although patients with milder forms of the disorder may be able to control their symptoms through dietary changes alone, the long-term results of Ménière's disease typically include progressive loss of hearing, increasing vertigo, or permanent tinnitus.

Special concerns

Although Ménière's disease is not fatal by itself, it can lead to injuries caused by falls or motor vehicle accidents (if the patient has a severe attack while driving). Although moderate **exercise** is beneficial, patients diagnosed with Ménière's should avoid occupations or sports that require a good sense of balance (e.g., house painting, construction work, or other jobs that require working on ladders; bicycle or horseback riding; mountain climbing; some forms of yoga, etc.) In addition, patients should check their house or apartment for loose rugs, inadequate lighting, unsafe stairs, or other features that could lead to slipping and falling in the event of a sudden attack. A small minority of patients are prevented by severe vertigo from working at any form of regular employment and must file disability claims.

Resources

BOOKS

Haybach, P. J. *Ménière's Disease: What You Need to Know.* Portland, OR: Vestibular Disorders Association, 2000.

"Ménière's Disease." Section 7, Chapter 85 in *The Merck Manual of Diagnosis and Therapy.* Edited by Mark H. Beers, MD, and Robert Berkow, MD. Whitehouse Station, NJ: Merck Research Laboratories, 1999.

Pelletier, Kenneth R., MD. *The Best Alternative Medicine,* Part II, "CAM Therapies for Specific Conditions: Ménière's Disease." New York: Simon & Schuster, 2002.

PERIODICALS

Hain, T. C., and M. Uddin. "Pharmacological Treatment of Vertigo." *CNS Drugs* 17 (2003): 85–100.

Li, John, MD, and Nicholas Lorenzo, MD. "Endolymphatic Hydrops." *eMedicine,* January 18, 2002. <www.emedicine.com/neuro/topic412.htm>.

Li, John, MD. "Inner Ear, Ménière Disease, Surgical Treatment." *eMedicine,* July 17, 2001. <www.emedicine.com/ent/topic233.htm>.

Morrison, A. W., and K. J. Johnson. "Genetics (Molecular Biology) and Ménière Disease." *Otolaryngologic Clinics of North America* 35 (June 2002): 497–516.

Radtke, A., T. Lempert, M. A. Gresty, et al. "Migraine and Ménière's Disease: Is There a Link?" *Neurology* 59 (December 10, 2002): 1700–1704.

Silverstein, H., and L. E. Jackson. "Vestibular Nerve Section." *Otolaryngologic Clinics of North America* 35 (June 2002): 655–673.

Silverstein, H., W. B. Lewis, L. E. Jackson, et al. "Changing Trends in the Surgical Treatment of Ménière's Disease: Results of a 10-Year Survey." *Ear, Nose, and Throat Journal* 82 (March 2003): 185–187, 191–194.

Usami, S., K. Takahashi, I. Yuge, et al. "Mutations in the COCH Gene are a Frequent Cause of Autosomal Dominant Progressive Cochleo-Vestibular Dysfunction, But Not of Ménière's Disease." *European Journal of Human Genetics* 11 (October 2003): 744–748.

Weisleder, P., and T. D. Fife. "Dizziness and Headache: A Common Association in Children and Adolescents." *Journal of Child Neurology* 16 (October 2001): 727–730.

OTHER

National Institute on Deafness and Other Communication Disorders (NIDCD) Health Information. *Ménière's Disease.* NIH Publication No. 98-3404. Bethesda, MD: NIDCD, 2001.

ORGANIZATIONS

American Academy of Otolaryngology—Head and Neck Surgery. One Prince Street, Alexandria, VA 22314. (703) 836-4444; TTY: (703) 519-1585. webmaster@entnet.org. <http://www.entnet.org>.

Ear Foundation. 1817 Patterson Street, Nashville, TN 37203. (615) 284-7807 or (800) 545-HEAR; Fax: (615) 284-7935. earfound@earfoundation.org. <http://www.theearfound.org>.

National Institute on Deafness and Other Communication Disorders (NIDCD), National Institutes of Health, 31 Center Drive, MSC 2320, Bethesda, MD 20892-2320. nidcdinfo@nidcd.nih.gov. <http://www.nidcd.nih.gov>.

Vestibular Disorders Association (VEDA). P. O. Box 4467, Portland, OR 97208-4467. (503) 229-7706. (800) 837-8428. veda@vestibular.org. <http://www.vestibular.org>.

Rebecca J. Frey, PhD

Meninges

Definition

Meninges (singular is meninx) is the collective term for the three membranes covering the brain and spinal cord. The meninges are composed of the dura mater (outer), the arachnoid (middle), and the pia mater (inner). In common usage, the membranes are often referred to as simply the dura, pia, and arachnoid.

Description

Dura is the Latin word for hard, while pia in Latin means soft. The dura mater was so-named because of its tough, fibrous consistency. The pia mater is thinner and more delicate than the dura mater, and is in direct contact with the neural tissue of the brain and spinal cord. Along with the arachnoid layer and the cerebrospinal fluid (CSF), the dura and pia membranes help cushion, protect, and nourish the brain and spinal cord.

Mater is Latin for mother, and thus refers to the membranes' protective and nourishing functions. Each of the meninges can also be classified as to the portion that covers the brain (e.g., dura mater cerebri or dura mater encephali), or that portion lining the spinal cord (e.g., pia mater spinalis). Arachnoid means "spidery," referring to the membrane's webbed appearance and consistency. The space between the arachnoid membrane and pia mater contains many fibrous filaments and blood vessels that attach the two layers.

Anatomy

The outer surface of the dura adheres to the skull, while the inner surface is loosely connected to the arachnoid layer. The exception is the spinal canal, where there is normally a thin layer of fat and a network of blood vessels between the dura and the bony portion of the vertebrae. There is normally no space between the dura and skull on one side, and the dura and arachnoid on the other. However, these are sometimes called "potential" spaces because abnormal conditions may create "actual" spaces there. Anything in the space between the dura and skull is called epidural (above the dura), while the space between the dura and arachnoid is considered subdural (below the dura).

There is normally an actual space between the arachnoid layer and the pia mater known as the subarachnoid space. As noted, it contains many fibrous filaments, known as trabeculae (little beams), joining and stabilizing the two layers. The importance of the subarachnoid space is that it contains the circulating CSF. It is this layer of fluid that helps to cushion the brain and protect it from sudden movements and impacts to the skull.

The pia mater has the appearance of a thin mesh, with a network of tiny blood vessels interlacing it. It is always in contact with the neural tissue of the brain and spinal cord, much like a skin. It follows all of the grooves, folds, and fissures of the brain's various lobes and prominences.

All of the meninges are composed of connective tissue, which is made up of relatively few cells, with an abundance of structural and supportive proteins.

Function

Given the singular importance of the **central nervous system** (CNS) to both basic and higher-level functions of the body, it is not surprising that a system evolved to help protect it. Thicker skull bones would certainly afford more protection against skull fracture and open head injury, but would come at the cost of greater weight for the spine to bear. If the head is struck, or strikes some other object, even unbreakable skull bones would not protect the brain from the injury that results as brain tissue impacts the inside of the skull (concussion). The layer of CSF that circulates in the subarachnoid space helps to lower this risk, although it cannot eliminate it. Wearing a sports helmet composed of a hard, plastic outer shell with firm padding inside simply mimics and augments the safety mechanism already present in the skull and outer lining of the brain.

The dura mater is the tough, but flexible, second line of defense for the brain after the skull. The flexibility of the dura is important in that most skull fractures, other than those involving severe penetrating injuries, will not result in loss of CSF through the injury site which, before the days of antibiotics and emergency medicine, would pose a serious risk for infection and death.

The arachnoid membrane provides a stable substrate and space through which the CSF can circulate, and also provides specialized tissue necessary for absorption of the CSF back into the bloodstream. The arachnoid trabeculae help to anchor the surrounding membranes and keep the subarachnoid space at a constant depth.

While the CSF is normally sterile and mostly inert—containing glucose, proteins, electrolytes (necessary minerals), and very few cells—the brain and spinal neurons nonetheless need some protection from direct contact with the fluid, which is provided by the pia mater. As blood vessels pass through the dura mater and then the subarachnoid space, they pierce the pia mater as they enter the CNS. The membrane follows the blood vessel down and becomes the external portion of the blood vessel wall.

CSF Production and Circulation

In a sense, the CSF can be thought of as a fourth layer of the meninges. The fluid is produced in, circulates through, and is reabsorbed by the meningeal layers, thus creating a self-contained system. The volume of fluid in adults is normally 100–150 ml. About 500 ml of new fluid is produced and reabsorbed each day, which means the CSF is "turned over" three times in 24 hours. It is important for the body to maintain CSF volume within the normal range, since there is limited space within the skull and spinal column. It is also important for the fluid to remain at a constant pressure. Increased fluid pressure typically leads to compression of the surrounding neural tissue, which then leads to increased fluid volume. Since the bones of the skull are not fused in a developing fetus or newborn infant, increased fluid pressure in the brain may cause the head to grow to an abnormally large size (see **Hydrocephalus**), called macrocephaly. The skull bones are fused after about 2 years of age, so increased fluid pressure and volume after that point will most likely result in compression of, and damage to, neural tissue.

The CSF is produced by a layer of densely packed capillaries and supporting cells known as the choroid plexus. It lines the upper portion of the lateral (cerebral), third, and fourth ventricles. Once produced, the CSF flows down through the fourth ventricle, and then through openings at the base of the brain and around the brain stem. Some of the fluid circulates down through the subarachnoid space encircling the length of the spinal cord, while the remainder flows up to the subarachnoid space around the brain.

Most of the fluid is absorbed back into the bloodstream through vessels lining branched projections from

Key Terms

Arachnoid membrane One of the three membranes that sheath the spinal cord and brain; the arachnoid is the middle membrane. Also called the arachnoid mater.

Cerebrospinal fluid The clear, normally colorless fluid that fills the brain cavities (ventricles), the subarachnoid space around the brain, and the spinal cord and acts as a shock absorber.

Choroid plexus Specialized cells located in the ventricles of the brain that produce cerebrospinal fluid.

Dura mater The strongest and outermost of three membranes that protect the brain, spinal cord, and nerves of the cauda equina.

Hydrocephalus An abnormal accumulation of cerebrospinal fluid within the brain. This accumulation can be harmful by pressing on brain structures, and damaging them.

Meningitis An infection or inflammation of the membranes that cover the brain and spinal cord. It is usually caused by bacteria or a virus.

Pia mater The innermost of the three meninges covering the brain.

Ventricles The four fluid-filled chambers, or cavities, found in the two cerebral hemispheres of the brain, at the center of the brain, and between the brain stem and cerebellum. They are linked by channels, or ducts, allowing cerebral fluid to circulate through them.

the arachnoid membrane called arachnoid villi, or granulations. These arachnoid granulations extend into the dura, primarily at points where large blood veins lie within the dural membrane itself. These veins traveling through the dura that drain blood and absorbed CSF from the brain are collectively known as the venous sinuses of the dura mater. The remainder of the CSF is absorbed through small lymph sacs scattered around the CNS known as perineural lymphatics.

Causes and symptoms

Infection/inflammation of the meninges is covered elsewhere (see Meningitis). Other abnormalities of the meninges typically involve situations in which a fluid occupies and expands the epidural, subdural, or subarachnoid spaces. For instance, blood accumulation that separates the dura from the inner side of the skull is known as an **epidural hematoma** (blood swelling). The same process occurrence between the dura and arachnoid layers is a **subdural hematoma**. Both of these conditions are most frequently caused by head trauma, but may also result from a bleeding disorder or defect in a cranial blood vessel (aneurysm).

A hemorrhage between the arachnoid membrane and the pia mater is called a subarachnoid bleed, and is usually caused by the rupture of a congenital aneurysm, hypertension, or trauma. Unlike conditions affecting the epidural and subdural spaces, a bleed into the subarachnoid space is less likely to affect its volume and increase pressure. A subarachnoid CSF infection (abscess), however, may cause increased pressure.

Meningitis may also cause bleeding into the subdural or epidural spaces, but more often results in the accumulation of fluid and pus, which are consequences of the body's response to the infection.

Resources
BOOKS
DeMyer, William. *Neuroanatomy*, 2nd ed. Baltimore: Williams & Wilkins, 1998.
Walker, Pam and Elaine Wood. *The Brain and Nervous System.* Farmington Hills: Lucent Books, 2003.
Weiner, William J. and Christopher G. Goetz, eds. *Neurology for the Non-Neurologist*, 4th ed. Philadelphia: Lippincott Williams & Wilkins, 1999.
Willett, Edward. *Meningitis.* Berkeley Heights: Enslow Publishers, Inc., 1999.

Scott J. Polzin, MS, CGC

Meningitis *see* **Encephalitis and meningitis**

Mental retardation

Definition

Mental retardation (MR) is a developmental disability that first appears in children under the age of 18. It is defined as a level of intellectual functioning (as measured by standard intelligence tests) that is well below average and results in significant limitations in the person's daily living skills (adaptive functioning).

Description

Mental retardation begins in childhood or adolescence before the age of 18. In most cases, it persists throughout adult life. A diagnosis of mental retardation is made if an individual has an intellectual functioning level well below average, as well as significant limitations in two or more adaptive skill areas. Intellectual functioning level is defined by standardized tests that measure the ability to reason in terms of mental age (intelligence quotient or IQ). Mental retardation is defined as an IQ score below 70–75; a normal score is 100. Adaptive skills refer to skills needed for daily life. Such skills include the ability to produce and understand language (communication); home-living skills; use of community resources; health, safety, leisure, self-care, and social skills; self-direction; functional academic skills (reading, writing, and arithmetic); and job-related skills.

In general, mentally retarded children reach such developmental milestones as walking and talking much later than children in the general population. Symptoms of mental retardation may appear at birth or later in childhood. The child's age at onset depends on the suspected cause of the disability. Some cases of mild mental retardation are not diagnosed before the child enters preschool or kindergarten. These children typically have difficulties with social, communication, and functional academic skills. Children who have a neurological disorder or illness such as encephalitis or meningitis may suddenly show signs of cognitive impairment and adaptive difficulties.

Mental retardation varies in severity. The *Diagnostic and Statistical Manual of Mental Disorders*, fourth edition, text revision (DSM-IV-TR), which is the diagnostic standard for mental healthcare professionals in the United States, classifies four degrees of mental retardation: mild, moderate, severe, and profound. These categories are based on the person's level of functioning.

Mild mental retardation

Approximately 85% of the mentally retarded population is in the mildly retarded category. Their IQ score ranges from 50–70, and they can often acquire academic skills up to about the sixth-grade level. They can become fairly self-sufficient and, in some cases, live independently, with community and social support.

Moderate mental retardation

About 10% of the mentally retarded population is considered moderately retarded. These people have IQ scores ranging from 35–55. They can carry out work and self-care tasks with moderate supervision. They typically acquire communication skills in childhood and are able to live and function successfully within the community in such supervised environments as group homes.

Severe mental retardation

About 3–4% of the mentally retarded population is severely retarded. They have IQ scores of 20–40. They may master very basic self-care skills and some communication skills. Many severely retarded individuals are able to live in a group home.

Profound mental retardation

Only 1–2% of the mentally retarded population is classified as profoundly retarded. These individuals have IQ scores under 20–25. They may be able to develop basic self-care and communication skills with appropriate support and training. Their retardation is often caused by an accompanying neurological disorder. Profoundly retarded people need a high level of structure and supervision.

AAMR classifications

The American Association on Mental Retardation (AAMR) has developed another widely accepted diagnostic classification system for mental retardation. The AAMR classification system focuses on the capabilities of retarded individuals rather than on their limitations. The categories describe the level of support required, including intermittent support, limited support, extensive support, and pervasive support. To some extent, the AAMR classification mirrors the DSM-IV-TR classification. Intermittent support, for example, is support that is needed only occasionally, perhaps during times of stress or crisis for the retarded person. It is the type of support typically required for most mildly retarded people. At the other end of the spectrum, pervasive support, which is life-long, daily support for most adaptive areas, would be required for profoundly retarded persons. The AAMR classification system refers to the "below-average intellectual function" as an IQ of 70–75 or below.

Demographics

The prevalence of mental retardation in North America is a subject of heated debate. It is thought to be 1–3% of the population, depending on the methods of assessment and criteria of assessment that are used. Many people believe that the actual prevalence is probably closer to 1%, and that the 3% figure is based on misleading mortality rates, cases that are diagnosed in early infancy, and the instability of the diagnosis across the age span. If the 1% figure is accepted, however, that means that 2.5 million mentally retarded people reside in the United States. Males are more likely than females to be mentally retarded at a 1.5:1 ratio.

Causes and symptoms

Causes

A variety of problems can lead to mental retardation. The three most common causes of mental retardation, accounting for about 30% of cases, are Down syndrome, fragile X, and fetal alcohol syndrome. In about 40% of cases, the cause of mental retardation cannot be found. The causes of mental retardation can be divided into broad classifications, including genetic factors, prenatal illnesses and exposures, childhood illnesses and injuries, and environmental factors.

GENETIC FACTORS About 30% of cases of mental retardation are caused by hereditary factors. Mental retardation may be caused by an inherited genetic abnormality such as fragile X syndrome. Fragile X, a defect in the chromosome that determines sex, is the most common inherited cause of mental retardation. Single-gene defects such as phenylketonuria (PKU) and other inborn errors of metabolism may also cause mental retardation if they are not discovered and treated early. An accident or mutation in genetic development may also cause retardation. Examples of such accidents are development of an extra chromosome 18 (trisomy 18) and Down syndrome. Down syndrome, also called mongolism or trisomy 21, is caused by an abnormality in the development of chromosome 21. It is the most common genetic cause of mental retardation.

PRENATAL ILLNESSES AND EXPOSURES Fetal alcohol syndrome (FAS) affects one in 3,000 children in Western countries. Fetal alcohol syndrome results from the mother's heavy drinking during the first 12 weeks (trimester) of pregnancy. Some studies have shown that even moderate alcohol use during pregnancy may cause learning disabilities in children. Drug abuse and cigarette smoking during pregnancy have also been linked to mental retardation. It is generally accepted that pregnant women should avoid all alcohol, tobacco, and recreational drugs.

Maternal infections and such illnesses as glandular disorders, rubella, toxoplasmosis, and cytomegalovirus (CMV) infection may cause mental retardation. When the mother has high blood pressure (hypertension) or blood poisoning (toxemia), the flow of oxygen to the fetus may be reduced, causing brain damage and mental retardation.

Birth defects that cause physical deformities of the head, brain, and **central nervous system** frequently cause mental retardation. Neural tube defect, for example, is a birth defect in which the neural tube that forms the spinal cord does not close completely. This defect may cause children to develop an accumulation of cerebrospinal fluid inside the skull (**hydrocephalus**). Hydrocephalus can cause learning impairment by putting pressure on the brain.

CHILDHOOD ILLNESSES AND INJURIES Hyperthyroidism, whooping cough, chicken pox, measles, and Hib disease (a bacterial infection) may cause mental retardation if they are not treated adequately. An infection of the membrane covering the brain (meningitis) or an inflammation of the brain itself (encephalitis) can cause swelling that in turn may cause brain damage and mental retardation. **Traumatic brain injury** caused by a blow to the head or by violent shaking of the upper body may also cause brain damage and mental retardation in children.

ENVIRONMENTAL FACTORS Ignored or neglected infants who are not provided with the mental and physical stimulation required for normal development may suffer irreversible learning impairment. Children who live in poverty and suffer from malnutrition, unhealthy living conditions, abuse, and improper or inadequate medical care are at a higher risk. Exposure to lead or mercury can also cause mental retardation. Many children have developed lead poisoning from eating the flaking lead-based paint often found in older buildings.

Symptoms

Low IQ scores and limitations in adaptive skills are the hallmarks of mental retardation. Aggression, self-injury, and mood disorders are sometimes associated with the disability. The severity of the symptoms and the age at which they first appear depend on the cause. Children who are mentally retarded reach developmental milestones significantly later than expected, if at all. If retardation is caused by chromosomal or other genetic disorders, it is often apparent from infancy. If retardation is caused by childhood illnesses or injuries, learning and adaptive skills that were once easy may suddenly become difficult or impossible to master.

Diagnosis

If mental retardation is suspected, a comprehensive physical examination and medical history should be done immediately to discover any organic cause of symptoms. Such conditions as hyperthyroidism and PKU are treatable. The progression of retardation can be stopped and, in some cases, partially reversed if these conditions are discovered early. If a neurological cause such as brain injury is suspected, the child may be referred to a **neurologist** or **neuropsychologist** for testing.

A complete medical, family, social, and educational history is compiled from existing medical and school records (if applicable) and from interviews with parents. Children are given intelligence tests to measure their learning abilities and intellectual functioning. Such tests include the Stanford-Binet Intelligence Scale, the Wechsler

Key Terms

Amniocentesis A test usually done between 16 and 20 weeks of pregnancy to detect any abnormalities in the development of the fetus. A small amount of the fluid surrounding the fetus (amniotic fluid) is drawn out through a needle inserted into the mother's womb. Laboratory analysis of this fluid can detect various genetic defects such as Down syndrome or neural tube defects.

Developmental delay The failure to meet certain developmental milestones such as sitting, walking, and talking at the average age. Developmental delay may indicate a problem in development of the central nervous system.

Down syndrome A genetic disorder characterized by an extra chromosome 21 (trisomy 21), mental retardation, and susceptibility to early-onset Alzheimer's disease.

Extensive support Ongoing daily support required to assist an individual in a specific adaptive area, such as daily help with preparing meals.

Hib disease An infection caused by *Haemophilus influenza*, type b (Hib). This disease mainly affects children under the age of five. In that age group, it is the leading cause of bacterial meningitis, pneumonia, joint and bone infections, and throat inflammations.

Inborn error of metabolism A rare enzyme deficiency; children with inborn errors of metabolism do not have certain enzymes that the body requires to maintain organ functions. Inborn errors of metabolism can cause brain damage and mental retardation if left untreated. Phenylketonuria is an inborn error of metabolism.

Limited support A predetermined period of assistance required to deal with a specific event, such as training for a new job.

Phenylketonuria (PKU) An inherited disease in which the body cannot metabolize the amino acid phenylalanine properly. If untreated, phenylketonuria can cause mental retardation.

Trisomy An abnormality in chromosomal development. In a trisomy syndrome, an extra chromosome is present so that the individual has three of a particular chromosome instead of the normal pair. An extra chromosome 18 (trisomy 18) causes mental retardation.

Ultrasonography A process that uses the reflection of high-frequency sound waves to make an image of structures deep within the body. Ultrasonography is routinely used to detect fetal abnormalities.

Intelligence Scales, the Wechsler Preschool and Primary Scale of Intelligence, and the Kaufman Assessment Battery for Children. For infants, the Bayley Scales of Infant Development may be used to assess motor, language, and problem-solving skills. Interviews with parents or other caregivers are used to assess the child's daily living, muscle control, communication, and social skills. The Woodcock-Johnson Scales of Independent Behavior and the Vineland Adaptive Behavior Scale are frequently used to evaluate these skills.

Treatment team

The treatment team will depend on the underlying cause of mental retardation. A neurologist, neuropsychologist, child psychiatrist, and/or development pediatrician may be helpful for nearly all cases of mental retardation, both to assess underlying cause and to plan for appropriate and helpful interventions. Other members of the treatment team will depend on the underlying cause of mental retardation, accompanying medical problems, and the severity of the deficits.

Treatment

Federal legislation entitles mentally retarded children to free testing and appropriate, individualized education and skills training within the school system from ages three to 21. For children under the age of three, many states have established early intervention programs that assess children, make recommendations, and begin treatment programs. Many day schools are available to help train retarded children in such basic skills as bathing and feeding themselves. Extracurricular activities and social programs are also important in helping retarded children and adolescents gain self-esteem.

Training in independent living and job skills is often begun in early adulthood. The level of training depends on the degree of retardation. Mildly retarded people can often acquire the skills needed to live independently and hold an outside job. Moderate to profoundly retarded persons usually require supervised community living in a group home or other residential setting.

Family therapy can help relatives of the mentally retarded develop coping skills. It can also help parents deal with feelings of guilt or anger. A supportive, warm home environment is essential to help the mentally retarded reach their full potential.

Prognosis

People with mild to moderate mental retardation are frequently able to achieve some self-sufficiency and to lead happy and fulfilling lives. To reach these goals, they need appropriate and consistent educational, community, social, family, and vocational supports. The outlook is less promising for those with severe to profound retardation. Studies have shown that these persons have a shortened life expectancy. The diseases that are usually associated with severe retardation may cause the shorter lifespan. People with Down syndrome will develop the brain changes that characterize **Alzheimer's disease** in later life and may develop the clinical symptoms of this disease as well.

Special concerns

Prevention

Immunization against diseases such as measles and Hib prevents many of the illnesses that can cause mental retardation. In addition, all children should undergo routine developmental screening as part of their pediatric care. Screening is particularly critical for those children who may be neglected or undernourished or may live in disease-producing conditions. Newborn screening and immediate treatment for PKU and hyperthyroidism can usually catch these disorders early enough to prevent retardation.

Good prenatal care can also help prevent retardation. Pregnant women should be educated about the risks of alcohol consumption and the need to maintain good nutrition during pregnancy. Such tests as amniocentesis and **ultrasonography** can determine whether a fetus is developing normally in the womb.

Resources

BOOKS

American Psychiatric Association. "Mental Retardation." In *Diagnostic and Statistical Manual of Mental Disorders*, 4th ed., text revision. Washington, DC: American Psychiatric Press, Inc., 2000.

Jaffe, Jerome H., M.D. "Mental Retardation." In *Comprehensive Textbook of Psychiatry*, edited by Benjamin J. Sadock, MD, and Virginia A. Sadock, MD. 7th edition. Philadelphia, PA: Lippincott Williams and Wilkins, 2000.

Julian, John N. "Mental Retardation." In *Psychiatry Update and Board Preparation*, edited by Thomas A. Stern, MD, and John B. Herman, MD. New York: McGraw Hill, 2000.

PERIODICALS

Bozikas,Vasilis, MD, et al. "Gabapentin for Behavioral Dyscontrol with Mental Retardation." *American Journal Psychiatry* June 2001: 965–966.

Margolese, Howard C., MD, et al. "Olanzapine-Induced Neuroleptic Malignant Syndrome with Mental Retardation." *American Journal Psychiatry* July 1999: 1115A–1116.

ORGANIZATIONS

American Association on Mental Retardation (AAMR). 444 North Capitol Street, NW, Washington, D.C. 20001. (800) 424-3688. <http://www.aamr.org>.

The Arc of the United States (formerly Association of Retarded Citizens of the United States). 1010 Wayne Avenue, Silver Spring, M.D. 20910. (301) 565-3842. <http://thearc.org>.

OTHER

National Information Center for Children and Youth and Disabilities. P.O. Box 1492,Washington, D.C. 20013. (800) 695-0285. <http://www.nichcy.org>.

Paula Anne Ford-Martin
Rosalyn Carson-DeWitt, MD

Meralgia paresthetica

Definition

Meralgia paresthetica is a condition characterized by numbness, tingling, or **pain** along the outer thigh.

Description

Meralgia paresthetica occurs when the lateral femoral cutaneous nerve, which supplies sensation to the outer part of the thigh, is compressed or entrapped at the point where it exits the pelvis. Usually, only one thigh is affected. Obese, diabetic, or pregnant people are more susceptible to this disorder. Tight clothing may exacerbate or cause the condition.

Demographics

Overweight individuals are more likely to develop meralgia paresthetica; men are more commonly affected than women. The disorder tends to occur in middle-aged individuals.

Causes and symptoms

Meralgia paresthetica is the result of pressure on the lateral femoral cutaneous nerve, and subsequent inflammation of the nerve. The point of pressure or entrapment is usually where the nerve exits the pelvis, running through the inguinal ligament. Being overweight, having diabetes or other risk factors for nerve disorders, wearing tight clothing or belts, previous surgery in the area of the lateral femoral cutaneous nerve, or injury (such as pelvic fracture) predispose individuals to meralgia paresthetica.

Symptoms of meralgia paresthetica include numbness, tingling, stinging, or burning pain along the outer thigh. The skin of the outer thigh may be particularly sensitive to touch, resulting in increased pain. Many people note that their symptoms are initiated or worsened by walking or standing.

Diagnosis

The diagnosis is usually evident based on the patient's description of symptoms and the physical examination. Neurological testing will usually reveal normal thigh-muscle strength and normal reflexes, but there will be numbness or extreme sensitivity of the skin along the outer aspect of the thigh.

Treatment team

Depending on its severity, meralgia paresthetica may be treated by a family medicine doctor, internal medicine specialist, **neurologist**, or orthopedic surgeon.

Treatment

Patients with meralgia paresthetica are usually advised to lose weight and to wear loose, light clothing. Sometimes medications (amitriptyline, **carbamazepine**, or **gabapentin**, for example) can ameliorate some of the symptoms. In patients with severe pain, temporary relief can be obtained by injecting lidocaine (a local anesthetic) and steroids (an anti-inflammatory agent) into the lateral femoral cutaneous nerve. In very refractory cases, surgery to free the entrapped lateral femoral cutaneous nerve may be required in order to improve symptoms.

Prognosis

Many cases of meralgia paresthetica resolve spontaneously, usually within two years of onset.

Resources

BOOKS

Pryse-Phillips, William, and T. Jock Murray. "Peripheral Neuropathies." In *Noble: Textbook of Primary Care Medicine*, edited by John Noble, et al. St. Louis: W. B. Saunders Company, 2001.

Verdugo, Renato J., et al. "Pain and temperature." In *Textbook of Clinical Neurology*, edited by Christopher G. Goetz. Philadelphia: W. B. Saunders Company, 2003.

PERIODICALS

Shapiro, B. E. "Entrapment and compressive neuropathies." *Medical Clinics of North America* 8, no. 3 (May 2003): 663–696

WEBSITES

National Institute of Neurological Disorders and Stroke (NINDS). *NINDS Meralgia Paresthetica Disease Information Page.* January 28, 2003 (June 3, 2004). <http://www.ninds.nih.gov/health_and_medical/disorders/meralgia_paresthetica.htm>.

Rosalyn Carson-DeWitt, MD

▌Metachromatic leukodystrophy

Definition

Metachromatic **leukodystrophy** (MLD) is a rare degenerative neurological disease, and is the most common form of the leukodystrophies, a group of disorders affecting the fatty covering that acts as an insulator around nerve fibers known as the myelin sheath. With destruction of the myelin sheath, progressive deterioration of muscle control and intellectual ability occurs. Metachromatic leukodystrophy is inherited as an autosomal recessive trait, meaning that that the disease is inherited from parents that are both carriers, but do not have the disorder. There are three forms of MLD, distinguished by the age of onset and by the molecular defect in the gene underlying the disease.

Description

The late infantile form of metachromatic leukodystrophy, which is the most common form, usually begins in the second year of life (ranges 1–3 years). After normal early development, the infant displays irritability and an unstable walk. As the disease progresses, physical and mental deterioration occur. Developmental milestones, such as language development, are not met, and muscle wasting eventually gives way to spastic movements, then profound weakness. **Seizures** usually occur, followed by paralysis.

The juvenile form of MLD usually begins between the ages of 4 and 10 (ranges 3–20 years), and presents with disturbances in the ability to walk (gait disturbances), urinary incontinence, mental deterioration, and emotional difficulties. Some scientists distinguish between early and late juvenile MLD. Late juvenile MLD is similar to the adult form of the disease. Adult MLD begins after the age of 20 (ranges 16–30 years) and presents mainly with emotional disturbances and psychiatric symptoms, leading to a diagnosis of psychosis. Disorders of movement and posture appear later. **Dementia** (loss of mental capacity), seizures, and decreased visual function also occur.

Key Terms

Autosomal recessive disorder A genetic disorder that is inherited from parents who are both carriers, but do not have the disorder. Parents with an affected recessive gene have a 25% chance of passing on the disorder to their offspring with each pregnancy.

Demyelination Loss of the myelin covering of some nerve fibers resulting in their impaired function.

Enzyme A protein produced by living cells that regulates the speed of the chemical reactions that are involved in the metabolism of living organisms, without itself being altered in the process.

Demographics

The frequency of MLD is estimated to be 1 in 40,000 persons in the United States. No differences have been identified on the basis of race, sex, or ethnic origin.

Causes and symptoms

MLD is caused by a deficiency of the enzyme arylsulfatase A (ARSA). Without properly functioning ARSA, a fatty substance known as sulfatide accumulates in the brain and other areas of the body such as the liver, gall bladder, kidneys, and/or spleen. The buildup of sulfatide in the **central nervous system** causes demyelination, the destruction of the myelin protective covering on nerve fibers. With progressive demyelination, motor skills and mental function diminish.

MLD is an autosomal recessive inherited disease and can be caused by mutations in two different genes, the ARSA and the prosaposin gene. Mutations in the ARSA gene are far more frequent. So far, about 50 mutations have been identified in ARSA gene.

Diagnosis

Diagnosis of MLD is suspected in a person displaying its symptoms. **Magnetic resonance imaging** may be used to identify lesions and atrophy (wasting) in the white matter of the brain that are characteristic of MLD. Urine tests usually show elevated sulfatide levels. Some psychiatric disorders coupled with difficulty walking or muscle wasting suggest the possibility of MLD. Blood testing can show a reduced activity of the ARSA enzyme.

Deficiency of the ARSA enzyme alone is not proof of MLD, because a substantial ARSA deficiency without any symptoms or clinical consequences is frequent in the general population. During diagnosis and genetic counseling, these harmless ARSA enzyme deficiencies must be distinguished from those causing MLD. The only diagnostic test that solves this problem and is definitive for MLD diagnosis is analysis of the genetic mutation.

Treatment team

The treatment team usually involves a **neurologist**, a pediatrician, an ophthalmologist, an orthopedist, a genetic counselor, a neurodevelopmental psychologist, a bone marrow transplant physician, a genetic and/or metabolic disease specialist, and also a physical and an occupational therapist.

Treatment

No effective treatment is available to reverse the course of MLD. Drug therapy is part of supportive care for symptoms such as behavioral disturbances, feeding difficulties, seizures, and constipation. Bone marrow transplantation has been tried and there is evidence that this treatment might slow the progression of the disease. In infants, during a symptom-free phase of the late infantile form, neurocognitive function may be stabilized, but the symptoms of motor function loss progress. Persons with the juvenile and adult forms of MLD and with mild or no symptoms are more likely to be stabilized with bone marrow transplantation. **Gene therapy** experimentation on animal models as a possible therapy is still under consideration, and there are not yet any gene therapy-related **clinical trials** for MLD.

Recovery and rehabilitation

MLD patients require follow-up evaluation and treatment. Physical therapists, occupational therapists, orthopedists, ophthalmologists, and neuropsychologists are often involved in helping maintain optimal function for as long as possible.

Clinical trials

As of early 2004, there is one open clinical trial for MLD sponsored by Fairview University and the National Institutes of Health: "Phase II Study of Allogeneic Bone Marrow or Umbilical Cord Blood Transplantation in Patients With Lysosomal or Peroxisomal Inborn Errors of Metabolism." Further information about the trial can be found at the National Institutes of Health clinical trials website <http://www.clinicaltrials.gov/ct/show/NCT00005894?order=1>.

Prognosis

In young children with the late infantile form of MLD, progressive loss of motor and cognitive functions is rapid. Death usually results within five years after the onset of clinical symptoms. In the early juvenile form of MLD, although progression is less rapid, death usually occurs within 10–15 years of diagnosis, and most young people with the disease die before the age of 20. Persons with the late juvenile form often survive into early adulthood, and patients with the adult form may have an even slower progression.

Special concerns

Genetic counseling is important to inform the family about the risk of occurrence of MLD in future offspring. Prenatal testing may be available on an experimental basis in some centers.

Resources

BOOKS

Icon Health Publications. *The Official Parent's Sourcebook on Metachromatic Leukodystrophy: A Revised and Updated Directory for the Internet Age.* San Diego: Icon International Publishers, 2002.

von Figura, K., V. Gieselman, and J. Jaeken. "Metachromatic leukodystrophy." In *The Metabolic and Molecular Bases of Inherited Disease,* 8th ed., C. Scriver, A. Beadet, D. Valle, W. Sly, et al, eds. New York: McGraw-Hill Professional, 2001.

PERIODICALS

Giesselmann, V. "Metachromatic leukodystrophy: recent research developments." *J Child Neurol.* 18, no. 9 (September 2003): 591–594.

OTHER

"NINDS Metachromatic Leukodystrophy Information Page." *National Institute of Neurological Disorders and Stroke.* (March 4, 2004). <http://www.ninds.nih.gov/ health_and_medical/disorders/meta_leu_doc.htm>.

ORGANIZATIONS

National Tay-Sachs and Allied Diseases Association. 2001 Beacon Street , Suite 204, Brighton, MA 02135. (617) 277-4463 or (800) 90-NTSAD (906-8723). info@ntsad.org. <http://www.ntsad.org>.

United Leukodystrophy Foundation. 2304 Highland Drive, Sycamore, IL 60178. (815) 895-3211 or (800) 728-5483; Fax: (815) 895-2432. ulf@tbcnet.com. <http://www.ulf.org>.

Igor Medica, MD, PhD

Methylphenidate *see* **Central nervous system stimulants**

Methylprednisolone *see* **Glucocorticoids**

Microcephaly

Definition

Microcephaly is a neurological disorder where the distance around the largest portion of the head (the circumference) is less than should normally be the case in an infant or a child. The condition can be evident at birth, or can develop within the first few years following birth. The smaller than normal head restricts the normal growth and development of the brain.

Description

The word microcephaly comes from the Greek *micros* meaning small, and *kephale* meaning head. The small head circumference that is a hallmark of microcephaly has been defined as that which is either two or three standard deviations (a statistical measure of variability) below the normal average head circumference for the age, gender, and race of the child. Put another way, the head size is markedly smaller than the expected size for about 97–99% of other children.

The condition can be present at birth or may develop during the first few years of life. In the latter situation, the growth of the head fails to keep to a normal pace. This produces a small head, relatively large face (since the face keeps growing at a normal rate), and a forehead that slopes backward. The smallness of the head becomes even more pronounced with age. An older child with microcephaly also has a body that is smaller and lighter than normal. This may be a consequence of the restricted brain development.

Demographics

Microcephaly is a rare neurological condition and occurs worldwide. Little detailed information on the prevalence of the disorder is available. Microcephaly does not appear to be more prevalent among any race or one gender.

Causes and symptoms

Microcephaly may have a genetic basis. If the gene defect(s) are expressed during fetal development, the condition is present at birth. This is the congenital form of the disorder. The microcephaly that develops after birth may still reflect genetically based developmental defects. As well, the delayed microcephaly can be caused if the normal openings in the skull close too soon after birth, preventing normal head growth. This condition is also referred to as **craniosynostosis**.

Other possible causes of microcephaly include infections during pregnancy (rubella, cytomegalovirus, toxoplasmosis), adverse effects of medication, and the

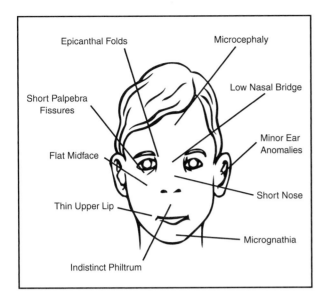

Epicanthal Folds
Microcephaly
Short Palpebra Fissures
Low Nasal Bridge
Flat Midface
Minor Ear Anomalies
Thin Upper Lip
Short Nose
Indistinct Philtrum
Micrognathia

Microcephaly and other abnormalities produced by fetal alcohol syndrome. (*EPD Photos.*)

excessive use of alcohol by the mother during pregnancy (fetal alcohol syndrome).

The damage from microcephaly comes because of the cramped interior of the skull. This lack of space exerts pressure on the growing brain. This causes impairment and delayed development of functions such as speech and control of muscles. The impaired muscle control can produce effects ranging from a relatively minor clumsiness in body movement to the more serious and complete loss of control of the arms and legs. A child can also be hyperactive and mentally retarded, although the latter is not always present. As a child grows older, **seizures** may occur.

It should be noted that at times it is diminished growth of the brain that results in microcephaly. Without proper brain growth, the surrounding skull does not expand and microcephaly results.

Diagnosis

Diagnosis of craniosynostosis and microcephaly is made by a physician, typically during examination after birth. A physician may also be alerted to the presence of microcephaly based on the appearance of the head at birth. Other clues in the few years after birth can be the failure to achieve certain developmental milestones, and the appearance of the distinctive facial appearance.

Treatment team

The medical treatment team can consist of family and more specialized physicians and nurses. Parents and caregivers play an important role in supportive care. As various developmental challenges present themselves,

physical therapists and special education providers may become part of the treatment team.

Treatment

In the case of craniosynostosis, surgery can be accomplished to reopen the prematurely closed regions of the skull. This allows the brain to grow normally. There is no such treatment for the congenital form of microcephaly. Treatment then consists of providing for the person's comfort and strategies to compensate for physical and mental delays.

Recovery and rehabilitation

Recovery from craniosynostosis can be complete if surgery is done at an early enough age. For a child with other forms of microcephaly, few treatment options are available. Emphasis, therefore, is placed upon maximizing mobility and mental development, rather than recovery. Speech therapists and audiologists can help with hearing and language development. Physical and occupational therapists provide aid in walking and adaptive equipment such as wheelchairs. Special education teachers coordinate educational goals and strategies based upon the child's abilities.

Clinical trials

Although as of April 2004, there are no ongoing **clinical trials** underway for the study or treatment of microcephaly, research is being done to explore and understand the mechanisms, particularly genetic, of brain and skull development. By understanding the nature of the developmental malfunctions, it is hoped that corrective or preventative strategies might be developed.

Prognosis

With surgery, the prognosis for children with craniosynostosis can be good. However the outlook for children with other forms of microcephaly is poor, and the likelihood of having normal brain function is likewise poor.

Special concerns

As microcephaly is often associated with chromosomal abnormalities, the specific genetic cause for a person's microcephaly should be determined, if possible. Genetic counseling is available to help parents with information about their child with microcephaly and to plan for future pregnancies.

Resources

BOOKS

Parker, J. N., and P. M. Parker. *The Official Parent's Sourcebook on Microcephaly: A Revised and Updated Directory for the Internet Age.* San Diego: Icon Health Publications, 2002.

PERIODICALS

Woods, C. G. "Human microcephaly." *Current Opinions in Neurobiology* (February 2004): 112–117.

OTHER

National Institute of Neurological Disorders and Stroke. *NINDS Microcephaly Information Page.* <http://www.ninds.nih.gov/health_and_medical/disorders/microcephaly.htm> (April 9, 2004).

ORGANIZATIONS

National Institute for Neurological Diseases and Stroke (NINDS). 6001 Executive Boulevard, Bethesda, MD 20892. (301) 496-5751 or (800) 352-9424. <http://www.ninds.nih.gov>.

National Institute for Child Health and Human Development (NICHD). 31 Center Drive, Rm. 2A32 MSC 2425, Bethesda, MD 20892-2425. (301) 496-5133; Fax: (301) 496-7101. <http://www.nichd.nih.gov>.

National Organization for Rare Disorders. 55 Kenosia Avenue, Danbury, CT 06813-1968. (203) 744-0100 or (800) 999-6673; Fax: (203) 798-2291. orphan@rarediseases.org. <http://www.rarediseases.org>.

March of Dimes Birth Defects Foundation. 1275 Mamaroneck Avenue, White Plains, NY 10605. (914) 428-7100 or (888) 663-4637; Fax: (914) 428-8203. askus@marchofdimes.com. <http://www.marchofdimes.com>.

Brian Douglas Hoyle, PhD

Migraine headache *see* **Headache**

Miller-Fisher syndrome *see* **Fisher syndrome**

Mini-strokes *see* **Transient ischemic attack**

Mitochondrial myopathies

Definition

Mitochondrial myopathies are a group of neuromuscular disorders that result from defects in the function of the mitochondrion, a small organelle located inside many cells that are responsible for fulfilling energy requirements of the tissue. These structures serve as "power plants" and are particularly important for providing energy for both muscle and brain function due to the large requirement for energy in these tissues.

People affected with one of these disorders usually have muscle symptoms such as weakness, breathlessness, **exercise** intolerance, heart failure, **dementia**, stroke-like symptoms, deafness, blindness, **seizures**, heavy eyelids or eye problems, and/or vomiting. Originally, mitochondrial myopathies were recognized based solely on clinical findings. Currently, there are genetic explanations that provide additional information that is usually consistent with the clinical diagnosis and can, in some cases, help determine the long-term prognosis. Mitochondrial myopathies can also result as secondary effects from other diseases.

Description

Myopathy means a disorder of the muscle tissue or muscle. Mitochondrial myopathies are, therefore, disorders of the muscle tissue caused by abnormalities of the mitochondria.

The following disorders are the most common mitochondrial myopathies, including:

• NARP: neuropathy, **ataxia** and retinitis pigmentosa

• KS: Kearns-Sayre syndrome

• Leigh's syndrome

• PEO: progressive external ophthalmoplegia

• MILS: maternally inherited Leigh's syndrome

• MELAS: mitochondrial encephalomyopathy, lactic acidosis, and strokelike episodes

• MERFF: **myoclonus epilepsy** with ragged-red fibers

• Pearson syndrome

• MNGIE: mitochondrial neurogastrointestinal **encephalopathy**

• LHON: Leber hereditary optic neuropathy

Demographics

The initial disease-causing or disease-related (pathogenic) alterations in mitochondrial DNA (mtDNA) were first identified in the early 1990s. Currently, more than 50 different single-base pathogenic mutations in the mtDNA sequence and more than 100 different pathogenic rearrangements within the genome have been identified. These include large deletions or duplications in the mtDNA sequence of bases. With the high mutation rate, it would seem that the prevalence of mitochondrial myopathies would be high; however, mitochondrial myopathies are relatively rare, having an incidence of

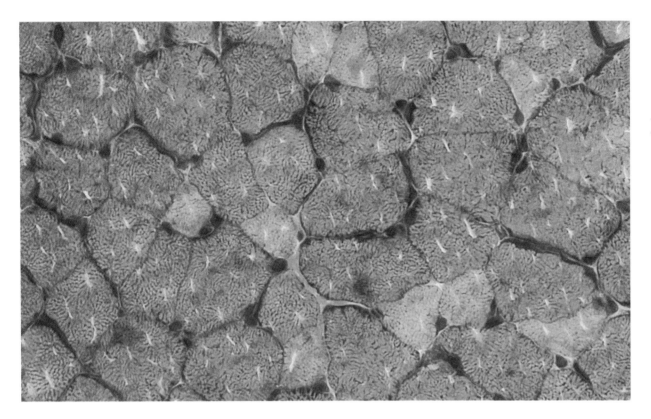

Fat accumulation in muscle. The focal ragged red fibers are consistent with mitochondrial myopathy.

approximately six out of every 100,000 individuals to as high as 16 out of 100,000 individuals. But there is evidence that, as part of the normal aging process, the accumulation of mtDNA mutations leads to neurological changes and abnormalities such as hearing loss or diabetes, which are normally considered to be associated with aging.

Causes and symptoms

In most cases, the primary defect in mitochondrial myopathies results from mutations in important genes that determine (encode) the structure of proteins that function in the mitochondria. Mutations can be found in DNA from the nucleus of the cell. This DNA is known as nuclear DNA, which is the DNA that most people consider with respect to human genetic diseases, but DNA is also found in the mitochondrial genome. Mitochondrial myopathies can be caused by defects in nuclear and mitochondrial DNA.

Mitochondrial DNA (mtDNA) is much smaller than nuclear DNA (nDNA). Nuclear DNA has approximately 3.9 billion base pairs in its entire sequence; mtDNA has only 16,500 pairs. Although mtDNA is much smaller in size, each cell contains anywhere from 2–100 mitochondria, and each mitochondria has 5–10 copies of its genome.

Unlike nDNA that is twisted into a double helix, mtDNA has a circular structure. Mitochondrial DNA also

has a high mutation rate, almost 20 times that of the nDNA. All of these factors are important in understanding the role of mtDNA mutations in the development of inherited or other mitochondrial myopathies.

A unique feature of mtDNA is that out of the more than 1,000 mtDNA genomes within the cell, a new mutation in one of the mtDNA genomes can be replicated each time the cell divides, thus increasing the number of defective mtDNA genomes. Because the distribution of the newly replicated mtDNA into the two daughter cells is random, one of the daughter cells may contain mtDNA that is not mutated (a condition referred to as homoplasmy), while the other daughter cell inherits both mutation genomes (known as heteroplasmy, or a mixture of mutated and normal genomes). Knowing the percentage of heteroplasmy for different mutations is often helpful in determining whether the disorder will manifest symptoms, as well as how severe they might be. As a result of the heteroplasmic nature of mitochondrial myopathies, the range of symptoms and severity of symptoms is often highly variable.

Mitochondrial myopathies are caused by mutations in either the nDNA or the mtDNA. These mutations generally affect tissues that have a high demand for metabolic energy production. Some disorders only affect a single organ, but many involve multiple organ systems. Generally, nDNA mutations result in clinical symptoms that develop during early childhood, while mtDNA mutations (either directly or as secondary effects from a nDNA mutation) lead to clinical manifestations that develop in late childhood or early adulthood. The genes that comprise the mtDNA genome encode proteins that function inside the mitochondria. For example, sugar broken down from food is used for fuel to manufacture a specific molecule, adenosine triphosphate (ATP), which is used by the cell to accomplish a variety of essential functions. ATP is produced by charged particles called electrons that come from digested food products to harness the energy. This is accomplished through five highly organized protein complexes. The first four complexes (complex I, II, III, and IV) are part of the electron transport chain and function to move the electrons towards the fifth complex (complex V), which produces the ATP molecule. A defect in any one of these complexes can lead to mitochondrial myopathies. Both DNA from the nucleus and the mitochondria are required to assemble the many subunits that make up these complexes.

The process of producing ATP requires oxygen. This is essentially why humans cannot live without it. In the absence of a properly functioning electron transport chain, precursor molecules as well as unused oxygen begin to accumulate. One molecule in particular, called lactic acid, accumulates normally during strenuous exercise when tissue demands for energy cannot be met, resulting in muscle **fatigue**. This occurs essentially by accumulation of lactic acid, or lactic acidosis. Persons with a deficiency in the electron transport chain, therefore, have symptoms similar to an athlete's muscle fatigue, but without the factor of strenuous exercise. Both muscle contraction and nerve cell stimulation requires ATP; thus, these cells are particularly sensitive to defects in mitochondrial function. Furthermore, oxygen that is not metabolized can be converted into toxic compounds called reactive oxygen species (ROS). ROS can lead to many symptoms that an individual with a mitochondrial myopathy will experience.

Inheritance and medical significance

Mitochondrial DNA is inherited almost entirely from the maternal sex cell (the egg). Therefore, mutations or alterations in the mtDNA can be transmitted from a maternal sex cell to all the mother's children, regardless of gender.

Heteroplasmy, or the condition of having both normal and mutated mtDNA genomes, has several clinically important implications. If mtDNA molecules are deleted, they are generally not transmitted from the mother to her offspring for reasons that are currently unclear. If the mtDNA is duplicated (or various sequences are repeated with the same sequences such that the total size of the genome increases by exactly the number of repeated bases) or there is a mutation that only affects one base in the sequence, there usually is some of the mutant mtDNA molecules that get transmitted. Additionally, a phenomenon called the mitochondrial genetic bottleneck occurs during the production of the mother's sex cells (eggs). This term refers to a reduction in the number of mtDNA molecules followed by an amplification of this reduced mtDNA that occurs during maturation of the mother's eggs. The result is considerable variability in the amount of mutated mtDNA molecules that each of the offspring inherits. However, in general, mothers that have a higher amount of mutated molecules are more likely to have offspring that are more severely affected compared to mothers that have a lower mutant load.

Inheritance and the nuclear genome

Not all mitochondrial proteins are produced by the mitochondrial genome. In fact, the majority is produced by the nuclear genome. Therefore, mitochondrial myopathies can be caused by mutations in both the nDNA and the mtDNA. This has important implications for genetic counselors that assess the recurrence risks in families with affected offspring. If the defect is of nuclear origin, it is typically recessive. In this case, there is a 25% chance of having an affected baby if both parents are carriers. There are also dominant disorders leading to mitochondrial myopathies that are characterized by a carrier parent passing on the mutant nuclear gene to 50% of the offspring. There are many mitochondrial myopathies that do not have a mtDNA mutation, and there are no nDNA mutations known.

Scientists are increasing their understanding of the intercommunication between the nucleus and the mitochondria. The identification of nDNA mutations that cause mitochondrial myopathies was first made when a nuclear gene involved in mtDNA replication was found to be defective in a disorder involving a patient with a mitochondrial myopathy.

Symptoms of mitochondrial myopathies are largely variable from person to person, even within the same family, and are dependent on the amount and type of genetic mutations present. These disorders can occur in infancy, childhood, or adulthood. In general, individuals with mitochondria dysfunction have abnormalities in the **central nervous system**. Defects can involve seizures, **movement disorders**, **headaches**, and cognitive (thought) disorders such as developmental delay or dementia (forgetfulness, senility). People with mitochondrial myopathies can also have hearing loss.

It is common that symptoms become apparent in a specific cluster of abnormalities and are thus considered a syndrome. For example, Kearns-Sayre syndrome can be recognized clinically due to similar symptoms that patients have. These symptoms include ocular abnormalities

Key Terms

Mitochondria A part of the cell that is responsible for energy production.

Mitochondrial DNA (mtDNA) The genetic material found in mitochondria, the organelles that generate energy for the cell. Because reproduction is by cloning, mtDNA is usually passed along female lines, as part of the egg's cytoplasm.

Myopathy A disorder of the muscle or muscle tissue.

Nucleic DNA (nDNA) The genetic material found in the nucleus of the cell.

(degeneration of the retina and external opthamaloplegia, or droopy eyelids), dysphagia (swallowing problems), progressive myopathy, and various central nervous system abnormalities such as hearing loss. Confirmation of this disorder can be performed by genetic analysis that looks for large deletions in mtDNA.

Due to the nature of the genetic and biophysical defects, mitochondrial myopathies have symptoms related to muscle weakness and atrophy. Droopy eyelids and loss of the ability to control eye movements indicate muscle wasting, which leads to paralysis, and compensatory attempts at correcting eye movements by tilting the head. Visual loss often occurs.

Muscle wasting, or myopathy, is not restricted to the eyes. The face and neck can also be affected, leading to incomprehensible speech and swallowing difficulties. Overall musculature wasting pervades many affected individuals, requiring wheelchairs and, in severe cases, assisted living requirements. Exercise-induced **pain** can also result.

Diagnosis

The diagnosis of mitochondrial myopathies is initially clinical, which means that it is based on the observable clinical manifestations that the patient shows versus results obtained from genetic analysis or laboratory tests. The physician will make careful observations of the affected child and interview the parents, in particular the mother, as it is common that she has the same mtDNA mutation, though usually at a lower percent load. Persons with mitochondrial myopathies are referred to a clinical geneticist for management and further evaluation, particularly in the absence of a confident clinical diagnosis. If there is a positive test after a genetic evaluation, genetic counseling is

critical for understanding the nature of the disease and the implications for future offspring.

Diagnostic criteria

Any multi-system progressive disorder should lead a physician to suspect a mitochondrial disorder. A diagnosis can be particularly difficult if there is only one symptom. The diagnostic criteria for mitochondrial myopathies involve phenotypic evaluation (or evaluation of observable traits), followed by laboratory evaluation. A clinical diagnosis can be confirmed by laboratory studies, muscle **biopsy**, and molecular genetic evaluation, in which a geneticist analyzes the mtDNA. If a mtDNA mutation is detected, diagnosis is much more straightforward. In the absence of a mtDNA mutation, diagnosis becomes difficult.

There are several classical clinical manifestations that warrant DNA studies, such as in the case of MELAS, MERRF or LHON. Other disorders such as MNGIE require nDNA studies. In the absence of specific clinical criteria characteristic of a mitochondrial myopathy, blood plasma or cerebral spinal fluid is measured for lactic acid concentration, ketone bodies, plasma acylcarnitines, and organic acids in the urine. These are metabolites that are typically abnormal in an individual with a mitochondrial myopathy. If they are abnormal, a muscle biopsy is performed. Molecular genetic testing can often confirm a clinical diagnosis with or without positive laboratory results.

Treatment team

Treatment for patients with mitochondrial myopathies is best performed by a **neurologist** and a clinical geneticist or specialist that has experience diagnosing, treating, and managing patients with mitochondrial myopathies.

Treatment

There is no cure for mitochondrial myopathies. Therefore, treatment is solely for the purposes of minimizing pain and symptoms, and increasing mobility. Due to the wide variability in the disorders, treatment is usually individualized. Although the diseases are rare, many of their clinical symptoms are common and treatable. There are medications and lifestyle modifications that can help treat conditions such as headaches, diabetes, stroke-like symptoms, and seizures that are often associated with mitochondrial myopathies.

Medications are tailored to reduce the specific symptoms that the patient is experiencing (anticonvulsant medication may be required, for example, for an individual suffering from seizures). Dietary supplements are often used, although they have not been investigated in long-term studies. Creatine, coenzyme Q 10, and carnitine are naturally occurring supplements that are thought to enhance ATP production.

Recovery and rehabilitation

Because there is no cure for mitochondrial myopathies, the focus is on maintaining optimum function for as long as possible, rather than recovery. Physical therapy helps extend the range of muscle movement. Occupational therapy helps with positioning and mobility devices, and trains the affected individual in strategies designed to accomplish self-care and activities of daily living. Speech therapy can help children and adults that have difficulty in speaking, as well as how to safely eat and swallow food. Hearing and visual aids (glasses) are often necessary and helpful.

Clinical trials

As of early 2004, there were few **clinical trials** to develop therapies to treat mitochondrial myopathies. There was one study to investigate the role of dichloroacetate to lower lactate levels in patients diagnosed with MELAS at the National Institutes of Health (NIH). Lactic acidosis has been shown to be associated with nerve cell and muscle cell impairment in patients that have MELAS. Decreasing the levels of lactate might help prevent severe lactic acidosis.

Prognosis

Mitochondrial myopathies are extremely variable in the symptoms produced, and so the prognosis for those affected with mitochondrial myopathies also varies. The adverse affects on muscle function are often progressive, and persons often show physical deterioration over time. Occasionally, affected persons are mentally delayed. It is difficult to determine the exact course that each individual will endure, and in many cases the symptoms are relatively mild. Life expectancy for a person with a mitochondrial myopathy depends on many different circumstances, including the percentage of mtDNA that is mutated, the type of mutation, and the tissue in which it is mutated. If it is a nDNA defect, the physical and developmental effects depend on the gene that is mutated, the location of the mutation in the gene, the importance this gene has on the function of the mitochondria, and whether there are compensatory mechanisms. Overall, the prognosis is dependent on the involvement of vital organs.

Special concerns

Perhaps one of the most problematic issues that patients with mitochondrial myopathies experience is the absence of a causative explanation for why the symptoms developed. This is especially challenging for determining recurrence risks for parents considering future pregnancies. Mitochondrial myopathic disorders can pose challenges for the entire family, especially since many affected children and adults are not born with the disorder, but the condition progressively worsens with time. Support groups are available through various national disease foundations and local community organizations.

Resources

BOOKS

Staff. *The Official Parent's Sourcebook on Mitochondrial Myopathies: A Revised and Updated Directory for the Internet Age.* San Diego: Icon Group International, 2002.

PERIODICALS

Chinnery, P. F., and D. M. Turnbull. "Epidemiology and Treatment of Mitochondrial Disorders." *Am J Med Genet* (2001) 106: 94–101.

Thorburn, D. R., and H. H. Dahl. "Mitochondrial Disorders: Genetics, Counseling, Prenatal Diagnosis and Reproductive Options." *Am J Med Genet* (2001) 106: 102–14.

OTHER

"Mitochondrial Myopathies: Facts About Mitochondrial Myopathies." *Muscular Dystrophy Association.* March 10, 2004 (May 23, 2004). <http://www.mdausa.org/publications/mitochondrial_myopathies.html>.

"NINDS Mitochondrial Myopathies Information Page." *National Institute of Neurological Disorders and Stroke.* March 10, 2004 (May 23, 2004). <http://www.ninds.nih.gov/health_and_medical/disorders/mitochon_doc.htm>.

ORGANIZATIONS

National Organization for Rare Disorders (NORD). P.O. Box 1968 (55 Kenosia Avenue), Danbury, CT 06813-1968. (203) 744-0100 or (800) 999-NORD (6673); Fax: (203) 798-2291. orphan@rarediseases.org. <http://www.rarediseases.org>.

United Mitochondrial Disease Foundation. 8085 Saltsburg Road Suite 201, Pittsburgh, PA 15239. (412) 793-8077; Fax: (412) 793-6477. info@umdf.org. <http://www.umdf.org>.

Bryan R. Cobb, PhD

Modafinil

Definition

Modafinil is a **central nervous system** (CNS) stimulant. It is primarily used to promote wakefulness and alertness in persons with **narcolepsy**, a condition that causes excessive sleepiness and cataplexy (episodes of sudden loss of muscle control).

Purpose

Modafinil is an improvement over amphetamines in the treatment of narcolepsy. It promotes wakefulness, but has less pronounced side effects than amphetamines. Modafinil acts to combat excessive daytime sleepiness (EDS) and cataplexy, the leading symptoms of narcolepsy, by stimulating sleep-suppressing peptides (orexins) in the brain.

Description

Although primarily indicated for the treatment of narcolepsy, modafinil is also used to treat some forms of **sleep apnea**. Experimentally, modafinil is being evaluated in the treatment of **Alzheimer's disease**, **depression**, **attention-deficit hyperactivity disorder** (**ADHD**), and **fatigue** associated with **multiple sclerosis**.

Recommended dosage

Modafinil is taken by mouth in tablet form. It is prescribed by physicians in varying dosages, and is usually taken once a day, in the morning.

Precautions

In some patients, modafinil may be habit forming. When taking the medication, it is important to follow physician instructions precisely. Modafinil may cause clumsiness and impair clarity of thinking. Persons taking this medication should not drive a car or operate machinery until they know how the stimulant will affect them. Patients should avoid alcohol while taking modafinil. It can exacerbate the side effects of alcohol and other medications.

Modafinil may not be suitable for persons with a history of liver or kidney disease, mental illness, high blood pressure, angina (chest **pain**), irregular heartbeats, or other heart problems. Before beginning treatment with modafinil, patients should notify their physician if they consume a large amount of alcohol, have a history of drug use, are pregnant, or plan to become pregnant. Patients who become pregnant while taking modafinil should inform their physician.

Side effects

Research indicates that modafinil is generally well tolerated. However, modafinil may case a variety of usually mild side effects. **Headache**, nausea, and upset stomach are the most frequently reported side effects of modafinil. Other possible side effects include excessive difficulty sleeping, nervousness, depression, diarrhea, dry mouth, runny nose, neck pain or stiffness, **back pain**, loss of appetite, and confusion.

Key Terms

Cataplexy A symptom of narcolepsy in which there is a sudden episode of muscle weakness triggered by emotions. The muscle weakness may cause the person's knees to buckle, or the head to drop. In severe cases, the patient may become paralyzed for a few seconds to minutes.

Narcolepsy A life-long sleep disorder marked by four symptoms: sudden brief sleep attacks, cataplexy (a sudden loss of muscle tone usually lasting up to 30 minutes), temporary paralysis, and hallucinations. The hallucinations are associated with falling asleep or the transition from sleeping to waking.

Orexin Another name for hypocretin, a chemical secreted in the hypothalmus that regulates the sleep/wake cycle. Narcolepsy is sometimes described as an orexin deficiency syndrome.

Other, uncommon side effects of modafinil can be potentially serious. Persons taking modafinil who experiences any of the following symptoms should immediately contact their physician: irregular heartbeat, unusually rapid heartbeat, shortness of breath, hives or rashes, chest pain, persistent or severe headache, and persistent fever, pain, or other sign of infection.

Interactions

Modafinil may have negative interactions with some anticoagulants (blood thinners), antidepressants, antifungals, antibiotics, and monoamine oxidase inhibitors (MAOIs). Seizure prevention medication, **diazepam** (Valium), **phenobarbital** (Luminal, Solfoton), phenytoin (Dilantin), propranolol (Inderal), and rifampin (Rifadin, Rimactane) may also adversely react with Modafinil.

Furthermore, modafinil may decrease the effectiveness of oral contraceptives (birth control pills). Patients should consult their physicians about using alternative methods of birth control while taking modafinil, and for at least one month after ending treatment.

Resources

BOOKS

Parker, James N., and Philip N. Parker. *The Official Patient's Sourcebook on Narcolepsy.* San Diego: ICON Health, 2002.

OTHER

"Drug Information, Modafinil (Systemic)." *MEDLINE Plus Health Information.* National Library of Medicine.

February 10, 2004 (May 23, 2004). <http://www.nlm.nih.gov/medlineplus/druginfo/uspdi/203466.html>.

ORGANIZATIONS

Center for Narcolepsy. 701B Welch Road—Room 146, Palo Alto, CA 94304-5742. (650) 725-6517; Fax: (650) 725-4913. <http://www-med.stanford.edu/school/Psychiatry/narcolepsy/>.

Adrienne Wilmoth Lerner

Key Terms

Balanced chromosome translocation A rearrangement of the chromosomes in which two chromosomes have broken and exchanged pieces without the loss of genetic material.

Cranial nerves The twelve nerves that originate in the brain, and control functions such as hearing, vision and facial expression.

Moebius syndrome

Definition

Moebius syndrome is a condition in which the facial nerve is underdeveloped, causing paralysis or weakness of the muscles of the face. Other nerves to the facial structures may also be underdeveloped.

Description

Moebius syndrome has been called "life without a smile" because the paralysis of the facial muscles, the most constant feature, leads to the physical inability to form a smile even when happy feelings are experienced.

Individuals with Moebius syndrome may also have abnormalities of their limbs, chest muscles, and tongue. The chance of **mental retardation** appears to be increased in people with Moebius syndrome, but most people with the disorder have normal intelligence.

Demographics

Moebius syndrome is extremely rare and does not seem to affect any particular ethnic group more than others. The families in which genes on chromosomes 3 and 10 were mapped were Dutch.

Causes and symptoms

Most cases of Moebius syndrome are isolated and do not appear to be genetic, but occurrence in multiple individuals within some families indicates that there are multiple genetic forms. The underlying problem is a defect in or absence of the sixth and seventh cranial nerves. The seventh or facial nerve normally controls facial expression. The abducens or sixth cranial nerve controls blinking and back-and-forth eye movement and is the second most commonly affected cranial nerve in Moebius syndrome. Additional cranial nerves affected in some patients control other eye movements and other functions such as hearing, balance, speech, and feeding.

The first sign of Moebius syndrome in newborns is an inability to suck, sometimes accompanied by excessive drooling and crossed eyes. Also seen at birth in some patients are abnormalities of the limbs, tongue, and jaw. Children also often have low muscle tone, particularly in the upper body. The lack of facial expression and inability to smile become apparent as children get older.

When cranial nerve palsy is associated with limb reduction abnormalities and the absence of the pectoralis muscles, the condition is known as Poland-Moebius or Möebius-Poland syndrome. Common limb abnormalities are missing or webbed fingers and clubfoot.

The prevalence of mental retardation in Moebius syndrome is uncertain. It has been estimated in the past to be between 10% and 50%, but these numbers are thought to be overestimates resulting from the lack of facial expression and drooling seen in people with Moebius syndrome. In one study of familial cases of Moebius syndrome, 3% were reported to be mentally retarded.

Diagnosis

Diagnosis of Moebius syndrome is made on the basis of clinical symptoms, especially the lack of facial expression. Because the exact genes involved in Moebius syndrome have not yet been identified, molecular genetic testing is not available.

Treatment team

Neurologists, neurosurgeons, and plastic surgeons may play a role in the treatment of a child with Moebius syndrome. Physical and speech therapists may help improve control over coordination, speech, and eating.

Treatment

The ability to smile has been restored in some cases of Moebius syndrome by surgery which transfers nerve and muscle from the thigh to the face. Other surgeries can be used to treat eye, limb, and jaw problems. In children with feeding problems, special bottles or feeding tubes are used.

Prognosis

Moebius syndrome does not appear to affect life span, and individuals who are treated for their symptoms can lead normal lives.

Resources

PERIODICALS

Kumar, Dhavendra. "Moebius Syndrome." *Journal of Medical Genetics* 27 (1990): 122–26.

ORGANIZATIONS

Moebius Syndrome Foundation (MSF). PO Box 993, Larchmont, NY 10538. (914) 834-6008. <http://www.ciaccess.com/moebius>.

Toni I. Pollin, MS, CGC
Rosalyn Carson-DeWitt, MD

Monomelic amyotrophy

Definition

Monomelic amyotrophy (MMA) is a rare disease of the nerves that control voluntary movements of the limbs.

Description

One of the **motor neuron diseases** (MND), degenerative conditions that involve the nerves of the upper or lower parts of the body, MMA is generally a benign disease associated with minimal disability. Onset of MMA primarily occurs between the ages of 15 and 25. The main features of the disease are wasting and weakness of a single upper or lower limb. Generally, MMA progresses slowly over a period of 2–4 years, and then reaches a stationary phase during which the disease remains stable for years.

Monomelic amyotrophy may also be known as benign focal amyotrophy, single limb atrophy, Hirayama syndrome or Sobue disease. Descriptive terms such as brachial monomelic amyotrophy (MMA confined to an arm) or monomelic amyotrophy of the lower limb (MMMA of a leg) may be used to specify the type of limb affected. O'Sullivan-McLeod syndrome, a variant of MMA, is a slowly progressive form of the disease that causes weakness and wasting of the small muscles of the hand and forearm.

Demographics

Monomelic amyotrophy occurs worldwide and is most prevalent in Asia, and especially in Japan and India. According to a report in 1984, MMA of the lower limb occurs in about four in a million people in India. There is a preponderance of males with MMA; estimates of the male to female ratio range from 5:1 to 13:1.

Causes and symptoms

As of 2004, the underlying cause or causes for MMA remain unresolved. Most cases are sporadic and occur in an individual without a family history of MMA. Numerous factors—such as viral infection, vascular insufficiency (inadequate blood supply) of the spinal cord, heavy physical activity, **radiation** injury, traumatic injury, and atrophy of the spinal cord—have been suggested as possible causes of MMA. There are a few reports of familial cases of MMA.

Symptoms of MMA appear slowly and steadily over a period of time. The main features of MMA are muscle weakness and atrophy (wasting) in a portion of one limb. The weakness and wasting progresses slowly and may spread to the corresponding limb on the opposite side of the body. Symptoms can develop elsewhere in the affected limb or another limb at the same time or later in the course of the disease. Patients may notice worsening of symptoms on exposure to the cold. Other symptoms of MMA include tremor, fasciculations, cramps, mild loss of sensation, excessive sweating, and an abnormal sympathetic skin response. It is rare that individuals with MMA experience significant functional impairment.

Diagnosis

Diagnosis of MMA is based on physical exam and medical history. Physical findings include reduced muscle girth (width around the arm or leg) and decreased strength in the affected limb. Tendon reflexes tend to be normal or sluggish. Cranial nerves, pyramidal tracts, sensory, cerebellar or extrapyramidal systems are not affected. Patients may report or display symptoms described above. They may also indicate difficulty carrying out activities of daily living such as writing, lifting, getting dressed, or walking.

Tests that may aid in diagnosis of MMA include **electromyography** (EMG), imaging studies such as **magnetic resonance imaging (MRI)** and computed tomography (**CT**) scans, and muscle **biopsy**. EMG shows chronic loss of nerve cells confined to specific areas of the affected limb. **MRI** has been reported to be a useful means of determining which muscles are affected in a given patient. Muscle biopsy shows evidence of atrophy of the neurons. EMG, muscle biopsy, or isometric strength testing may also reveal significant findings in seemingly normal muscles of the affected and the contralateral limb.

Treatment

There is no cure for MMA. The goal of treatment, which is largely supportive, is to help patients optimize function and manage any disability associated with the disorder. Treatment primarily consists of rehabilitation measures such as physical therapy and occupational therapy. Severe muscle weakness (present in a minority of cases) may require orthopedic intervention such as splinting.

Treatment team

In addition to routine health care through their primary care practitioners, individuals with MMA generally see specialists in neurology and rehabilitation. Some patients with MMA may receive comprehensive services through a **muscular dystrophy** association (MDA) clinic or another type of neuromuscular clinic. Given the rarity of MMA, the potential for rehabilitation in this disorder is unknown.

Recovery and rehabilitation

Rehabilitation for MMA consists of physical and occupational therapy. The goal of these therapies is to make full use of the patient's existing functions. Physical therapy can help a patient with MMA to strengthen muscles in a weak arm or leg. Occupational therapy can teach patients to use adaptive techniques and devices that may help compensate for difficulty with everyday tasks such as writing, buttoning, or tying shoes. Depending upon the degree of weakness in the affected limb, a person with MMA may need to use the unaffected limb for activities previously performed by the now atrophied limb.

Clinical trials

As of 2004, there were no **clinical trials** for patients with MMA. As more is learned about how MMA or related motor neuron diseases develop, it is hoped that novel therapies may be developed in the future.

Prognosis

MMA is generally a benign condition. Disability associated with MMA is typically mild. In the majority of cases, the disorder usually ceases to progress within five years of onset. People with MMA can expect to have a normal life span.

Special concerns

Initially, symptoms of MMA can be similar to early signs of other, more serious neurological disorders such as **amyotrophic lateral sclerosis** (ALS or Lou Gehrig's disease) and **spinal muscular atrophy**. For this reason, periodic neurological evaluation may be recommended to be sure that no symptoms of these or other motor neuron diseases develop.

Key Terms

Electromyography   A diagnostic test that records the electrical activity of muscles. In the test, small electrodes are placed on or in the skin; the patterns of electrical activity are projected on a screen or over a loudspeaker. This procedure is used to test for muscle disorders, including muscular dystrophy.

Fasciculations   Small involuntary muscle contractions visible under the skin.

Sympathetic skin response   Minute change of palmar and plantar electrical potential.

Resources

BOOKS

Parker, James N., and Philip M. Parker, eds. *The Official Parent's Sourcebook on Monomelic amyotrophy: A Revised and Updated Directory for the Internet Age.* San Diego, CA: ICON Health Publications, 2002.

PERIODICALS

Gourie-Devi, M., and A. Nalani. "Long-term follow-up of 44 patients with brachial monomelic amyotrophy." *Acta Neurol Scand* 107 (March 2003): 215–20.

Hirayama, K., Y. Toyokura, and T. Tsubaki. "Juvenile muscular atrophy of unilateral upper extremity: A new clinical entity." *Psychiatr Neurol Jpn* 61 (1959): 2190–9.

Kiernan, M. C., A. K. Lethlean, and P. W. Blum. "Monomelic amyotrophy: non progressive atrophy of the upper limb." *J Clin Neurosci* 6 (July 1999): 353–355.

Munchau, A., and T. Rosenkranz. "Benign monomelic amyotrophy of the lower limb-case report and review of the literature." *European Neurology* 43 (2000): 238–40.

Riggs, J. E., S. S. Schochet, and L. Gutman. "Benign focal amyotrophy. Variant of chronic spinal muscular atrophy." *Archives of Neurology* 41 (1984): 678–679.

Sobue, I., N. Saito, and K. Ando. "Juvenile type of distal and segmental muscular atrophy of upper extremities." *Ann Neurol* 3 (1978): 429–33.

WEBSITES

The Muscular Dystrophy Association (MDA). *The Spinal Muscular Atrophies.* <http://www.mdausa.org/research/munsat.html>.

The National Institute of Neurological Disorders and Stroke (NINDS). *NINDS Motor Neuron Diseases Information Page.* <http://www.ninds.nih.gov/health_and_medical/disorders/motor_neuron_diseases.htm.htm>.

The National Institute of Neurological Disorders and Stroke (NINDS). *NINDS Monomelic Amyotrophy Information Page.* <http://www.ninds.nih.gov/health_and_medical/disorders/monomelic_amyotrophy.htm>.

ORGANIZATIONS

Muscular Dystrophy Association. 3300 East Sunrise Drive, Tucson, AZ 85718. (520) 529-2000 or (800) 572-1717; Fax: (520) 529-5300. mda@mdausa.org. <http://www.mdausa.org>.

National Organization for Rare Disorders. P.O. Box 1968, 55 Kensonia Avenue, Danbury, CT 06813. (203) 744-0100 or (800) 999-NORD; Fax: (203) 798-2291. orphan@rarediseases.org. <http://www.rarediseases.org>.

Dawn J. Cardeiro, MS, CGC

Motor neuron diseases

Definition

Motor neuron diseases are a group of progressive disorders involving the nerve cells responsible for carrying impulses that instruct the muscles in the upper and lower body to move. Motor neuron diseases are varied and destructive in their effect. They commonly have distinctive differences in their origin and causation, but a similar result in their outcome for the patient: severe muscle weakness. **Amyotrophic lateral sclerosis** (ALS), **spinal muscular atrophy, poliomyelitis,** and **primary lateral sclerosis** are all examples of motor neuron diseases.

Description

A motor neuron is one of the largest cells in the body. It has a large cell body with many extensions reaching out in 360° from the cell body (soma). These extensions are called dendrites and are chemically able to receive instructions from adjacent neurons. These instructions are received in the form of an impulse stimulation of a particular protein channel on the dendrite by a neurotransmitter termed acetycholine (ACh). Extending from the soma of the motor neuron is a long portion of the cell called the axon. When conditions are favorable, an electrical signal passes down the axon to a region of the cell identified as the axon terminals. These terminals also branch in many directions and have, at their tips, a region called the synaptic end bulb. This region releases ACh that crosses a small gap until it reaches a protein on another dendrite.

When motor neurons line up in a tract, they allow an electrical signal to spread from the brain to the intended muscle. There are a tremendous number of nerve tracts that extend to all the muscles of the body that are responsible for contraction and relaxation of all types of muscles, including smooth and cardiac, as well as skeletal muscle. When the motor neuron is affected or damaged and it cannot perform at peak performance, the muscles of the body

are affected. Often, a disorder of the motor neurons results in progressive muscle atrophy (shrinking and wasting) of some, if not all, the muscles of the body. Muscle twitching (fasciculation) is common among these disorders. Motor neuron diseases are difficult to treat, debilitating to movement and, in some cases, fatal.

Amyotrophic lateral sclerosis (ALS) is a disorder that generally involves either the lower or upper motor systems of the body. In advanced stages, both regions of the body are affected. This disease is commonly known as Lou Gehrig's disease after the famous baseball player who died from the condition. It is caused by sclerosis (a hardening of the surrounding fibrous tissues) in the corticospinal tracts. Associated with the sclerosis is a loss of the tissue of the anterior horns (gray matter) in the spinal cord, including the brainstem. Lou Gehrig's disease is characterized by a wasting of the muscles that, in turn, produces weakness. The bulbar, or facial/mouth muscles can initially become involved, which may lead to slurring of speech and drooling. The significance of this involvement is that, with rapid progression, the patient may not be able to swallow properly. This may lead to the risk of choking and other difficulties with obtaining nutrition and proper respiration. Death from complications of ALS is common within five years.

Spinal muscular atrophies (SMAs) are a wide group of genetic disorders characterized by primary degeneration of the anterior horn cells of the spinal cord, resulting in progressive muscle weakness. Spinal muscular atrophies affect only lower motor neurons. In babies and children, many SMAs are rapidly progressive with paralysis of the legs, trunk, and eventually, the respiratory muscles. In teenagers and adults, SMAs are usually slowly progressive. **Kennedy's disease,** an X-linked (carried by women and passed on to male offspring) SMA, features similar wasting of facial muscles as seen in ALS, with characteristic difficulty speaking and swallowing.

Primary lateral sclerosis (PLS) is a rare motor neuron disease that resembles ALS. Primary lateral sclerosis often begins after age 50, and results in slowly progressive weakness and stiffness in the leg muscles, clumsiness, and difficulty maintaining balance. Symptoms worsen over a period of years. Muscle spasms in the legs may also occur, but in PLS, there is no evidence of the degeneration of spinal motor neurons or muscle wasting (amyotrophy) that occurs in ALS.

Unlike most motor neuron diseases, poliomyelitis results from infection with a virus. Contamination occurs through fecal or oral exposure. Once inside the body, the virus uses the cells of the gastrointestinal tract to enter the bloodstream and move throughout the body. Eventually, the poliovirus invades the nerve cells of the spinal cord and

Key Terms

Atrophy   Shrinking or wasting of muscles or tissues.

Amyotrophy   A type of neuropathy resulting in pain, weakness, and/or wasting in the muscles.

Contractures   Abnormal, usually permanent contraction of a muscle due to atrophy of muscle fibers, extensive scar tissue over a joint, or other factors.

Dysarthria   Imperfect articulation of speech due to muscular weakness resulting from damage to the central or peripheral nervous system.

Dysphagia   Difficulty swallowing.

Fasciculations   Fine muscle tremors or twitches.

Gait   Posture and manner of walking.

Motor neuron   A neuron conducting impulses outwards from the brain or spinal cord with the specific job of controlling a muscle movement.

kills the motor neurons. When the motor neurons are destroyed, the muscles they connect to become damaged and weaken. The result is varying degrees of paralysis, including difficulty swallowing, walking, breathing, and control of speech.

Demographics

Motor neuron diseases are uncommon, as about one person in 50,000 is diagnosed with a motor neuron disease in the United States each year. In total, about 5,500 people in the United States each year receive a diagnosis of a motor neuron disease.

About 20,000 Americans are living with ALS and nearly 4,500 new cases are reported annually. The peak age for onset is around 55 years of age, but younger patients have been observed. Spinal muscular atrophies and primary lateral sclerosis are rare diseases.

The occurrence of poliomyelitis is seen in records of epidemics that were intricately documented in the last 100 years. A description of an epidemic in recent times in the United States discussed a low of 4,197 cases in the early 1940s to a high of 42,033 in 1949. By 1952, the number of case had reached over 58,000. In 1955, a vaccine was developed that used weakened forms of the virus. This vaccine and the subsequent Sabin vaccine nearly wiped out polio in the world. The Americas were declared free of polio in the 1990s. In 2002, there were less than 500 cases worldwide, and in 2003, that number decreased to less than 100 cases. It is expected that by the end of the year

2005, the disease will be eradicated. Although new cases have begun to appear in regions of Africa and India, the World Health Organization (WHO) is keeping track of the outbreaks, and scientists are hopeful that poliomyelitis will soon disappear from the list of motor neuron diseases.

Causes and symptoms

Causes of many motor neuron diseases are unknown, and others have varying causes according to the specific motor neuron disease. Most cases of ALS occur sporadically for an unknown reason, however, up to 10% of ALS cases are inherited. Most spinal muscular atrophies are inherited. A virus causes poliomyelitis. Additionally, environmental factors and toxins are under study as causes or triggers for motor neuron diseases.

Muscle weakness is the symptom common to all motor neuron diseases. Muscles of the legs are most often affected, leading to clumsiness, unstable gait, or lower limb paralysis. Muscle cramps and fasciculations (twitching) occur with most motor neuron diseases. Facial muscles may also be affected, leading to difficulty with speech (**dysarthria**). Later in the course of some motor neuron diseases, the muscles involved with swallowing and breathing may be impaired (dysphagia).

Diagnosis

Diagnosis of motor neuron disease is often based upon symptoms and exclusion of other neurological diseases. Nerve conduction studies can help distinguish some forms of **peripheral neuropathy** from motor neuron disease. Electromyelogram (EMG), a test measuring the electrical activity in muscles, can support the diagnosis of ALS and some other motor neuron diseases. Although computed tomography (**CT**) **scans** and **magnetic resonance imaging (MRI)** scans are often normal in persons with motor neuron disease, they may help exclude spinal malformations or tumors that could be responsible for similar symptoms. A muscle **biopsy** can exclude myopathies. Diagnosis of primary lateral sclerosis is especially difficult and often delayed, as it is frequently misdiagnosed as ALS. Polio may be diagnosed by recovering the virus from a stool or throat culture, examining antibodies in the blood or, rarely, by spinal fluid analysis. Finally, molecular genetic studies can aid in the diagnosis of spinal muscular trophies and the small percentage of inherited ALS cases.

Treatment team

Caring for a person with a motor neuron disease requires a network of health professionals, community resources, and friends or family members. A **neurologist** usually makes the diagnosis, and the neurologist and primary physician coordinate ongoing treatment and symptom relief. Physical, occupational, and respiratory therapists provide specialized care, as do nurses. Social service and mental health consultants organize support services.

Treatment

There are few specific treatments for motor neuron diseases, and efforts focus on reducing the symptoms of muscle spasm and **pain** while maintaining the highest practical level of overall health. Riluzole, the first drug approved by the U.S. Food and Drug Administration for the treatment of ALS, has extended the life of ALS patients by several months and also extended the time a person with ALS can effectively use his or her own muscles to breathe.

Other medications used to treat persons with motor neuron disease are designed to relieve symptoms and improve the quality of life for patients. These include medicines to help with **depression**, excess saliva production, sleep disturbances, and constipation.

Recovery and rehabilitation

Recovery from motor neuron diseases depends on the type of disease and the amount of muscle degeneration present. In diseases such as ALS, the emphasis is placed upon maintaining mobility and function for as long as possible, rather than recovery. With all motor neuron diseases, physical therapy can teach exercises to help with range of motion and prevent contractures (stiff muscles at the joints). Occupational therapy provides assistive devices for mobility such as wheelchairs, positioning devices, braces, and other orthotics for performing daily activities such as reaching and dressing. Respiratory therapists and speech therapists help prevent pneumonia by maintaining lung function and promoting safe eating strategies. Speech therapists also help with alternate forms of communication if facial muscles are involved.

Recovery from polio may be complete or only partial, depending on the degree of lower motor neuron damage. Years or decades after recovering from polio, persons may again experience muscle weakness and pain. This is known as postpolio syndrome. Vigorous **exercise** has been shown to cause additional weakness in postpolio syndrome, and physicians recommend energy conservation and lifestyle changes for these patients.

Clinical trials

The National Institutes of Health (NIH) has more than 20 **clinical trials** scheduled for 2004–05 for the study of motor neuron diseases, including one trial designed to evaluate a new drug, Minocycline, in the treatment of ALS. Details and up-to-date information about patient recruiting can be found at the NIH Website for clinical trails at <http://www.clinicaltrials.gov>.

Prognosis

The prognosis of persons with motor neuron diseases depends on the type of the disease and the amount and progression of muscle degeneration. Most persons with ALS die from complications of respiratory failure within five years of developing symptoms. About one out of 10 persons with ALS live a decade or longer with the disease. The prognosis for a person with spinal muscular atrophy varies greatly, according to the severity of the disease. Some forms result in immobility and death within a few years, while others impede movement, but do not affect a normal lifespan.

Special concerns

It is important to remember that even in the most severe motor neuron diseases, a person's personality, intelligence, reasoning ability, or memory are not impaired. The person with motor neuron disease also retains the senses of sight, smell, hearing, taste, and in the unaffected areas, touch.

Resources
BOOKS
Kunci, Ralph W. *Motor Neuron Disease.* Philadelphia: W.B. Saunders, 2002.
Oliver, David. *Motor Neuron Disease: A Family Affair.* London: Sheldon Press, 1995.
Silver, Julie. *Postpolio Syndrome.* Philadelphia: Hanley & Belfus, 2003.
Wade, Mary Dodson. *ALS—Lou Gehrig's Disease.* Berkeley Heights, NJ: Enslow Publishers, 2001.

OTHER
"NINDS Motor Neuron Diseases Information Page." *National Institute of Neurological Disorders and Stroke.* May 15, 2004 (June 1, 2004). <http://www.ninds.nih.gov/health_and_medical/disorders/motor_neuron_diseases.htm>.

ORGANIZATIONS
ALS Association (ALSA). 27001 Agoura Road, Suite 150, Calabasas Hills, CA 91301-5104. (818) 880-9007 or (800) 782-4747; Fax: (818) 880-9006. info@alsa-national.org. <http://www.alsa.org>.
Families of SMA. PO Box 196, Libertyville, IL 60048-0196. (800) 886-1762; Fax: (847) 367-7623. sma@fsma.org. <http://www.fsma.org>.
Primary Lateral Sclerosis Newsletter. 101 Pinta Court, Los Gatos, CA 95032. (408) 356-8227; Fax: (408) 356-8227. 73112.611@compuserve.com.

Brook Ellen Hall, PhD

Movement disorders

Definition

Movement disorders are a group of diseases and syndromes affecting the ability to produce and control movement.

Description

Though it seems simple and effortless, normal movement in fact requires an astonishingly complex system of control. Disruption of any portion of this system can cause a person to produce movements that are too weak, too forceful, too uncoordinated, or too poorly controlled for the task at hand. Unwanted movements may occur at rest. Intentional movement may become impossible. Such conditions are called movement disorders.

Abnormal movements themselves are symptoms of underlying disorders. In some cases, the abnormal movements are the only symptoms. Disorders causing abnormal movements include:

- **Parkinson's disease**
- Parkinsonism caused by drugs or poisons
- Parkinson-plus syndromes (**progressive supranuclear palsy**, **multiple system atrophy**, and cortical-basal ganglionic degeneration)
- Huntington's disease
- Wilson's disease
- inherited ataxias (**Friedreich's ataxia**), **Machado-Joseph disease**, and spinocerebellar ataxias)
- **Tourette syndrome** and other tic disorders
- essential tremor
- **restless legs syndrome**
- **dystonia**
- **stroke**
- **cerebral palsy**
- encephalopathies
- intoxication
- poisoning by carbon monoxide, cyanide, methanol, or manganese.

Causes and symptoms

Causes

Movement is produced and coordinated by several interacting brain centers, including the motor cortex, the **cerebellum**, and a group of structures in the inner portions of the brain called the basal ganglia. Sensory information provides critical input on the current position and velocity of body parts, and spinal nerve cells (neurons) help prevent opposing muscle groups from contracting at the same time.

To understand how movement disorders occur, it is helpful to consider a normal voluntary movement, such as reaching to touch a nearby object with the right index finger. To accomplish the desired movement, the arm must be lifted and extended. The hand must be held out to align with the forearm, and the forefinger must be extended while the other fingers remain flexed.

THE MOTOR CORTEX Voluntary motor commands begin in the motor cortex located on the outer, wrinkled surface of the brain. Movement of the right arm is begun by the left motor cortex, which generates a large volley of signals to the involved muscles. These electrical signals pass along upper motor neurons through the midbrain to the spinal cord. Within the spinal cord, they connect to lower motor neurons, which convey the signals out of the spinal cord to the surface of the muscles involved. Electrical stimulation of the muscles causes contraction, and the force of contraction pulling on the skeleton causes movement of the arm, hand, and fingers.

Damage to or death of any of the neurons along this path causes weakness or paralysis of the affected muscles.

ANTAGONISTIC MUSCLE PAIRS This picture of movement is too simple, however. One important refinement to it comes from considering the role of opposing, or antagonistic, muscle pairs. Contraction of the biceps muscle, located on the top of the upper arm, pulls on the forearm to flex the elbow and bend the arm. Contraction of the triceps, located on the opposite side, extends the elbow and straightens the arm. Within the spine, these muscles are normally wired so that willed (voluntary) contraction of one is automatically accompanied by blocking of the other. In other words, the command to contract the biceps provokes another command within the spine to prevent contraction of the triceps. In this way, these antagonist muscles are kept from resisting one another. Spinal cord or brain injury can damage this control system and cause involuntary simultaneous contraction and **spasticity**, an increase in resistance to movement during motion.

THE CEREBELLUM Once the movement of the arm is initiated, sensory information is needed to guide the finger to its precise destination. In addition to sight, the most important source of information comes from the "position sense" provided by the many sensory neurons located within the limbs (proprioception). Proprioception is what allows you to touch your nose with your finger even with your eyes closed. The balance organs in the ears provide important information about posture. Both postural and proprioceptive information are processed by a structure at the rear of the brain called the cerebellum. The cerebellum sends out electrical signals to modify movements as they

Key Terms

Botulinum toxin Any of a group of potent bacterial toxins or poisons produced by different strains of the bacterium *Clostridium botulinum*. The toxins cause muscle paralysis, and thus force the relaxation of a muscle in spasm.

Cerebral palsy A movement disorder caused by a permanent brain defect or injury present at birth or shortly after. It is frequently associated with premature birth. Cerebral palsy is not progressive.

Computed tomography (CT) An imaging technique in which cross-sectional x rays of the body are compiled to create a three-dimensional image of the body's internal structures.

Encephalopathy An abnormality in the structure or function of tissues of the brain.

Essential tremor An uncontrollable (involuntary) shaking of the hands, head, and face. Also called familial tremor because it is sometimes inherited, it can begin in the teens or in middle age. The exact cause is not known.

Fetal tissue transplantation A method of treating Parkinson's and other neurological diseases by grafting brain cells from human fetuses onto the basal ganglia. Human adults cannot grow new brain cells but developing fetuses can. Grafting fetal tissue stimulates the growth of new brain cells in affected adult brains.

Hereditary ataxia One of a group of hereditary degenerative diseases of the spinal cord or cerebellum. These diseases cause tremor, spasm, and wasting of muscle.

Huntington's disease A rare hereditary condition that causes progressive chorea (jerky muscle movements) and mental deterioration that ends in dementia. Huntington's symptoms usually appear in patients in their 40s. There is no effective treatment.

Levodopa (L-dopa) A substance used in the treatment of Parkinson's disease. Levodopa can cross the blood-brain barrier that protects the brain. Once in the brain, it is converted to dopamine and thus can replace the dopamine lost in Parkinson's disease.

Magnetic resonance imaging (MRI) An imaging technique that uses a large circular magnet and radio waves to generate signals from atoms in the body. These signals are used to construct images of internal structures.

Parkinson's disease A slowly progressive disease that destroys nerve cells in the basal ganglia and thus causes loss of dopamine, a chemical that aids in transmission of nerve signals (neurotransmitter). Parkinson's is characterized by shaking in resting muscles, a stooping posture, slurred speech, muscular stiffness, and weakness.

Positron emission tomography (PET) A diagnostic technique in which computer-assisted x rays are used to track a radioactive substance inside a patient's body. PET can be used to study the biochemical activity of the brain.

Progressive supranuclear palsy A rare disease that gradually destroys nerve cells in the parts of the brain that control eye movements, breathing, and muscle coordination. The loss of nerve cells causes palsy, or paralysis, that slowly gets worse as the disease progresses. The palsy affects ability to move the eyes, relax the muscles, and control balance.

Restless legs syndrome A condition that causes an annoying feeling of tiredness, uneasiness, and itching deep within the muscle of the leg. It is accompanied by twitching and sometimes pain. The only relief is in walking or moving the legs.

Tourette syndrome An abnormal condition that causes uncontrollable facial grimaces and tics and arm and shoulder movements. Tourette syndrome is perhaps best known for uncontrollable vocal tics that include grunts, shouts, and use of obscene language (coprolalia).

Wilson's disease An inborn defect of copper metabolism in which free copper may be deposited in a variety of areas of the body. Deposits in the brain can cause tremor and other symptoms of Parkinson's disease.

progress, "sculpting" the barrage of voluntary commands into a tightly controlled, constantly evolving pattern. Cerebellar disorders cause inability to control the force, fine positioning, and speed of movements (**ataxia**). Disorders of the cerebellum may also impair the ability to judge distance so that a person under- or overreaches the target (dysmetria). Tremor during voluntary movements can also result from cerebellar damage.

THE BASAL GANGLIA Both the cerebellum and the motor cortex send information to a set of structures deep within the brain that help control involuntary components of movement (basal ganglia). The basal ganglia send output messages to the motor cortex, helping to initiate movements, regulate repetitive or patterned movements, and control muscle tone.

Circuits within the basal ganglia are complex. Within this structure, some groups of cells begin the action of other basal ganglia components and some groups of cells block the action. These complicated feedback circuits are not entirely understood. Disruptions of these circuits are known to cause several distinct movement disorders. A portion of the basal ganglia called the substantia nigra sends electrical signals that block output from another structure called the subthalamic nucleus. The subthalamic nucleus sends signals to the globus pallidus, which in turn blocks the thalamic nuclei. Finally, the thalamic nuclei send signals to the motor cortex. The substantia nigra, then, begins movement and the globus pallidus blocks it.

This complicated circuit can be disrupted at several points. For instance, loss of substantia nigra cells, as in Parkinson's disease, increases blocking of the thalamic nuclei, preventing them from sending signals to the motor cortex. The result is a loss of movement (motor activity), a characteristic of Parkinson's.

In contrast, cell loss in early Huntington's disease decreases blocking of signals from the thalamic nuclei, causing more cortex stimulation and stronger but uncontrolled movements.

Disruptions in other portions of the basal ganglia are thought to cause tics, **tremors**, dystonia, and a variety of other movement disorders, although the exact mechanisms are not well understood.

Some movement disorders, including Huntington's disease and inherited ataxias, are caused by inherited genetic defects. Some diseases that cause sustained muscle contraction limited to a particular muscle group (focal dystonia) are inherited, but others are caused by trauma. The cause of most cases of Parkinson's disease is unknown, although genes have been found for some familial forms.

Symptoms

Abnormal movements are broadly classified as either hyperkinetic—too much movement—and hypokinetic—too little movement. Hyperkinetic movements include:

- Dystonia: sustained muscle contractions, often causing twisting or repetitive movements and abnormal postures. Dystonia may be limited to one area (focal) or may affect the whole body (general). Focal dystonias may affect the neck (cervical dystonia or torticollis), the face (one-sided or **hemifacial spasm**, contraction of the eyelid or **blepharospasm**, contraction of the mouth and jaw or oromandibular dystonia, simultaneous spasm of the chin and eyelid or Meige syndrome), the vocal cords (laryngeal dystonia), or the arms and legs (writer's cramp, occupational cramps). Dystonia may be painful as well as incapacitating.

- Tremor: uncontrollable (involuntary) shaking of a body part. Tremor may occur only when muscles are relaxed or it may occur only during an action or holding an active posture.

- Tics: involuntary, rapid, nonrhythmic movement or sound. Tics can be controlled briefly.

- **Myoclonus**: a sudden, shock-like muscle contraction. Myoclonic jerks may occur singly or repetitively. Unlike tics, myoclonus cannot be controlled even briefly.

- **Chorea**: rapid, nonrhythmic, usually jerky movements, most often in the arms and legs.

- Ballism: like chorea, but the movements are much larger, more explosive and involve more of the arm or leg. This condition, also called ballismus, can occur on both sides of the body or on one side only (hemiballismus).

- Akathisia: restlessness and a desire to move to relieve uncomfortable sensations. Sensations may include a feeling of crawling, itching, stretching, or creeping, usually in the legs.

- Athetosis. slow, writhing, continuous, uncontrollable movement of the arms and legs.

Hypokinetic movements include:

- Bradykinesia: slowness of movement.

- Freezing: inability to begin a movement or involuntary stopping of a movement before it is completed.

- Rigidity: an increase in muscle tension when an arm or leg is moved by an outside force.

- Postural instability: loss of ability to maintain upright posture caused by slow or absent righting reflexes.

Diagnosis

Diagnosis of movement disorders requires a careful medical history and a thorough physical and neurological examination. Brain imaging studies are usually performed. Imaging techniques include computed tomography scan (**CT scan**), **positron emission tomography (PET)**, or **magnetic resonance imaging (MRI)** scans. Routine blood and urine analyses are performed. A lumbar puncture (spinal tap) may be necessary. Video recording of the abnormal movement is often used to analyze movement patterns and to track progress of the disorder and its treatment. Genetic testing is available for some forms of movement disorders.

Treatment

Treatment of a movement disorder begins with determining its cause. Physical and occupational therapy may help make up for lost control and strength. Drug therapy can help compensate for some imbalances of the basal ganglionic circuit. For instance, levodopa (L-dopa) or related compounds can substitute for lost dopamine-producing cells in Parkinson's disease. Conversely, blocking normal dopamine action is a possible treatment in some hyperkinetic disorders, including tics. Oral medications can also help reduce overall muscle tone. Local injections of **botulinum toxin** can selectively weaken overactive muscles in dystonia and spasticity. Destruction of peripheral nerves through injection of phenol can reduce spasticity. All of these treatments may have some side effects.

Surgical destruction or inactivation of basal ganglionic circuits has proven effective for Parkinson's disease and is being tested for other movement disorders. Transplantation of fetal cells into the basal ganglia has produced mixed results in Parkinson's disease.

There are several alternative therapies that can be useful when treating movement disorders. The progress made will depend on the individual and his/her condition. Among the therapies that may be helpful are **acupuncture**, homeopathy, touch therapies, postural alignment therapies, and biofeedback.

Prognosis

The prognosis for a patient with a movement disorder depends on the specific disorder.

Resources

BOOKS

Martini, Frederic. *Fundamentals of Anatomy and Physiology.* Englewood Cliffs, NJ: Prentice Hall, 1989.

Watts, Ray L., and William C. Koller, eds. *Movement Disorders: Neurologic Principles and Practice.* New York: McGraw-Hill, 1997.

ORGANIZATIONS

Worldwide Education and Awareness for Movement Disorders. One Gustave L. Levy Place, Box 1052, New York, NY 10029. (800) 437-6683. <http://www.wemove.org>.

Richard Robinson

Moyamoya disease

Definition

Moyamoya disease is a rare disorder of blood vessels in the brain known as internal carotid arteries (ICA). The condition is characterized by stenosis (narrowing) or occlusion (blockage) of one or both ICA with subsequent formation of an abnormal network of blood vessels adjacent to the ICA.

Description

Moyamoya disease was first described in Japan in 1955. The term *moyamoya*, a Japanese word that means "puff of smoke," describes the appearance of the abnormal vessels that form adjacent to the internal carotid arteries. Alternate names for the disorder include spontaneous occlusion of the circle of Willis, and basal occlusive disease with telangiectasia.

Moyamoya disease can occur in children (juvenile type) or in adults (adult type). Children tend to be less than age 10 and adults are usually between ages 30 and 49. Affected individuals typically present with signs of **stroke** or other types of cerebral ischemia (decreased blood flow to an area of the brain due to obstruction in an artery), cerebral hemorrhage (bleeding), or **seizures** (mainly in children). Symptoms in an affected child or adult may include disturbed consciousness, speech deficits, sensory and cognitive impairment, involuntary movements, or vision problems. Options for treatment for people with moyamoya disease consist of medications and brain surgery. Without treatment, repeated strokes, transient ischemic attacks, brain hemorrhages, or seizures can lead to serious cognitive impairment, physical disability, or death.

Demographics

Moyamoya disease occurs worldwide and is most prevalent in Asia, and especially in Japan. According to a report in 1998, more than 6000 cases had been described. The disease occurs in about one in a million people per year. Estimates of disease incidence in Japan are as much as ten times greater. Slightly more females than males are affected. The male-to-female ratio has been reported to be around 2:3. Approximately 10% of cases of moyamoya disease are familial.

Causes and symptoms

The cause of moyamoya disease is unknown. Possible explanations for the disorder include injuries to the brain, infection, multifactorial inheritance, genetic factors, or other causes. For example, moyamoya disease has been associated with meningitis, **radiation** therapy to the skull in children, and genetic conditions such as Down syndrome, **neurofibromatosis**, and sickle cell anemia. Also, there have been reports linking a region on chromosome 3 (named MYM1) and a region on chromosome 17 (named MYM2) to moyamoya disease in some families.

The initial symptoms of moyamoya disease are somewhat different in children and adults. In children, there is ischemia due to stenosis and occlusion of the circle of

Willis, a ring of arteries at the base of the brain. In children, the disease tends to cause repeated "mini-strokes" known as transient ischemic attacks (TIAs) or, less often, seizures. The TIAs usually manifest as weakness of one side of the body (hemiparesis), speech disturbances, and sensory deficits. TIAs may be made worse by hyperventilation, such as with intense crying. Involuntary movements may occur. **Mental retardation** may be present.

Adults with moyamoya disease typically present with bleeding in the brain (cerebral hemorrhage) or strokes. Cerebral hemorrhage occurs as a result of breakdown of the coexisting blood vessels that formed earlier in life due to stenosis or occlusion of the ICA. The cerebral hemorrhages are commonly located in the thalamus, basal ganglia, or deep white matter of the brain. Symptoms can include disturbance of consciousness and/or hemiparesis. Adult patients with moyamoya disease may go on to have further hemorrhages and strokes which can result in significant and irreversible brain damage.

Diagnosis

A diagnosis of moyamoya disease is based on findings from neuroradiologic studies and on clinical signs consistent with this diagnosis. Neuroradiologic studies used to establish the diagnosis of moyamoya disease include cerebral **angiography**, **magnetic resonance imaging (MRI)**, magnetic resonance angiography (MRA), and computed tomography (**CT**) **scan**. Cerebral angiography is the most common means of confirming a diagnosis of moyamoya disease. There are reports indicating that MRI and MRA, which are less invasive procedures, may be used instead of cerebral angiography. CT scan findings tend to be non-specific and not as useful as CA, MRI, and MRA in making the diagnosis.

Characteristic brain findings in moyamoya disease include narrowing or occlusion of the end portion of one or both internal carotid arteries, an abnormal network or blood vessels at the base of the brain, and presence of these findings on both sides of the brain. In about 10% of cases, cerebral **aneurysms** may also be found. Nuclear medicine studies such as Xenon-enhanced CT, **positron emission tomography (PET)**, or single photon emission computed tomography (SPECT) may be performed in order to evaluate cerebral blood flow (CBF) patterns. The information obtained from CBF studies helps the **neurologist** and/or neurosurgeon to devise a treatment plan.

Treatment

There is no cure for moyamoya disease. Early treatment is important to avoid mental and physical impairment. Treatment options include medications and surgical revascularization.

Medications. Individuals having TIAs and stroke may be given antiplatelet drugs, vasodilators, or anticoagulants to help prevent future attacks. Steroid therapy may be prescribed for a person who has involuntary movements. For a patient with a cerebral hemorrhage, treatment may include management of hypertension, if present.

Surgery. The purpose of revascularization surgery in moyamoya disease is to augment or redirect blood flow in the brain. Surgical revascularization has been reported to improve cerebral blood flow, to reduce ischemic attacks, and, in children, to increase IQ. The optimal method of surgery depends on the patient's history and clinical status. There are various direct and indirect methods of restoring blood supply in the brain. Examples of direct bypass surgery include techniques known as superficial temporal artery to middle cerebral artery bypass, and extracranial-intracranial bypass to anterior or posterior cerebral artery. Examples of indirect bypass surgery include techniques known as encephaloduroarteriosynangiosis, encephalomyosynangiosis, and encephaloarteriosynangiosis.

Treatment team

Management of moyamoya disease requires a multidisciplinary approach. In addition to the patient's primary health care professionals, medical professionals involved in the care of patients with moyamoya disease generally include specialists in neurology, neurosurgery, neuroradiology, and anesthesiology. Specialists in orthopedic surgery, ophthalmology, rehabilitation, physical therapy, occupational therapy, speech therapy, and mental health may also be involved in the care of affected individuals. Psychological counseling and contact with other affected patients may assist families in coping with this condition, especially given it's rarity.

Recovery and rehabilitation

The potential for rehabilitation in moyamoya disease depends in part on the degree of impairment caused by complications such as strokes, cerebral hemorrhages, and seizures. Interventions such as physical, occupational, and speech therapy may be recommended for management of problems such as hemiparesis, speech problems, and sensory deficits. Some patients may require assistance with daily living. In cases in which there is significant disability, consideration may be given to in-home nursing care or placement in a residential care facility that can provide 24-hour care and support services.

Clinical trials

As of 2004, there were no **clinical trials** specifically for patients with moyamoya disease. As more is learned about the causes of moyamoya disease, it is hoped that novel therapies may be developed in the future. As of 2004, one laboratory listed on the GeneTests web site (www.genetests.org) was conducting genetic research on moyamoya disease. Interested patients may discuss the feasibility of participating in this research with their physician.

Prognosis

As of 2004, the prognosis for moyamoya disease was not well defined. The prognosis depends in part on the extent of brain injury present at the time of diagnosis and the success of treatment. For example, a person who had a major stroke or cerebral hemorrhage may already be permanently impaired, both physically and mentally. Reports of clinical outcome after treatment are mixed. Some individuals experience improvement of symptoms while others continue to show progressive decline. Moyamoya disease tends to be more progressive in children than in adults. In those patients who don't stabilize clinically, significant disability or death may occur.

Special concerns

Children with moyamoya disease may have learning disabilities or mental retardation. They may also experience physical disabilities that impact academic performance. Such children may be eligible to have an Individual Education Plan (IEP). An IEP provides a framework from which administrators, teachers, and parents can meet the educational needs of a child with special learning needs. Depending upon severity of symptoms and the degree of learning difficulties, some children with moyamoya disease may be best served by special education classes or a private educational setting.

Resources

BOOKS

Ikezaki, Kiyonobu and Christopher M. Loftus, eds. *Moyamoya Disease*. Rolling Meadows, IL: American Association of Neurological Surgeons, 2001.

Parker, James N., and Philip M. Parker, eds. *The Official Parent's Sourcebook on Moyamoya Disease: A Revised and Updated Directory for the Internet Age*. San Diego, CA: ICON Health Publications, 2002.

PERIODICALS

Ikezaki, K. "Rational approach to treatment of moyamoya disease in childhood." *Journal of Child Neurology* 15 (November 2000): 350–6.

Kobayashi, E., N. Saeki, H. Oishi, S. Hirai, and A. Yamaura. "Long-term natural history of hemorrhagic moyamoya disease in 42 patients." *Journal of Neurosurgery* 93 (December 2000): 976–80.

Lamphere, K. "Moyamoya disease. An uncommon cause of stroke in the young." *Adv Nurse Pract* 11 (2003): 63–6.

Shetty-Alva, N., and S. Alva. "Familial moyamoya disease in Caucasians." *Pediatric Neurology* 23 (November 2000): 445–7.

Yonekawa, Y., and N. Kahn. "Moyamoya disese." *Advances in Neurology* 92 (2003): 113–118.

WEBSITES

The National Institute of Neurological Disorders and Stroke (NINDS). *Moyamoya Disease Information Page*. <http://www.ninds.nih.gov/health_and_medical/disorders/moyamoya.htm>.

Online Mendelian Inheritance In Man (OMIM). *Moyamoya Disease 1*. <http://www.ncbi.nlm.nih.gov:80/entrez/dispomim.cgi?id=252350htm>.

ORGANIZATIONS

Children's Hemiplegia and Stroke Association (CHASA). 4101 West Green Oaks Blvd., PMB #149, Arlington, TX 76016. (817) 492-4325. info5@chasa.org. <http://www.hemikids.org>.

Families with Moyamoya Support Network. 4900 McGowan Street SE, Cedar Rapids, IA 52403.

National Stroke Association. 9707 East Easter Lane, Englewood, CO 80112-3747. (303) 649-9299 or 800-STROKES (787-6537); Fax: (303) 649-1328. info@stroke.org. <http://www.stroke.org>.

Dawn J. Cardeiro, MS, CGC

Mucopolysaccharidoses

Definition

The mucopolysaccharidoses (MPS) are a number of metabolic disorders that follow a chronic and progressive course and involve many body systems.

Description

Though the symptoms and severity vary for each MPS disorder, common features include enlarged organs (organomegaly), dysostosis multiplex (abnormal bone formation), and a characteristic facial appearance. Hearing, vision, breathing, heart function, joint mobility, and mental capacity may also be affected. As of 2003, seven types of MPS have been classified. The MPS disorders are caused by absent or insufficient production of proteins known as lysosomal enzymes The specific enzyme that is deficient or absent distinguishes one type of MPS from another. However, before these enzymes were identified, the signs and symptoms expressed by an affected individual led to the diagnosis. The discovery of these enzymes resulted in a reclassification of some of the MPS disorders. These conditions are often referred to as MPS I, MPS II, MPS III, MPS IV, MPS VI, MPS VII, and MPS IX and may also referred to by their original names, which are Hurler (MPS I H), Hurler-Scheie (MPS I H/S), Scheie (MPS I S), Hunter (MPS II), Sanfilippo (MPS III), Morquio (MPS IV), Maroteaux-Lamy (MPS VI), Sly (MPS VII), and Hyaluronidase deficiency (MPS IX).

Demographics

The MPS syndromes are considered to be rare. Sanfilippo syndrome appears to be the most common MPS with a reported incidence of one in 70,000. The incidence of Hyaluronidase deficiency is not yet known. The incidence of the remaining six classes of MPS are estimated to be: one in 100,000 for Hurler syndrome; one in 500,000 for Scheie syndrome; one in 115,000 for Hurler/Scheie disease; one in 100,000 (male live births) for Hunter syndrome (mild and severe combined); one in 100,000 to one in 300,000 for Morquio syndrome (types A and B included); one in 215,000 for Maroteaux-Lamy syndrome; and less than one in 250,000 for Sly syndrome. These figures are general; more exact figures have been reported for individual MPS disorders in certain countries.

Causes and symptoms

All of the MPS are genetic conditions. MPS I, MPS III, MPS IV, MPS VI, MPS VII, and MPS IX are inherited in an autosomal recessive manner which means that affected individuals have two altered or non-functioning genes, one from each parent, for a specific enzyme that is needed to break down mucopolysaccharides. MPS II (Hunter syndrome) is inherited in an X-linked manner which means that the gene for MPS II is located on the X chromosome, one of the two sex chromosomes. Hunter syndrome primarily affects males because they have only one X chromosome and therefore lack a second, normal copy of the gene responsible for the condition. Carriers for

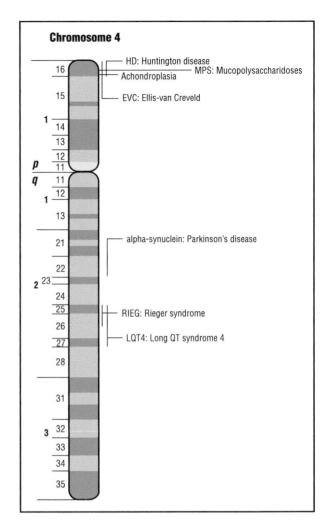

Mucopolysaccharidoses, on chromosome 4. *(Gale Group.)*

the autosomal recessive forms of MPS have one normal copy and one non-working copy of the MPS gene in question. Female carriers of the X-linked MPS (MPS II) have one X chromosome with a normal gene for the condition (the IDS gene) and one X chromosome with a non-working IDS gene.

The enzymes that are deficient in the MPS disorders normally break down a type of mucopolysaccharide (a long chain of sugar molecules) in the body known as glycosaminoglycans (GAGs). Glycosaminoglycans are essential for building the bones, cartilage, skin, tendons, and other tissues in the body. Normally, the human body continuously breaks down and builds GAGs. There are several enzymes involved in breaking down each GAG and a deficiency or absence of any of the essential enzymes can cause one or more GAGs to accumulate in the tissues and organs in the body. When too much GAG is stored, organs and tissues can be damaged or not function properly. The accumulating material is stored in cellular structures called lysosomes, and these disorders are also known as lysosomal storage diseases.

MPS I

Mutations in the alpha-L-iduronidase (IDUA) gene located on chromosome 4 cause the MPS I disorders (Hurler, Hurler-Scheie, and Scheie syndromes). Initially, these three disorders were believed to be separate because each was associated with different physical symptoms and prognoses. However, once the underlying cause of these conditions was identified, it was recognized that all three were variants of the same disorder.

MPS I H (HURLER SYNDROME) Individuals with Hurler syndrome tend to have the most severe form of MPS I. Hurler syndrome may also be referred to as severe MPS I. Infants with Hurler syndrome appear normal at birth and typically begin to develop normally. Symptoms of Hurler syndrome are often evident within the first year or two after birth. Many of these infants may initially grow faster than expected, but their growth slows and typically stops by age three. Facial features also begin to appear coarse; affected children develop a short nose, flatter face, thicker skin, and a protruding tongue. Additionally, their heads become larger and they develop more hair on their bodies with the hair becoming coarser. Affected children with Hurler syndrome lose previously attained skills (milestones) and eventually suffer from profound **mental retardation**. Progressive abnormal development of all bones of the body (dysostosis multiplex) occurs in all children with Hurler syndrome. Children usually develop joint contractures (stiff joints), kyphosis (a "hunchback" curve of the spine), and broad hands with short fingers. Many of these children experience breathing difficulties, and respiratory infections are common. Other common problems include heart valve dysfunction, cardiomyopathy (weakness of the heart muscle), hepatosplenomegaly (enlarged spleen and liver), clouding of the cornea, hearing loss, and **carpal tunnel syndrome**. Children with Hurler syndrome typically die within the first ten years of life.

MPS I H/S (HURLER-SCHEIE SYNDROME) Hurler-Scheie syndrome is felt to be the intermediate form of MPS I, meaning that the symptoms are not as severe as those in individuals who have Hurler syndrome but not as mild as those with Scheie syndrome. Hurler-Scheie syndrome may also be referred to as intermediate MPS I. Individuals with Hurler-Scheie syndrome tend to be shorter than expected and may develop some of the physical features seen in Hurler syndrome, but usually they are not as severe. Intellectual ability varies; individuals have normal or near normal intelligence. The prognosis for children with Hurler-Scheie syndrome is variable with some individuals dying during childhood and others living to adulthood.

MPS I S (SCHEIE SYNDROME) Scheie syndrome is considered the mild form of MPS I. Individuals with Scheie syndrome usually have normal intelligence, but there have been some reports of affected individuals developing psychiatric problems. Common physical problems include corneal clouding, heart abnormalities, and orthopedic difficulties involving the hands and back. Individuals with Scheie syndrome do not develop the facial features seen with severe MPS I. Usually life span is normal.

MPS II (Hunter syndrome)

Mutations in the iduronate-2-sulphatase (IDS) gene cause both forms of MPS II (mild and severe). Nearly all individuals with Hunter syndrome are male, because the gene that causes the condition is located on the X chromosome. The severe form is associated with progressive mental retardation and physical disability, with most individuals dying before age 15. Males with the mild form of Hunter syndrome usually have have normal or near normal intelligence. They tend to develop physical differences similar to males with the severe form, but not as quickly. Most males with Hunter syndrome develop joint stiffness, chronic diarrhea, enlarged liver and spleen, heart valve problems, hearing loss, kyphosis, and tend to be shorter than expected. Men with mild Hunter syndrome can have a normal life span and some have had children.

MPS III (Sanfilippo syndrome)

MPS III is a variable condition with symptoms beginning to appear between ages two and six years of age. The condition is characterized by developmental delay, behavioral problems, and mild physical problems (as compared to other types of MPS). Specific problems include: **seizures**, sleeplessness, thick skin, joint contractures, enlarged tongues, cardiomyopathy, hyperactivity, and mental retardation. The life expectancy in MPS III is also variable. On average, individuals with MPS III live until adolescence. Initially, the diagnosis of MPS III, like the other MPS conditions, was clinical; the diagnosis was made by observation of certain physical characteristics. It was later discovered that a deficiency in one of four enzymes could lead to the developmental delay and physical symptoms associated with MPS III. Each type of MPS III is now subdivided into four groups, labeled A-D, according to the specific enzyme deficiency. All four of these enzymes help to break down the same GAG, heparan sulfate.

MPS IIIA (SANFILIPPO SYNDROME TYPE A) MPS IIIA is caused by a deficiency of the enzyme heparan sulfate sulfamidase, due to mutations in the SGSH gene on chromosome 17. Type IIIA is felt to be the most severe of the four types, in which symptoms appear and death occurs at an earlier age.

Key Terms

Carpal tunnel syndrome A condition caused by compression of the median nerve in the carpal tunnel of the hand, characterized by pain.

Cornea The clear, dome-shaped outer covering of the eye that lies in front of the iris and pupil. The cornea lets light into the eye.

Gene A building block of inheritance, which contains the instructions for the production of a particular protein, and is made up of a molecular sequence found on a section of DNA. Each gene is found on a precise location on a chromosome.

Hydrops fetalis A condition in which a fetus or newborn baby accumulates fluids, causing swollen arms and legs and impaired breathing.

Metabolic Refers to the chemical reactions in living organisms.

Mucopolysaccharide A complex molecule made of smaller sugar molecules strung together to form a chain. It is found in mucous secretions and intercellular spaces.

Mutation A permanent change in the genetic material that may alter a trait or characteristic of an individual, or manifest as disease. This change can be transmitted to offspring.

MPS IIIB (SANFILIPPO SYNDROME TYPE B) MPS IIIB is due to a deficiency in N-acetyl-alpha-D-glucosaminidase due to mutations in the NAGLU gene, also located on chromosome 17. This type of MPS III is not felt to be as severe as Type IIIA and the characteristics vary. Type IIIB is the most common of the four types of MPS III in southeastern Europe.

MPS IIIC (SANFILIPPO SYNDROME TYPE C) A deficiency in the enzyme acetyl-CoA-alpha-glucosaminide acetyltransferase causes MPS IIIC. This is considered a rare form of MPS III. The gene involved in MPS IIIC is believed to be located on chromosome 14.

MPS IIID (SANFILIPPO SYNDROME TYPE D) MPS IIID is caused by a deficiency in the enzyme N-acetylglucosamine-6-sulfatase, due to mutations in the GNS gene located on chromosome 12. This form of MPS III is also rare.

MPS IV (Morquio syndrome)

Morquio syndrome is characterized by severe skeletal deformities and their secondary effects on the nervous system. Intelligence is usually normal. One of the earliest symptoms seen in this condition is a difference in the way the child walks. Skeletal abnormalities can be extreme and include dwarfism, kyphosis (outward-curved spine), prominent breastbone, flat feet, and genu-valgum (knock-knees). A bone deformity known as odontoid hypoplasia (improper formation of the bones that stabilize the head and neck) can result in compression of the spinal cord, a potentially serious and life-threatening complication. As with several of the MPS disorders, Morquio syndrome was originally diagnosed by the presence of particular signs and symptoms. However, it is now known that the deficiency of two different enzymes can result in MPS IV. These two types of MPS IV are called MPS IV A and MPS IV B. MPS IV is variable in its severity. MPS IV A is the classic (typical) or the severe form of the condition and is caused by a deficiency in the enzyme galactosamine-6-sulphatase. The gene involved with MPS IV A (GALNS) is located on chromosome 16. MPS IV B is considered the milder form of the condition. The enzyme, beta-galactosidase, is deficient in MPS IV B. The gene involved with MPS IV B (GLB1) is located on chromosome 3.

MPS VI (Maroteaux-Lamy syndrome)

MPS VI is caused by deficiency of the enzyme N-acetylglucosamine-4-sulphatase (arylsulfatase B), due to mutations in the ARSD gene located on chromosome 5. Affected individuals may have a mild or severe form of the condition. Typically, the nervous system and intelligence are not affected. Individuals with a more severe form of MPS VI can develop airway obstruction, **hydrocephalus** (extra fluid accumulating in the brain), and abnormal growth and formation of the bones. Additionally, individuals with a severe form of MPS VI are more likely to die while in their teens. With a milder form of the condition, individuals tend to be shorter than expected for their age, develop corneal clouding, and live longer.

MPS VII (Sly syndrome)

MPS VII, an extremely rare form of MPS, results from a deficiency of the enzyme beta-glucuronidase due to mutations in the GUSB gene on chromosome 7. MPS VII is also highly variable, but symptoms are generally similar to those seen in individuals with Hurler syndrome. In severe cases, infants may be born with *hydrops fetalis*.

MPS IX (Hyaluronidase deficiency)

MPS IX is a condition that was first described in 1996 and has been grouped with the other MPS conditions by some researchers. MPS IX is caused by the deficiency of the enzyme hyaluronidase due to mutations in the HYAL1 gene on chromosome 3. In the few individuals described with this condition, the symptoms are variable, but some develop soft-tissue masses (growths under the skin). Also, these individuals are shorter than expected for their age.

Diagnosis

Identification of symptoms is usually the first step in making an MPS diagnosis. Doctors will then use laboratory tests to establish an accurate diagnosis. They may first use a screening test that looks for glycosaminoglycans in the urine. The definitive diagnosis of an MPS is made using a biochemical test that measures the specific enzyme (known to be reduced or absent) in the individual's tissues or bodily fluids. Genetic testing may also be used to confirm a suspected diagnosis and, in some cases, to provide limited information about potential disease severity. Genetic testing is accomplished by looking for specific changes known as mutations in the gene responsible for the MPS disorder. Genetic testing is available for all of the MPS disorders except MPS IIIC, MPS IVB, and MPS IX. If the gene mutation(s) have been found in an affected individual, the same genetic test may be used for carrier screening in unaffected family members, such as adult siblings, and for prenatal diagnosis. If the DNA mutations are not found or if genetic testing is not available, carrier screening and prenatal diagnosis may be accomplished using biochemical methods. Preimplantation genetic diagnosis (PGD) is available on a research basis for MPS I and MPS II. More information on PGD for these types of MPS can be found by contacting the Reproductive Genetics Institute at (773) 472-4900 or at rgi@flash.net.

Treatment team

Treatment of MPS disorders requires a multidisciplinary approach. In addition to the patient's primary health care professionals, medical professionals involved in the care of patients with an MPS usually includes specialists in neurology, neurosurgery, ophthalmology (eyes), otolaryngology (ear-nose-throat), audiology (hearing), cardiology, pulmonology (lungs), anesthesiology, gastroenterology, nutrition, orthopedic surgery, rehabilitation (physical, occupational, and speech therapy) and genetics. Some patients with MPS may receive comprehensive services through a specialty clinic such as metabolic or neurogenetics clinic. A genetic specialist, such as a clinical geneticist or a genetic counselor, may be helpful to the patient and family, especially at the time of diagnosis or prior to genetic testing. Psychological counseling and MPS support groups may also assist families in coping with this condition.

Treatment

Treatment of the MPS disorders primarily consists of supportive care and management of complications. Bone marrow transplant (BMT) and enzyme replacement are two promising therapies that offer the possibility of altering the course of these conditions. Due to the progressive nature of the MPS disorders, regular evaluations by primary care providers and specialists is required to detect problems early. Treatment for the most common problems found in the MPS disorders is listed below.

Symmtomatic care and treatment

HYDROCEPHALUS Hydrocephalus (increased fluid in the ventricles of the brain) commonly occurs in MPS I, MPS II, MPS VI, and MPS VII due to a blocked circulation of cerebral spinal fluid in the brain. If the hydrocephalus is detected early, a surgical procedure known as ventriculoperitoneal shunting or a VP shunt may afford the affected individual with a better outcome. Periodic **CT** or **MRI** scans may be recommended to monitor for hydrocephalus in a child with MPS. In MPS III, enlarged ventricles (spaces in the brain) may occur but here the enlargement is thought to be due to cortical atrophy (loss of brain cells). It has been reported that shunting may decrease behavior problems associated with this form of MPS.

SEIZURES Seizures are a problem found in severe forms of MPS and especially in MPS III (Sanfilippo syndrome). Patients with seizures are given a type of prescription medication known as an anticonvulsant.

VISION AND HEARING Regular evaluation by an ophthalmologist is recommended to look for common eye problems including changes in the retina, glaucoma, and corneal clouding. Retinal degeneration, an eye problem that leads to night blindness and loss of peripheral vision, is common in MPS I, MPS II, and MPS III. Adding a night light to a hall or bedroom may help with this. Glaucoma is especially common in MPS I and is usually treated with medications. Corneal clouding is found in MPS I, MPS IV, MPS VI and MPS VII. People with corneal clouding have photophobia (the inability to tolerate bright light). Caps with a visor or sunglasses may be recommended to help reduce this problem. Corneal transplantation is possible for people with significantly reduced vision yet transplants may not always result in improved vision in the long term.

Hearing problems are common in the MPS disorders. Regular hearing evaluations are important so that children with hearing loss can be treated early. Hearing aids may provide some degree of improvement. Recurrent otitis media (middle ear infections) significantly contribute to hearing loss in individuals with MPS. Prescription medications are used to treat otitis media. Ventilating tubes in the ears may be used to minimize the long term effects of these infections.

CARDIOVASCULAR Many individuals with MPS show some signs of heart disease. Common problems include abnormal heart valves, narrowing of the blood vessels in the heart, and weak heart muscles (cardiomyopathy). Patients with MPS I H and the severe form of MPS II usually have damage to the mitral valve. In MPS I H/S, MPS IS, MPS IV, and MPS VI, aortic valvular disease is more common. Medications may be prescribed for congestive heart failure and hypertension associated with underlying heart disease. Valve replacement surgery is possible and has been reported in the MPS disorders.

AIRWAY DISEASE Obstruction of the airway is a common and significant problem for individuals with MPS. This problem can be due to a narrowed trachea (wind pipe), thickened vocal cords, large adenoids or tonsils, decreased rib movement with breathing, and a large tongue. A condition known as obstructive **sleep apnea** (temporary cessation of breathing while asleep) is the most common airway problem in MPS. Treatment for sleep apnea may include: removal of adenoids and tonsils, CPAP or BiPAP treatment, or a tracheostomy. CPAP (continuous positive airway pressure) and BiPAP (bilevel positive airway pressure) are treatments that help to keep the airway open at nighttime. A tracheostomy, an permanent opening through the neck into the trachea, may be needed in severe cases of sleep apnea.

FEEDING PROBLEMS For many individuals with MPS, neurological problems eventually lead to significant problems with chewing and swallowing. Surgical placement of gastrostomy tube (G-tube) or a jejunostomy tube (J-tube) may be recommended when feeding problems cause weight loss, choking, gagging, or episodes of pneumonia.

SKELETAL DEFORMITIES Bony problems, especially of the neck, spine, and hips may require orthopedic intervention. Problems of the cervical spine due to odontoid hypoplasia (improper formation bones that stabilize the head and neck) can be quite serious. Odontoid hypoplasia can lead to slippage of the bones in the neck and compression of the spine in the cervical (neck) region. In severe cases, this spinal cord compression may result in nerve damage, paralysis or death. Odontoid hypoplasia is common in MPS IV (Morquio syndrome). Treatment includes regular monitoring with MRI or X-rays and cervical fusion surgery for severe cases. Other bony problems seen in the MPS disorders include progressive scoliosis or kyphosis (curvatures of the spine) and hip dysplasia (abnormal hip joint). Bracing and sometimes surgery may be used to treat spine curvature. A surgical procedure known as spinal fusion may be considered in patients with significant curvature. Patients with hip dysplasia may be given non-steroidal anti-inflammatory medications.

CARPAL TUNNEL SYNDROME Carpal tunnel syndrome is a common problem in MPS. Although many individuals with MPS may not have typical symptoms (numbness, tingling, **pain**), the carpal tunnel syndrome can and may be severe. Treatment options include splinting, anti-inflammatory medications and surgery.

Bone marrow transplantation (BMT)

Bone marrow transplants have been used to treat children with MPS I, MPS II, MPS III, and MPS VI. Some success has been achieved with BMT in MPS I and in MPS VI; however, this treatment is not a cure and is considered experimental due to the associated risks, including death. Some children who have undergone BMT have shown reduced progression of some disease symptoms. It remains uncertain whether BMT can prevent brain damage. BMT is not recommended as a treatment for MPS II or MPS III.

Enzyme replacement therapy

Enzyme replacement therapy is available for MPS I. A pharmaceutical form of alpha-L-iduronidase known as laronidase is available in the United States. More information may be obtained at<http://www.aldurazyme.com>. Enzyme therapy may be an option in the future for individuals with MPS IV.

Recovery and rehabilitation

Rehabilitation for the MPS disorders consists of physical, occupational, and possibly speech therapy. For example, physical therapy may help preserve joint function for individuals with joint stiffness. Joint stiffness is present in all of the MPS disorders except MPS IV and MPS IX. In physical therapy, patients may undergo range-of-motion exercises (passive bending and stretching of the arms and legs). Also, physical therapy after neck, spine or knee surgery can help patients (who could walk prior to surgery) to walk again. Occupational therapy can teach patients to use adaptive techniques and devices that may help compensate for loss of mobility and/or for loss of speech. Speech therapy may be indicated for individuals with MPS; however, this intervention may not be useful in cases in which the mental condition is rapidly deteriorating.

Hyperactivity can be a severe problem in individuals with MPS, especially in MPS III and MPS II. Medications may or may not be successful in treating this problem. Behavior modification programs may be helpful for some hyperactive MPS children. It may also be necessary to adapt the house and yard to the child.

Clinical trials

As of December 2003, there were four **clinical trials** related to the MPS disorders that were recruiting patients. A phase II/II trial to determine whether the administration of iduronate-2-sulfatase enzyme is safe and efficacious in patients with MPS II will be conducted in the United States, Brazil, Germany and England. Information on this trial can be found at <http://www.clinicaltrials.gov> or by contacting Transkaryotic Therapies at 617-613-4499. A phase III trial to evaluate the ability of recombinant human arylsulfatase B enzyme to enhance endurance in patients with Mucopolysaccharidosis VI (MPS VI) will be conducted in the United States. Information on this trial can be found at <http://www.clinicaltrials.gov> or by contacting BioMarin Pharmaceuticals at 415-884-6700. A phase II study of allogeneic bone marrow or umbilical cord blood transplantation in patients with mucopolysaccharidosis I will be conducted in the United States. Information on this trial can be found at <http://www.clinicaltrials.gov> or by contacting the Study Chair at the Fairview University Medical Center in Minneapolis, Minnesota, at 612-624-5407. A phase II study of bone marrow or umbilical cord blood transplantation in patients with lysosomal or peroxisomal inborn errors of metabolism. Information on this trial can be found at <http://www.clinicaltrials.gov> or by contacting the Study Chair at the Fairview University Medical Center in Minneapolis, Minnesota at 612-624-5407.

Prognosis

Life expectancy for individuals with an MPS is extremely varied. In severe forms of MPS, affected individuals may die in infancy such as in the severe cases of Sly syndrome, or they may die in in childhood or adolescence such as in Hurler syndrome and severe Hunter syndrome. In milder forms of MPS such as Scheie syndrome, mild Hunter syndrome individuals can live well into adulthood. Life spans for individuals with Sanfillipo syndrome, Maroteaux-Lamy syndrome, Morquio syndrome and mild Sly syndrome are quite variable. As more MPS I patients utilize enzyme replacement therapy, new information about prognosis and life span for this disorder will be learned.

Special concerns

Many individuals with an MPS condition have problems with airway constriction. This constriction may be so serious as to create significant difficulties in administering general anesthesia. Therefore, it is recommended that surgical procedures be performed under local anesthesia whenever possible. If general anesthesia is needed, it should be administered by an anesthesiologist experienced in the MPS disorders.

Children and families affected by an MPS may benefit from social services. A social worker may be able to help families obtain Social Security, Medicaid, or other assistance available from agencies that specialize in the care of persons with disabilities. A child with MPS may benefit from an Individual Education Plan (IEP). An IEP provides a framework from which administrators, teachers, and parents can meet the educational needs of a child with MPS.

Resources

BOOKS

Neufeld, Elizabeth F. and Joseph Muenzer. "The Mucopolysaccharidoses." Chapter 136. In *The Metabolic and Molecular Bases of Inherited Disease*, 8th ed., Vol. 3, edited by Charles R. Scriver, Arthur L. Beaudet, William S. Sly, and David Valle. New York: McGraw-Hill Medical Publishing Division, 2001.

Parker, James N., and Philip M. Parker, eds. *The Official Parent's Sourcebook on Mucopolysachharidoses: A Revised and Updated Directory for the Internet Age.* San Diego, CA: ICON Health Publications, 2002.

PERIODICALS

Froissart, R., I. Moreira da Silva, N. Guffon, D. Bozon, and I. Maire. "Mucopolysaccharidosis type II-genotype/phenotype aspects." *Acta Paediatrica Supplement* 91 (2002): 82–87.

Gulati, M. S., and M. A. Agin. "Morquio syndrome: a rehabilitation perspective." *Journal of Spinal Cord Medicine* 19 (January 1996): 12–16.

Kakkis, E. D. "Enzyme replacement therapy for the mucopolysaccharide storage disorders." *Expert Opinion on Investigational Drugs* 11 (May 2002): 675–685.

Robertson, S. P., G. L. Klug, and J. G. Rogers. "Cerebrospinal fluid shunts in the management of behavioral problems in Sanfilippo syndrome." *European Journal of Pediatrics* 157 (August 1998): 653–655.

Vougioukas, V. I., A. Berlis, M. V. Kopp, R. Korinthenberg, J. Spreer, and V. van Velthoven. "Neurosurgical interventions in children with Maroteaux-Lamy syndrome. Case report and review of the literature." *Pediatric Neurosurgery* 35 (July 2001): 35–38.

WEBSITES

Online Mendelian Inheritance in Man (OMIM). National Center for Biotechnology Information. <http://www.ncbi.nlm.nih.gov/Omim/>.

The National Institute of Neurological Disorders and Stroke (NINDS). *Mucopolysaccharidoses Information Page.* <http://www.ninds.nih.gov/health_and_medical/disorders/mucopolysaccharidoses.htm>.

OTHER

The National MPS Society. *MPS Disorder booklets.* 45 Packard Drive, Bangor, ME: The National MPS Society, 2001-2003. <http://www.mpssociety.org/lib-health.html>.

ORGANIZATIONS

Canadian Society for Mucopolysaccharide and Related Diseases. PO Box 64714, Unionville, Ontario L3R-OM9, CA. (904) 479-8701 or (800) 667-1846. rldillio@interlog.com. <http://www.mpssociety.ca>.

National MPS Society, Inc. 45 Packard Drive, Bangor, ME 04401. (207) 947-1445; Fax: (207) 990-3074. info@mpssociety.org. <http://www.mpssociety.org>.

Society for Mucopolysaccharide Diseases. 46 Woodside Road, Amersham, Buckinghamshire HP6-6AJ, UK. (149) 443-4252; Fax: (149) 443-4252. mps@mpssociety.co.uk. <http://www.mpssociety.co.uk>.

Dawn J. Cardeiro, MS, CGC

Multi-infarct dementia

Definition

Multi-infarct **dementia** is one form of dementia that occurs when small blood vessels in the brain are blocked by blood clots or fatty deposits. The blockage interrupts the flow of blood to regions of the brain (a **stroke**), which, if sustained, causes the death of cells in numerous areas of the brain. Another form of multi-infarct dementia is inherited.

Description

Blockage or narrowing of small blood vessels by blood clots or by deposits of fat can impede the flow of blood through the vessel. Deprivation of the essential blood is catastrophic for the regions that are supplied by the vessels. In the brain, such vessel blockage can cause the death of brain cells. This event is also called a stroke. The stroke-related cell death affects the functioning of the brain.

Multi-infarct dementia is the most common form of dementia (the loss of cognitive brain due to disease or injury) due to changes in blood vessels. **Alzheimer's disease** is the most common of these so-called vascular dementias. The term multi-infarct is used because there are many areas in the brain where cell damage or death occurs. Besides dementia, multi-infarct dementia can cause stroke, headaches of migraine-like intensity, and behavioral disturbances.

An inherited form of multi-infarct dementia is designated as CADASIL, which is an acronym for cerebral autosomal dominant arteriopathy with subcortical infarcts and leukoencephalopathy.

Demographics

Multi-infarct dementia usually begins between the ages of 60–75 years. For as-yet-undetermined reasons, it affects men more than women. Multi-infarct dementia is the second most common cause of dementia in older people after Alzheimer's disease, accounting for up to 20% of all progressively worsening dementias.

CADASIL occurs in young male and female adults. It has been diagnosed in Americans, Africans, and Asians, and may occur in other racial groups.

Causes and symptoms

The root cause of multi-infarct dementia is usually small blood clots that lodge in blood vessels in the brain, which results in the death of brain cells. Over time, the series of small strokes (also known as mini-strokes, transient ischemic attacks, or TIAs) magnifies the brain cell damage. Blood clots can result from an elevated blood pressure. Indeed, it is uncommon for someone affected with multi-infarct dementia not to have a history of high blood pressure.

There are a variety of symptoms caused by the brain cell loss. These include mental confusion, problems retaining information even for a short time, loss of recognition of surroundings that are familiar (which can lead to getting lost in previously familiar territory), loss of control of urination and defecation, moving with a rapid shuffling motion, difficulty in following instructions, rapid swings in emotion, and difficulty performing tasks that were previously routine. These symptoms appear in a stepwise manner, from less to more severe. As well, the initial symptoms can be so slight as to be unrecognized, disregarded, or rationalized as being due to other causes such as a temporarily stressful period. These early problems include a mild weakness in an arm or a leg, slurred speech, or **dizziness** that only lasts for a few days. As more blood vessels become blocked with the occurrence of more strokes, the more severe symptoms associated with mental decline become apparent.

CADASIL is characterized by a series of strokes, which is thought to be triggered by genetically determined deficiencies of small cerebral arteries. The defects affect blood flow to the brain in a similar fashion as occurs in multi-infarct dementia. The symptoms associated with CADASIL range from migraines to a slowly progressing series of symptoms that is similar to the symptoms that develop in multi-infarct dementia.

Diagnosis

Multi-infarct dementia is diagnosed based on the history of symptoms, especially of high blood pressure and strokes. A physician will look for several features during the examination, which include arm or leg weakness, speech difficulties, or dizziness. Tests that can be performed in the doctor's office include taking a blood pressure reading, recording the heartbeat (an electroencephalogram, or EEG), and obtaining blood for laboratory analysis. Ultrasound studies of the carotid artery may also be performed.

Diagnosis most often involves the non-destructive imaging of the brain by means of computed tomography (**CT**) or **magnetic resonance imaging (MRI)** to reveal blood clots or the characteristic damaged regions of the brain.

Key Terms

Dementia   A chronic loss of mental capacity due to an organic cause.

Infarct   Tissue death due to lack of oxygen resulting from a blood clot, plaque, or inflammation that blocks an artery.

Transient ischemic attack (TIA)   A temporary, stroke-like event that lasts for only a short time and is caused by a blood vessel that is temporarily blocked.

Diagnosis can also be aided by an examination by a psychologist or a psychiatrist to test a person's degree of mental reasoning, ability to learn and retain new information, and attention span. Symptoms can be similar to those of Alzheimer's disease, which can complicate and delay the diagnosis of both disorders. Indeed, a person can have both disorders at the same time, as their causes are different.

Treatment team

A person with multi-infarct dementia can benefit from a support network that includes a family physician, **neurologist**, pharmacist, nurses, and supportive family members and other care givers. Community resources are also important, such as assisted living facilities, adult day or **respite** care centers, and local agencies on aging.

Treatment

There is no specific treatment for multi-infarct dementia, as the damage to the brain cells cannot be reversed. Treatment typically involves trying to limit further deterioration. This focuses on establishing and/or maintaining a lower blood pressure, which lessens the tendency of blood clot formation. Those people who are diabetic will be treated for this condition, as diabetes can contribute to stroke. Other factors that can be involved in lessening blood pressure include maintaining a target cholesterol level, **exercise**, avoiding smoking, and moderation in alcohol consumption.

Aspirin is known to reduce the tendency of the blood to clot. Some physicians will prescribe aspirin or similarly acting drugs for this purpose. As well, those with high cholesterol may benefit from a diet change and/or the use of cholesterol-lowering drugs such as statins. In some people, surgery that removes blockages in the main blood vessel to the brain (the carotid artery) can be done. Other surgical treatments that increase blood flow through vessels include angioplasty and stenting to increase arterial flow to the brain.

Recovery and rehabilitation

As damage to the brain cannot be reversed, the focus for a person with multi-infarct dementia is placed upon prevention of further brain tissue injury, and maintaining optimum independent functioning.

Clinical trials

As of May 2004, there were no **clinical trials** underway or in the process of recruiting patients for either multi-infarct dementia or CADASIL. However, research is being funded by agencies such as the National Institute of Neurological Disorders and Stroke and is aimed at understanding the development of dementia. The hope is that the diagnosis of dementias will be improved. Ultimately, the goal is to reverse or prevent the disorder.

Prognosis

The outlook for people with multi-infarct dementia is poor. While some improvement in mental faculty may occur, this is typically of short-term duration. Over longer time, mental decline is inevitable and marked.

Special concerns

A person with multi-infarct dementia is often reliant on family and friends for daily care and support. Family and caregivers can help by stimulating a person's mental activity and prompting the individual to recall past experiences. Eventually, around-the-clock care may become necessary to provide a safe and stimulating environment.

Resources
BOOKS

Bird, T. D. "Memory Loss and Dementia." In *Harrison's Principles of Internal Medicine, 15th Edition*, edited by Franci, A. S., E. Daunwald, and K. J. Isrelbacher. New York: McGraw Hill, 2001.

Mace Nancy L. *The 36-Hour Day: A Family Guide to Caring for Persons with Alzheimer Disease, Related Dementing Illnesses, and Memory Loss in Later Life.* New York: Warner Books, 2001.

OTHER

"Multi-Infarct Dementia." *National Mental Health Association.* May 14, 2004 (June 1, 2004). <http://www.nmha.org/infoctr/factsheets/102.cfm>.

"Multi-Infarct Dementia Fact Sheet." *Alzheimer's Disease Education & Referral Center (ADEAR).* May 15, 2004 (June 1, 2004). <http://www.alzheimers.org/pubs/mid.htm>.

"NINDS Multi-Infarct Dementia Information Page." *National Institute of Neurological Disorders and Stroke.* May 14, 2004 (June 1, 2004). <http://www.ninds.nih.gov/health_and_medical/disorders/multi-infarctdementia.doc>.

ORGANIZATIONS

National Institute for Neurological Diseases and Stroke (NINDS). P.O. Box 5801, Bethesda, MD 20824. (301) 496-5751. (800) 352-9424. <http://www.ninds/nih.gov>.

National Institute on Aging (NIA). 31 Center Drive, Rm. 5C27 MSC 2292, Bethesda, MD 20892-2292. (301) 496-1752 or (800) 222-2225. niainfo@nih.gov. <http://www.nia.nih.gov>.

National Institute of Mental Health (NIMH). 6001 Executive Blvd. Rm. 8184, MSC 9663, Bethesda, MD 20892-9663. (301) 443-4513 or (866) 615-6464; Fax: (301) 443-4279. nimhinfo@nih.gov. <http://www.nimh.nih.gov>.

Brian Douglas Hoyle, PhD

Multifocal motor neuropathy

Definition

Multifocal motor neuropathy is a rare condition in which the muscles in the body become progressively weaker over months to years.

Description

Multifocal motor neuropathy is often mistaken for the more catastrophic, inevitably fatal condition called **amyotrophic lateral sclerosis** (ALS). Unlike ALS, however, multifocal motor neuropathy can be treated; therefore, distinguishing between these two conditions is crucial.

Demographics

Multifocal motor neuropathy is a very rare condition, affecting only about 1 per 100,000 people in the population. Men are about three times as likely to be affected as women. Most patients are between the ages of thirty and fifty when symptoms are noted, with the average age of onset being 40 years.

Causes and symptoms

Multifocal motor neuropathy is thought to result from an autoimmune disorder; that is, the body's immune system accidentally misidentifies markers on the body's own nerve cells as foreign. The immune system then begins to produce cells that attack and injure or destroy either the nerve cells or the myelin sheath wrapped around the nerve cells. Because the myelin sheath allows messages to be conducted down a nerve quickly, injury to the sheath or to the nerve itself results in slowed or faulty nerve conduction.

Symptoms of multifocal motor neuropathy usually begin with gradually progressive weakness of the hands. Leg and foot weakness may follow, as well as decreased muscle volume (called muscle wasting), muscle cramps, and involuntary twitching and cramping of muscles. The weakness is asymmetric; that is, a muscle group on only one side of the body may be affected. Over time, numbness or tingling of affected areas may occur, although sensation is not lost.

Diagnosis

Diagnosis of multifocal motor neuropathy usually requires both a careful physical examination, as well as electromyographic (EMG) testing. Physical examination will reveal weakness and decreased muscle size, abnormal reflexes, muscle twitches, and totally normal sensation. EMG involves inserting a needle electrode into a muscle, and measuring the electrical activity within the muscle at rest and during use. A characteristic pattern of abnormal nerve conduction and muscle contraction will be noted on EMG.

Blood tests will usually reveal the presence of antibodies (immune cells) directed against ganglioside, a component of nerve cells.

Treatment team

Patients with multifocal motor neuropathy are usually cared for by neurologists.

Treatment

Treatment for multifocal motor neuropathy involves using intravenous immunoglobulin (IVIg) to dampen down the immune system's overactivity. If IVIg is not successful, then the immunosuppressant drug cyclophosphamide may be administered.

In very mild, early cases, treatment may not be necessary. If the condition progresses or prompts serious disability, treatment may be necessary. Treatment may then be required intermittently, if the condition progresses again.

Prognosis

Muscle strength usually begins to improve within three to six weeks of the initiation of treatment. Early treatment of multifocal motor neuropathy usually results in sufficient symptom resolution to prevent any permanent disability. Over many years, however, many patients will note a continued, slow progression of muscle weakness.

Resources

BOOKS

Asbury, Arthur K., and Stephen L. Hauser. "Guillain-Barré Syndrome and Other Immune-mediated Neuropathies." In *Harrison's Principles of Internal Medicine*, edited by Eugene Braunwald, et al. NY: McGraw-Hill Professional, 2001.

Griffin, John W. "Immune Mediated Neuropathies." In *Cecil Textbook of Internal Medicine*, edited by Lee Goldman, et al. Philadelphia: W. B. Saunders Company, 2000.

Shields, Robert W., and Asa J. Wilbourn. "Demyelinating disorders of the peripheral nervous system." In *Textbook of Clinical Neurology*, edited by Christopher G. Goetz. Philadelphia: W. B. Saunders Company, 2003.

WEBSITES

National Institute of Neurological Disorders and Stroke (NINDS). *NINDS Multifocal Motor Neuropathy Information Page.* November 1, 2003 (June 3, 2004). <http://www.ninds.nih.gov/health_and_medical/disorders/multifocal_neuropathy.htm>.

Rosalyn Carson-DeWitt, MD

Multiple sclerosis

Definition

Multiple sclerosis is an inflammatory demyelinating disease of the **central nervous system**. The disease results in injury to the myelin sheath (the fatty matter that covers the axons of the nerve cells), the oligodendrocytes (the cells that produce myelin) and, to a lesser extent, the axons and nerve cells themselves. The symptoms of multiple sclerosis vary, depending in part on the location of plaques (areas of thick scar tissue) within the central nervous system. Common symptoms include weakness and **fatigue**, sensory disturbances in the limbs, bladder or bowel dysfunction, problems with sexual function, and **ataxia** (loss of coordination). Although the disease may not be cured or prevented at this time, treatments are available to reduce severity and delay progression.

Description

Multiple, or disseminated, sclerosis (MS) is a slowly progressive disease of the central nervous system (CNS), that comprises the brain and spinal cord. In 1868, French physician Jean-Martin Charcot (1825–1893) produced his lectures on "Sclerose en plaques," providing the first detailed clinical description of the disease. The cause of multiple sclerosis is unknown, and it cannot be prevented or cured. Great progress, however, is being made in treating and identifying underlying mechanisms that trigger the disease. The primary characteristic of MS is the destruction of myelin, a fatty insulation covering the nerve fibers. The end results of this process, called demyelination, are multiple patches of hard, scarred tissue called plaques. Another important feature in the disease is destruction of axons, the long filaments that carry electric impulses away from a nerve cell, which is now considered to be a major factor in the permanent disability that occurs with MS.

Multiple sclerosis is usually characterized by a relapsing remitting course in the early stages, with full or nearly full recovery initially. In the early stages, there may be little damage to axons. Over time, the disease enters an irreversible progressive phase of neurological deficit. Each relapse causes further loss of nervous tissue and progressive dysfunction. In some cases there may be chronic progression without remission or acute disease rapidly leading to death.

MS is a diverse disease. No two affected persons are the same and each will experience different combinations of symptoms with differing severity. The most common form is relapsing-remitting multiple sclerosis (RRMS), which affects 80–85% of people with MS. These patients develop disease relapses, often without a specific trigger, but possibly associated with infections. Disease relapses can last between 24 hours and several months, and the person may, or may not, completely recover. The disease is stable between relapses, although affected persons can have residual symptoms and disability.

After several years, the majority (70%) of persons with MS will develop secondary progressive multiple sclerosis (SPMS), whereby they experience a progressive neurological deterioration. They may still suffer from superimposed relapses. A subcategory of RRMS patients (around 20%) has benign MS. These patients have rare and mild relapses and a long course of disease with minimal or no disability. If patients have a steady neurological decline from the onset, without relapses, they are described as having primary-progressive multiple sclerosis (PPMS). This comprises approximately 15–20% of people with the disease

A fourth, rare type of MS is progressive-relapsing multiple sclerosis (PRMS), which is considered a variant of PPMS with similar prognosis. In patients with PRMS, there is a gradual neurological decline from the beginning. It is similar to PPMS, but has superimposed, acute relapses.

Demographics

According to the National Multiple Sclerosis Society, approximately 400,000 Americans acknowledge having MS, and every week about 200 people are diagnosed. Worldwide, MS may affect 2.5 million individuals. The usual age of onset is within the third and fourth decades, although the disease can begin in childhood and also above the age of 60 years. Overall, MS occurs more frequently in women than in men, and the female-to-male ratio is approximately of 2:1. This female predominance is less defined in patients with PPMS, which typically develops at a later age.

There is a variation in the worldwide distribution of MS, with the highest prevalence in the northern and central Europe, northern North America and southeastern

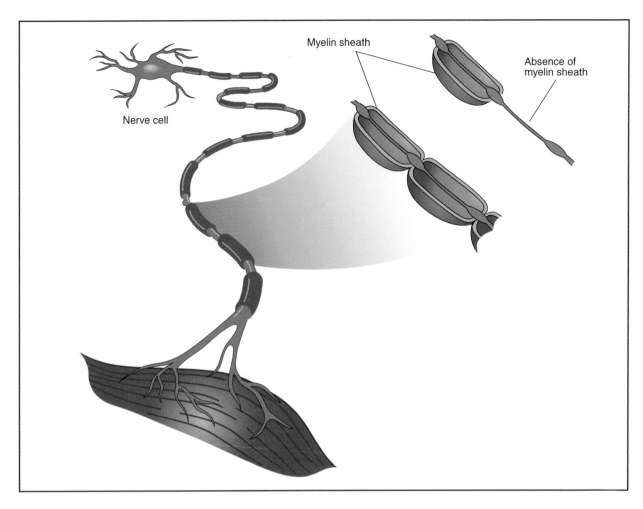

MS results in injury to the myelin sheath that covers the axons of the nerve cells, the cells that produce myelin (oligodendrocytes), and, to a lesser extent, the axons and nerve cells themselves. (*Illustration by Electronic Illustrators Group.*)

Australia. Clusters, or areas with more than the expected amount, occur. There are also racial differences, with a low prevalence in Asians and Africans or people of African descent, and a higher frequency in Caucasians, especially of northern European descendent. MS is rare between the equator and latitudes 30°–35° north and south. The prevalence of MS increases proportionally with increased distance from the equator. There is no satisfactory explanation of this phenomenon, although certain variables have been researched. These include environmental factors, such as climate, humidity, hours of daily sunshine, resistance to certain viruses, and even consumption of cow's milk.

Causes and symptoms

The causes of multiple sclerosis remain unknown, but it is widely accepted that susceptibility to MS is determined by a complex interaction between susceptibility genes and environment. The most popular current theory is that the disease occurs in people with a genetic susceptibility, who are exposed to some environmental assault (a virus or a toxin) that disrupts the blood-brain barrier, a protective membrane that controls the passage of substances from the blood into the central nervous system. Most researchers consider MS to be an autoimmune disease-one in which the body, through its immune system, launches a defensive attack against its own tissues. Immune factors converge in the nerve cells and trigger inflammation and an autoimmune attack on myelin and axons. Still, a number of disease patterns have been observed in MS patients, and some experts believe that MS may prove to be not a single disorder, but may represent several diseases with different causes.

Components of myelin such as myelin basic protein have been the focus of much research because, when injected into laboratory animals, they can precipitate experimental allergic encephalomyelitis (EAE), a chronic relapsing brain and spinal cord disease that resembles MS. The injected myelin probably stimulates the immune system to produce anti-myelin T-cells that attack the animal's own myelin.

Increasing scientific evidence suggests that genetics may play a role in determining a person's susceptibility to MS. No specific gene has been identified and it seems to have a mode of inheritance that involves multiple genes. Twin studies have shown an increased risk of 30% in identical twins, and around 5% in fraternal twins. First-degree relatives of a person with MS have a two or three percent increased risk, which, although small, is higher than in the general population. Further indications that more than one gene is involved in MS susceptibility comes from studies of families in which more than one member has MS.

Several research teams found that people with MS inherit certain regions on individual genes more frequently than people without MS. Of particular interest is the human leukocyte antigen (HLA) or major histocompatibility complex region on chromosome 6. HLAs are genetically determined proteins that influence the immune system. Another interesting candidate is CD24, which has shown to be essential for the induction of EAE in mice. CD24 is a cell surface protein with expression in a variety of cell types that can participate in the rise of MS, including activated T-cells.

An infectious cause of MS has been indicated by some studies as well as by similarities to infectious demyelinating diseases. However, infectious agents more likely shape the immune response that may induce the disease under special circumstances. Evidence is mounting that infection with the Epstein-Barr virus (EBV), which can cause mononucleosis, may also increase the risk of developing multiple sclerosis later in life. Researchers have shown that people with multiple sclerosis tend to carry higher levels of antibodies to the Epstein-Barr virus and that they seem to be at higher risk for the disease. Some of the immune cells that become programmed to attack the Epstein-Barr virus may begin to attack myelin as well.

Environmental factors, other than infectious agents, for which there is some evidence of an association with MS, include toxins, low sunlight exposure, diet factors, and trauma.

Almost any neurological deficit can occur in MS, but there are several signs and symptoms that are characteristic and their presence should suggest MS as a possible diagnosis, particularly in a young adult.

Vision disorders such as optic neuritis can occur. Optic neuritis (ON) is an inflammation of the optic nerve characterized by acute or subacute loss of vision usually in one, but occasionally in both eyes. The visual loss evolves over a period of hours or days. Vision returns to normal within two months, but may deteriorate in later years. Previous history of optic neuritis in a person who develops a neurological illness will strongly support the diagnosis of MS.

Cognitive (thought) impairment is thought to affect 40–70% of MS patients and can be present even in the early stages of MS. Approximately one-third of people with MS have some degree of memory loss. Other areas of cognitive function particularly affected in the MS patient include sustained attention, verbal fluency, and spatial perception. **Dementia** (loss of intellectual function) is often common in the latter stages of MS.

Many MS patients are temperature sensitive. In hotter weather or during a period of raised body temperature, their MS symptoms worsen. Most frequently, vision is affected and muscle weakness occurs.

About two-thirds of MS patients experience **pain** at some point during the course of the disease and 40% are never pain free. MS causes many pain syndromes; some are acute, while others are chronic. Some worsen with age and disease progression. Pain syndromes associated with MS are trigeminal (facial) pain, powerful spasms and cramps, optic neuritis pain, pressure pain, stiffened joints, and a variety of sensations including feelings of itching, burning, and shooting pain.

The Lhermitte's sign can occur, which is actually more of a symptom than a sign. A tingling or electric-like sensation down the back and legs is felt upon flexing the neck. The symptom is non-specific, but occurs more frequently in MS than in any other condition and provides an important clue to the correct diagnosis.

Urinary incontinence affects up to 90% of people with multiple sclerosis and usually occurs before major physical disability is apparent. Bladder problems are due to plaques in the spinal cord. If demyelination occurs in both controlling pathways, the bladder will neither store urine nor empty it properly. Constipation affects about 40% of people with MS. Bowel incontinence and urgency of defecation can also occur in about half of people with MS.

Fatigue is a common complaint in MS. Characteristics of fatigue include muscle weakness, coordination problems, ataxia, transient deafness, changes in taste or smell and numbness of the extremities. **Spasticity** occurs in up to 90% of MS patients and it can be painful and distressing. Spasticity is characterized by weakness, loss of dexterity, and the inability to control specific movements. It is usually more severe in the legs and torso.

Sexual dysfunction is common among people with multiple sclerosis. If MS damages the nerve pathways from the brain to the sexual organs via the spinal cord, sexual response can be directly affected. Physicians and people with MS often neglect to deal with this aspect of the

Key Terms

Autoimmune disease   One of a group of diseases, like rheumatoid arthritis and systemic lupus erythematosus, in which the immune system is overactive and has lost the ability to distinguish between self and non-self. The body's immune cells turn on the body, attacking various tissues and organs.

Axon   A long, threadlike projection that is part of a neuron (nerve cell).

Myelin   A fatty sheath surrounding nerves throughout the body that helps them conduct impulses more quickly.

disease, and both treatments and strategies for success are available.

Depression is common in MS; some studies show that over 50% of people with MS have depression at some point in their lifetime. There is also an increased risk of suicide. If depression is present, it should be treated prior to initiating MS therapy. Depression in those with MS is treated in the same way as the general population.

Diagnosis

MS diagnosis is based upon an individual's history of clinical symptoms and neurological examination. A qualified physician, often a **neurologist**, must thoroughly review all symptoms experienced by an individual to suspect MS. Other conditions with similar symptoms must be ruled out, often requiring various tests.

The diagnosis of MS is usually made in a young adult with relapsing and remitting symptoms referable to different areas of CNS white matter. Diagnosis is more difficult in a patient with the recent onset of neurological complaints or with a primary progressive clinical course.

Laboratory studies include blood work to exclude collagen vascular disease, infections (ie, **Lyme disease**, syphilis), endocrine abnormalities, vitamin B-12 deficiency, sarcoidosis, and **vasculitis**. The examination of cerebrospinal fluid (CSF) has been used to support the diagnosis of MS. The presence of myelin basic protein in the CSF of an MS patient may be highly suggestive of activity of the MS process, but its absence does not rule out active disease.

A newer neuroimaging technique, magnetic resonance spectroscopy (MRS), has been useful in following NAA (N-acetyl-aspartate) levels in patients with multiple sclerosis. NAA is an amino acid found in neurons and axons of the mature brain. In patients with relapsing-remitting MS, NAA levels are reduced, suggesting axonal loss; however, in patients with secondary progressive MS with more disability, the NAA levels are reduced more significantly. In fact, patients with MS had lower levels of NAA even in areas of the brain previously thought to be unaffected, when compared with levels in normal persons.

Magnetic resonance imaging (MRI) remains the imaging procedure of choice for diagnosing and monitoring disease progression in the brain and spinal cord. This test can show brain abnormalities in 90–95% of patients and spinal cord lesions in up to 75% of cases, especially in elderly patients. However, MRI alone cannot be used to diagnose MS. Evoked potential tests that measure how quickly and accurately a person's nervous system responds to certain stimulation have been the most useful neurophysiological studies for evaluation of MS.

At the onset, MS may be mistaken for other inflammatory diseases of the central nervous system, such as Behçet disease, antiphospholipid syndrome or **acute disseminated encephalomyelitis** (ADEM). Pseudotumoral MS may be reminiscent of lymphoma, other tumors (glial tumors), or infectious diseases (like Lyme disease, HTLV1 infection or abcess). Recurrent relapses of neurological impairment may also be mistaken for cavernomatosis. In most cases, MRI findings, cerebrospinal fluid analysis, evoked potentials, the association with systemic signs and the relapsing remitting nature of the disease allow physicians to exclude other diseases, and to arrive at a diagnosis of MS.

Treatment team

The multidisciplinary team usually includes specialists in neurology, urology, ophthalmology, neuropsychology, and social work.

Treatment

The three goals of drug therapy in the treatment of MS are management of acute episodes, prevention of disease progression, and treatment of chronic symptoms. Specific symptoms that may be treated include muscle spasticity, lack of co-ordination, tremor, fatigue, pain, bladder and bowel dysfunctions, sexual dysfunction and depression.

Exacerbations (episodes of worsening symptoms) can be defined as temporary flare-ups, sometimes referred to as attacks or relapses. Most relapses show a degree of spontaneous recovery, but treatment is offered for those relapses that have a severe impact on function. Steroids are the treatment of choice for relapses, usually methyl-prednisolone given orally or by intravenous infusion. Before starting steroids, infection should be excluded because steroids have immunosuppressant action and can exacerbate the infection.

Disease modifying treatments are aimed at slowing disease progression. The two current types of immunomodulatory agents used as a first line treatment are interferon beta and glatiramer acetate. Interferon beta has proved effective with RRMS and SPMS. There is currently no evidence for improvement with PPMS. Discontinuation of the treatment may be necessary because of intolerance to side effects, when a pregnancy is planned, or when it is no longer effective. Glatiramer is the appropriate treatment to reduce relapse frequency in patients with RRMS and it should not be used for both PPMS and SPMS. Stopping criteria for glatiramer are the same of interferon beta.

A number of treatments are available for managing MS chronic symptoms and complications, each one with specific drugs. Indeed, symptomatic treatment, along with supportive measures and rehabilitation, are a major part of the MS treatment.

Recovery and rehabilitation

When recovering from a symptom flare-up or learning to cope with a change in mobility, rehabilitation through physical therapy can be of great value training patients to improve mobility and to decrease spasticity and strengthen muscles. Some of those who have a physically demanding or highly stressful job may choose to make a career change, in which case vocational training is helpful.

Occupational therapy helps in assessing the patient's functional abilities in completing activities of daily living, assessing fine motor skills, and evaluating for adaptive equipment and assistive technology needs. Speech therapists assess the patient's speech, language, and swallowing and may work with the patient on compensatory techniques to manage cognitive problems.

Clinical trials

The National Institute of Neurological Disorders and Stroke (NINDS) is recruiting patients to evaluate the safety, tolerability, and effect of the drug Rolipram on MS. The NINDS is also recruiting patients with relapsing-remitting or secondary progressive multiple sclerosis to examine the safety and effectiveness of Zenapax (a laboratory-manufactured antibody) in treatment of MS. More information is available at the website: <http://www.clinicaltrials.gov>, a clinical trial service sponsored by the United States government.

Prognosis

It is generally very difficult to predict the course of MS. The disorder varies greatly in each individual, but most people with MS can expect to live 95% of the normal life expectancy. Some studies have shown that people who have few attacks in the first several years after diagnosis, long intervals between attacks, complete recovery from attacks, and attacks that are sensory in nature (i.e., numbness or tingling) tend to fare better. People who have early symptoms of tremor, difficulty in walking, or who have frequent attacks with incomplete recoveries, or more lesions visible on MRI scans early on, tend to have a more progressive disease course.

Special concerns

People with should avoid caffeine-containing beverage, which can actually be dehydrating. The diet should also be rich in fiber, particularly from whole grains, fruits and vegetables to increase digestive motility and reduce constipation. Maintenance of weight in the normal range is also desirable in order to diminishes stress on the joints and skeletal muscles.

Gait difficulty (difficulty with walking) may worsen during pregnancy, and assistive devices for walking or a wheelchair are useful at this time. During pregnancy, bladder and bowel problems may also be aggravated in women with MS who already have these dysfunctions.

Resources

BOOKS

O'Connor, Paul. *Multiple Sclerosis: The Facts You Need.* Firefly Books, 1999.

Warren, Sharon, and Kenneth Warren. *Multiple Sclerosis.* World Health Organization, 2001.

PERIODICALS

Myles, Mary L. "The ongoing battle against multiple sclerosis." *Canadian Journal of Diagnosis* (June, 2003): 108–117.

OTHER

"About MS." *Multiple Sclerosis Association of America.* <http://www.msaa.com> (February 12, 2004).

National Institute of Neurological Disorders and Stroke. *NINDS Multiple Sclerosis Information Page.* <http://www.ninds.nih.gov/health_and_medical/disorders/multiple_sclerosis.htm> (February 12, 2004).

National Multiple Sclerosis Society. *Living with MS.* <http://www.nationalmssociety.org> (February 1, 2004).

ORGANIZATIONS

The National Multiple Sclerosis Society. 733 Third Avenue, 6th floor, New York, NY 10017. (212) 986-3240 or (800) 344-4867; Fax: (212) 986-7981. nat@nmss.org. <http://www.nationalmssociety.org>.

Marcos do Carmo Oyama
Iuri Drumond Louro

Multiple system atrophy

Definition

Multiple system atrophy (MSA) is a neurodegenerative disease characterized by parkinsonism, cerebellar dysfunction, and autonomic disturbances.

Description

MSA causes a wide range of symptoms, in keeping with its name of "multiple system" atrophy. Parkinsonian symptoms include tremor, rigidity and slowed movements; cerebellar symptoms include incoordination and unsteady gait; and autonomic symptoms include **orthostatic hypotension** (drop in blood pressure upon standing) and urinary incontinence. Because of this wide variety of symptoms, it was originally thought of as three distinct diseases: **striatonigral degeneration** (parkinsonian symptoms), **olivopontocerebellar atrophy** (cerebellar symptoms) and Shy-Drager syndrome (autonomic symptoms). Further study showed the overlap among these conditions was best explained by considering them as a single disease with symptoms clustered into three groups. Historically, confusion about the disease was made even worse because olivopontocerebellar atrophy is also the name of an unrelated genetically inherited disease. It is hoped that widespread use of the name MSA will clear up some of this confusion.

Demographics

Because MSA is often misdiagnosed, figures on its prevalence are not known with certainty. It is estimated there are between 25,000 and 100,000 people in the United States with MSA. Onset is usually in the early fifties, and men are slightly more likely to be affected than women.

Causes and symptoms

The cause or causes of MSA are unknown. No genes have been found for MSA. Some evidence indicates that toxins may be responsible, but no specific agents have been identified. The brains of MSA patients reveal that cells called glia undergo characteristic changes. Glia are supportive cells for neurons, brain cells that conduct electrical signals. In MSA, glia develop tangles of proteins within them, called glial cytoplasmic inclusions. It is not known whether these actually cause MSA, or are caused by some other problem that is the real culprit.

The symptoms of MSA fall into three separate areas-parkinsonism, cerebellar symptoms, and autonomic disturbances. The distribution and severity of individual symptoms varies among patients. MSA is a progressive disease, and symptoms worsen over time.

Key Terms

Atrophy   The progressive wasting and loss of function of any part of the body.

Cerebellum   The part of the brain involved in the coordination of movement, walking, and balance.

Neurodegeneration   The deterioration of nerve tissues.

Parkinsonism is the initial symptom in almost half of all patients. The classic symptoms of **Parkinson's disease** (**PD**)—tremor, stiffness or rigidity, and slowed movements—are seen in MSA, although tremor is not as common, and is jerkier than the tremor of PD.

Cerebellar symptoms are the initial feature in very few MSA patients, but occur in about half of patients at some point during the disease. The **cerebellum** is an important center for coordination, and degeneration of the cerebellum in MSA leads to loss of balance, incoordination in the limbs, and loss of smooth eye movements. A person with cerebellar dysfunction in MSA typically walks with a wide stance to improve stability, and may lose the hand-eye coordination that makes so many simple activities possible.

Autonomic symptoms refer to those involving the autonomic nervous system. The autonomic nervous system controls a variety of "automatic" body functions, including blood pressure, heart rate, sweating, and bladder function. Autonomic symptoms are the initial complaint in half or more of all MSA patients. The most common initial problem is urinary dysfunction in women, and erectile dysfunction in men. Urinary dysfunction may be incontinence, or inability to void the bladder. Other autonomic symptoms include lack of sweating, constipation, and fecal incontinence.

Orthostatic hypotension is a common autonomic symptom. It refers to a significant drop in blood pressure shortly after standing. It can cause **dizziness**, lightheadedness, **fainting**, weakness, **fatigue**, yawning, slurred speech, **headache**, neck ache, cognitive impairment, and blurred vision.

Other symptoms may also occur in MSA. These may include:

- vocal cord paralysis, leading to hoarseness
- swallowing difficulty
- **sleep apnea**
- spasticity

- myoclonus
- Raynaud's phenomenon (cold extremities)

Diagnosis

The diagnosis of MSA is difficult, because it is easily mistaken in its earlier stages for Parkinson's disease, which is much more common. Autonomic disturbance also occurs in PD, but is much more pronounced in MSA. MSA is the more likely diagnostic choice when disease progression is rapid, and when the patient responds mildly or poorly to levodopa, the mainstay of PD treatment. Some centers use **electromyography** of the anal sphincter (the muscles surrounding the anus) in order to confirm the diagnosis of MSA. Abnormal results indicate MSA rather than PD, although this method is not universally recognized as valid.

Neuroimaging may be used to rule out other causes of similar symptoms, such as lesions in the brain or normal pressure **hydrocephalus**.

Treatment team

The treatment team includes the **neurologist**, possibly a **movement disorders** specialist, a urologist, and a speech/language pathologist.

Treatment

There are no treatments that halt or slow the degeneration of brain cells that causes MSA. Treatment is aimed at relieving symptoms.

Treatment of parkinsonian symptoms is attempted with standard PD drugs, namely levodopa and the dopamine agonists. Unfortunately, these are rarely as effective in MSA as they are in PD, although about one-third of patients have at least a moderate response. In the best case, treatment relieves stiffness, tremor and slowed movements, allowing increased activities of daily living.

Orthostatic hypotension is treated with medications to increase retention of fluids (fludrocortisone), compressive stockings to keep blood from pooling in the legs, increasing fluids, and increasing salt intake. Midodrine, a drug that helps maintain blood pressure is often prescribed.

A urologist may be needed to define the type of urinary dysfunction the patient has, and to manage treatment. A bedside commode or condom catheter may be helpful for urge incontinence, or inability to hold urine once the urge to urinate occurs. If incomplete voiding is the problem, intermittent catheterization may be needed. Detrusor hyperreflexia, in which the bladder muscle undergoes spasms, may be treated with drugs to reduce these spasms.

Male erectile dysfunction may be treated with sildenafil or other medications.

Anhidrosis, or lack of sweating, can be dangerous in an active patient, because of the risk of overheating. Awareness of the problem and avoidance of prolonged **exercise** are helpful.

Gait **ataxia** may require a mobility aid, such as a cane, walker, or eventually a wheelchair.

Speech and swallowing problems are dealt with by a speech/language pathologist, who may work with the patient to develop swallowing strategies, and instruct in the use of assistive communication devices. Sleep apnea may be treated with continuous positive airway pressure ventilation.

Clinical trials

Clinical trials for MSA are usually directed toward better diagnosis, or symptomatic treatment. Until researchers develop a better understanding of the causes of the disease, little progress can be expected in development of treatments to slow its progression.

Prognosis

The average survival after diagnosis is 9-10 years. Death usually occurs from pneumonia or suddenly from insufficient respiration, due to degeneration of the respiratory centers in the brain.

Special concerns

Resources

PERIODICALS

Wenning, G. K., et al. "Multiple System Atrophy." *Lancet Neurology* 3 (2004): 93-103.

WEBSITES

Shy-Drager Syndrome/Multiple System Atrophy Support Group. <www.shy-drager-syndrome.org>.
WE MOVE. <www.wemove.org>.

Richard Robinson

Muscle-nerve biopsy *see* **Biopsy**

Muscular dystrophy

Definition

Muscular dystrophies (MD) are inherited disorders characterized by progressive weakness and degeneration of the skeletal or voluntary muscles which control movement, without a central or peripheral nerve abnormality. The muscles of the heart and other involuntary muscles are also affected in some forms of MD, and a few forms involve other organs as well. The major forms of muscular dystrophy include myotonic, Duchenne, Becker, limb-girdle, facioscapulohumeral, congenital, oculopharyngeal, distal, Emery-Dreifuss and Fukuyama muscular dystrophy.

Description

The commonest form of these inherited disorders is the Duchenne muscular dystrophy (DMD). The disorder was originally described in the mid-nineteenth century by the English physician Edward Meryon. At a meeting of the Royal Medical and Chirurgical Society in 1851, and later published in the transactions of the society, he described in detail the clinical presentation of Duchenne muscular dystrophy, beginning in early childhood with progressive muscle wasting and weakness and leading to death in late adolescence. Furthermore, his detailed histological studies led him to conclude that the muscle membrane or sarcolemma was broken down and destroyed.

Duchenne muscular dystrophy will usually produce symptoms between the ages of three and seven in young boys. It begins with a weakness in the pelvic area first and then progresses to the shoulder muscles. As the disorder escalates, the muscles enlarge although the muscle tissue is weak. The heart muscle will also enlarge, creating problems with the heartbeat that can be detected on an electrocardiogram. In most cases, the affected child has a waddling walk, often falls, has difficulty rising from a sitting position, has a difficult time climbing stairs, is unable to fully extend the arms and legs, and may develop scoliosis (an abnormally curved spine). In most cases, children with DMD are confined to a wheel chair between the ages of ten and twelve.

Most people with Becker muscular dystrophy (BMD) first experience difficulties between the ages of five and fifteen years, although onset in the third or fourth decade or even later can occur. By definition, patients with BMD are able to walk beyond age fifteen, while patients with DMD are typically in a wheelchair by the age of twelve. Patients with BMD have a reduced life expectancy, but most survive into the fourth or fifth decade. **Mental retardation** may occur in BMD, but it is not as common as in DMD. Cardiac (heart muscle) involvement occurs in BMD and may result in heart failure.

Myotonic muscular dystrophy (MMD) affects the muscles in the hands and feet. Limb-girdle muscular dystrophy (LGMD) begins late in childhood affecting mainly the muscles of the shoulders and hips. Facioscapulohumeral muscular dystrophy (FSHD) affects only the muscles of the upper arms, face and shoulder girdle. Landouzy-Dejerine muscular dystrophy (LDMD), which is transmitted by an autosomal dominant gene, affects the face, shoulder and lower leg muscles.

Other disorders related to muscular dystrophy include Steinert's disease, Thomsen's disease, and Pompe's disease. Steinert's disease affects both males and females, causing the muscles to be unable to relax after contracting, while Thomsen's disease causes a stiffness of the legs, hands and eyelids. Pompe's disease, which is a glycogen storage disease, affects the liver, heart, nerves and muscles.

Demographics

United States

The incidence of muscular dystrophy varies, depending on the specific type. Duchenne muscular dystrophy is the most common condition. It is inherited on the X chromosome, primarily affects boys, and is the most severe type of the disease. Although women with the defective gene are carriers, they usually show no symptoms. DMD has an inheritance pattern of 1 case per 3,500 live male births, and one-third of cases are due to spontaneous new mutations.

Becker muscular dystrophy is the second most common form, with an incidence of 1 case per 30,000 live male births. Like DMD, BMD is linked to the X chromosome. Other types of MD are rare. Limb-girdle muscular dystrophy includes several different illnesses, which can be inherited by both males and females, as can facioscapulohumeral muscular dystrophy.

International

The incidence of muscular dystrophies internationally is similar to that of the United States, however some types are especially frequent in certain populations and are rare elsewhere. For example, autosomal dominant distal muscular dystrophy occurs more often in Scandinavia than elsewhere, Fukuyama muscular dystrophy in Japan, oculopharyngeal muscular dystrophy in French Canada, and several autosomal recessive LGMD in communities in Brazil, North America, and the Middle East.

Causes and symptoms

All types of muscular dystrophy are inherited. They are caused by a defect in one or more of the genes that control muscle structure and function. Some types are inherited as a dominant gene abnormality, while others are inherited as a recessive gene abnormality or an X-linked recessive gene abnormality. In an X-linked recessive gene abnormality, the gene is on the X chromosome, one of the pair of chromosomes that determine a person's sex.

Both DMD and BMD are inherited X-linked recessive diseases affecting primarily skeletal muscle and the myocardium (heart muscle). Dystrophin, a large protein that stabilizes the plasma membrane during muscle contractions, is absent in DMD and reduced in BMD. This results

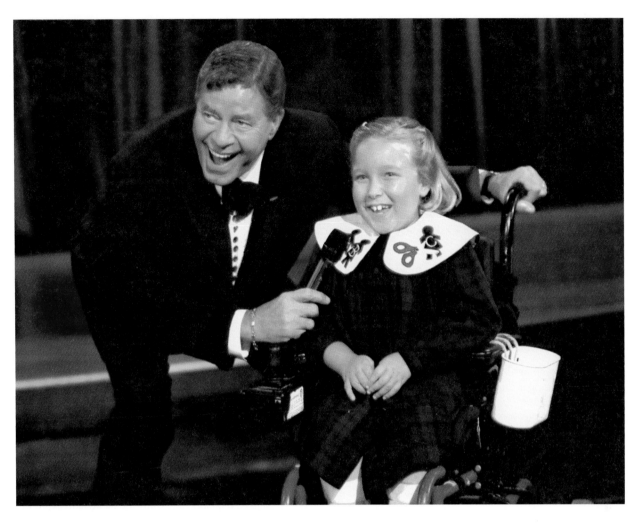

Jerry Lewis, talking with Sarah Schwegel, MDA National Goodwill Ambassador, during the Muscular Dystrophy Association Labor Day Telethon. *(Reproduced by permission of the Muscular Dystrophy Association.)*

in an unstable muscle cell membrane and impaired function in the cell. Muscle fibers continually deteriorate and regenerate until the capacity for repair is no longer sufficient. Muscle fiber tissue is eventually replaced by fat and connective tissue. The abnormal gene for DMD and BMD is on the short arm of the X chromosome at position Xp21.

Two types of MMD are well recognized: noncongenital (NC-MMD, not present at birth) and congenital (C-MMD, present at birth). In MMD, a DNA sequence within the gene on chromosome 19q 13.3, is repeated many times, leading to an enlarged, unstable area of the chromosome. Called a triplet repeat mutation, the flawed gene grows by sudden leaps when transmitted from generation to generation, causing the disease to occur at a younger age and in a more severe form (a phenomenon called anticipation). C-MMD patients have been shown to have substantially more repeats than those found in NC-MMD patients.

In FSHD, the abnormal gene is known to be near the end of chromosome 4. Exact DNA testing for diagnostic purposes is not yet available except in some cases, a detailed genetic analysis of a particular family can be accomplished.

Genetic studies with LGMD have identified one form linked to chromosome 15q, another form to chromosome 2p, and two more severe forms to 13ql2 and 17ql2-q21.

Symptoms can first appear during early childhood or late in adult life, depending on the type of muscular dystrophy.

• Duchenne muscular dystrophy—Symptoms usually begin between ages two and four. Because of a progressive weakening of leg muscles, the child falls frequently and has difficulty getting up from the ground. The child also has trouble walking or running normally. By age 12, most patients are unable to walk and are limited to a wheelchair. As the illness progresses, there also is an abnormal curvature of the spine.

• Becker muscular dystrophy—Symptoms are similar to those of DMD, but they are milder and begin later, usually between ages five and fifteen.

• Myotonic muscular dystrophy—Muscle myotonia may develop soon after birth or begin as late as early adulthood, and especially affects the hands, wrists and tongue. There also is wasting and weakening of facial muscles, neck muscles, and muscles of the wrists, fingers and ankles. Involvement of the tongue and throat muscles causes speech problems and difficulty swallowing. If the diaphragm and chest muscle also are involved, there may be breathing problems.

• Limb-girdle muscular dystrophy—Symptoms begin in late childhood or early adulthood. They include progressive muscle weakness in the shoulders and hips, together with breathing problems (if the diaphragm is involved). If illness also affects the heart muscle, there may be heart failure or abnormal heart rhythms.

• Facioscapulohumeral muscular dystrophy—Symptoms may begin during infancy, late childhood, or early adulthood. Usually, the first sign is facial weakness with difficulty smiling, whistling and closing the eyes. Later, there is difficulty raising the arms or flexing the wrists and/or ankles.

Diagnosis

The diagnosis of muscular dystrophy is made with a physical examination and diagnostic testing by the child's physician. During the examination, the child's physician obtains a complete prenatal and birth history and asks if other family members are known to have MD. In addition to a clinical history and a physical exam, others exams may be suggested:

• Serum creatine kinase—Measurement of serum (a blood component) concentration of creatine kinase is a simple and inexpensive diagnostic test for severe forms of dystrophy known to be associated with high concentrations of creatine in the blood. In DMD, serum creatine kinase values are raised from birth, and testing in newborns for early diagnosis could reduce the possibility of further affected boys in a family and improve medical assistance before the onset of symptoms.

• Electromyography—This test is important in the establishment of the myopathic (muscle disease not caused by nerve dysfunction) nature of the disease and for the exclusion of neurogenic (from the nerves) causes of weakness, including peripheral nerve disorders. Because **electromyography** is an invasive technique involving a

needle stick, it is becoming less favored in the investigation of children, but it still has an important role in the diagnosis of adult disease.

• Muscle histology—The one unifying feature of the dystrophies is their similar muscle histological (in the tissues) findings, such as variation in muscle fiber size, muscle fiber death, invasion by macrophages (a versatile immune cell), and ultimately, replacement by fat and connective tissue. This picture is aggravated in the more severe forms of dystrophy, such as Duchenne type. However, in FSHD and LGMD, inflammatory changes in tissues are often the main features.

• Immunohistochemistry and mutation analysis—In some muscular dystrophies, certain proteins are deficient in muscle tissue. Immunohistochemistry involves methods of detecting the presence of these specific proteins in muscle cells or tissues. A diagnosis can be made when these protein deficiencies are identified. Analysis of genetic mutations associated with muscular dystrophies is also important for genetic counseling and prenatal diagnosis.

Treatment team

There are many professionals available to help the child with muscular dystrophy, depending on the patient's needs. These include physicians, orthopedic surgeons (bone specialists), physical therapists, orthotists (specialists on equipment to maintain posture and mobility), occupational therapists, dietitians, nurses, **social workers**, psychologists, teachers, religious advisers, staff from the Muscular Dystrophy Association, parents, and other persons with MD.

Physical therapy involves a program of stretching exercises to maintain muscle length and the flexibility of joints. Physical therapists also work with orthotists. Night splints, calipers, swivel walkers, and braces are some of the aids employed. Physical therapists are the main professionals involved in teaching parents the appropriate exercises and in making sure that any mobility aids are comfortable. Both physical therapy and hydrotherapy (water therapy) contribute significantly to mobility and respiratory function.

Treatment

Although there is no known cure for muscular dystrophy, **exercise** and physical therapy are recommended to maintain mobility for as long as possible. Corticosteroid drugs and gene therapies are being studied to help relieve the symptoms.

Specific treatment for muscular dystrophy is determined by the child's physician based on age, overall

Key Terms

Autosomal dominant disorder A genetic disorder caused by a dominant mutant gene that can be inherited by either parent.

Autosomal recessive disorder A genetic disorder that is inherited from parents that are both carriers, but do not have the disorder. Parents with an affected recessive gene have a 25% chance of passing on the disorder to their offspring with each pregnancy.

Dystrophin A large protein that stabilizes the plasma membrane of a muscle cell during muscle contractions. Dystrophin is absent or reduced in the most common forms of muscular dystrophy.

Electromyography A test used to detect nerve function. It measures the electrical activity generated by muscles.

Immunohistochemistry A method of detecting the presence of specific proteins in cells or tissues.

Macrophage A large, versatile immune cell that acts as a scavenger, engulfing dead cells, foreign substances, and other debris.

Mutation A permanent, heritable change in a gene or chromosome structure.

Myopathy Refers to a disorder of the muscle, usually associated with weakness.

Myotonia Abnormally long muscular contractions.

health, medical history, extent of the condition, type of condition, child's tolerance for specific medications, procedures or therapies.

Drug therapies

In children with Duchenne muscular dystrophy, corticosteroids (such as prednisone) may be prescribed to temporarily delay progression of their illness; however, some patients cannot tolerate this medication because of side effects. Powerful medications that suppress the immune system have been reported to help some patients, but their use is controversial. In patients with MMD, myotonia (abnormally long muscular contractions) may be treated with medications such as **carbamazepine** or phenytoin.

Gene therapy

With advances in molecular biology techniques, another method of treatment currently under intense investigation is somatic **gene therapy**. The idea is to introduce healthy immature cells into affected muscles, which would fuse and stimulate production of enough dystrophin to reverse the degeneration already taking place. Although this has been achieved successfully in mice, the benefit may not translate into humans. The mice cannot demonstrate muscle strength, and the laboratory-raised mice were not able to mount a rejection response that may occur in humans.

Other therapies

The orthopedic problems in children with MD lead to progressive weakness with walking difficulties, soft-tissue contractures, and spinal deformities. The role of the orthopedic surgeon is to correct deformities and help maintain the child's ambulatory status for as long as possible. The modalities available to obtain these goals include: functional testing; physical therapy; use of orthoses (specialized aids); fracture management; soft tissue, bone, and spinal surgeries; use of a wheelchair when indicated; and genetic and/or psychological testing.

Recovery and rehabilitation

To date, there is no known treatment, medicine, or surgery that will cure MD, or stop the muscles from weakening. The goal of treatment is to prevent deformity and allow the child to function as independently as possible at home and in the community.

Physical therapy

In general, patients are given supportive care, together with leg braces and physical therapy to maximize their ability to function in daily life. Stretching limbs to avoid tightened tendons and muscles is particularly important. When tightness of tendons develops (called contractures), surgery can be performed. When chest muscles are involved, respiratory therapy may be used to delay the onset of breathing problems. In addition, people with MD are given age-appropriate dietary therapy to help them avoid obesity. Obesity is especially harmful to patients with MD because it places additional strain on their already weak muscles. Unfortunately, many MD patients are at a high risk of obesity because their limited physical activity prevents them from exercising.

Wheelchair prescription

If the person with MD becomes nonambulatory, wheelchair mobility is essential. The wheelchair should complement the patient's lifestyle, providing comfort, safety, and functionality. Special attention should be given to the frame, seat, backrest, front rigging, rear wheels, and casters because of the functional weakness and contractures in the upper and lower extremities of patients with limb-girdle dystrophy. An accessible home and work environment and personal or public transportation with safe restraint systems for the wheelchair are also important.

Additional resources

Specific planning for vocational needs and desires may be coordinated with therapists. Resources within the community, such as the Parks and Recreation Department for activity programs, may be explored. Educational institutions, from public schools to community colleges and universities, have resources that may be used. Adaptive physical education program and Disabled Student Services generally are available for persons with MD.

Clinical trials

There are numerous open **clinical trials** for MD:

- An open-label pilot study of Oxatomide in steroid-naive DMD, sponsored by Cooperative International Neuromuscular Research Group;

- An open-label pilot study of Coenzyme Q10 in steroid-treated DMD, sponsored by Cooperative International Neuromuscular Research Group;

- Study of Inherited Neurological Disorders, sponsored by National Institute of Neurological Disorders and Stroke (NINDS);

- Study of Albuterol and Oxandrolone in Patients With FSHD, sponsored by the Food and Drug Administration Office of Orphan Products Development.

Updated information on clinical trials is available at the National Institutes of Health website for clinical trials at <www.clinicaltrials.org>.

Prognosis

The prognosis varies according to the type of MD and its progression. Some patients have only mild symptoms with a normal lifespan, whereas others have severe symptoms and die at a young age. For example, children with DMD often die before age 18 because of respiratory failure, heart failure, pneumonia or other problems. In persons with BMD, death tends to occur later. Some examples of complications associated with MD that lead to permanent, progressive disability are:

- deformities, such as scoliosis and joint contractures

- decreased mobility

- decreased ability to perform daily self-care tasks, such as bathing and dressing

- mental impairment (varies)

- cardiomyopathy (weakened heart muscle)

- respiratory failure

Special concerns

Genetic counseling is an important aspect of the care and evaluation of patients with DMD and BMD and their family members. A minority of female carriers have MD symptoms, but even in these symptomatic patients, correct diagnosis requires appropriate testing. In families in which an affected male has a known deletion or duplication of the dystrophin gene, testing for carrier status is performed accurately by testing possible carriers for the same mutation, the absence of which would exclude them as a carrier.

Resources

BOOKS

Parker, James N., and Philip M. Parker. *The 2002 Official Patient's Sourcebook on Muscular Dystrophy.* San Diego: Icon Group International, 2002.

Siegel, Irwin M. *Muscular Dystrophy in Children: A Guide for Families.* Gardena, CA: Scb Distributors, 1999.

Thompson, Charlotte. *Raising a Child with a Neuromuscular Disorder: A Guide for Parents, Grandparents, Friends, and Professionals* New York: Oxford Press, 1999.

Wolfson, Penny. *Moonrise: One Family, Genetic Identity, and Muscular Dystrophy.* New York: St. Martin's Press, 2003.

PERIODICALS

Emery, A. "The muscular dystrophies." *The Lancet* 359 (February 2002): 687–695.

OTHER

"Facts About Duchenne and Becker Muscular Dystrophies (DMD and BMD)" Muscular Dystrophy Association. (March 20, 2004). <http://www.mdausa.org/publications/fa-dmdbmd.html>.

"NINDS Muscular Dystrophy (MD) Information Page" National Institute of Neurological Disorders and Stroke. (March 20, 2004). <http://www.ninds.nih.gov/health_and_medical/disorders/md.htm>.

ORGANIZATIONS

Muscular Dystrophy Association. 3300 East Sunrise Drive, Tucson, AZ 85718-3208. (520) 529-2000 or (800) 572-1717; Fax: (520) 529-5300. mda@mdausa.org. <http://www.mdausa.org/>.

Muscular Dystrophy Family Foundation. 2330 North Meridien Street, Indianapolis, IN 46208. (317) 923-6333 or (800) 544-1213; Fax: (317) 923-6334. mdff@mdff.org. <http://www.mdff.org/>.

Parent Project for Muscular Dystrophy Research. 1012 North University Blvd., Middletown, OH 45042. (413) 424-0696 or (800) 714-KIDS (5437); Fax: (513) 425-9907. ParentProject@aol.com. <http://www.parentprojectmd.org/>.

Francisco de Paula Careta
Iuri Drumond Louro, MD, PhD

Myasthenia, congenital

Definition

Congenital myasthenia is an inherited disorder that results in muscle weakness caused by a malfunction at the neuromuscular junction, the area where nerve cells communicate to muscle cells.

Description

Congenital myasthenia is caused by a number of genetic defects that affect the ability of a nerve impulse to move from nerve to nerve, and from the nerve to muscle. The genetic abnormalities can be present in the fetus at the moment of conception or may occur during fetal development. This genetic cause of the disease separates the congenital form of myasthenia from **myasthenia gravis** and **Lambert-Eaton myasthenic syndrome**, both of which are caused by the malfunctioning of the immune system.

Demographics

Congenital myasthenia occurs in the young, and occurs with equal frequency in boys and girls. Symptoms tend to appear within the first two years of life. It is common to have siblings who are affected. The disease is extremely rare, occurring in only one to two per million live births.

Causes and symptoms

The root of congenital myasthenia are defects in various genes that play a role in the transmission of nerve impulses. At least a dozen genetic defects have been identified as causes of congenital myasthenic syndromes so far. The defects can affect the manufacture or the release of acetylcholine, a neurotransmitter, or molecule that acts as a communication bridge between adjacent nerves.

As a result of the varying genetic roots of the disease, different congenital myasthenic syndromes exist. These can produce different effects in those who are affected. The symptoms, which usually begin in infancy or toddlerhood, can include a poor sucking response, drooping eyelids (a condition called ptosis), eyes that appear to wander or float (ophthalmoplegia), weakness in facial muscles that is apparent as an abnormal appearance, weakness in the arms and legs, breathing difficulty, delayed development of muscle skills, and a feeling of **fatigue**. Usually, a parent may notice that the infant is experiencing delays in developmental milestones that require coordinated muscle strength, such as sitting up alone, crawling, or walking. All or just a few of these symptoms can be present in a person with congenital myasthenia. As well, the severity of the symptoms can vary from person to person. Some children

---

Key Terms

Myasthenia Muscular weakness, or a group of chronic muscular diseases characterized by muscle weakness.

Neuromuscular junction The junction between a nerve fiber and the muscle it supplies.

Ophthalmoplegia Paralysis of the motor nerves of the eye, resulting in wandering or floating eye movements.

---

may be severely impaired, while others lead near normal lives. Even though children display symptoms, their parents may not be similarly affected.

Diagnosis

The disease is usually diagnosed in the early years of childhood by the abnormal appearance of the face and/or by the noticeable weakening of the arms or legs. A test of muscle strength known as the tensilon test that is considered to be accurate in diagnosis of other forms of myasthenia is usually not specific for congenital myasthenia. Congenital myasthenia is often misdiagnosed as myasthenia gravis or other neuromuscular diseases.

Accurate diagnosis of congenital myasthenia requires specialized testing. These include testing specific nerves to determine if the nerves fatigue more quickly than is normal. While at least a dozen genes that are responsible for the disease are known, genetic testing technology is not currently routinely available. Only a handful of centers in the United States are able to test the anconeus and intercostal muscles to detect the abnormal genes. However, as such technology becomes routine (i.e., gene chips), genetic testing will no doubt become one of the principle means of diagnosis.

Treatment team

Treatment can involve the family physician, a **neurologist**, family members, and physical therapists. The latter can provide exercises that assist in maximizing muscular strength.

Treatment

Treatment for most types of congenital myasthenia typically involves the use of drugs that help promote the transmission of nerve impulses. Drugs that retard the breakdown of acetylcholine can be used. An example of an acetylcholinesterase is mestinon. Other drugs that show merit in some cases include guanidine, ephedrine sulfate,

---

and albuterol. People may build up a tolerance to ephedrine, which decreases its effectiveness.

Recovery and rehabilitation

As there is no recovery from congenital myasthenia, treatment is aimed at maximizing muscle function through drug therapy and physical therapy.

Clinical trials

As of mid-2004, there were no **clinical trials** underway or in the planning stages specific for congenital myasthenia. However, agencies such as the National Institute for Neurological Diseases and Stroke continue to fund research that seeks to better understand the underlying genetic bases of congenital myasthenia, and to discover more effective means of increasing nerve signal transmission. Updated information on clinical trials related to congenital myasthenia can be located at the National Institutes of Health website for clinical trials at www.clinicaltrials.org.

Prognosis

With accurate diagnosis, most types of congenital myasthenia can be improved or at least stabilized by the use of drug therapy. More severe forms of the disease may weaken respiratory muscles and result in a reduced lifespan.

Resources

BOOKS

Thompson, Charlotte. *Raising a Child with a Neuromuscular Disorder: A Guide for Parents, Grandparents, Friends, and Professionals.* New York: Oxford Univ. Press, 1999.

OTHER

"Congenital Myasthenic Syndromes MDA Fact Sheet." <http://www.mdausa.org/disease/fasheet_cms.html>. *Muscular Dystrophy* (May 6, 2004).

"NINDS Congenital Myasthenia Information Page." *National Institute for Neurological Diseases and Stroke.* (May 4, 2004). <http://www.ninds.nih.gov/health_and_medical/disorders/congenital_myasthenia.htm>.

ORGANIZATIONS

National Institute for Neurological Diseases and Stroke (NINDS). P.O. Box 5801, Bethesda, MD 20824. (301) 496-5751. (800) 352-9424. <http://www.ninds/nih.gov>.

National Organization for Rare Disorders (NORD). 55 Kenosia Avenue, Danbury, CT 06813-1968. (203) 744-0100 or (800) 999-6673; Fax: (203) 798-2291. orphan@rarediseases.org. <http://www.rarediseases.org>.

Myasthenia Gravis Foundation of America, Inc. 1821 University Ave. W., Suite S256, St. Paul, MN 55104. (651) 917-6256 or (800) 541-5454; Fax: (651) 917-1835. mgfa@myasthenia.org. <http://www.myasthenia.org>.

Brian Douglas Hoyle, PhD

Myasthenia gravis

Definition

Myasthenia gravis (MG) is a chronic autoimmune disease characterized by **fatigue** and muscular weakness, especially in the face and neck, that results from a breakdown in the normal communication between nerves and muscles caused by the deficiency of acetylcholine at the neuromuscular (nerve-muscle) junctions. MG is the most common primary disorder of neuromuscular transmission.

Description

MG is a chronic autoimmune neuromuscular disease characterized by varying degrees of weakness of the skeletal (voluntary) muscles of the body. The hallmark of this disease is muscle weakness that increases during periods of activity and improves after periods of rest. Muscles that control eye and eyelid movements, facial expression, chewing, talking, and swallowing are often, but not always, involved. The muscles that control breathing and neck and limb movements may also be affected.

Myasthenia gravis can be classified according to which skeletal muscles are affected. Within a year of onset, approximately 85–90% of affected persons develop generalized MG, which is characterized by weakness in the trunk, arms, and legs. About 10–15% of patients have weakness only in muscles that control eye movement. This type is called ocular myasthenia gravis.

Other types of MG include congenital MG, an inherited condition caused by a genetic defect, and transient neonatal, which occurs in infants born from mothers who have MG. Congenital MG develops at or shortly after birth and causes generalized symptoms.

Demographics

Myasthenia gravis occurs in all ethnic groups and both genders. The prevalence of MG in the United States is estimated to be 14 per 100,000 population, which equals approximately 36,000 cases in the United States. However, this disease is probably under diagnosed and the prevalence may be higher. Previous studies showed that women are more often affected than men. The most common age at onset is the second and third decades in women

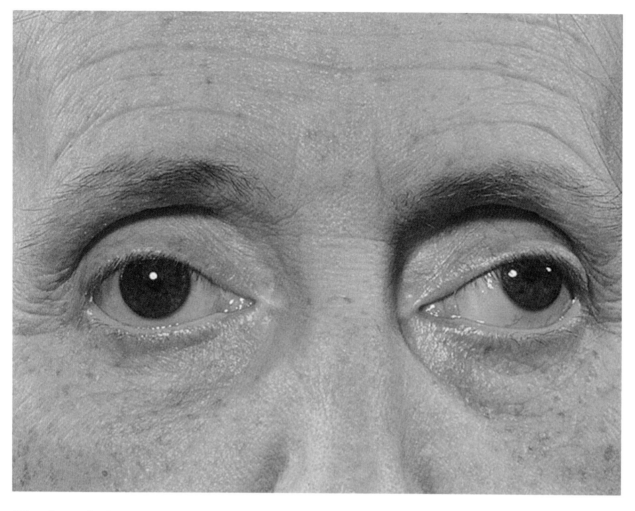

Although myasthenia gravis may affect any voluntary muscle, muscles that control eye and eyelid movement, facial expression, and swallowing are most frequently affected. *(Custom Medical Stock Photo. Reproduced by permission.)*

and the seventh and eighth decades in men. As the population ages, the average age of onset has increased correspondingly, and now males are considered to be more often affected than females, and the onset of symptoms is usually after age 50.

Causes and symptoms

Myasthenia gravis is an autoimmune disease caused by abnormal antibodies carried in the blood stream. Nerves release a chemical called acetylcholine (ACh) that activates receptors on muscles to trigger contraction. The normal neuromuscular junction releases ACh from the motor nerve terminal in discrete packages (quanta). The ACh quanta diffuse across the synaptic cleft and bind to receptors on the folded muscle end-plate membrane. Stimulation of the motor nerve releases many ACh quanta that depolarize the muscle end-plate region and then the muscle membrane, causing muscle contraction.

The myasthenia antibodies interfere with this process by binding to specific sites on the surface of the muscles, the post-synaptic muscle membrane is distorted and simplified, having lost its normal folded shape. The most common antibodies are directed against the muscle acetylcholine receptor (AChR). ACh is released normally, but its effect on the post-synaptic membrane is reduced. The post-junctional membrane is less sensitive to applied ACh, and the probability that any nerve impulse will cause a muscle action potential is reduced.

Ten percent of patients with MG have a tumor in the thymus, (a thymoma) that is usually benign, and 70% have changes (germinal centers) that indicate an active immune response. These are areas within lymphoid tissue where B-cells interact with helper T-cells to produce antibodies. Because the thymus is the central organ for immunological self-tolerance, it is reasonable to suspect that thymic abnormalities cause the breakdown in tolerance that leads to an immune-mediated attack on AChR in this disease. The thymus contains all the necessary elements for the beginnings of MG: myoid cells that express the AChR antigen, antigen presenting cells, and immunocompetent T-cells. However, it is still uncertain whether the role of the thymus in the pathogenesis of disease is primary or secondary.

There are very rare genetic abnormalities that cause problems similar to myasthenia gravis. These diseases are called congenital or inherited myasthenias and usually are present in infants. MG is not directly inherited, nor is it contagious. Occasionally, the disease may occur in more than one member of the same family. Rarely, children may show signs of congenital (present at birth) myasthenia or congenital myasthenic syndrome. These are not autoimmune disorders, but are caused by defective genes that control proteins in the acetylcholine receptor or in acetylcholinesterase. In neonatal myasthenia that develops in 10–20% of infants born to mothers who have MG, the fetus may acquire immune proteins (antibodies) from a mother affected with MG. Generally, cases of neonatal myasthenia are transient and the child's symptoms usually disappear within few weeks after birth.

Although MG may affect any voluntary muscle, muscles that control eye and eyelid movement, facial expression, and swallowing are most frequently affected. The onset of the disorder may be sudden. Symptoms often are not immediately recognized as myasthenia gravis. In most cases, the first noticeable symptom is weakness of the eye muscles. In others, difficulty in swallowing and slurred speech may be the first signs. The degree of muscle weakness involved in this disease varies greatly among patients, ranging from a localized form, limited to eye muscles (ocular myasthenia), to a severe or generalized form in which many muscles, sometimes including those that control breathing, are affected. Symptoms, which vary in type and severity, may include a drooping of one or both eyelids (ptosis), blurred or double vision (diplopia) due to weakness of the muscles that control eye movements, unstable or waddling gait, weakness in arms, hands, fingers, legs, and neck, a change in facial expression, difficulty in swallowing and shortness of breath, and impaired speech (**dysarthria**).

Diagnosis

A delay in diagnosis of one or two years is not unusual in cases of MG. Because weakness is a common symptom of many other disorders, the diagnosis is often missed in people who experience mild weakness or in those individuals whose weakness is restricted to only a few muscles. The first steps of diagnosing MG include a review of the individual's medical history, and physical and neurological examinations. The signs a physician must look for are impairment of eye movements or muscle weakness without any changes in the individual's ability to feel things. If the physician suspects MG, several tests are available to confirm the diagnosis.

The Edrophonium Chloride (Tensilon) Test

This approach requires the intravenous administration of edrophonium chloride or Tensilon(r), a drug that temporarily increases the levels of acetylcholine at the neuromuscular junction. In people with myasthenia gravis involving the eye muscles, the drug will chloride will briefly relieve weakness.

Antibodies Against Acetylcholine Receptor (AChR)

In general, an elevated concentration of AChR binding antibodies in a patient with compatible clinical features confirms the diagnosis of MG, but normal antibody concentrations do not exclude the diagnosis.

Repetitive Nerve Stimulation (RNS)

This test records weakening muscle responses when the nerves are repetitively stimulated, and helps to differentiate nerve disorders from muscle disorders. Repetitive stimulation of a nerve during a **nerve conduction study** may demonstrate faults of the muscle action potential (CMAP) due to impaired nerve-to-muscle transmission. A significant decrement to RNS in either a hand or shoulder muscle is found in about 60% of patients with MG.

Single fiber electromyogram (SFEMG)

SFEMG is the most sensitive clinical test of neuromuscular transmission and shows increased jitter in some muscles in almost all patients with myasthenia gravis. Jitter is greatest in weak muscles, but may be abnormal even in muscles with normal strength. Patients with mild or purely ocular (eye) muscle weakness may have increased jitter only in facial muscles. Increased jitter is a nonspecific sign of abnormal neuromuscular transmission and can also be seen in other motor diseases.

Computed tomography (CT) or magnetic resonance imaging (MRI)

Computed tomography (**CT**) or **magnetic resonance imaging (MRI)** may be used to identify an abnormal thymus gland or the presence of a thymoma. Pulmonary function testing, which measures breathing strength, helps to predict whether respiration may fail and lead to a myasthenic crisis.

Treatment team

The treatment team is normally composed of a **neurologist**, a nutritionist (dietary advice), a speech pathologist, a pulmonologist, a geneticist, a neurologist, a dentist, a otolaryngologist, a physical therapist, and nurses.

Treatment

Treatment regimens for myasthenia gravis are practical rather than curative. Treatment decisions are based on knowledge of the natural history of disease in each patient and the predicted response to a specific form of therapy. Treatment goals must be individualized according to the severity of disease, the patient's age and sex, and the degree of functional impairment. The response to any form of treatment is difficult to assess because the severity of symptoms fluctuates. Spontaneous improvement, even remissions, occur without specific therapy, especially during the early stages of the disease.

Cholinesterase inhibitors

Cholinesterase inhibitors result in increased ACh accumulation at the neuromuscular junction and prolongs its effect. These drugs cause considerable improvement in some patients and little to none in others. Pyridostigmine bromide (Mestinon) and neostigmine bromide (Prostigmin) are the most commonly prescribed cholinesterase inhibitors. No fixed dosage schedule suits all patients. The need for cholinesterase inhibitors varies from day to day and during the same day in response to infection, menstruation, emotional stress, and hot weather. Different muscles respond differently; with any dose, certain muscles become stronger, others do not change, and still others become weaker. Adverse effects of cholinesterase inhibitors include gastrointestinal complaints: queasiness, loose stools, nausea, vomiting, abdominal cramps, and diarrhea.

Thymectomy

Thymectomy (removal of the thymus) is recommended for most people with myasthenia gravis. The greatest benefit from the surgery generally occurs two to five years afterwards. However, the response is relatively unpredictable and significant impairment may continue for months or years after surgery. The best responses to thymectomy are in young people early in the course of the disease, but improvement can occur even after 30 years of symptoms. Persons with disease onset after the age of 60 rarely show substantial improvement from thymectomy. Patients with thymomas (tumor on the thymus) do not respond as well to thymectomy as do patients without them.

Corticosteroids

Marked improvement or complete relief of symptoms occurs in more than 75% of people treated with prednisone, and some improvement occurs in most of the rest. Much of the improvement occurs in the first six to eight

Key Terms

Acetylcholine A chemical called a neurotransmitter that functions primarily to mediate activity of the nervous system and skeletal muscles.

Neuromuscular Involving both the muscles and the nerves that control them.

Thymoma A tumor that originates in the thymus, a small gland located in the upper chest just below the neck, that produces hormones necessary for the development of certain components of the immune system.

weeks of therapy, but strength may increase to total remission in the months that follow. The best responses occur in patients with recent onset of symptoms, but patients with chronic disease may also respond. The severity of disease does not predict the ultimate improvement. Patients with thymoma have an excellent response to prednisone before or after removal of the tumor. About one-third of patients become weaker temporarily after starting prednisone, usually within the first seven to ten days, but this temporary weakness lasts for only a few days. The major disadvantages of chronic corticosteroid therapy are the side effects, such as weight gain and fluid retention.

Immunosuppressant drugs

Azathioprine reverses symptoms in most patients with myasthenia gravis, but the benefits are delayed by four to eight months. Once improvement begins, it is maintained for as long as the drug is given. Symptoms recur two to three months after the drug is discontinued or the dose is reduced below therapeutic levels. Patients who experience no improvement on corticosteroids may respond to azathioprine, and the reverse is also true. Sometimes, people with MG respond better to treatment with both drugs than to either one alone. Because the response to azathioprine is delayed, both drugs may be started simultaneously with the intent of rapidly tapering prednisone when azathioprine becomes effective. Approximately one-third of patients have mild dose-dependent side effects that may require dose reductions, but do not require stopping treatment.

Cyclosporine is sometimes beneficial in treating MG. Most patients with myasthenia gravis improve within two months after starting cyclosporine and improvement is maintained as long as therapeutic doses are given. Maximum improvement is achieved six months or longer after starting treatment. After achieving the maximal response, the dose is gradually reduced to the minimum that maintains improvement. Toxicity to the kidneys and hypertension are important adverse reactions of cyclosporine. Many drugs interfere with cyclosporine metabolism and should be avoided or used with caution.

Cyclophosphamide is also given intravenously and orally for the treatment of myasthenia gravis. More than half of patients receiving cyclophosphamide experience a dramatic improvement in their symptoms after one year; however, side effects are common. Life-threatening infections are an important risk for all persons taking immunosuppressant drugs.

Plasma exchange

Plasma exchange is used as a short-term intervention for patients with sudden worsening of myasthenic symptoms, to rapidly improve strength before surgery, and as a chronic intermittent treatment for patients who are refractory to all other treatments. The need for plasma exchange and its frequency of use is determined by the clinical response in the individual patient. Almost all patients with acquired MG improve temporarily following plasma exchange. Maximum improvement may be reached as early as after the first exchange or as late as the fourteenth. Improvement lasts for weeks or months and then the effect is lost unless the exchange is followed by thymectomy or immunosuppressive therapy. Most patients who respond to the first plasma exchange will respond again to subsequent courses. Repeated exchanges do not have a cumulative benefit.

Intravenous immune globulin (IVIG)

Immune globulin given intravenously results in improvement in more than half of MG patients, usually beginning within one week of therapy and lasting for several weeks or months.

Recovery and rehabilitation

Physical and occupational therapists provide strategies to help people with myasthenia gravis maintain daily activities during almost all phases of the disease. As the progression of symptoms occurs over months or years, these strategies adapt to the changing needs of the person with myasthenia gravis. For example, wheelchairs, specialized eating utensils, and positioning aids might be required during the progressive phase. When improvement is made, shower stools, rolling carts for carrying shopping items, and exercises to promote maintenance of posture can all help avoid fatigue. While the symptoms of the disease may go into remission, recovery is not said to be complete, as symptoms may recur. The longer the person remains in remission; however, the greater is the chance that the disease will not recur

Clinical trials

As of February 2004, there were two open **clinical trials** for MG, both sponsored by the Rush University Medical Center in Chicago, Illinois:

• Study of CellCept in the Treatment of MG: This is a multicenter, placebo-controlled study testing CellCept and prednisone as the initial form of immunotherapy in the treatment of MG. The purpose of the study is to determine if the combination of these two medications provides better control of MG symptoms compared with prednisone alone.

• Study of Etanercept Among Individuals With MG: The purpose of the study is to determine if Etanercept improves muscle strength in patients with MG.

Up-to-date information on clinical trials can be found at the United States government website for clinical trials located at <www.clinicaltrials.org>.

Prognosis

Symptoms of myasthenia gravis usually progress to maximum severity within three years. After that time, persons with MG normally stabilize or improve. With treatment, the outlook for most patients with MG is bright: they will have significant improvement of their muscle weakness and they can expect to lead normal or nearly normal lives.

Many people's MG symptoms may go into remission temporarily and muscle weakness may disappear completely, so that medications can be discontinued. Stable, long-lasting complete remissions are the goal of thymus removal (thymectomy). In a few cases, the severe weakness of MG may cause a crisis (respiratory failure), which requires immediate emergency medical care. Advances in medical care have reduced the mortality rate from respiratory failure in myasthenia gravis patients to approximately three percent. Patients over the age of 40, those with a short history of severe disease, and those with thymoma tend to have less significant improvement.

Special concerns

Myasthenia gravis cannot be prevented, but avoiding the following triggers may help patients prevent exacerbations (worsening of symptoms):

• emotional stress

• exposure to extreme temperatures

• fever

• illness (e.g., respiratory infection, pneumonia, tooth abscess)

• low levels of potassium in the blood (hypokalemia; caused by diuretics, frequent vomiting)

• some medications, such as muscle relaxants, **anticonvulsants**, and certain antibiotics

Resources

BOOKS

Henderson, Ronald E. *Attacking Myasthenia Gravis.* Seattle: Court Street Press, 2002.

Icon Health Publications. *The Official Patient's Sourcebook on Myasthenia Gravis: A Revised and Updated Directory for the Internet Age.* San Diego: Icon Grp. Int., 2002.

OTHER

National Institute of Neurological Disorders and Stroke. "Myasthenia Gravis Fact Sheet." <http://www.ninds.nih.gov/health_and_medical/pubs/myasthenia_gravis.htm> (February 11, 2004).

ORGANIZATIONS

Myasthenia Gravis Foundation of America, Inc. 5841 Cedar Lake Road Suite 204, Minneapolis, MN 55416. (952) 545-9438 or (800) 541-5454; Fax: (952) 646-2028. myastheniagravis@msn.com. <http://www.myasthenia.org>.

Beatriz Alves Vianna
Iuri Drumond Louro

Myelinoclastic diffuse sclerosis *see*
Schilder's disease

Myoclonic encephalopathy of infants *see*
Opsoclonus myoclonus

Myoclonus

Definition

Myoclonus is a brief, rapid, shock-like jerking movement.

Description

Myoclonus can be a symptom of a separate disorder, or can be the only or primary neurological finding, in which case it is termed "essential myoclonus." Myoclonus may occur in **epilepsy**, or following many different types of brain injury, such as lack of oxygen, **stroke**, trauma, or poisoning. Myoclonus can occur in one or more limbs, or may be generalized, involving much of the body.

Demographics

Because myoclonus is so often part of another disorder, the prevalence of myoclonus is not known with certainty. One study indicates that the prevalence of all types

---

Key Terms

Hypoxia   A condition characterized by insufficient oxygen in the cells of the body.

---

of myoclonus may be approximately 10 per 100,000 population.

Causes and symptoms

Myoclonus can be a symptom of a very wide variety of disorders. A partial list includes:

• epilepsy (several types)
• **Tay-Sachs** disease and other storage diseases
• spinocerebellar degenerative diseases
• **Hallervorden-Spatz** syndrome
• **Huntington's disease**
• **multiple system atrophy**
• **corticobasal degeneration**
• **Creutzfeldt-Jakob disease**
• brain infections, including HIV
• focal brain damage, including from stroke or tumor
• heat stroke
• electrical shock
• **hypoxia** (oxygen deprivation)
• toxins and drugs

Myoclonus also occurs normally, as a person falls asleep or while sleeping. This type of myoclonus is not associated with disease.

Diagnosis

The diagnosis of myoclonus is not difficult, and depends on careful patient description of the symptoms. Much more effort is devoted to determining the underlying cause. Blood tests, neuroimaging studies, genetic tests, **electroencephalography** (EEG) and other types of studies may be performed in order to determine the underlying disorder.

Treatment team

Myoclonus is treated by a **neurologist**.

Treatment

If an underlying disorder can be identified, this is treated with the expectation that successful treatment may diminish the myoclonus. In many cases this is not possible, however. Alternatively, the underlying disorder may be discovered, but may be impossible to treat. Such is the case with hypoxic myoclonus, or damage done by a stroke or trauma.

Several medications can be used to reduce the severity or frequency of the myoclonus. Valproic acid and clonazepam are the two most widely used drugs. Anticholinergic drugs, such as benztropine or trihexyphenidyl, may be useful. **Anticonvulsants** may be helpful, as may **benzodiazepines**, depending on the type of myoclonus. **Deep brain stimulation** has been reported to help at least one patient. **Botulinum toxin** injection may be useful in focal myoclonus.

Recovery and rehabilitation

Treatment of myoclonus is rarely entirely successful. The patient is likely to have some residual myoclonus even with the most successful treatments. Nonetheless, treatment may reduce frequency and severity, allowing more normal function.

Prognosis

Myoclonus is not a life-threatening disorder, but may continue to have a significant impact on quality of life and activities of daily living.

Resources
WEBSITES
Myoclonus Research Foundation. <http://www.myoclonus.com/index.htm>.
WE MOVE. <http://www.wemove.org>.

Richard Robinson

Myofibrillar myopathy

Definition

Myofibrillar myopathies (MFMs) are a group of skeletal muscle diseases that are frequently associated with involvement of the heart muscle. Myofibrillar myopathies can be hereditary or occur sporadically (spontaneously). The hallmark of myofibrillar disease is the abnormal accumulation of the protein desmin in the muscles, causing progressive weakness.

Description

The term myofibrillar **myopathy** was proposed in 1996 as a broad term for an abnormal pattern of muscle deterioration associated with the excess accumulation of multiple proteins that include desmin. Desmin, the main muscle intermediate fiber of the cytoskeleton (the fibrous network that provides structure for the cell), is a protein in cardiac, skeletal, and smooth muscles. This protein interacts with other proteins to form a network that maintains the structure of the cell.

The main features of myofibrillar myopathies include shoulder and hip muscle deterioration, often called "limb-girdle" myopathy, along with weakness of muscles farther away from the center of the body, called distal muscle weakness. The muscles involved often include the heart, and complications such as conduction blocks, arrhythmias, and congestive heart failure are often experienced.

Most persons with myofibrillar myopathy develop the disorder due to an autosomal-dominant or autosomal-recessive inheritance pattern, which means that males and females are equally affected, and there is a 50% chance of passing on the disorder in each pregnancy. In an autosomal-recessive inheritance pattern, the affected gene is recessive and one parent is its carrier. The risk of a child being affected with myofibrillar myopathy in an autosomal-recessive inheritance pattern is 25% for each pregnancy. A lesser number of myofibrillar myopathy cases are sporadic, meaning no inheritance pattern can be found.

The pattern of weakness in this condition is often similar to patients with the other limb-girdle muscular dystrophies, but some patients have more weakness in the hands and ankles in addition to the more typical shoulder and hip weakness. Myofibrillar myopathy, like limb-girdle **muscular dystrophy**, slowly worsens over time, but the rate of progression is variable and some affected persons remain functional for many years.

Desmin-related myopathy (DRM) is a subgroup of myofibrillar myopathy and is the most clearly recognized type among this group. DRM was originally described as a skeletal and cardiac myopathy characterized by abnormal accumulation of desmin within muscle fibers. This definition focused attention on desmin as a key molecule associated with a diverse group of clinically and pathologically related disorders.

Demographics

The true incidence of myofibrillar myopathy is unknown, but it is very rare. Both sexes are affected equally in MFM, since inheritance is usually autosomal recessive or autosomal dominant.

Causes and symptoms

Two gene mutations have been described in myofibrillar myopathy. Mutations on chromosome 2 in the gene for desmin are transmitted in an autosomal-dominant or autosomal-recessive inheritance pattern. Mutations on chromosome 11 in the gene for αBC (alpha-B-crystallin) are transmitted in an autosomal-dominant inheritance pattern, which can also cause a desmin storage myopathy.

Key Terms

Cardiomyopathy A disease of the heart muscle that leads to generalized deterioration of the muscle and its pumping ability.

Cytoskeleton A network of filaments that give structure and shape to the cell.

Desmin A protein that provides part of the structure to heart, skeletal, and smooth muscle cells.

Limb-girdle myopathy A muscular dystrophy-type disorder characterized by weakness in the muscles of the shoulders, trunk, and pelvic girdle, often progressing to respiratory or cardiac failure.

Myopathy A disorder of the muscles.

Defects in the function of desmin, as well as in other proteins, cause fragility of the myofibrils (structures in muscles that help them contract). In the heart, normal desmin protects the structural integrity of myofibrils during repeated muscle contractures over time. When desmin accumulates in abnormal amounts and locations of the heart muscle cell, myofibrils degrade and lose their ability to contract efficiently, resulting in weakness and inefficient pumping ability of the heart.

Myofibrillar myopathy becomes apparent in early to middle adulthood when muscle weakness in the lower extremities and gait (manner of walking) disturbances develop. The myopathy slowly progresses to also involve respiratory, facial, and heart muscles. Occasionally, this pattern is reversed and the heart muscle shows weakness before the skeletal muscles. Symptoms of alterations in the heart include abnormal rhythms that may cause **fainting** or, rarely, sudden death.

Diagnosis

Diagnostic difficulties arise from the fact that the disease has many variations: in some cases, myofibrillar myopathy is a relentlessly progressive skeletal disorder with no signs of cardiac involvement, while in others, cardiomyopathy (weak heart muscle action) is the leading or even exclusive feature. Respiratory muscle insufficiency may also be a major factor in myofibrillar myopathy and is a leading cause of death.

Most of the known genetic mutations responsible for myofibrillar myopathy are autosomal dominant, but some are autosomal recessive. A significant number of the mutations also occur spontaneously without inheritance pattern. For this reason, genetic testing is critical for establishing an accurate diagnosis. The true prevalence of myofibrillar myopathy may be assessed only when most or all persons with characteristic symptoms are tested genetically.

Electromyography (EMG) and nerve conduction studies (NCSs) should be performed in all persons in whom a myofibrillar myopathy is suspected. EMG and NCSs are important to exclude causes of weakness that result from nerve malfunction, including peripheral nerve disorders. Because electromyography involves inserting a needle into a muscle, it is becoming less favored in investigating muscle weakness in children, but it still has an important role in the diagnosis of the adult disease. In myofibrillar myopathy, **nerve conduction study** findings are normal and EMG findings are either normal or show typical patterns of myopathies.

Muscle **biopsy** is an important part of the diagnostic approach because it shows myofibrillar myopathy's histologic features (i.e., its organization and effect on tissue structure). In the typical diagnostic sequence, muscle biopsy is done first, then genetic studies are pursued.

Treatment team

The treatment team of hereditary muscle diseases, depending on the needs of a particular patient, includes a **neurologist**, pulmonologist, cardiologist, orthopedic surgeon, physiatrist, physical therapist, orthotist, and genetic counselors.

Because the diagnosis of hereditary myopathy is often difficult, interpretation of muscle biopsy, laboratory tests, and electrodiagnostic studies should be performed by a clinician experienced in the diagnosis and treatment of neuromuscular diseases.

Treatment

No specific treatment is available for any of the myofibrillar myopathies, but aggressive supportive care is essential to preserve muscle activity, to allow for maximal functional ability, and to prolong life expectancy.

The primary concerns are preventing and correcting skeletal abnormalities (e.g., scoliosis, foot deformities, and contractures) and maintaining ambulation. Aggressive use of passive stretching, bracing, and orthopedic procedures allows the affected person to remain independent for as long as possible.

Complications with the heart and lungs are the other chief concern. Early intervention to treat cardiac and respiratory insufficiency, at times requiring intermittent positive pressure ventilation (BiPAP/CPAP), can help improve function and prolong life expectancy.

Orthopedic surgery may be needed to help correct or prevent contractures (rigid muscles near joints), foot deformities, and scoliosis.

While no dietary restrictions are indicated for persons with myopathies, the diet should be tailored to the caloric needs of the patient. This may include restricting calories, especially in children with minimal mobility.

Recovery and rehabilitation

To date, there is no known treatment, medicine, or surgery that will cure MFM or stop the muscles from weakening. The goal is to prevent deformity and allow the patient to function as independently as possible. Since myofibrillar myopathy is a life-long condition that is not correctable, management includes focusing on preventing or minimizing deformities and maximizing the patient's functional ability at home and in the community.

In general, patients are given supportive care, together with leg braces and physical therapy, to maximize their ability to function in daily life. Stretching limbs to avoid tightened tendons and muscles is particularly important.

Clinical trials

As of mid-2004, there were no **clinical trials** recruiting participants specific for myofibrillar myopathy.

Prognosis

Myofibrillar myopathies are among a large group of related but distinct diseases. In general, it is expected that there will be slow progression of weakness, which worsens in affected muscles, then spreads, and progresses with time.

Heart muscle weakness and the tendency to have abnormal electrical activity of the heart can increase the risk of palpitations, fainting, and sudden death. Most patients with this group of diseases live into adulthood, but do not reach their full life expectancy.

Special concerns

Genetic counseling is often helpful to assist patients with family-planning decisions.

Vigorous physical activity is often impossible (or impractical) for patients with significant weakness, but activities like swimming, water aerobics, and low-resistance **exercise** equipment are often tolerated very well. The goal of these activities should be to increase the number of calories burned, but not to build strength.

Maintaining ambulation and functional ability with the aggressive use of physical therapy and bracing is highly recommended. Children and young adults are often encouraged continue with school in regular classes, with modifications designed to meet their specific physical needs.

Resources within the community may be explored. Educational institutions have resources that may be used.

Adaptive physical education programs and disabled student services are generally available for qualified individuals. Access and mobility concerns in the community invariably touch upon the adjustment issues faced by individuals with a progressive disability.

Resources

BOOKS

Emery, Alan E. H. *Muscular Dystrophy: The Facts.* Oxford, UK: Oxford University Press, 2000.

Parker, James N., and Philip M. Parker, eds. *The 2002 Official Patient's Sourcebook on Muscular Dystrophy.* San Diego: Icon Group International, 2002.

PERIODICALS

Selcen, D., et al. "Myofibrillar Myopathy: Clinical, Morphological and Genetic Studies in 63 Patients." *Brain* 127 (February 2004): 439–451.

OTHER

"Myofibrillar Myopathy; MDA-Ask the Experts." *Muscular Dystrophy Association.* July 2001. (May 4, 2004 [June 2, 2004].) <http://www.mdausa.org/experts/question.cfm?id=428>.

"Myopathy, Desmin Storage." *WebMD Health.* May 4, 2004 (June 2, 2004). <http://webcenter.health.webmd.netscape.com/hw/health_guide_atoz/nord1008.asp>.

ORGANIZATIONS

National Institute of Arthritis and Musculoskeletal and Skin Diseases (NIAMS). Bldg. 31, Rm. 4C05, Bethesda, MD 20892-2350 or (877) 22-NIAMS (226-4267); Fax: (301) 496-8188. NIAMSInfo@mail.nih.gov. <http://www.nih.gov/niams>.

Muscular Dystrophy Association. 3300 East Sunrise Drive, Tucson, AZ 85718-3208. (520) 529-2000 or (800) 572-1717; Fax: (520) 529-5300. mda@mdausa.org. <http://www.mdausa.org/>.

American Heart Association. 7272 Greenville Avenue, Dallas, TX 75231-4596. (214) 373-6300 or (800) 242-8721; Fax: (214) 373-0268. inquire@heart.org. <http://www.americanheart.org>.

Francisco de Paula Careta
Iuri Drumond Louro, MD, PhD

Myopathy

Definition

Myopathy is a general term referring to any skeletal muscle disease or neuromuscular disorder. Myopathy can be acquired or inherited, and can occur at birth or later in life. Myopathies can result from endocrine disorders, metabolic disorders, muscle infection or inflammation, drugs, and mutations in genes.

Description

Skeletal muscle diseases, or myopathies, are disorders with structural changes or functional impairment of the muscle. These conditions can be differentiated from other diseases of the motor unit by characteristic clinical and laboratory findings. The main symptom is muscle weakness that can be either intermittent or persistent. Different myopathy types exist with different associated causes. The main types include congenital myopathy, **muscular dystrophy**, **inflammatory myopathy**, and drug-induced myopathy.

Congenital myopathy (CM) is a term used for muscle disorders present at birth. According to this definition, the CMs could include hundreds of distinct neuromuscular syndromes and disorders. In general, this disease causes loss of muscle tone and muscle weakness in infancy and delayed motor skills, such as walking, later in childhood. Four distinct disorders are classified as CMs: central core disease, nemaline rod myopathy, centronuclear (myotubular) myopathy, and multicore myopathy.

Muscular dystrophy (MD) refers to a group of genetic diseases characterized by progressive weakness and degeneration of the skeletal or voluntary muscles that control movement. The muscles of the heart and some other involuntary muscles are also affected in some forms of MD, and a few forms involve other organs as well. The major forms of MD include myotonic, Duchenne, Becker, limb-girdle, facioscapulohumeral, congenital, oculopharyngeal, distal, and Emery-Dreifuss.

Inflammatory myopathies (IM) are a group of muscle diseases involving the inflammation and degeneration of skeletal muscle tissues. They are thought to be autoimmune disorders. In IMs, inflammatory cells surround, invade, and destroy normal muscle fibers as though they were defective or foreign to the body. This eventually results in discernible muscle weakness. This muscle weakness is usually symmetrical and develops slowly over weeks to months or even years. The IMs include **dermatomyositis**, **polymyositis**, and **inclusion body myositis**.

Drug induced myopathy (DIM) is a muscle disease caused by toxic substances that produce muscle damage. The toxic substances may act directly on muscle cells, but muscle damage can also be secondary to electrolyte disturbances, excessive energy requirements, or the inadequate delivery of oxygen and nutrients due to muscle compression. Drug use may also result in development of an immunologic reaction directed against the muscle.

Muscle damage can be generalized or local, as occurs when a drug is injected into a muscle.

Demographics

Worldwide, CMs account for about 14% of all myopathies. Central core disease accounts for 16% of cases; nemaline rod myopathy for 20%; centronuclear myopathy for 14%; and multicore myopathy for 10%. Prevalence of MD is higher in males. In the United States, Duchenne and Becker MD occur in approximately one in 3,300 boys. Overall incidence of MD is about 63 per one million people.

Worldwide incidence of IM is about five to 10 per 100,000 people. These disorders are more common in women. Incidence and prevalence of DIM are unknown. Myopathy caused by corticosteroids is the most common disorder, and it is more common in women.

Causes and symptoms

CMs and MDs are caused by a genetic defect. In both conditions, mutations have been identified in genes that encode for muscle proteins. The loss or dysfunction of these proteins presumably leads to the specific morphological feature in the muscle and to clinically noticeable muscle disease. For example, in Becker dystrophy, there is a less-active form of dystrophin (a protein involved in the complex interactions of the muscle membrane and extracellular environment) that may not be effective as a gateway regulator, allowing some leakage of intracellular substances, resulting in the myopathy.

The causes of IM are not known. An autoimmune process is likely, as these conditions are often associated with other autoimmune diseases and because they respond to immunosuppressive medication. Muscle **biopsy** typically shows changes attributed to destruction by infiltrating lymphocytes (white blood cells).

In DIMs, there are a number of causative agents. Drugs such as lipid-lowering agents (statins, clofibrate and gemfibrizol), agents that cause hypokalemia (diuretics, theophylline, amphotericin B), lithium, succinylcholine, antibiotics (trimethoprim, isoniazid), **anticonvulsants** (valproic acid, **lamotrigine**, prolonged propofol infusion), vasopressin, colchicine, episilon, aminocaproic acid, high dose alfa-interferon, and illicit drugs (cocaine, heroin, phencyclidine, amphetamines) are possible myopathy inducers.

Although symptoms depend on the type of myopathy, some generalizations can be made. Skeletal muscle weakness is the hallmark of most myopathies. In most myopathies, weakness occurs primarily in the muscles of the shoulders, upper arms, thighs, and pelvis (proximal muscles). In some cases, the distal muscles of the hands and

Key Terms

Autoimmune disorder A large group of diseases characterized by abnormal functioning of the immune system that produces antibodies against its own tissues.

Congenital Present at birth.

Myopathy Disease of the muscle, most often associated with weakness.

feet may be involved during advanced stages of the disease. Other typical symptoms of muscle disease include the following:

- muscle aching
- muscle cramping
- muscle pain
- muscle stiffness
- muscle tenderness
- muscle tightness

Initially, individuals may feel fatigued during very light physical activity. Walking and climbing stairs may be difficult because of weakness in the pelvic and leg muscles that stabilize the trunk. Patients often find it difficult to rise from a chair. As the myopathy progresses, there may be muscle wasting.

Diagnosis

Generally, diagnosis involves several outpatient tests to determine the type of myopathy. Sometimes it is necessary to wait until the disease progresses to a point at which the syndrome can be identified.

A blood serum enzyme test measures how much muscle protein is circulating in the blood. Usually, this is helpful only at the early stages of the disease, when the sudden increase of muscle protein in the blood is conspicuous. Antibodies found in the blood might indicate an IM. DNA may be collected to evaluate whether one of the known genetic defects is present.

An electromyogram (EMG) measures the electrical activity of the muscle. It involves placing a tiny needle into the muscle and recording the muscular activity on a monitor (oscilloscope). This helps identify which muscles are weakened.

A muscle tissue biopsy involves surgically removing a very small amount of tissue to be examined under the microscope and analyzed for abnormalities.

Treatment team

A multidisciplinary team is involved in the treatment of myopathy patients. This team may include a **neurologist**, a rheumatologist, an orthopedic surgeon, a pulmonologist, a cardiologist, an orthopedist, a dermatologist, and a genetic counselor. It can also include physical and occupational therapists.

Treatment

Treatment depends on the cause, and goals are to slow progression of the disease and relieve symptoms. Treatments range from drug therapy for MD and IM to simply avoiding situations that work the muscles too hard. Some physicians recommend that patients keep their weight down (a lighter body demands less work from the muscles) and avoid overexerting their muscles. For MD, the corticosteroids deflazacort and prednisone seem to be the most effective medications. Calcium supplements and antidepressants may be prescribed to counteract the side effects. The IMs are usually treated with drugs that suppress the action of the immune system such as methotrexate, cyclosporine, and azathioprine, all of which have potentially serious side effects. For CM, treatment involves supportive measures to help patients cope with the symptoms.

Recovery and rehabilitation

Physical therapy can prevent weakening in a patient's healthy muscles, however, it cannot restore already weakened muscles. Occupational and respiratory therapy help patients learn how to use special equipment that can improve their quality of life.

Clinical trials

There are numerous open **clinical trials** for myopathies, including:

- Study and Treatment of Inflammatory Muscle Diseases and Infliximab to Treat Dermatomyositis and Polymyositis, sponsored by National Institute of Arthritis and Musculoskeletal and Skin Diseases (NIAMS)

- Diagnostic Evaluation of Patients with Neuromuscular Disease and Screening Protocol for Patients with Neurological Disorders with Muscle Stiffness, sponsored by National Institute of Neurological Disorders and Stroke (NINDS)

- Physiologic Effects of PRMS & Testosterone in the Debilitated Elderly, sponsored by Department of Veterans Affairs Medical Research Service

- Myositis in Children, sponsored by National Institute of Environmental Health Sciences (NIEHS)

More updated information on clinical trials can be found on the National Institutes of Health clinical trials website at <www.clinicaltrials.gov>.

Prognosis

The prognosis for persons with myopathy varies. Some individuals have a normal life span and little or no disability. In others, however, the disorder may be progressive, severely disabling, life threatening, or fatal. If the underlying cause of the disorder can be treated successfully, the prognosis is usually good. Progressive myopathies that develop later in life usually have a better prognosis than conditions that develop during childhood. Persons with Duchenne MD rarely live beyond their middle to late 20s, and persons with Becker MD may live until middle age.

Special concerns

If the cardiac muscle is affected in later disease stages, abnormal heart rhythms or heart muscle insufficiency (cardiomyopathy) may develop. Cardiomyopathy patients are at risk for congestive heart failure.

When muscles involved in breathing weaken, there may be significant breathing difficulties and increased risk for pneumonia, flu, and other respiratory infections. In severe cases, patients may require a respirator. When swallowing muscles are affected, persons are at increased risk for choking and malnutrition.

Resources

BOOKS

Vinken, Pierre J., et al. *Myopathies.* New York: Elsevier Health Sciences, 1992.

Askanas, Valerie, et al. *Inclusion-Body Myositis and Myopathies.* New York: Cambridge University Press, 1998.

PERIODICALS

Mastaglia, F. L., M. Garlepp, B. Phillips, and P. Zilko. "Inflammatory myopathies: clinical, diagnostic and therapeutic aspects." *Muscle & Nerve* 27 (April 2003): 407–425.

OTHER

"NINDS Myopathy Information Page." *National Institute of Neurological Disorders and Stroke.* <http://www.ninds.nih.gov/health_and_medical/disorders/myopathy.htm> (March 15, 2004).

"Facts about Duchenne and Becker Muscular Dystrophies (DMD and BMD)." *Muscular Dystrophy Association.* <http://www.mdausa.org/publications/fa-dmdbmd.html> (March 15, 2004).

ORGANIZATIONS

National Institute of Arthritis and Musculoskeletal and Skin Diseases (NIAMS): National Institutes of Health. Bldg. 31, Rm. 4C05, Bethesda, MD 20892-2350. (301) 496-8188 or (877) 22-NIAMS (226-4267). NIAMSInfo@mail.nih.gov. <http://www.nih.gov/niams>.

Muscular Dystrophy Association. 3300 East Sunrise Drive, Tucson, AZ 85718-3208. (520) 529-2000 or (800) 572-1717; Fax: (520) 529-5300. mda@mdausa.org. <http://www.mdausa.org/>.

Greiciane Gaburro Paneto
Iuri Drumond Louro, MD, PhD

Myotonic dystrophy

Definition

Myotonic dystrophy is an inherited disorder that affects muscle tone, and hair loss and can involve varying degrees of impaired cognitive abilities. It is inherited as a dominant disorder, which means that individuals that carry the defective gene have the disease. The amount of symptoms exhibited in persons with myotonic dystrophy varies.

Description

Physical limitations resulting from myotonic dystrophy can be significant, involving muscle weakness and difficulty lifting items and performing certain routine daily tasks. There are many cases in which affected persons experience mental delays, and this usually correlates with the extent of the genetic defect. Myotonic dystrophy is a progressive disorder in terms of muscle weakness and muscle wasting.

Demographics

Myotonic dystrophy is relatively rare, occurring approximately once in 8,000 people. There is also a more rare, severe congenital form that occurs with an incidence of about 1 in 100,000.

Causes and symptoms

Myotonic dystrophy involves many different tissues within the body, including the eye, the heart, the endocrine system, and the **central nervous system**. The clinical manifestations in myotonic dystrophy span from mild to severe, leading to three separate categories with somewhat overlapping characteristics: mild, classical, and congenital (in which the clinical manifestations are evident at birth).

Mild myotonic dystrophy

In the mild form, persons usually develop cataracts and experience mild muscle tone dysfunction (myotonia). They normally do not experience clinical manifestations until they reach 20 years of age. Some patients do not develop symptoms until 70 years of age.

Classical myotonic dystrophy

In the classical form, patients can have generalized weakness, myotonia that is more severe than the mild form, cataracts, balding, and heart rhythm disturbances. The age of onset can be from 10 years until they are 30 years old.

Congenital myotonic dystrophy

Symptoms in the congenital form of myotonic dystrophy are evident at birth. Affected infants show muscle weakness, respiratory defects, and eventually, **mental retardation**. There are cases that appear after birth but before 10 years of age, although the symptoms might be slight and remain unnoticed. Congenital myotonic dystrophy is almost always inherited from the mother; however, inheritance from the father has occurred. Mental retardation is thought to be associated with early respiratory failure and the effects of the mutated gene on the brain.

Causes of myotonic dystrophy

Myotonic dystrophy is caused by a DNA alteration the in the Myotonin-protein kinase (DMPK) gene. This gene has been found to localize to specialized structures of the heart and skeletal muscle. Normal function is important for intercellular conduction and impulse transmission. It interacts with a variety of proteins that are important in signaling neurological messages. The abnormal gene product leads to disease but the mechanism is complex and in some tissues, it is relatively unclear. The alteration in the DNA leads to abnormal RNA processing, an important step in the production of proteins. This abnormal processing is felt to result in functional alterations of this protein that can lead to disease.

Diagnosis

Myotonic dystrophy is diagnosed clinically in individuals that have a specific type of muscle weakness. This is confirmed with molecular genetics testing, where the DMPK is analyzed. This gene is located on chromosome 19q13.2-13.3. Within the gene, there is a DNA sequence that is a string of three letters in the DNA alphabet (GTC, which are abbreviations for the nucleotides guanine, thymine, and cytosine) that are normally repeated up to 37 times. CTG repeats repeated greater than 50 times alters the function of the protein and can lead to disease. Individuals that have repeats from 38–49 times are considered to have permutations and in this range they generally do not produce symptoms, but their children are at risk for having repeats that expand into the disease causing range. Patients have more symptoms when they have repeat sizes

---

---

greater than 50. DNA testing is 100% sensitive (able to determine the defect) and widely available. Prenatal diagnosis to determine if a fetus is affected is also available.

Myotonic dystrophy is suspected by physicians if patients experience muscle weakness in the lower legs, hands, neck, and face. The will experience a characteristic sustained muscle contraction whereby they have difficulty in quickly releasing their hand grip during a handshake. They also develop cataracts. Newborns usually have generalized and facial muscle weakness, club foot, and respiratory difficulties. Their muscles usually appear hypotonic (floppy).

Treatment team

A general practitioner may not see very many cases of myotonic dystrophy during his career, but may be the first physician to observe a patient. Usually, a **neurologist** and a geneticist are consulted. Depending on the age of onset, the extent of professional help varies. When the age of onset is a birth or infancy, a cardiologist and a pulmonologist will be necessary to evaluate and heart or respiratory deficiencies, respectively. These individuals usually also require special education, depending on the extent of the cognitive deficits.

Treatment

There is no specific treatment that has been identified to help the muscle weakness or prevent muscle wasting in myotonic dystrophy. Ankle and/or leg braces can be used to help support the muscles as the disease worsens. Heart problems, cataracts, and other abnormalities can often be treated. There are also medications that can help relieve the myotonia.

Recovery and rehabilitation

Although patients with this disorder do not recover, occupational and physical therapy is felt to be of benefit in many cases to help maintain optimum function for as long as possible.

Clinical trials

As of May 2004, the National Institute of Arthritis and Musculoskeletal and Skin Diseases (NIAMS) and the National Institute of Neurological Disorders and Stroke (NINDS) were recruiting patients for a registry that will connect people with myotonic dystrophy with researchers studying these diseases. (Contact information: Colleen M. Donlin-Smith, MA, telephone: 585-275-6372, email: Colleen_DonlinSmith@urmc.rochester.edu; Eileen Eastwood, telephone 585-275-6372; email: Eileen_Eastwood@urmc.rochester.edu).

Prognosis

The prognosis for patients that are diagnosed with the mild form of the disease is quite good. They usually do not have mental retardation and can live a close to normal lifespan. Affected individuals that have the classic form have a more severe prognosis. They have more clinical manifestations and lifespan usually ranges 48–55 years. The congenital form is the most severe, although patients live, on average, until they are 45 years old. They have more severe mental retardation, respiratory deficits, and have clinical manifestations at birth.

Special concerns

As this disorder can be inherited, genetic counseling for at-risk families is recommended. Offspring of an affected individual, regardless of gender, have a 50% chance of inheriting the mutant gene. It is important to recognize that expanded repeats within the gene can expand even more in the gametes (sex cells—sperm or egg) from individuals with expansions, resulting in the transmission of even longer trinucleotide repeat genes. This expansion leading to longer repeats is associated with more severe disease that is observed in the parent. Therefore, affected individuals are more likely to have more offspring with a more serious form of the disorder. Premutation carriers, or individuals that have repeats that do not usually cause disease but are likely to expand in their offspring, should be identified (if possible) in cases where there is a family history of the disorder. These individuals are at risk for having affected offspring, although they may not themselves have the disorder.

Resources

BOOKS

Nussbaum, Robert L., Roderick R. McInnes, and Huntington F. Willard. *Genetics in Medicine.* Philadelphia: Saunders, 2001.

Rimoin, David L. *Emery and Rimoin's Principles and Practice of Medical Genetics.* London; New York: Churchill Livingstone, 2002.

PERIODICALS

Cobo, A. M., J. J. Poza, L. Martorell, A. Lopez de Munain, J. I. Emparanza, and M. Baiget. "Contribution of molecular analyses to the estimation of the risk of congenital myotonic dystrophy." *J Med Genet* 32 (1995): 105–108.

Redman, J. B., R. G. Fenwick Jr, Y. H. Fu, A. Pizzuti, C. T. Caskey. "Relationship between parental trinucleotide GCT repeat length and severity of myotonic dystrophy in offspring." *JAMA* 269 (1993): 1960–1965.

OTHER

"Myotonic Dystrophy; General Information." *International Myotonic Dystrophy Association.* <http://www.myotonicdystrophy.org/General%20Information.htm> (May 6, 2004).

"Myotonic Dystrophy." *Gene and Disease.* <http://www.ncbi.nlm.nih.gov/books/bv.fcgi?call=bv.View..ShowSection&rid=gnd.section.164> (May 5, 2004).

ORGANIZATIONS

Muscular Dystrophy Association (MDA). 3300 East Sunrise Drive, Tucson, AZ 85718-3208. (800) 572-1717 or (520) 529-2000; Fax: (520) 529-5300. mda@mdausa.org. <www.mdausa.org>.

Muscular Dystrophy Campaign. 7-11 Prescott Place, London SW4 6BS, UK. (+44) 0 020 7720 8055; Fax: (+44) 0 020 7498 0670. info@muscular-dystrophy.org. <http://www.muscular-dystrophy.org>.

Bryan Richard Cobb, PhD

Narcolepsy

Definition

Narcolepsy is a disorder marked by excessive daytime sleepiness, uncontrollable sleep attacks, and cataplexy (a sudden loss of muscle tone, usually lasting up to half an hour).

Description

Narcolepsy is the second-leading cause of excessive daytime sleepiness (after obstructive **sleep apnea**). Persistent sleepiness and sleep attacks are the hallmarks of this condition. The sleepiness has been compared to the feeling of trying to stay awake after not sleeping for two or three days.

People with narcolepsy fall asleep suddenly—anywhere, at any time, even in the middle of a conversation. These sleep attacks can last from a few seconds to more than an hour. Depending on where the sleep attacks occur, they may be mildly inconvenient or even dangerous to the person, particularly if they occur while driving. Some people continue to function outwardly during the sleep episodes, such as continuing a conversation or putting things away. But when they wake up, they have no memory of the event.

Sleep researchers have identified several different types of sleep in humans. One type of sleep is called rapid eye movement (REM) sleep, because the person's eyes move rapidly back and forth underneath the closed eyelids. REM sleep is associated with dreaming. Normally, when people fall asleep, they experience 90 minutes of non-REM sleep, which is then followed by a phase of REM sleep. People with narcolepsy, however, enter REM sleep immediately. In addition, REM sleep occurs inappropriately throughout the day in patients with narcolepsy.

Demographics

There has been debate over the incidence of narcolepsy. It is thought to affect between one in every 1,000–2,000 Americans. The known prevalence in other countries varies, from one in 600 in Japan to one in 500,000 in Israel. The reasons for these demographic differences are not clear. In about 8–12% of cases, people diagnosed with narcolepsy know of other family members with similar symptoms.

Causes and symptoms

One of the causes of narcolepsy is a genetic mutation. In 1999, researchers identified the gene that causes the disorder. The narcolepsy gene allows cells in the hypothalamus (the part of the brain that regulates sleep behavior) to receive messages from other cells. As a result of the mutation, the cells cannot communicate properly, and abnormal sleeping patterns develop.

Researchers are also looking into the possibility that narcolepsy may be caused by some kind of autoimmune disorder. This theory suggests that the person's immune system accidentally turns against the specific area of the brain that controls alertness and sleep, injuring or destroying it.

The disorder sometimes runs in families, but most people with narcolepsy have no family members with the disorder. Researchers believe that the inheritance of narcolepsy is similar to that of heart disease, in which several genes play a role in being susceptible to the disorder. But heart disease does not usually develop without an environmental trigger of some sort.

While the symptoms of narcolepsy usually appear during a person's late teens or early 20s, the disease may not be diagnosed for many years. Most often, the first symptom is an overwhelming feeling of **fatigue**. After several months or years, cataplexy and other symptoms of the disorder appear.

Cataplexy is the most dramatic symptom of narcolepsy, affecting 75% of people with the disorder. During attacks, the knees buckle and the neck muscles go slack. In extreme cases, the person may become paralyzed and fall to the floor. This loss of muscle tone is temporary, lasting from a few seconds to half an hour, but it is frightening.

Key Terms

Cataplexy A symptom of narcolepsy marked by a sudden episode of muscle weakness triggered by strong emotions. The muscle weakness may cause the person's knees to buckle, or the head to drop. In severe cases, the patient may become paralyzed for a few seconds to minutes.

Hypnagogic hallucinations Dream-like auditory or visual hallucinations that occur while a person is falling asleep.

Hypothalamus A part of the forebrain that controls heartbeat, body temperature, thirst, hunger, blood pressure, blood sugar levels, and other functions.

Polysomnogram A machine that is used to diagnose

sleep disorders by measuring and recording a variety of body functions related to sleep, including heart rate, eye movements, brain waves, muscle activity, breathing, changes in blood oxygen concentration, and body position.

Rapid eye movement (REM) sleep A type of sleep during which the person's eyes move back and forth rapidly underneath their closed eyelids. REM sleep is associated with dreaming.

Sleep paralysis An abnormal episode of sleep in which the patient cannot move for a few minutes, usually occurring while falling asleep or waking up. Sleep paralysis is often found in patients with narcolepsy.

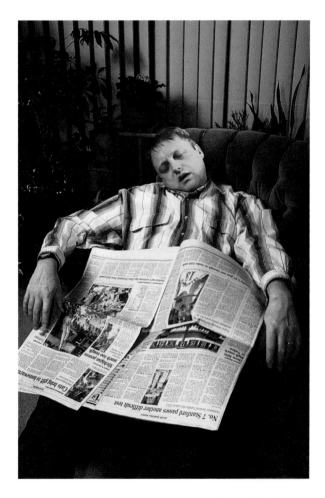

A narcoleptic has lost consciousness while reading the paper. *(© Bannor/Custom Medical Stock Photo. Reproduced by permission.)*

The attacks can occur at any time, but are often triggered by strong emotions such as anger, joy, or surprise.

Other symptoms of narcolepsy include:

- sleep attacks: short, uncontrollable sleep episodes throughout the day
- sleep paralysis: a frightening inability to move shortly after awakening or dozing off
- auditory or visual hallucinations: intense, sometimes terrifying experiences at the beginning or end of a sleep period
- disturbed nighttime sleep: tossing and turning, nightmares, and frequent awakenings during the night

Diagnosis

The diagnosis of narcolepsy can be made by a general practitioner familiar with the disorder as well as by a psychiatrist. If a person comes to the doctor with reports of both excessive daytime sleepiness and cataplexy, a diagnosis may be made on the patient's history alone. Laboratory tests, however, can confirm a diagnosis of narcolepsy. These tests may include an overnight polysomnogram, which is a test in which sleep is monitored with a variety of electrodes that record information about heart rate, eye movements, brain waves, muscle activity, breathing, changes in blood oxygen concentration, and body position. A multiple sleep latency test, which measures sleep latency (onset) and how quickly REM sleep occurs, may also be used. People who have narcolepsy usually fall asleep in less than five minutes.

If the diagnosis is still open to question, a genetic blood test can reveal the existence of certain substances in people who have a tendency to develop narcolepsy. Positive test results suggest, but do not prove, that the patient has narcolepsy.

Narcolepsy is a complex disorder, and it is often misdiagnosed. Many people with the disorder struggle with symptoms for an average of 14 years before being correctly diagnosed.

Treatment team

Sleep disorder specialists are experts in management of narcolepsy. Other team members may include neurologists, psychiatrists, or psychologists.

Treatment

There is no cure for narcolepsy. It is not progressive, and it is not fatal, but it is a chronic disorder. The symptoms can be managed with lifestyle adjustments and/or medication.

People with narcolepsy must plan their days carefully. Scheduling regular naps (either several short, 15-minute naps or one long nap in the afternoon) can help boost alertness and wakefulness. A full eight hours of nighttime sleep should also be a goal. **Exercise** can often help people with narcolepsy feel more alert and energetic, although they should avoid exercising within a few hours of bedtime. Substances that contain alcohol, nicotine, and caffeine should be avoided because they can interfere with refreshing sleep and with daytime alertness.

Medications for narcolepsy may include the use of antidepressants (tricyclic antidepressants or selective serotonin-reuptake inhibitors [SSRIs]) to treat such symptoms of the disorder as cataplexy, hypnagogic hallucinations, and/or sleep paralysis.

Stimulants (amphetamines) may also be used to help individuals with narcolepsy stay awake and alert.

With the recent discovery of the gene that causes narcolepsy, researchers are hopeful that other treatments can be designed to relieve the symptoms of the disorder.

Clinical trials

A number of **clinical trials** are underway to investigate a number of drugs that may help improve daytime sleepiness in narcolepsy patients. For more information visit <http://www.clinicaltrials.gov>.

Prognosis

Narcolepsy is not a degenerative disease, and patients do not develop other neurologic symptoms. Narcolepsy can, however, interfere with a person's ability to work, play, drive, socialize, and perform other daily activities. In severe cases, the disorder prevents people from living a normal life, leading to **depression** and a loss of independence.

Resources

PERIODICALS

Mignot, E. "Genetics of Narcolepsy and Other Sleep Disorders." *American Journal of Human Genetics* 60 (1997): 1289–1302.

Siegel, Jeremy M. "Narcolepsy." *Scientific American* (January 2000).

ORGANIZATIONS

American Academy of Sleep Medicine. 6301 Bandel Rd. NW, Suite 101, Rochester, MN 55901. (507) 287-6008. (March 23, 2004). <http://www.aasmnet.org>.

American Sleep Disorders Association. 1610 14th St. NW, Suite 300, Rochester, MN 55901. (507) 287-6006.

Narcolepsy Network. P. O. Box 42460, Cincinnati, OH 45242. (973) 276- 0115.

National Center on Sleep Disorders Research. Two Rockledge Centre, 6701 Rockledge Drive, Bethesda, MD 20892. (301) 435-0199.

National Sleep Foundation. 1522 K St., NW, Suite 500, Washington, DC 20005. (202) 785-2300. (March 23, 2004). <http://www.sleepfoundation.org>.

Stanford Center for Narcolepsy. 1201 Welch Road, Room P-112, Stanford, CA 94305. (415) 725-6517.

University of Illinois Center for Narcolepsy Research. 845 S. Damen Ave., Chicago, IL 60612. (312) 996-5176.

OTHER

Stanford Researchers Nab Narcolepsy Gene For Sleep Disorders. Stanford University Medical Center. Cited August 5, 1999 (March 23, 2004). <http://www.stanford.edu/%7Edement/ngene.html>.

Rosalyn Carson-DeWitt, MD

Neostigmine *see* **Cholinergic stimulants**

Nerve compression

Definition

Nerve compression is the restriction in the space around a nerve that can occur due to several reasons. Functioning of the nerve is compromised.

Description

There are a variety of circumstances that cause nerve compression. Despite this variety, the resulting damage to the nerve produces a similar diminished functioning of the nerve.

Demographics

The incidence of brachial plexus palsy, usually a result of birth injury to the nerves that conduct signals from the spine to the shoulder and resulting in a limp or paralyzed arm, is low, on the order of one to two births out of every 1,000. Brachial plexus palsy is associated with a difficult labor, especially compression on the baby's shoulders. Intervention or assistance during labor can lessen the chance of the physical trauma that causes the nerve damage. However, the condition cannot be totally eliminated, especially in times where an emergency response is needed to speed the birth of a fetus in distress.

Meralgia parasthetica, a condition involving compression of the lateral femoral cutaneous nerve, results in paresthesia, or tingling, numbness, and burning **pain** in the outer side of the thigh. Meraglia paresthetica has traditionally affected men more than women. The condition is not rare, but its overall prevalence is unknown. **Meralgia paresthetica** may occur after abdominal surgery or significant weight gain, in military members who often march, soccer players, or for no apparent reason in the general population. Other nerve compression maladies such as **carpal tunnel syndrome** can be quite common.

Causes and symptoms

There are a variety of conditions that lead to nerve compression, according to the affected nerve.

Carpal tunnel syndrome

In carpal tunnel syndrome, the nerves that pass through the wrist are pinched due to the enlargement of local tendons and ligaments. The enlargement occurs due to inflammation, which can be associated with the strain of performing a repetitive task such as typing. Carpal tunnel syndrome is also associated with maladies like diabetes, and with the restricted space that can develop in the wrist as weight is gained during pregnancy or in someone who is obese. The enlargement of the tendons and ligaments restricts the space available for the nerves that reach to the finger and also for the muscle that connects to the base of the thumb. As a consequence, the ability of the nerve to properly transmit impulses to the muscles in the fingers and thumb is affected.

The initial symptoms of carpal tunnel syndrome tend to be felt at night because the hand is at rest. The symptoms can be a burning or a tingling numbness in the fingers, in particular the thumb, along with the index and middle fingers. As well, the reduced transmission of nerve impulses to the muscles decrease muscle strength. It can become difficult to grip an object or make a fist.

Thoracic outlet syndrome

In **thoracic outlet syndrome**, nerve compression can occur as a result of stresses on the neck and shoulders that cause these areas to impinge on local nerves. While the underlying cause of the syndrome is not clear, there seems to be an association between thoracic outlet syndrome and physical labor, in particular the repeated lifting

of heavy objects onto the shoulders, causing the shoulders to pull back and down. Reaching for objects that are positioned above shoulder level can also be irritating to muscles in the shoulders and the upper arms. Swelling and inflammation of the muscles can compress nerves between the neck and shoulders.

The symptoms of thoracic outlet syndrome include weakness of the arms, pain, and numbness of the arms and fingers. In more extreme cases, the sense of touch and ability to sense temperature changes can be lost in the fingers.

Brachial plexus palsy

Palsy is a term meaning the inability to purposely move a body part. Brachial plexus palsy refers to paralysis that is associated with compression and tearing of a group of nerves called the brachial plexus. These nerves are a connection between the spinal cord and the nerves that run into the arms neck, and shoulders. The nerves can become compressed and even torn when the neck is stretched. This can occur in an infant born following a difficult delivery, which can occur if the baby is large, in a breech position, or if the period of labor is long. In these situations, the baby's neck can be abnormally flexed. The abnormal position damages the brachial plexus nerves.

The brachial plexus affects certain segments of the spinal cord. When viewed in a x ray, the spinal cord is reminiscent of Lego blocks stacked on each other. Each 'block' represents a segment. Typically, brachial nerves that originate from upper segments of the spinal column (segments C5 and C6) are affected. This condition is also called Erb's palsy. Less commonly, nerves associated with lower segments (C7 and T1) can be deranged. This condition is called Klumke's paralysis. In some cases, all the nerves of the brachial plexus can be affected.

The causes of nerve damage can also involve injuries to the shoulder, arm, and the collarbone (clavicle). The main symptom of brachial plexus palsy, paralysis in an arm, is evident immediately after birth. A newborn will lie with the affected arm by its side, with the elbow extended. While the other arm will be capable of a normal range of motion, the affected arm will be immobile.

Meralgia paresthetica

This painful condition is due to the pinching of the lateral femoral cutaneous nerve as the nerve exits the pelvis. The nerve can become pinched as the position of the pelvic region changes due to weight gain, injury, pregnancy, or extended periods of standing of walking (i.e., military marching). The affected nerve becomes compressed as it crosses a region of the pelvis called the iliac crest. As well, the nerve can be rubbed during the pelvic motions that occur with walking. This friction increases the nerve damage.

A person with meralgia paresthetica experiences an ache, numbness, tingling, or burning sensations in their thigh. The ache can be mild or severe, and generally eases during rest and returns with resumption of activity.

Cubital tunnel syndrome

This syndrome results from pressure that compresses the ulnar nerve. The ulnar nerve is one of the main nerves of the hand, which connects the muscles of the forearm and hand with the spinal cord. The nerve passes across the back of the elbow behind a bump called the medial epicondyle. The sensation that is described as the funny bone is actually the transient sensation that occurs when the ulnar nerve is compressed in a bump.

Cubital tunnel syndrome is a more protracted from of the nerve compression. It results from the stretching or pushing of the nerve against the medial epicondyle when the elbow is bent. The condition is aggravated over time by the bending of the elbow. Symptoms of cubital tunnel syndrome are typically a numb feeling in the ring finger and small finger, weakness in muscles of the hand and forearm, and elbow pain. Without intervention, more serious nerve damage can occur.

Diagnosis

Carpal tunnel syndrome is diagnosed based on the pattern of the symptoms, the location of the symptoms, and a history of repetitive activity that might predispose to the syndrome. Similarly, thoracic outlet syndrome is diagnosed by the location of the symptoms and a person's work history (i.e., a job involving a lot of lifting).

The diagnosis of brachial plexus palsy is prominently based on the visual observation of the motion difficulties experienced by the newborn. X rays may be taken to discount any other injuries such as fractures of the spine, clavicle (collarbone), humerus (the large bone in the upper arm), or a dislocation of the shoulder.

Meralgia paresthetica is diagnosed by the nature of the symptoms and the occupation of the person. For example, hip and thigh pain in a soldier can alert a clinician to the possibility of this malady. As well, people usually experience tenderness in a specific spot over a ligament in the hip, and symptoms can be made worse by extending the hip in the Nachlas test.

Diagnosis of meralgia paresthetica needs to rule out other maladies to the pelvis and spine, as well as diabetes mellitus. For example, damage to spinal discs will impair reflexes, while reflexes are normal in meralgia paresthetica.

Cubital tunnel syndrome is diagnosed by the type and location of the symptoms.

Key Terms

Palsy Paralysis or uncontrolled movement of controlled muscles.

Paresthesia Abnormal physical sensations such as numbness, burning, prickling, or tingling.

Treatment team

Treatment often involves the family physician, family members, and physical and occupational therapists. In severe cases, a surgeon may be consulted for many types of nerve compression.

Treatment

Carpal tunnel syndrome responds to immobilization of the affected area. Often, a person will wear a splint that keeps the wrist from flexing. This reduces the strain and pressure on the nerves. Another option is to administer anti-inflammatory drugs or injections of cortisone. These compounds help reduce the swelling in the wrist. In a small number of cases of carpal tunnel syndrome, surgery can be a useful option. The ligament that connects to the bottom of the wrist is cut.

Persons with thoracic outlet syndrome are put on a planned program of **exercise** therapy designed to relieve the inflammation. Avoiding the repetitive activities that caused the muscle inflammation, at least temporarily, is a must. Re-design of the workplace so that heavy objects do not have to be placed above shoulder level can be a wise strategy. Anti-inflammatory drugs may be prescribed. Finally, if these efforts have not produced a satisfactory response, surgery may be an option.

Treatment for brachial plexus palsy consists of physical therapy that relieves the strain on the affected nerves. The therapy usually involves a gentle range of motions and the use of electrical stimulation of the muscles that are associated with the damaged nerves. Keeping the muscles supple and strong is an important part of the treatment. When a nerve has been more seriously damaged, surgery may be necessary to repair the tear or other damage. This is usually evident within three months of birth. Surgery can involve the grafting of a new section of nerve to replace the damaged and now-defective region of the original nerve.

Treatment for meralgia paresthetica can involve relief of the stress on the pelvis through weight loss or modifying the activity that causes the stress. Treatment for cubital tunnel syndrome can involve the use of medications that reduce inflammation. These include non-steroidal anti-inflammatory medications such as aspirin and ibuprofen.

Some people gain relief by wearing a special brace while sleeping that prevents the elbow from bending.

Recovery and rehabilitation

Rehabilitation and recovery from carpal tunnel syndrome can be complete for some people. Avoiding the activity that inflamed the wrist can help ensure that the inflammation and nerve injury does not reoccur. Other people do recover, but more slowly. For others, the syndrome becomes a chronic concern.

Recovery from brachial plexus palsy ranges from limited to complete. Most recovery occurs by two years of age. The Erb's type of palsy is a milder form, and recovery can occur in three to four months. With the more serious Klumke's paralysis, 18–24 months of physical therapy can be required to achieve significant improvement.

Clinical trials

Rather than specific **clinical trials**, research is ongoing to try to better understand the triggers for the various nerve compression syndromes, and to find better and more efficient rehabilitation techniques. In the United States, organizations including the National Institute of Arthritis and Musculoskeletal and Skin Diseases fund such research.

Prognosis

For carpal tunnel syndrome, the outlook for many people is quite good. Once the inflammation has been dealt with, avoiding the cause of the irritation can prevent a reoccurrence of the trouble. However, for about 1% of those with carpal tunnel syndrome, permanent injury develops.

The prognosis for brachial plexus palsy varies upon the nature of the nerve damage. Some cases resolve quickly and completely without intervention, others require extended time and therapy, and in the worst-cases, impaired use of an arm can be permanent.

Meralgia paresthetica due to pregnancy, obesity, and diabetes may resolve completely when the condition is properly treated. Other mechanically-related causes of the malady can be less successfully treated. In the latter case, modification of life-style may be needed.

Most people with cubital tunnel syndrome respond well to conservative treatment, although surgery is necessary for some. For those resulting to surgery, permanent elbow numbness may result.

Resources

OTHER

"Cubital Tunnel Syndrome." (May 4, 2004). *e-hand.com.* <http://www.e-hand.com/hw/hw007.htm>.

"Meralgia Paresthetica." (May 6, 2004). *eMedicine.com.* <http://www.emedicine.com/neuro/topic590.htm>.

"NINDS Carpal Tunnel Syndrome Information Page." (May 6, 2004). National Institute of Neurological Diseases and Stroke. <http://www.ninds.nih.gov/health_and_medical/disorders/carpal_doc.htm>.

"What is thoracic outlet syndrome?" *Canadian Centre for Occupational Health and Safety.* (May 6, 2004). <http://www.ccohs.ca/oshanswers/diseases/thoracic.html>.

ORGANIZATIONS

National Institute for Neurological Diseases and Stroke (NINDS). P.O. Box 5801, Bethesda, MD 20824. (301) 496-5751 or (800) 352-9424. <http://www.ninds/nih.gov>.

National Chronic Pain Outreach Organization (NCPOA). P.O. Box 274, Millboro, VA 24460. (540) 862-9437; Fax: (540) 862-9485. ncpoa@cfw.org. <http://www.chronic-pain.org>.

National Institute of Arthritis and Musculoskeletal and Skin Diseases (NIAMS). 31 Centre Dr., Rm. 4Co2 MSC 2350, Bethesda, MD 20892-2350. (301) 496-8190 or (877) 226-4267. info@mail.nih.gov. <http://www.niams.nih.gov>.

American Chronic Pain Association (ACPA). P.O. Box 850, Rocklin, CA 95677-0850. (916) 632-0922 or (800) 533-3231; Fax: ACPA@pacbell.net. <http://www.theacpa.org>.

Brian Douglas Hoyle, PhD

Nerve conduction study

Definition

A nerve conduction study is a test that measures the movement of an impulse through a nerve after the deliberate stimulation of the nerve.

Purpose

The ability of a nerve to swiftly and properly transmit an impulse down its length, and to pass on the impulse to the adjacent nerve or to a connection muscle in which it is embedded, is vital to the performance of many activities in the body.

When proper functioning of nerves does not occur, as can happen due to accidents, infections, or progressive and genetically based diseases, the proper treatment depends on an understanding of the nature of the problem. The nerve conduction study is one tool that a clinician can use to assess nerve function. Often, the nerve conduction study is performed in concert with a test called an electromyogram. Together, these tests, along with other procedures that comprise what is known as electrodiagnostic testing, provide vital information on the functioning of nerves and muscles.

Description

Nerve cells consist of a body, with branches at one end. The branches are called axons. The axons are positioned near an adjacent nerve or a muscle. Nerve impulses pass from the axons of one nerve to the next nerve or muscle. The impulse transmission speed can be reduced in damaged nerves.

Surrounding a nerve is a tough protective coat of a material called myelin. Nerve damage can involve damage or loss of myelin, damage to the nerve body, or damage to the axon region. The nerve conduction study, which was devised in the 1960s, can detect the loss of nerve function due to these injuries, and, from the nature of the nerve signal pattern that is produced, offer clues as to the nature of the problem.

Depending on the nature of the nerve damage, the pattern of signal transmission can be different. For example, in a normal nerve cell, sensors placed at either end of the cell will register the same signal pattern. But, in a nerve cell that is blocked somewhere along its length, these sensors will register different signal patterns. In another example, in a nerve cell in which transmission is not completely blocked, the signal pattern at the axon may be similar in shape, but reduced in intensity, to that of the originating signal, because not as much of the signal is completing the journey down the nerve cell.

Diseases of the nerve itself mainly affect the size of the responses (amplitudes); diseases of the myelin mainly affect the speed of the responses.

Nerve conduction studies are now routine, and can be done in virtually any hospital equipped with the appropriate machine and staffed with a qualified examiner. The nerve conduction study utilizes a computer, computer monitor, amplifier, loudspeaker, electrical stimulator, and filters. These filters are mathematical filters that can distinguish random, background electrical signals from the signal produced by an activated nerve. When the study is done, small electrodes are placed on the skin over the muscles being tested. Generally, these muscles are located in the arms or legs. Some of the electrodes are designed to record the electrical signal that passes by them. Other electrodes (reference electrodes) are designed to monitor the quality of the signals to make sure that the test is operating properly. If monitoring of the test is not done, then the results obtained are meaningless.

After the electrodes are in place, a small electrical current can be applied to the skin. The electrical stimulation is usually done at several points along the nerve, not just at a single point. This is done because conduction of

---

Key Terms

Axon The long, slender part of a nerve cell that carries electrochemical signals to another nerve cell.

Electromyogram (EMG) Aa diagnostic used test to evaluate nerve and muscle function.

Nerve impulse The electrochemical signal carried by an axon from one neuron to another neuron.

Neuron A nerve cell.

---

an impulse through a nerve is not uniform. Some regions of a nerve conduct more slowly than other regions. By positioning the stimulating electrodes at several sites, a more accurate overall measurement of conduction velocity is obtained.

The electrical current activates nerves in the vicinity, including those associated with the particular muscle. The nerves are stimulated to produce a signal. This is known as the "firing" of the nerve. The nerve signal, which it also electric, can be detected by some of the electrodes and conveyed to the computer for analysis.

The analysis of the nerve signal involves the study of the movement of the signal through the nerve and from the nerve to the adjacent muscle. Using characteristics such as the speed of the impulse, and the shape, wavelength, and height of the signal wave, an examiner can assess whether the nerve is functional or defective.

Risks

A nerve conduction study can be done quite quickly. A person will experience some discomfort from the series of small electrical shocks that are felt. Otherwise, no damage or residual effects occur.

Normal results

Analysis of the results of a nerve conduction study

Under normal circumstances, the movement of the electrical impulse down the length of a nerve is very fast, on the order of 115–197 ft/sec (35–60 m/sec).

A number of aspects of the nerve impulse are measured in nerve conduction studies. The first aspect (or parameter) is known as latency. Latency is the time between the stimulus (the applied electrical current) and the response (the firing of the nerve). In damaged nerves, latency is typically increased.

Another parameter is known as the amplitude. Electrical signals are waves. The distance from the crest of one wave to the bottom of the trough of the adjacent wave is the amplitude. Impulses in damaged nerves can have an abnormal amplitude, or may show different amplitudes in the undamaged and damaged sections of the same nerve.

The area under a wave can also vary if not all muscle fibers are being stimulated by a nerve or if the muscle fibers are not all reacting to a nerve impulse at the same time. The speed of a nerve impulse (the conduction velocity) can be also be determined and compared to data produced by a normally functioning nerve.

A number of other, more technically complex parameters can also be recorded and analyzed. A skilled examiner can tell from the appearance of the impulse waves on the computer monitor whether or not a nerve or muscle is functioning normally, and can even begin to gauge the nature of a problem. Examples of maladies that can be partially diagnosed using the nerve conduction study include **Guillain-Barré syndrome**, **amyotrophic lateral sclerosis** (ALS, or Lou Gehrig's disease, Charcot's disease), and **multifocal motor neuropathy**.

Conditions affecting the nerve conduction study

The nerve conduction study does not produce uniform results from person to person. Various factors affect the transmission of a nerve impulse and the detected signal.

Temperature affects the speed of impulse movement. Signals move more slowly at lower temperatures, due to the tighter packing of the molecules of the nerve. This variable can be minimized during the nerve conduction study by maintaining the skin temperature at 80–85° Fahrenheit (27–29° Celcius). Use of a controlled temperature also allows study runs done at different times to be more comparable, which can be very useful in evaluating whether muscle or nerve problems are worsening or getting better.

The speed of nerve impulse transmission changes as the body ages. In infants, the transmission speed is only about half that seen in adults. By age five, most people have attained the adult velocity. A gradual decline in conduction velocity begins as people reach their 20s, and continues for the remainder of life. Another factor that influences conduction velocity is the length of the nerve itself. An impulse that has to travel a longer distance will take longer. Some nerves are naturally longer than others. Measurement of nerve conduction takes into account the length of the target nerve.

Resources

OTHER

"Electromyography (EMG) and Nerve Conduction Studies." *WebMD.* May 1, 2004 (June 2, 2004). <http://my.webmd.com/hw/health_guide_atoz/hw213852.asp>.

"Nerve conduction velocity." *Medline Plus.* National Library of Medicine. May 3, 2004 (June 2, 2004). <http://www.nlm.nih.gov/medlineplus/print/ency/article/003927.htm>.

"Nerve Conduction Velocity Test." *MedicineNet.com.* May 1, 2004 (June 2, 2004). <http://www.medicinenet.com/Nerve_Conduction_Velocity_Test/article.htm>.

Brian Douglas Hoyle, PhD

Neurodegeneration with brain iron accumulation *see* **Pantothenate kinase-associated neurodegeneration**

Neurofibromatosis

Definition

Neurofibromatosis (NF) is a genetic condition in which fleshy tumors called neurofibromas grow throughout the body. Neurofibromatosis was first written up in the medical literature in 1882 by a German physician, Dr. Friedrich Daniel von Recklinghausen.

Description

Neurofibromas are tumors that are composed of the fibrous substance that covers nerve cells. These neurofibromas grow along the nerves in the body (the peripheral nerves), and cause skin and bone abnormalities. Furthermore, while neurofibromas initially start out as benign (non-cancerous) growths, 3–5% of all neurofibromas are converted into malignant (cancerous) tumors. Neurofibromatosis patients are also at risk of developing other types of cancerous tumors of the nervous system.

Neurofibromatosis is divided into two types, NF1 and NF2. NF1, also called Von Recklinghausen disease or peripheral neurofibromatosis, is the most common. Visible skin signs of NF1 tend to be present at birth, or certainly by about age 10. NF1 causes predominantly skin and bone changes, as well as problems due to the growing neurofibromas exerting damaging pressure on peripheral nerves. NF2, also called central neurofibromatosis or bilateral acoustic neurofibromatosis, is less common. Its predominant problem involves neurofibromas growing on the eighth cranial nerve (also known as the acoustic or auditory nerve). These tumors interfere with the functioning of the cranial nerve VIII, causing serious hearing impairment or even profound deafness, as well as a variety of symptoms due to pressure on adjacent nerves that serve the head and neck areas.

Demographics

NF1 occurs in one out of 4,000 births; NF2 occurs in one out of 40,000 births. Males and females are equally affected. In the United States, about 100,000 people are identified as having either NF1 or NF2.

Causes and symptoms

Neurofibromatosis is a genetic disease that is inherited in an autosomal dominant fashion, meaning that only one parent with neurofibromatosis is required to pass on the disease to offspring. Half of all cases of neurofibromatosis is inherited from a parent with the disorder; the other half of cases of neurofibromatosis does not have a history of the disease in a parent. They are considered to have developed the disease due to a spontaneous mutation, which can then be passed on to the patient's own offspring. When one parent has neurofibromatosis, each child has a 50% chance of inheriting the condition.

Neurofibromatosis 1

Patients with NF1 are most often diagnosed in childhood or even infancy. The most common characteristics of NF1 include:

• cafe-au-lait macules (light brown, flat skin patches)

• freckles in the armpit and groin areas (axillary and inguinal freckling)

• neurofibromas on and under the skin, ranging from millimeters to inches (centimeters) in size (an individual may have anywhere from several to thousands of these soft, rubbery, flesh-colored tumors)

• Lisch nodules, tumors within the iris of the eye

• vision problems, probably due to gliomas (tumors made of cells called glial cells that serve a supportive function within the **central nervous system**) located within or exerting pressure on the optic nerves

• learning problems or frank mental retardation

• scoliosis (side-to-side curvature of the spine)

• high blood pressure

• short adult height

• early (precocious) puberty

• increased risk of malignant brain and spinal cord tumors, kidney tumors (Wilms' tumor), adrenal tumors (pheochromocytoma), leukemia (cancer of blood cells), and tumors of the tendons, muscles, or connective tissue (rhabdomyosarcoma)

Neurofibromatosis 2

The most common characteristics of NF2 include:

• hearing problems due to neurofibromas in both acoustic nerves

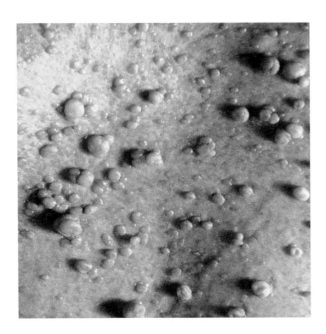

Neurofibromatosis. Visible are large and small smooth, round, protruding growths scattered across a patient's back. *(Photograph by Michael English, M.D. Custom Medical Stock Photo. Reproduced by permission.)*

• cataracts, the abnormal clouding of the lens of the eye

• **headache, pain** or numbness in the face

• problems with balance and coordination when walking, resulting in unsteadiness

• ringing in the ears (tinnitus)

• cafe-au-lait macules (many fewer than in NF1)

• neurofibromas on and under the skin (many fewer than in NF1)

Diagnosis

NF1 is diagnosed when the patient has at least two of the following criteria:

• six or more cafe-au-lait macules that measure more than 0.2 in (5 mm) in children before puberty, or that measure more than 0.6 in (15 mm) in patients after puberty

• demonstration of two or more neurofibromas

• axillary or inguinal freckling

• presence of optic glioma

• presence of two or more Lisch nodules, diagnosed through slit-lamp examination (a slit-lamp is a microscope with an extremely strong light that can be focused into a slit in order to examine the eye)

• bone abnormalities such as defects of the skull bone (sphenoid wing) or abnormal thinning of the usually dense outer layer of the long thigh, leg, or arm bones

- a parent, sibling, or child who has been diagnosed with NF1

NF2 is diagnosed when the patient has at least one of the following criteria:

- gadolinium-enhanced **magnetic resonance imaging (MRI)** scan or other appropriate imaging study that demonstrates tumors of the two cranial nerves VIII

- a parent, sibling, or child who has been diagnosed with NF2, and has either a diagnosed tumor on one cranial nerve VIII or at least two of the following: neurofibroma, meningioma (tumor of the membrane that covers the spinal cord and brain [meninges]), glioma (tumor composed of the supportive cells called glial cells), schwannoma (tumor composed of the schwann cells that normally wrap around nerves throughout the body, creating a sheath that both insulates the nerves and allows nerve conduction to occur more quickly), or a specific type of cataract called a juvenile posterior subcapsular lenticular opacity

Treatment team

Treatment of neurofibromatosis requires a multidisciplinary team approach, with neurologists, ophthalmologists, otolaryngologists (ENTs), neurosurgeons, general surgeons, plastic surgeons, orthopedic surgeons, and dermatologists all collaborating. Depending on the kinds of challenges that the specific patient faces, other team members may include speech and language specialists, learning specialists, occupational therapists, and physical therapists.

Treatment

There is no known cure for either NF1 or NF2. Regular examinations are important in order to catch new developments early, such as the advent of high blood pressure, malignant transformation of a neurofibroma, or development of cataracts.

Treatment is purely supportive and depends on the specific manifestations of the disease in a given patient. For example, a patient with scoliosis may require bracing; patients with cataracts may require surgery; patients with auditory nerve tumors may require traditional scalpel surgery or gamma-knife surgery (also called stereotactic radiosurgery, this is a technique that allows a very focused, very high dose of **radiation** to be delivered to a carefully designated tissue location). Optic gliomas may be treated with radiation therapy. Any tumors that are impinging on nerves and causing symptoms or tumors that have undergone malignant transformation may require surgical removal, while tumors that are purely problematic from a cosmetic standpoint may be left alone.

Clinical trials

A variety of **clinical trials** are underway, including studies of several types of drugs such as drug R115777, tipifarnib, pirfenidone, and combination methotrexate/vinblastine therapy, each of which may be useful in shrinking tumors associated with neurofibromatosis. Information about these trials are available through the National Cancer Institute.

Prognosis

Even within the same family, the manifestations and severity of neurofibromatosis can differ widely.

Special concerns

Genetic counseling is crucial for families with a history of neurofibromatosis to help ascertain the risk of future offspring being born with neurofibromatosis.

Resources

BOOKS

Barkovich, A. James, and Ruben I. Kuzniecky. "Neurocutaneous Syndromes." *Cecil Textbook of Medicine*, edited by Lee Goldman. Philadelphia: W. B. Saunders Company, 2003.

Berg, Bruce O. "Chromosomal Abnormalities and Neurocutaneous Disorders>" *Textbook of Clinical Neurology*, edited by Christopher G. Goetz. Philadelphia: W. B. Saunders Company, 2003.

Haslam, Robert H. A. "Neurocutaneous Syndromes." *Nelson Textbook of Pediatrics*, edited by Richard E. Behrman, et al. Philadelphia: W. B. Saunders Company, 2004.

WEBSITES

National Institute of Neurological Disorders and Stroke (NINDS). *Neurofibromatosis Fact Sheet*. (April 27, 2004). <http://www.ninds.nih.gov>.

ORGANIZATIONS

National Cancer Institute (NCI). 9000 Rockville Pike, Bethesda, MD 20892. gillesan@exchange.nih.gov or prpl@mail.cc.nih.gov.

The National Neurofibromatosis Foundation, Inc. 95 Pine Street, 16th Floor, New York, NY 10005. (212) 344-NNFF (6633) or (800) 323-7938. nnff@nf.org. <http://www.nf.org>.

Rosalyn Carson-DeWitt, MD

Neuroleptic malignant syndrome

Definition

Neuroleptic malignant syndrome is a rare, potentially life-threatening disorder that is usually precipitated by the use of medications that block the neurotransmitter called

Key Terms

Acoustic nerve The cranial nerve VIII, involved in both hearing and balance.

Axillary Referring to the armpit.

Cataracts Abnormal clouding or opacities within the lens of the eye.

Gamma-knife surgery A technique of focusing very intense radiation on an extremely well-defined area of abnormal tissue requiring treatment, thus allowing a very high dose of radiation to be used with less damage to neighboring, normal tissue.

Glial cell A type of cell in the nervous system that provides support for the nerve cells.

Glioma A tumor made up of abnormal glial cells.

Inguinal Referring to the groin area.

Iris In the eye, the colored ring that is located behind the cornea and in front of the lens.

Leukemia Cancer of a blood cell.

Lisch nodule A benign growth within the iris of the eye.

Macule A small, flat area of abnormal color on the skin.

Meninges The three-layered membranous covering of the brain and spinal cord.

Meningioma A tumor made up of cells of the lining of the brain and spinal cord (meninges).

Neurofibromas Soft, rubbery, flesh-colored tumors made up of the fibrous substance that covers peripheral nerves.

Pheochromocytoma A tumor of the adrenal glands that causes high blood pressure.

Posterior subcapsular lenticular opacity A type of cataract in the eye.

Rhabdomyosarcoma A tumor of the tendons, muscles, or connective tissue.

Schwann cell Cells that cover the nerve fibers in the body, providing both insulation and increasing the speed of nerve conduction.

Scoliosis Side-to-side curvature of the spine.

Sphenoid A bone of the skull.

Tinnitus The abnormal sensation of hearing a ringing or buzzing noise.

Wilms' tumor A childhood tumor of the kidneys.

---

dopamine. Most often, the drugs involved are those that treat psychosis, called neuroleptic medications. The syndrome results in dysfunction of the autonomic nervous system, the branch of the nervous system responsible for regulating such involuntary actions as heart rate, blood pressure, digestion, and sweating. Muscle tone, body temperature, and consciousness are also severely affected.

Description

Most cases of neuroleptic malignant syndrome develop between four to 14 days of the initiation of a new drug or an increase in dose. However, the syndrome can begin as soon as hours after the first dose or as long as years after medication initiation.

A variety of factors may increase an individual's risk of developing this condition, including:

- high environmental temperatures
- dehydration
- agitation or catatonia in a patient
- high initial dose or rapid dose increase of neuroleptic, and use of high-potency or intramuscular, long-acting (depot) preparations
- simultaneous use of more than one causative agent

- sudden discontinuation of medications for **Parkinson's disease**
- past history of organic brain syndromes, **depression**, or bipolar disorder
- past episode of neuromuscular malignant syndrome (risk of recurrence may be as high as 30%)

Because of heightened awareness of this syndrome and improved monitoring for its development, mortality rates have dropped from 20–30% down to 5–11.6%.

Demographics

Neuroleptic malignant syndrome is thought to affect about 0.02–12.2% of all patients using neuroleptic medications. Because more men than women take neuroleptic medications, the male-to-female ratio is about 2:1.

Causes and symptoms

Neuroleptic malignant syndrome occurs due to interference with dopamine activity in the **central nervous system**, either by depletion of available reserves of dopamine or by blockade of receptors that dopamine usually stimulates.

Neuroleptic malignant syndrome most commonly affects patients who are using neuroleptic or antipsychotic medications, including prochlorperazine (Compazine), promethazine (Phenergan), olanzapine (Zyprexa), clozapine (Clozaril), and risperidone (Risperdal). Other medications that block dopamine may also precipitate the syndrome, including metoclopramide (Reglan), amoxapine (Ascendin), and lithium. Too-fast withdrawal of drugs used to treat Parkinson's disease (levodopa, bromocriptine, and **amantadine**) can also precipitate neuroleptic malignant syndrome.

Symptoms of the disorder include:

- extremely high body temperature (hyperthermia), ranging from 38.6° to 42.3° C or 101° to 108° F

- heavy sweating

- fast heart rate (tachydardia)

- fast respiratory rate (tachypnea)

- rapidly fluctuating blood pressure

- impaired consciousness

- tremor

- rigid, stiff muscles (termed "lead pipe rigidity")

- catatonia (a fixed stuporous state)

Without relatively immediate, aggressive treatment, coma and complete respiratory and cardiovascular collapse will take place, followed by death.

Diagnosis

Diagnosis requires a high level of suspicion when characteristic symptoms appear in a patient treated with agents known to cause neuroleptic malignant syndrome.

The usual diagnostic criteria for neuroleptic malignant syndrome includes the presence of hyperthermia (temperature over 38° C or 101° F) with no other assignable cause, muscle rigidity, and at least five of the following signs or symptoms: impaired mental status, tremor, fast heart rate, fast respiratory rate, loss of bladder or bowel control, fluctuating blood pressure, metabolic acidosis, fluctuating blood pressure, excess blood acidity (metabolic acidosis), increased blood levels of creatanine phosphokinase (normally found in muscles and released into the bloodstream due to muscle damage), heavy sweating, drooling, or increased white blood cell count (leukocytosis).

Treatment team

Neuroleptic malignant syndrome usually requires treatment in an intensive care unit, with appropriate specialists, including intensivists, pulmonologists, cardiologists, psychiatrists.

Treatment

Treatment must be aggressive. Supportive treatment should include hydration with fluids, cooling, and supplemental oxygen. Causative medications should be immediately discontinued, and medications that restore dopamine levels (bromocriptine, amantadine) administered. Dantrolene can be given to more quickly resolve muscle rigidity and hyperthermia. **Benzodiazepines**, such as lorazepam, may help agitated patients, and may also help relax rigid muscles. Benzodiazepines may also aid in the reversal of catatonia. In severe or intractable cases of catatonia or psychosis that remains after other symptoms of neuroleptic malignant syndrome have resolved, electroconvulsive therapy may be required.

Prognosis

With quick identification of the syndrome and immediate supportive treatment, the majority of patients recover fully, although mortality rates are still significant. Signs that may warn of a poor prognosis include temperature over 104° F and kidney failure. In patients whose syndrome was precipitated by the use of oral medications, symptoms may last for seven to 10 days. In patients whose syndrome was precipitated by the use of long-acting, intramuscular preparation, symptoms may continue as long as 21 days.

Special concerns

Patients with a history of neuroleptic malignant syndrome are also at increased risk for a similar malignant hyperthermia syndrome that is precipitated by the administration of surgical anesthetics.

Resources
BOOKS

Saper, Clifford B. "Autonomic disorders and their management." *Cecil Textbook of Medicine*, edited by Lee Goldman. Philadelphia: W. B. Saunders Company, 2003.

Kompoliti, Katie, and Stacy S. Horn. "Drug-induced and iatrogenic neurological disorders." *Ferri's Clinical Advisor: Instant Diagnosis and Treatment*, edited by Fred F. Ferri. St. Louis: Mosby, 2004.

Olson, William H. ldquo;Neuroleptic malignant syndrome." *Nelson Textbook of Pediatrics*, edited by Richard E. Behrman, et al. Philadelphia: W. B. Saunders Company, 2004.

WEBSITES

National Institute of Neurological Disorders and Stroke (NINDS). *NINDS Neuroleptic Malignant Syndrome Information Page.* January 23, 2002 (June 4, 2004). <http://www.ninds.nih.gov/health_and_medical/disorders/neuroleptic_syndrome.htm>.

Key Terms

Autonomic nervous system The divisions of the nervous system that control involuntary functions, such as breathing, heart rate, blood pressure, digestion, glands, smooth muscle.

Bipolar disorder A psychiatric illness characterized by both recurrent depression and recurrent mania (abnormally high energy, agitation, irritability).

Catatonia A fixed, motionless stupor.

Creatanine phosphokinase A chemical normally found in the muscle fibers, and released into the bloodstream when the muscles undergo damage and breakdown.

Depot A type of drug preparation and administration that involves the slow, gradual release from an area of the body where the drug has been injected.

Depression A psychiatric disorder in which the mood is low for a prolonged period of time, and feelings of hopelessness and inadequacy interfere with normal functioning.

Dopamine A brain neurotransmitter involved in movement.

Hyperthermia Elevated body temperature.

Leukocytosis An elevated white blood cell count.

Metabolic acidosis Overly acidic condition of the blood.

Neuroleptic Referring to a type of drug used to treat psychosis.

Neurotransmitter A chemical that transmits information in the nervous system.

Organic brain syndrome A brain disorder that is caused by defective structure or abnormal functioning of the brain.

Parkinson's disease A disease caused by deficient dopamine in the brain, and resulting in a progressively severe movement disorder (tremor, weakness, difficulty walking, muscle rigidity, fixed facial expression).

Receptor An area on the cell membrane where a specific chemical can bind, in order to either activate or inhibit certain cellular functions.

Tachycardia Elevated heart rate.

Tachypnea Elevated breathing rate.

ORGANIZATIONS

Neuroleptic Malignant Syndrome Information Service. PO Box 1069 11 East State Street, Sherburne, NY 13460. (607) 674-7920 or (888) 667-8367; Fax: (607) 674-7910. gillesan@exchange.nih.gov or info@nmsis.org. <http://www.nmsis.org/index.shtml>.

Rosalyn Carson-DeWitt, MD

Neurologist

Definition

A neurologist is a physician who has undergone additional training to diagnose and treat disorders of the nervous system.

Description

The training a neurologist receives enables the individual to recognize nervous system malfunctions, to accurately diagnose the nature of the dysfunction (such as disease or injury), and to treat the malady. While many people associate a neurologist with treating brain injuries, this is just one facet of a neurologist's responsibility and expertise. Diseases of the spinal cord, nerves, and muscles that affect the operation of the nervous system can also be addressed by a neurologist.

The training that is necessary to become a neurologist begins with the traditional medical background. From there, the medical doctor trains for several more years to acquire expertise in the structure, functioning, and repair of the body's neurological structures, including the area of the brain called the cerebral cortex, and how the various regions of the cortex contribute to the normal and abnormal functioning of the body.

Typically, a neurologist's educational path begins with premed studies at a university or college. These studies can last up to four years. Successful candidates enter medical school. Another four years of study is required for a degree as a doctor of medicine (MD). Following completion of the advanced degree, a one-year internship is usually undertaken in internal medicine; sometimes, internships in transitional programs that include pediatrics and emergency-room training are chosen. Finally, another training period of at least three years follows in a neurology residency program. The latter program provides specialty experience in a hospital and can include research. Postdoctoral fellowships lasting one year or more offer additional opportunities for further specialization.

After completion of the more than decade-long training, medical doctors can become certified as neurologists through the American Board of Psychiatry and Neurology. Those with an osteopathy background can be certified through the American Board of Osteopathic Neurologists and Psychiatrists. Most neurologists belong to professional organizations such as the American Academy of Neurology (AAN), which is dedicated to setting practice standards, supporting research, providing continuing education, and promoting optimum care for persons with neurological disorders. Numerous professional publications specialize in neurology, including *Neurology Today*, *Neurology*, *Brain*, and *Archives of Neurology*.

A neurologist can sometimes be a patient's principle physician. This is true when the patient has a neurological problem such as **Parkinson's** or **Alzheimer's disease** or **multiple sclerosis**. As well, an important aspect of a neurologist's daily duties is to offer advice to other physicians on how to treat neurological problems. A family physician might consult a neurologist when caring for patients with **stroke** or severe **headache**.

When a neurologist examines a patient, details such as vision, physical strength and coordination, reflexes, and sensations like touch and smell are probed to help determine if the medical problem is related to nervous system damage. More tests might be done to help determine the exact cause of the problem and how to treat the condition. While neurologists can recommend surgery, they do not actually perform the surgery. That is the domain of the neurosurgeon.

One well-known neurologist is the English-born physician and writer Oliver Sacks (1933–). In addition to maintaining a clinical practice, Sacks has authored numerous popular books that describe patients' experiences with neurological disorders and neurologists' experiences in treating them. Another notable neurologist was Alois Alzheimer (1864–1915). A German neurologist, he first observed and identified the symptoms of what is now known as Alzheimer's disease.

Resources

BOOKS

Bluestein, Bonnie Ellen. *Preserve Your Love for Science: Life of William A Hammond, American Neurologist.* Cambridge, UK: Cambridge University Press, 1991.

Restak, Richard. *The Brain Has a Mind of Its Own: Insights from a Practicing Neurologist.* Three Rivers, MI: Three Rivers Press, 1999.

Sacks, Oliver. *The Man Who Mistook His Wife for a Hat: And Other Clinical Tales.* Carmichael, CA: Touchstone Books, 1998.

OTHER

"What Is a Neurologist?" *Neurology Channel* Healthcommunities.com. May 6, 2004 (June 2, 2004). <http://www.neurologychannel.com/aneurologist.shtml>.

ORGANIZATIONS

American Board of Psychiatry and Neurology, Inc. 500 Lake Cook Road, Suite 335, Deerfield, IL 60015-5249. (847) 945-7900 or (800) 373-1166; Fax: (847) 945-1146. <http://www.abpn.com>.

American Academy of Neurology. 1080 Montreal Avenue, Saint Paul, MN 55116. (651) 695-2717 or (800) 879-1960; Fax: (651) 695-2791. memberservices@aan.com. <http://www.aan.com>.

Brian Douglas Hoyle, PhD

Neuromuscular blockers

Definition

Neuromuscular blocking agents are a class of drugs primarily indicated for use as an adjunct to anesthesia. Neuromuscular blocking drugs relax skeletal muscles and induce paralysis.

Purpose

Neuromuscular blockers are indicated for a wide variety of uses in a hospital setting, from surgery to trauma care. In surgery, they are used to prepare patients for intubation before being placed on a ventilator and to suppress the patient's spontaneous breathing once on a ventilator.

Description

Neuromuscular blockers relax skeletal muscle tone by blocking transmission of key **neurotransmitters** through the neuron receptors at the neuromuscular junction (NMJ). They are divided into two major categories, depolarizing and non-depolarizing neuromuscular blockers, corresponding to the manner in which they exert their therapeutic effect. Depolarizing neuromuscular blocking agents mimic the effects of the neurotransmitter acetylcholine (ACh) and change the interaction between ACh and neuron receptors. Blockade occurs because membranes surrounding the neuromuscular junction become unresponsive to typical ACh-receptor interaction. Non-depolarizing neuromuscular blockers bind to receptors to prevent transmission of impulses through ACh neurotransmitters.

Neuromuscular blockers are primarily used in a clinical or hospital setting. In the United States, they are known by several generic and brand names, including atracurium (Tracurium), cisatracurium (Nimbex), doxacurium (Neuromax), mivacurium (Mivacron), pancuronium (Pavulon), pipecuronium (Arduan), rocuronium (Zemeron), succinylcholine (Anectine), tubocurarine, and vecuronium (Norcuron).

A physician will decide which neuromuscular blocking agent, or combination of neuromuscular blocker and other type of anesthesia, is appropriate for an individual patient. During surgical anesthesia, neuromuscular blockers are administered after the induction of unconsciousness, in order to avoid patient distress at the inability to purposefully move muscles. Neuromuscular blockers can be used on pediatric patients.

Recommended dosage

Neuromuscular blocking agents are most often administered though an intravenous (IV) infusion tube. Typically, the time in which the medicines begin to exert their effects and duration of action are more predictable when neuromuscular blocking agents are administered via IV. Dosages vary depending on the neuromuscular blocking agent used and the duration of action desired. The age, weight, and general health of an individual patient can also affect dosing requirements.

Depolarizing and non-depolarizing agents are grouped together into three categories based on the time in which they begin to exert their anesthetic effects, causing muscle relaxation or paralysis and desensitization, and the duration of those effects (duration of action). Short-acting neuromuscular blockers begin to work within 30 seconds to two-and-a-half minutes and have a typical duration of action ranging from five to twenty minutes. Short-acting agents include mivacurium, rocuronium, and succinylcholine. Intermediate-acting agents exert their effects within two to five minutes and typically last for twenty to sixty minutes. Atracurium, cisatracurium, pancuronium, and vecuronium are intermediate-acting neuromuscular blockers. Long-acting neuromuscular blocking agents take effect within two-and-a-half to six minutes and last as long as 75–100 minutes. Doxacurium, pipecuronium, and tubocurarine are long-acting neuromuscular blocking agents.

The duration of action of any neuromuscular blocking agent can be prolonged by administering smaller supplemental (maintenance) doses via IV following the initial blockade-creating dose.

Precautions

Each neuromuscular blocking agent has its own particular precautions, contraindications, and side effects. However, many are common to all neuromuscular blockers. Neuromuscular blocking agents may not be suitable for persons with a history of lung diseases, **stroke**, increased intracranial pressure, increased intraocular (within the eye) pressure as in glaucoma, liver or kidney disease, decreased renal function, diseases or disorders affecting the muscles, angina (chest **pain**), and irregular heartbeats and other heart problems. Neuromuscular blockers are not typically used on patients with recent, severe burns, elevated potassium levels, or severe muscle trauma. There is an increased risk of seizure in patients with seizure disorders such as **epilepsy**.

Neuromuscular blockers can be administered to patients who have suffered a **spinal cord injury** resulting in paraplegia (paralysis) immediately following the injury. But further use of neuromuscular blockers is typically avoided 10–100 days after the initial trauma.

Patients who are obese or have increased plasma cholinesterase activity may exhibit increased resistance to neuromuscular blocking agents. Some **cholinergic stimulants** that act as **cholinesterase inhibitors**, including medications used in the treatment of **Alzheimer's disease**, may enhance neuromuscular blockade and prolong the duration of action of neuromuscular blockers.

With careful supervision, neuromuscular blocking agents can be used in pediatric patients. However, rare but serious complications such as bradycardia (decreased heart rate) are more likely to develop in children than in adults.

Placental transfer (passing of the medication to the fetus) of neuromuscular blocking agents is minimal. Histamine release is associated with neuromuscular blocking agents tubocurare and succinylcholine. Complications such as bronchospasm, decreased blood pressure, and blood clotting problems could arise in patients especially sensitive or susceptible to changes in histamine levels.

Side effects

In some patients, neuromuscular blockers may produce mild or moderate side effects. Anesthesiologists (specialists in administering anesthesia and treating pain) may notice a slight red flushing of the face as neuromuscular blockers are administered to the patient. After completion of the surgical procedure, **headache**, nausea, muscle soreness, and muscle weakness are the most frequently reported side effects attributed to neuromuscular blockers. Most of these side effects disappear or occur less frequently after a few hours or days.

With depolarizing neuromuscular blocking agents, fasciculations (involuntary muscle contractions) may occur before the onset of muscle relaxation or paralysis. Some patients report generalized muscle soreness or pain after taking a neuromuscular blocking agent that causes fasciculations. Women and middle-aged patients reported this side effect more frequently.

Key Terms

Acetylcholine   The neurotransmitter, or chemical that works in the brain to transmit nerve signals, involved in regulating muscles, memory, mood, and sleep.

Fasciculations   Fine tremors of the muscles.

Neuromuscular junction   The junction between a nerve fiber and the muscle it supplies.

Neurotransmitter   Chemicals that allow the movement of information from one neuron across the gap between the adjacent neuron.

Other, uncommon side effects or complications associated with neuromuscular blockers can be serious or may indicate an allergic reaction. As neuromuscular blockers are most frequently used in trauma, surgical, and intensive hospital care, physicians may be able to counteract the following side effects or complications as they occur:

• bradycardia

• cessation of breathing

• severe bronchospasm

• prolonged numbness in the extremities

• extended paralysis

• jaw rigidity

• skeletal muscle atrophy or trauma

• impaired blood clotting

• severe decrease in blood pressure

• chest pain or irregular heartbeat

Interactions

Neuromuscular blocking agents may have negative interactions with some anticoagulants, **anticonvulsants** (especially those also indicated for use as skeletal muscle relaxants), antihistamines, antidepressants, antibiotics, pain killers (including non-prescription medications) and monoamine oxidase inhibitors (MAOIs).

Cholinergic stimulants, some insecticides, diuretics (furosemide), local anesthetics, magnesium, antidepressants, anticonvulsants, aminoglycoside antibiotics, high estrogen levels, and metoclopramide (Reglan) may affect the duration of action of neuromuscular blocking agents.

Resources

BOOKS

Omoigui, Erowid. *The Anesthesia Drugs Handbook.* St. Louis: Mosby, 1995.

PERIODICALS

Hunter, Jennifer M. "New Neuromuscular Blocking Drugs." *New England Journal of Medicine* 332, no. 25 (1995): 1691–1699.

Adrienne Wilmoth Lerner

Neuromyelitis optica *see* **Devic syndrome**

Neuronal ceroid lipofuscinosis *see* **Batten disease**

Neuronal migration disorders

Definition

Neuronal migration disorders are a diverse group of congenital brain abnormalities that arise specifically from defective formation of the **central nervous system**. During early brain development, neurons are born and move over large distances to reach their targets and thereby give rise to the different parts of the brain. The control of this process is highly orchestrated and dependent on the expression of various environmental and genetic factors that continue to be discovered in genetic studies of mice and humans. The critical role neuronal migration plays in brain development is evident from the variety of gross malformations that can occur when it goes wrong. Defective neuronal migration leads to a broad range of clinical syndromes, and most affected patients will have a combination of **mental retardation** and **epilepsy**.

Description

Neuronal migration disorders include **lissencephaly** as part of the agyria-pachygyria-band spectrum, cobblestone lissencephaly, periventricular heterotopia, and other variants such as Zellweger and Kallman syndrome. Patients may have only focal collections of abnormally located neurons known as heterotopias. The common factor in these disorders is a defect in neuronal migration, a key process in brain development that occurs during weeks 12 to 16 of gestation. Some disorders such as polymicrogyria and **schizencephaly** are presumably due to abnormal neuronal migration due to studies showing heterotopias in other parts of the brain, but the exact relationship is unclear. Early in brain development, neurons are born in specific locations in the brain and migrate to their final destinations to create distinct brain regions. Each step of this process, from starting, continuing, and stopping migration, is controlled by distinct molecular mechanisms that are regulated by the activity of genes. Defects in these genes lead to the various presentations of neuronal migration disorders seen in clinical practice.

Lissencephaly

Lissencephaly is the most extreme example of defective neuronal migration. In lissencephaly or agyria, neuronal migration fails globally, causing the brain to appear completely smooth and have abnormal layering in the cortex. Various genes have been associated with varying levels of severity of lissencephaly giving rise to a spectrum of disorders ranging from classical lissencephaly to milder forms such as double cortex syndrome or pachygyria. Classical or type I lissencephaly differs from type II or cobblestone lissencephaly. In cobblestone lissencephaly, the defect is presumably an overmigration of neurons past their targets, giving rise to the abnormally bumpy surface.

Periventricular heterotopia

Periventricular heterotopia is a disorder where neurons fail to begin the process of migration. Neurons are generated near the ventricular zone but do not start the process of migration to their destinations. Instead, they are stuck and collect around the ventricles, giving rise to the distinct appearance on brain imaging.

Other neuronal migration disorders

Zellweger syndrome is a disorder of neuronal migration that may consist of abnormally large folds (pachygyria) and heterotopias spread throughout the brain. It is thought to be due to a defect in peroxisome metabolism, a pathway by which cells break down waste products. The relationship between this metabolic defect and neuronal migration is unclear at this time. Kallman syndrome is a disorder where cells fail to migrate to the portion of the brain controlling smell as well as the hypothalamus, a region that controls hormone secretion. The mechanism underlying this disease is unclear.

Schizencephaly is grouped as a neuronal migration disorder although the exact etiology is unknown. Schizencephaly is an example of abnormal neuronal migration that may occur locally rather than globally. In schizencephaly, an early insult to the brain in the form of an infection, **stroke**, or genetic defect leads to abnormal migration of neurons in a portion of the brain and subsequent lack of developed brain tissue, giving rise to the characteristic brain clefts that define this syndrome. Schizencephaly may show a wide range of presentations, with bilateral clefts that vary in size and extent of involvement.

Polymicrogyria refers to an abnormal amount of small convolutions (gyri) in affected areas of the cerebral cortex and is believed to be a neuronal migration disorder, although the exact etiology is unknown.

Demographics

Neuronal migration disorders are rare overall, but the exact incidence is unknown. Patients may have very mild degrees of the different disorders and may not be diagnosed if they do not manifest symptoms, making the actual incidence difficult to determine.

Causes and symptoms

The majority of neuronal migration disorders seen in clinical practice are thought to be genetic in cause. Much of what is known about neuronal migration disorders to date has been discovered from intense research identifying the genes affected in individuals with these diseases. The widespread abnormal expression of defective genes leads to the global nature of the disorders, contrary to acquired developmental brain insults, which lead to more localized defects. Several genes have been implicated in causing the various disorders, and they continue to be identified. The most well characterized genes include DCX on the X chromosome, responsible for double cortex syndrome, and LIS1 on chromosome 17, the first gene identified for lissencephaly. Cobblestone lissencephaly is associated with abnormalities in fukutin, a gene responsible for Fukuyama **muscular dystrophy**, a syndrome consisting of muscle weakness and cobblestone lissencephaly. Periventricular heterotopia is associated with abnormalities of the filamin1 gene on the X chromosome. DCX, LIS1, and filamin1 are genes responsible for controlling the mechanics of cell movement during neuronal migration. Schizencephaly has been associated with abnormalities in EMX2, a transcription factor gene whose role in neuronal migration is as yet unidentified. Neuronal migration disorders can also be associated with early insults to the brain from infections or damage from stroke.

Most neuronal migration disorders present with some combination of epilepsy, mental retardation, and abnormalities in head size, known as **microcephaly**. Some patients, such as those with small heterotopias, may have no symptoms at all since the severity of the defect is very mild. Patients may also have **cerebral palsy** or abnormalities in muscle tone. Depending on the severity of the malformation, the level of mental retardation may vary from mild to severe. Patients with lissencephaly are usually severely delayed, have failure to thrive, and are microcephalic. They may also have accompanying eye problems. Patients with double cortex syndrome or schizencephaly may have milder symptoms and may only present with **seizures**. Schizencephaly may have associated complications of increased fluid pressure in the brain, known as **hydrocephalus**. Periventricular heterotopia and polymicrogyria may present with only seizures. Some neuronal migration disorders such as lissencephaly may be part of a larger syndrome affecting other body parts such as the muscle, eyes, or face.

Diagnosis

Diagnosis is usually made by neuroimaging. **CT scan** or **MRI** of the brain will show the characteristic abnormality. MRI has better resolution and may detect polymicrogyria or small heterotopias more easily than CT. Genetic testing is available for patients with lissencephaly to identify whether the DCX or LIS1 gene is defective. Knowledge of the genes affected allows for counseling and family planning. Laboratory tests are not useful in diagnosis.

Treatment team

Management of neuronal migration disorders involves a pediatrician, pediatric **neurologist** and physical therapists. With symptoms of later onset, an adult neurologist may be involved in treating symptoms of seizures. Rehabilitation specialists may help in prescribing medications for cerebral palsy or increased muscle tone. A case manager may be involved in coordinating care and resources.

Treatment

There are no known cures for the various neuronal migration disorders at this time. The majority of treatments are directed towards symptoms caused by the malformed brain. Seizures may be treated with anticonvulsant medications. Refractory seizures may respond to neurosurgical removal of abnormal brain tissue. Neurosurgery may be required to relieve hydrocephalus, by placement of a shunt. Increased muscle tone may respond to injections of **botulinum toxin** or muscle relaxants. Patients may require feeding through a tube due to inability to swallow normally.

Recovery and rehabilitation

Due to the congenital nature of neuronal migration disorders, most patients do not recover from their symptoms. The course of disease tends to be static. Physical and occupational therapists may help treat symptoms of weakness or increased tone that limit mobility and daily hand use.

Clinical trials

A clinical trial is currently under way and is funded by the National Institutes of Health to identify genes responsible for neuronal migration disorders such as lissencephaly and schizencephaly. For contact information for the Walsh Lab Site, see Resources below.

Prognosis

There is no known cure for any of the neuronal migration disorders. Due to the congenital nature of the diseases, the symptoms tend to be static and do not improve. The prognosis varies for each individual depending on the extent of the defect and the accompanying neurologic deficits. Most individuals with severe malformations such as classical lissencephaly or bilateral schizencephaly will die at an early age due to failure to thrive or infections such as pneumonia. Their cognitive development stays at the three month level. Patients with milder forms such as unilateral schizencephaly, periventricular heterotopia, or subcortical band heterotopia may have mild mental retardation and seizures only and live a normal life span.

Special concerns

Educational and Social Needs

Due to developmental disability, children with neuronal migration disorders who survive beyond the age of two may benefit from special education programs. Various state and federal programs are available to help individuals and their families with meeting these needs.

Resources

BOOKS

"Congenital Anomalies of the Nervous System." In *Nelson Textbook of Pediatrics*, 17th edition, edited by Richard E. Behrman, Robert M. Kliegman, and Hal B. Jenson. Philadelphia, PA: Saunders 2004.

Menkes, John H., and Harvey Sarnat, eds. *Childhood Neurology*, 6th edition. Philadelphia: Lippincott Williams & Wilkins, 2000.

PERIODICALS

Gleeson, J. G. "Neuronal Migration Disorders." *Mental Retardation and Developmental Disabilities Research Reviews* 7 (2001): 167–171.

Guerrini, R., and R. Carrozzo. "Epilepsy and Genetic Malformations of the Cerebral Cortex." *American Journal of Medical Genetics* 106 (2001): 160–173.

Kato, M., and W. B. Dobyns. "Lissencephaly and the molecular basis of neuronal migration." *Human Molecular Genetics* 12 (2003): R89–R96.

Ross, M. E., and C. A. Walsh. "Human Brain Malformations and Their Lessons for Neuronal Migration." *Annual Review of Neuroscience* 24 (2001): 1041–1070.

WEBSITES

Cephalic Disorders Information Page. National Institutes of Neurological Disorders and Stroke (NINDS). <http://www.ninds.nih.gov/health_and_medical/pubs/cephalic_disorders.htm>.

ORGANIZATIONS

March of Dimes Birth Defects Foundation. 1275 Mamaroneck Avenue, White Plains, NY 10605. (914) 428-7100 or

(888) 663-4637; Fax: (914) 428-8203. askus@ marchofdimes.com. <http://www.marchofdimes.com>.

Peter T. Lin, MD

Neuropathologist

Definition

A pathologist is a medical doctor who is specialized in the study and diagnosis of the changes that are produced in the body by various diseases. A neuropathologist is a specialized pathologist who is concerned with diseases of the **central nervous system** (the brain and spinal cord). Often a neuropathologist is concerned with the diagnosis of brain tumors.

A neuropathologist is also an expert in the various aspects of diseases of the nervous system and skeletal muscles. This range of disease includes degenerative diseases, infections, metabolic disorders, immunologic disorders, disorders of blood vessels, and physical injury. A neuropathologist functions as the primary consultant to neurologists and neurosurgeons.

Description

A neuropathologist is a medical doctor who has pursued specialized training. Aspects of this training include neurology, anatomy, cell biology, and biochemistry. Typically, a patient will not see a neuropathologist. Rather, the specialist works in the background, in the setting of the laboratory, to assist in the patient's diagnosis. In the path that leads to the diagnosis of a tumor, disease, or other malady, a neuropathologist typically becomes involved at the request of a **neurologist**. It is the neurologist who suspects a problem or seeks to confirm the presence of a tumor, based on tests such as **magnetic resonance imaging (MRI)** or a computed assisted tomography (CAT) scan. The neurologist can obtain some of the tissue of concern in a procedure known as a **biopsy**, as well as obtaining fluid or cell samples.

It is this material that is sent to the pathology lab where the neuropathologist seeks to identify the nature of the problem. The diagnosis of brain and spinal cord related damage often involves a visual look at the samples using the extremely high magnification of the electron microscope. The neuropathologist can assess from the appearance of the sample whether the sample is unaffected or damaged. For example, in brain tissue obtained from a patient with suspected **Alzheimer disease**, the neuropathologist will look for evidence of the presence of

amyloid plaques, which are caused by abnormal folding of protein. As well, the neuropathologist will look for other diagnostic signs that support or do not support the suspected malady.

In the case of a tumor, part of a neuropathologist's responsibility is to identify the tumor and grade it as malignant or benign. This is no small task, as there are literally hundreds of different types of tumors. The correct identification greatly aids the subsequent treatment process and the patient's prognosis.

The neuropathological analysis of a tumor is concerned mainly with two areas. The first is the origin of the tumor in the brain. Determining the tumor's origin aids in naming the tumor. Secondly, the neuropathologist determines if the tumor displays signs of rapid growth. The speed of growth of the tumor can be quantified as a grade. A result such as "grade three astrocytoma" is very informative to the neurologist. Even if the neuropathologist determines that a brain or spinal cord tumor is benign, the location of the tumor may still pose serious health risks, and this important determination is also usually made by the neuropathologist.

Another important tool that a neuropathologist uses to examine tissue samples is histology. The treatment of a thin section of a sample with specific compounds that will bind to and highlight (stain) regions of interest in the specimen allows the neuropathologist to determine if the stained regions are normal or abnormal in character. The histological stains can be applied to a section that has been sliced from the sample at room temperature or at a very low temperature. The use of frozen sections can help preserve structural detail in the specimen that might otherwise be changed at a higher temperature.

The assessment of a stained specimen by the neuropathologist is typically done by examining the material using a light microscope. This type of microscope does not magnify the specimen nearly as much as does the electron microscope. But such high-power magnification is not necessary to detect the cellular changes in the stained specimen. By carefully selecting the stain regimen, a skilled neuropathologist can reveal much detail about a specimen. Histological examinations can also be done much more quickly and easily than electron microscopic examinations. Saving time can be important in diagnosis and treatment, especially when dealing with brain tumors.

Finally, one of the consultative duties of a neuropathologist can also include legal testimony. Their expert knowledge can be useful in court cases in which the mental state or functional ability of a person is an important consideration.

Resources

BOOKS

Nelson, James S. *Principles and Practice of Neuropathology.* New York: Oxford University Press, 2003.

OTHER

Department of Neurology, University of Debrecen, Hungary. *Neuroanatomy and Neuropathology on the Internet.* <http://www.neuropat.dote.hu/> (February 10, 2004).

ORGANIZATIONS

American Association of Neuropathologists (AANP). 2085 Adelbert Rd., Cleveland, OH 44106. (216) 368–2488; Fax: (216) 368–8964. aanp@cwru.edu. <http://www.aanp-jnen.com>.

Brian Douglas Hoyle, PhD

Neuropathy, hereditary *see* **Charcot-Marie-Tooth disorder**

Neuropsychological testing

Definition

Clinical neuropsychology is a field with historical origins in both psychology and neurology. The primary activity of neuropsychologists is assessment of brain functioning through structured and systematic behavioral observation. Neuropsychological tests are designed to examine a variety of cognitive abilities, including speed of information processing, attention, memory, language, and executive functions, which are necessary for goal-directed behavior. By testing a range of cognitive abilities and examining patterns of performance in different cognitive areas, neuropsychologists can make inferences about underlying brain function. Neuropsychological testing is an important component of the assessment and treatment of **traumatic brain injury**, **dementia**, neurological conditions, and psychiatric disorders. Neuropsychological testing is also an important tool for examining the effects of toxic substances and medical conditions on brain functioning.

Description

As early as the seventeenth century, scientists theorized about associations between regions of the brain and specific functions. The French philosopher Descartes believed the human soul could be localized to a specific brain structure, the pineal gland. In the eighteenth century, Franz Gall advocated the theory that specific mental qualities such as spirituality or aggression were governed by discrete parts of the brain. In contrast, Pierre Flourens contended that the brain was an integrated system that governed cognitive functioning in a holistic manner. Later discoveries indicated that brain function is both localized and integrated. Paul Broca and Karl Wernicke furthered understanding of localization and integration of function when they reported the loss of language abilities in patients with lesions to two regions in the left hemisphere of the brain.

The modern field of neuropsychology emerged in the twentieth century, combining theories based on anatomical observations of neurology with the techniques of psychology, including objective observation of behavior and the use of statistical analysis to differentiate functional abilities and define impairment. The famous Soviet **neuropsychologist** Alexander Luria played a major role in defining neuropsychology as it is practiced today. Luria formulated two principle goals of neuropsychology: to localize brain lesions and analyze psychological activities arising from brain function through behavioral observation. American neuropsychologist Ralph Reitan emphasized the importance of using standardized psychometric tests to guide systematic observations of brain-behavior relationships.

Before the introduction of neuroimaging techniques like the computed tomography (CAT or **CT**) scan and **magnetic resonance imaging (MRI)**, the primary focus of neuropsychology was diagnosis. Since clinicians lacked non-surgical methods for directly observing brain lesions or structural abnormalities in living patients, neuropsychological testing was the only way to determine which part of the brain was affected in a given patient. Neuropsychological tests can identify syndromes associated with problems in a particular area of the brain. For instance, a patient who performs well on tests of attention, memory, and language, but poorly on tests that require visual spatial skills such as copying a complex geometric figure or making designs with colored blocks, may have dysfunction in the right parietal lobe, the region of the brain involved in complex processing of visual information. When a patient complains of problems with verbal communication after a **stroke**, separate tests that examine

Key Terms

Abstraction Ability to think about concepts or ideas separate from specific examples.

Battery A number of separate items (such as tests) used together. In psychology, a group or series of tests given with a common purpose, such as personality assessment or measurement of intelligence.

Executive functions A set of cognitive abilities that control and regulate other abilities and behaviors. Necessary for goal-directed behavior, they include the ability to initiate and stop actions, to monitor and change behavior as needed, and to plan future behavior when faced with novel tasks and situations.

Hemisphere One side of the brain, right or left.

Psychometric Pertaining to testing and measurement of mental or psychological abilities. Psychometric tests convert an individual's psychological traits and attributes into a numerical estimation or evaluation.

Syndrome A group of symptoms that together characterize a disease or disorder.

production and comprehension of language help neuropsychologists identify the location of the stroke in the left hemisphere. Neuropsychological tests can also be used as screening tests to see if more extensive diagnostic evaluation is appropriate. Neuropsychological screening of elderly people complaining of memory problems can help identify those at risk for dementia versus those experiencing normal age-related memory loss.

As neuropsychological testing came to play a less vital role in localization of brain dysfunction, clinical neuropsychologists found new uses for their skills and knowledge. By clarifying which cognitive abilities are impaired or preserved in patients with brain injury or illness, neuropsychologists can predict how well individuals will respond to different forms of treatment or rehabilitation. Although patterns of test scores illustrate profiles of cognitive strength and weakness, neuropsychologists can also learn a great deal about patients by observing how they approach a particular test. For example, two patients can complete a test in very different ways yet obtain similar scores. One patient may work slowly and methodically, making no errors, while another rushes through the test, making several errors but quickly correcting them. Some individuals persevere despite repeated failure on a series of

test items, while others refuse to continue after a few failures. These differences might not be apparent in test scores, but can help clinicians choose among rehabilitation and treatment approaches.

Performance on neuropsychological tests is usually evaluated through comparison to the average performance of large samples of normal individuals. Most tests include tables of these normal scores, often divided into groups based on demographic variables like age and education that appear to affect cognitive functioning. This allows individuals to be compared to appropriate peers.

The typical neuropsychological examination evaluates sensation and perception, gross and fine motor skills, basic and complex attention, visual spatial skills, receptive and productive language abilities, recall and recognition memory, and executive functions such as cognitive flexibility and abstraction. Motivation and personality are often assessed as well, particularly when clients are seeking financial compensation for injuries, or cognitive complaints that are not typical of the associated injury or illness.

Some neuropsychologists prefer to use fixed test batteries like the Halstead-Reitan battery or the Luria-Nebraska battery for all patients. These batteries include tests of a wide range of cognitive functions, and those who advocate their use believe that all functions must be assessed in each patient in order to avoid diagnostic bias or failure to detect subtle problems. The more common approach today, however, is to use a flexible battery based on hypotheses generated through a clinical interview, observation of the patient, and review of medical records. While this approach is more prone to bias, it has the advantage of preventing unnecessary testing. Since patients often find neuropsychological testing stressful and fatiguing, and these factors can negatively influence performance, advocates of the flexible battery approach argue that tailoring test batteries to particular patients can provide more accurate information.

Resources
BOOKS

Lezak, Muriel Deutsh. *Neuropsychological Assessment.* 3rd edition. New York: Oxford University Press, 1995.

Mitrushina, Maura N., Kyle B. Boone, and Louis F. D'Elia. *Handbook of Normative Data for Neuropsychological Assessment.* New York: Oxford University Press, 1999.

Spreen, Otfried and Esther Strauss. *A Compendium of Neuropsychological Tests: Administration, Norms, and Commentary.* 2nd Edition. New York: Oxford University Press, 1998.

Walsh, Kevin and David Darby. *Neuropsychology: A Clinical Approach.* 4th edition. Edinburgh: Churchill Livingstone, 1999.

ORGANIZATIONS

American Psychological Association. Division 40, 750 First Street, NE, Washington, DC 20002-4242. <http://www.div40.org/>.

International Neuropsychological Society. 700 Ackerman Road, Suite 550, Columbus, OH 43202. <http://www.acs.ohio-state.edu/ins/>.

National Academy of Neuropsychology. 2121 South Oneida Street, Suite 550, Denver, CO 80224-2594. <http://nanonline.org/>.

Danielle Barry, MS
Rosalyn Carson-DeWitt, MD

Neuropsychologist

Definition

A clinical psychologist is a licensed or certified professional who holds a doctoral degree in psychology and works in the area of prevention and treatment of emotional and mental disorders. A neuropsychologist is typically a clinical psychologist with additional training and experience in neuropsychology, an area of psychology that focuses on brain-behavior relationships.

Description

Neuropsychologists are licensed professionals within the field of psychology. Most have a doctorate (PhD) in psychology with additional years of post-doctoral training in clinical neuropsychology. The graduate education and training for neuropsychologists emphasizes **brain anatomy**, brain function, and brain injury or disease. The neuropsychologist also learns how to administer and interpret certain types of standardized tests that can detect effects of brain dysfunction. Neuropsychologists may receive certification from the American Board of Clinical Neuropsychology (ABCN), the member board of the American Board of Professional Psychology (ABPP) that administers the competency exam in the specialty of clinical neuropsychology.

Neuropsychologists are not medical doctors; they are consultants who work closely with physicians, teachers, and other professionals to assess an individual's brain functioning. With the aid of standardized tests, neuropsychologists help to diagnose and assess patients with a variety of medical conditions that impact intellectual, cognitive, or behavioral functioning. They may also provide psychotherapy or other therapeutic interventions.

Neuropsychologists usually work in private practice or in institutional settings such as hospitals or clinics. Most neuropsychologists are in clinical practice; that is, their primary responsibilities include evaluation and treatment of patients. A neuropsychologist's practice may include pediatric neuropsychology, a specialty that concerns the relationship between learning and behavior and a child's brain, and forensic neuropsychology, an area that deals with determination of disability for legal purposes. In addition to seeing patients, neuropsychologists may also engage in professional activities such as teaching, research, and administration.

Reasons for referral

Neuropsychological evaluation is generally warranted for patients who show signs of problems with memory or thinking. Such problems may manifest as changes in language, learning, organization, perception, coordination, or personality. These symptoms can be due to a variety of medical, neurological, psychological, or genetic causes. Examples of conditions that may prompt a referral to a neuropsychologist include **stroke**, brain trauma, **dementia** (such as **Alzheimer's disease**), **seizures**, psychiatric illness, toxic exposures (such as to lead), or an illness that increases the chance of brain injury (such as diabetes or alcoholism).

Neuropsychological evaluation

The purpose of a neuropsychological evaluation is to provide useful information about an individual's brain functioning. Such information may help a physician, teacher, or other professional:

• make or confirm a diagnosis

• find problems with brain functioning

• determine individual thinking skill strengths and weaknesses

• guide treatment decisions such as rehabilitation, special education, vocational counseling, or other services

• track changes in brain functioning over time

Neuropsychological evaluation can reveal abnormalities or even subtle difference in brain functioning that may not be detected by other means. For example, testing can help determine if a person's mild memory changes represent the normal aging process or if they signify a neurological disorder such as Alzheimer's disease.

During the evaluation, a neuropsychologist may take a medical history, review medical records, and administer and interpret a series of standardized tests. Though the time required to conduct a neuropsychological exam varies, the exam can last six to eight hours and may span the course of several visits. The standardized tests used in

Key Terms

Psychotherapy Psychological counseling that seeks to determine the underlying causes of a patient's depression. The form of this counseling may be cognitive/behavioral, interpersonal, or psychodynamic.

a neuropsychological assessment involve answering questions ("paper and pencil" or computerized tests) or performing hands-on activities at a table. The goal of testing is to evaluate how well the brain functions when it performs certain tasks. A trained examiner, also called a technician, may give or score the tests. Testing does not include x rays, electrodes, needles, or other invasive procedures. Tests used may examine one or more of the following areas:

• general intellect

• attention, memory, and learning

• reasoning and problem-solving

• planning and organization

• visual-spatial skills (perception)

• language

• sensory skills

• motor functions

• academic skills

• emotions

• behavior

• personality

Neuropsychologists tailor their services to the patient's needs and the reason for referral. For example, in a child who is having difficulty reading, the neuropsychologist will try to determine if this difficulty is related to a problem with attention, language, auditory processing, or another cause.

The neuropsychologist's conclusions about an individual's brain functioning may complement findings from brain imaging studies such as a computerized topography (CT) scan or **magnetic resonance imaging (MRI)**, or the results of blood tests. Depending on the circumstances, a neuropsychologist may treat the patient with interventions such as cognitive rehabilitation, behavior management, or psychotherapy. A neuropsychologist may also recommend

referrals to other health care specialists, including neurologists, psychiatrists, psychologists, **social workers**, nurses, special education teachers, therapists, or vocational counselors.

Resources

BOOKS

Stringer, A. Y., and E. L. Cooley. *Pathways to Prominence: Reflections of Twentieth Century Neuropsychologists.* Philadelphia: Psychology Press, 2001.

Joseph, R. *Neuropsychiatry, Neuropsychology, and Clinical Neuroscience: Emotion, Evolution, Cognition, Language, Memory, Brain Damage, and Abnormal Development.* Baltimore: Lippincott, Williams & Wilkins, 1996.

PERIODICALS

Division 40, American Psychological Association. "Definition of a Clinical Neuropsychologist." *The Clinical Neuropsychologist* 3 (1989): 22.

Sweet, J. J., E. A. Peck, C. Abromowitz, and S. Etzweiler. "National Academy of Neuropsychology/Division 40 of the American Psychological Association Practice Survey of Clinical Neuropsychology in the United States, Part I: Practitioner and Practice Characteristics, Professional Activities, and Time Requirements." *The Clinical Neuropsychologist* 16 (2002): 109–127.

Therapeutics and Technology Subcommittee of the American Academy of Neurology. "Assessment: Neuropsychological Testing of Adults. Considerations for Neurologists." *Neurology* 47 (1996): 592–599.

WEBSITES

National Academy of Neuropsychology (NAN). *Neuropsychological Evaluation Brochure.* 2001 (April 27, 2004). <http://www.nanonline.org/paio/PaioResHandout.shtm>.

National Academy of Neuropsychology (NAN). *Neuropsychological Evaluation Information Sheet.* 2001 (April 27, 2004). <http://www.nanonline.org/paio/PaioResHandout.shtm>.

National Academy of Neuropsychology (NAN). *Pediatric Neuropsychological Evaluation Information Sheet: For Parents.* 2001 (April 27, 2004). <http://www.nanonline.org/paio/PaioResHandout.shtm>.

National Academy of Neuropsychology (NAN). *Pediatric Neuropsychological Evaluation Information Sheet: For Physicians.* 2001 (April 27, 2004). <http://www.nanonline.org/paio/PaioResHandout.shtm>.

Public Interest Advisory Committee, Division 40 (Clinical Neuropsychology), American Psychological Association. *Pediatric Neuropsychology Brochure.* 2000 (April 27, 2004). <http://www.nanonline.org/paio/PaioResHandout.shtm>.

Public Interest Advisory Committee, Division 40 (Clinical Neuropsychology), American Psychological Association.

Clinical Neuropsychology Brochure. 2000 (April 27, 2004). <http://www.nanonline.org/paio/PaioResHandout.shtm>.

ORGANIZATIONS

National Academy of Neuropsychology. 2121 South Oneida Street, Suite 550, Denver, CO 80224-2594. (303) 691-3694. office@nanonline.org. <http://www.NANonline.org>.

American Psychological Association, Division 40—Clinical Neuropsychology Homepage. 750 First Street NE, Washington, DC 20002-4242. (202) 336-6013; Fax: (202) 218-3599. kcooke@apa.org. <http://www.div40.org>.

Dawn Cardeiro, MS, CGC

Neurosarcoidosis

Definition

Neurosarcoidosis refers to an autoimmune disorder of unknown cause, which causes deposition of inflammatory lesions called granulomas in the **central nervous system**.

Description

Sarcoidosis is a multisystem disease of unknown cause. It is thought that the disorder is caused by an inflammatory reaction in the body which forms a lesion called a granuloma. Neurosarcoidosis is characterized by formation of granulomas in the central nervous system. The granulomas consist of inflammatory cells (lymphocytes, mononuclear phagocytes) which function during inflammatory reactions. The disorder is often unrecognized since most patients do not exhibit symptoms. Typically the disease is diagnosed by routine chest x ray. If symptoms are present they usually include respiratory problems (shortness of breath, cough) since the lungs are affected most frequently.

Neurological description

Patients can have a broad range of clinical signs and symptoms that typically could involve mononeuropathy, **peripheral neuropathy**, or central nervous system involvement. Mononeuropathy problems can include facial nerve palsy, impaired taste and smell, blindness (or other eye problems such as double vision, visual field defects, blurry vision, dry/sore eyes), or speech problems (impaired swollowing or hoarseness). Patients can also develop vertigo, weakness of neck muscles and tongue deviation and atrophy.

Peripheral nerve involvement

Neurosarcoidosis can cause damage to peripheral nerves that can affect motor nerves (responsible for movement of muscles) and sensory nerves (responsible for sensation). Symptoms of sensory loss include loss of sensation and abnormal sensation (numb, painful, tingling sensations) over the thorax (chest) and the areas where stockings and gloves are usually worn. Motor neurosarcoidosis is characterized by weakness that can progress to immobility and joint stiffness.

Central nervous system (CNS) involvement can affect the pituitary gland, **cerebellum**, or cerebral cortex. The spinal cord is rarely involved. Signs and symptoms of CNS involvement can include polyuria, polydipsia, obesity, impotence, amenorrhea, confusion/amnesia (short and long term memory), meningitis, and **seizures** (focal seizures).

Demographics

Sarcoid disorders are more prevalent in African Americans, and in the United States there seems to be a variable prevalence within different states. The prevalence is much higher in the southeastern United States among both Caucasian and African Americans. The prevalence is high in Puerto Rico, reaching approximately 175 cases per 100,000 persons. The frequency for neurological involvement for all cases of sarcoid disease is 5%. However, neurological involvement has been reported to occur in up to 5% to 16% of cases. Internationally the incidence of sarcoid varies widely. In Spain the incidence is low (0.04 per 100,000) whereas in Sweden the incidence is high, representing 64 cases per 100,000 persons. Studies reveal the prevalence in London is 27 per 100,000 and 97 per 100,000 among Irish men. In the Caribbean, studies indicate that the prevalence is as high as 200 per 100,000 in men from the West Indies and 13% of individuals from Martinique.

There does not seem to be a racial predilection for the development of sarcoid neuropathy. Sarcoid disease is uncommon in Chinese, Inuits, Southeast Asians, Canadian Indians, New Zealand Maoris and native Japanese. Death from neurosarcoidosis is unusual. About 66% of patients with neurosarcoidosis have self-limited monophasic illness. Approximately 33% have a chronic remitting and relapsing course. Neurosarcoidosis commonly occurs in adults aged 25-50 years. Neurosarcoidosis is not common in children, but if it does occur, it affects children age 9-15 years. The clinical signs in children are different than in adults. When neurosarcoidosis is present in children over the age of eight, there is usually a triad of signs which include arthritis, uveitis, and cutaneous nodules. In children ocular (eye) problems occur in approximately 100% of cases, which typically manifest as iritis and/or anterior vitreitis. For all cases, if the nervous system is involved it usually occurs within two years of disease onset.

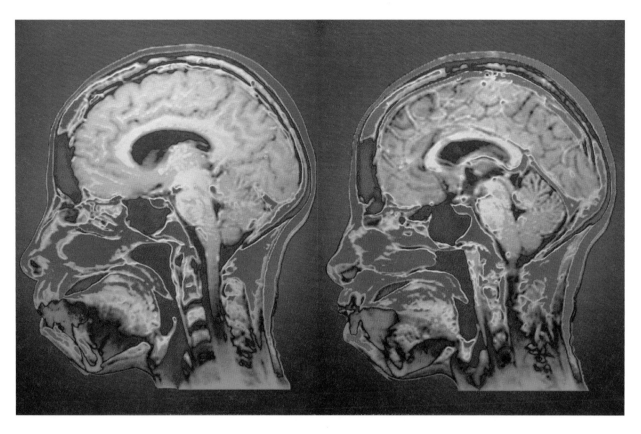

Cerebral MRIs of a 52-year-old patient with neurosarcoidosis. The MRIs show the presence of numerous granulomas in the meninges and cisterns. *(Phototake, Inc. All rights reserved.)*

Causes and symptoms

The causes of sarcoid disease are not clear. Current evidence suggests that sarcoidosis is due to the abnormal proliferation of a certain cell called a T-helper cell, which functions to help immune cells attack a foreign substance. The abnormal proliferation of T-helper cells is thought to result from an exaggerated response to a foreign substance or to self cells (a condition referred to as autoimmunity, in which for unknown reasons, the body's natural defense cells attack normal cells in organs).

During physical examination patients may exhibit weakness, absence of tendon reflexes, lack of sensation in a stocking and glove distribution, atrophy of muscles, and focal mononueropathies that may affect the cranial nerves (causing problem with hearing, vision, smell, balance, or paralysis of facial muscles). Some patients may develop Heerfordt syndrome characterized by fever, uveitis, swelling of the parotid gland, and facial palsy.

Diagnosis

Blood analysis is essential since patients may have increased erythrocyte sedimentation rate (ESR) or anemia (hypochromic microcytic type). Blood analysis can provide information concerning multiple organs (kidney, liver, blood) and this is important since sarcoidosis is a multisystem disease (affects many different organs in the body). **CT** and **MRI** scans are important in assessing neurosarcoidosis. MRI is the imaging tool of choice in cases of neurosarcoidosis, because of the high quality superior images obtained. The presence of a mass or lesion in the CNS can be visualized by MRI images. To confirm the diagnosis it is necessary to take a **biopsy** of either muscle or nerve tissue. Examination of the tissue specimen with a microscope reveals the characteristic granuloma within tissues.

Treatment team

The effects of neurosarcoidosis can involve several symptoms from different organ systems. The treatment team consists of a **neurologist**, neurosurgeon, endocrinologist, rheumatologist, and pulmonologist.

Treatment

There is no definitive treatment, but corticosteroids remain the standard treatment. The most commonly used oral corticosteroid is prednisone, which works to decrease inflammatory actions in the body that are responsible for granuloma formation. Doses are usually tapered down.

Key Terms

Amenorrhea The absence or abnormal stoppage of menstrual periods.

Anterior vitreitis Inflammation of the corpus vitreum, which surrounds and fills the inner portion of the eyeball between the lens and the retina.

Atrophy The progressive wasting and loss of function of any part of the body.

Iritis Inflammation of the iris, the membrane in the pupil, the colored portion of the eye. It is characterized by photophobia, pain, and inflammatory congestion.

Mononeuropathy Disorder involving a single nerve.

Pituitary gland The most important of the endocrine glands (glands that release hormones directly

into the bloodstream), the pituitary is located at the base of the brain. Sometimes referred to as the "master gland," it regulates and controls the activities of other endocrine glands and many body processes including growth and reproductive function. Also called the hypophysis.

Polydipsia Excessive thirst.

Polyuria Excessive production and excretion of urine.

Uveitis Inflammation of all or part the uvea. The uvea is a continuous layer of tissue which consists of the iris, the ciliary body, and the choroid. The uvea lies between the retina and sclera.

Vertigo A feeling of dizziness together with a sensation of movement and a feeling of rotating in space.

Additionally, patients can be given immunosuppressant agents (e.g., cyclosporine) which can suppress autoimmune responses (which are responsible for granuloma formation). Surgery is rare and reserved for cases that require removal of a mass (space-occupying lesion) in the brain.

Recovery and rehabilitation

Neurosarcoidosis is a slowly chronic disease with a progressive course, which is fatal in about 50% of patients. Follow-up visits with a neurologist every three to six months are advisable. During visits the neurologist will monitor progress and make recommendations.

Clinical trials

There are several studies currently active concerning sarcoidosis. The National Heart, Lung and Blood Institute Drug study are conducting clinical research trials with patients who have lung involvement (pulmonary sarcoidosis). Contact Pauline Barnes, RN (1-877-644-5864) or visit their website: <http://www.sarcoidresearch.org>.

Prognosis

Spontaneous resolution of neurosarcoidosis can occur but it is not common. Many patients with neurosarcoidosis have a slow chronic and progressive course with intermittent exacerbations. Neurosarcoidosis responds to steroid therapy, but long-term outcome of neurologic impairment is unknown.

Special concerns

Sarcoidosis is difficult to diagnose, and sometimes a delay can cause patients to get sicker before proper treatment is initiated. On rare occasions a patient may even die because the diagnosis was not suspected. Caution must be taken to exclude other diseases before a final diagnosis is made. Additionally, before corticosteroid therapy is initiated, the clinician must rule out an infectious cause.

Resources
BOOKS

Goldman, Lee et al. *Cecil's Textbook of Medicine* 21st ed. Philadelphia: WB. Saunders Company, 2000.

Noble, John., et al eds. *Textbook of Primary Care Medicine* 3rd ed. St. Louis: Mosby, Inc., 2001.

PERIODICALS

Nikhar, N.K. *Sarcoidosis and Neuropathy* .

Suleman, Amer. *Neurosarcoidosis.*

WEBSITES

National Organization for Rare Disorders (NORD). <http://www.rarediseases.org>.

ORGANIZATIONS

Sarcoidosis Research Institute. 3475 Central Avenue, Memphis, TN 38111. (901) 766-6951; Fax: (901) 744-7294. paula@sarcoidosisresearch.org. <http://www.sarcoidosisresearch.org>.

Laith Farid Gulli, M.D.
Nicole Mallory, M.S.,PA-C

Neurotransmitters

Definition

Neurotransmitters are chemicals that allow the movement of information from one neuron across the gap between it and the adjacent neuron. The release of neurotransmitters from one area of a neuron and the recognition of the chemicals by a receptor site on the adjacent neuron causes an electrical reaction that facilitates the release of the neurotransmitter and its movement across the gap.

Description

The transmission of information from one neuron to another depends on the ability of the information to traverse the gap (also known as the synapse) between the terminal end of one neuron and the receptor end of an adjacent neuron. The transfer is accomplished by neurotransmitters.

In 1921, an Austrian scientist named Otto Loewi discovered the first neurotransmitter. He named the compound "vagusstoff," as he was experimenting with the vagus nerve of frog hearts. Now, this compound is known as acetylcholine.

Neurotransmitters are manufactured in a region of a neuron known as the cell body. From there, they are transported to the terminal end of the neuron, where they are enclosed in small membrane-bound bags called vesicles (the sole exception is nitric oxide, which is not contained inside a vesicle, but is released from the neuron soon after being made). In response to an action potential signal, the neurotransmitters are released from the terminal area when the vesicle membrane fuses with the neuron membrane. The neurotransmitter chemical then diffuses across the synapse.

At the other side of the synapse, neurotransmitters encounter receptors. An individual receptor is a transmembrane protein, meaning part of the protein projects from both the inside and outside surfaces of the neuron membrane, with the rest of the protein spanning the membrane. A receptor may be capable of binding to a neurotransmitter, similar to the way a key fits into a lock. Not all neurotransmitters can bind to all receptors; there is selectivity within the binding process.

When a receptor site recognizes a neurotransmitter, the site is described as becoming activated. This can result in depolarization or hyperpolarization, which acts directly on the affected neurons, or the activation of another molecule (second messenger) that eventually alters the flow of information between neurons.

Depolarization stimulates the release of the neurotransmitter from the terminal end of the neuron. Hyperpolarization makes it less likely that this release will occur.

This dual mechanism provides a means of control over when and how quickly information can pass from neuron to neuron. The binding of a neurotransmitter to a receptor triggers a biological effect. However, once the recognition process is complete, its ability to stimulate the biological effect is lost. The receptor is then ready to bind another neurotransmitter.

Neurotransmitters can also be inactivated by degradation by a specific enzyme (e.g., acetylcholinesterase degrades acetylcholine). Cells known as astrocytes can remove neurotransmitters from the receptor area. Finally, some neurotransmitters (norepinephrine, dopamine, and serotonin) can be reabsorbed into the terminal region of the neuron.

Since Loewi's discovery of acetylcholine, many neurotransmitters have been discovered, including the following partial list:

- Acetylcholine: Acetylcholine is particularly important in the stimulation of muscle tissue. After stimulation, acetylcholine degrades to acetate and choline, which are absorbed back into the first neuron to form another acetylcholine molecule. The poison curare blocks transmission of acetylcholine. Some nerve gases inhibit the breakdown of acetylcholine, producing a continuous stimulation of the receptor cells, and spasms of muscles such as the heart.

- Epinephrine (adrenaline) and norepinephrine: These compounds are secreted principally from the adrenal gland. Secretion causes an increased heart rate and the enhanced production of glucose as a ready energy source (the "fight or flight" response).

- Dopamine: Dopamine facilitates critical brain functions and, when unusual quantities are present, abnormal dopamine neurotransmission may play a role in **Parkinson's disease**, certain addictions, and schizophrenia.

- Serotonin: Synthesized from the amino acid tryptophan, serotonin is assumed to play a biochemical role in mood and mood disorders, including anxiety, **depression**, and bipolar disorder.

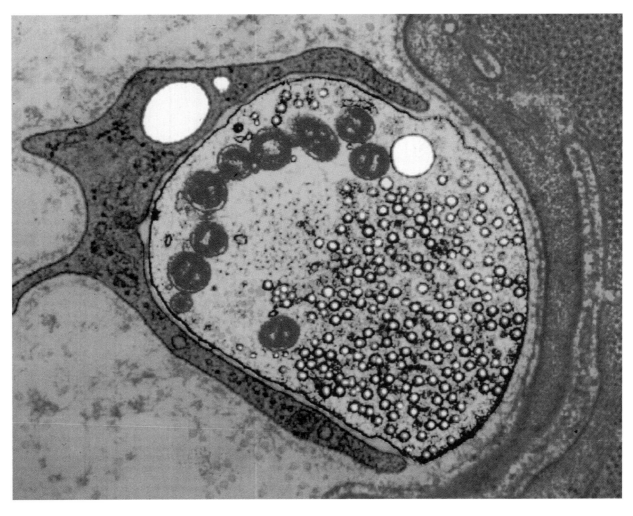

Nerve teminal synapses with muscle fiber (red). *(© Don Fawcett/Photo Researchers, Inc. Reproduced by permission.)*

- Aspartate: An amino acid that stimulates neurons in the **central nervous system**, particularly those that transfer information to the area of the brain called the cerebrum.

- Oxytocin: A short protein (peptide) that is released within the brain, ovary, and testes. The compound stimulates the release of milk by mammary glands, contractions during birth, and maternal behavior.

- Somatostatin: Another peptide, which is inhibitory to the secretion of growth hormone from the pituitary gland, of insulin, and of a variety of gastrointestinal hormones involved with nutrient absorption.

- Insulin: A peptide secreted by the pancreas that stimulates other cells to absorb glucose.

As exemplified above, neurotransmitters have different actions. In addition, some neurotransmitters have different effects depending upon which receptor to which they bind. For example, acetylcholine can be stimulatory when bound to one receptor and inhibitory when bound to another receptor.

Resources

BOOKS

Alberts, B., A. Johnson, J. Lewis, M. Raff, K. Roberts, and P. Walter. *Molecular Biology of the Cell.* New York: Garland Publishers, 2002.

OTHER

King, M. W., Indiana State University. *Biochemistry of Neurotransmitters.* <http://www.indstate.edu/theme/mwking/nerves.html> (January 20, 2004).

Washington State University. "Neurotransmitters and Neuroactive Peptides." *Neuroscience for Kids.* <http://faculty.washington.edu/chudler.chnt1.html> (January 22, 2004).

Brian Douglas Hoyle, PhD

Nevus cavernosus *see* **Cerebral cavernous malformation**

Niemann-Pick disease

Definition

Niemann-Pick disease (NPD) is a term that defines a group of diseases that affect metabolism and which are caused by specific genetic mutations. Currently, there are three categories of Niemann-Pick diseases: type A (NPD-A), the acute infantile form; type B (NPD-B), a less common, chronic, non-neurological form; and type C (NPD-C), a biochemically and genetically distinct form of the disease.

Description

NPD-A is a debilitating neurodegenerative (progressive nervous system dysfunction) childhood disorder characterized by failure to thrive, enlarged liver, and progressive neurological deterioration, which generally leads to death by three years of age. In contrast, NPD-B patients have an enlarged liver, no neurological involvement, and often survive into adulthood. NPD-C, although similar in name to types A and B, is very different at the biochemical and genetic level. People with NPD-C are not able to metabolize cholesterol and other lipids properly within the cells. Consequently, excessive amounts of cholesterol accumulate in the liver and spleen. The vast majority of children with NPD-C die before age 20, and many before the age of 10. Later onset of symptoms usually leads to a longer life span, although death usually occurs by age forty.

Demographics

Both Niemann-Pick disease types A and B occur in many ethnic groups; however, they occur more frequently among individuals of Ashkenazi Jewish descent than in the general population. NPD-A occurs most frequently, and it accounts for about 85% of all cases of the disease. NPD-C affects an estimated 500 children in the United States.

Causes and symptoms

All forms of NPD are inherited autosomal recessive disorders, requiring the presence of an inherited genetic mutation in only one copy of the gene responsible for the disease. Both males and females are affected equally. Types A and B are both caused by the deficiency of a specific enzyme known as the acid sphingomyelinase (ASM). This enzyme is ordinarily found in special compartments within cells called lysosomes and is required to metabolize a certain lipid (fat). If ASM is absent or not functioning properly, this lipid cannot be metabolized and is accumulated within the cell, eventually causing cell death and the malfunction of major organs and systems.

NPD-C disease is a fatal lipid storage disorder characterized by cholesterol accumulation in the liver, spleen, and **central nervous system**. Mutations in two independent genes result in the clinical features of this disease.

Symptoms of all forms of NPD are variable; no single symptom should be used to include or exclude NPD as a diagnosis. A person in the early stages of the disease may exhibit only a few of the symptoms, and even in the later stages not all symptoms may be present.

NPD-A begins in the first few months of life. Symptoms normally include feeding difficulties, abdomen enlargement, progressive loss of early motor skills, and cherry red spots in the eyes.

NPD-B is biochemically similar to type A, but the symptoms are more variable. Abdomen enlargement may be detected in early childhood, but there is almost no neurological involvement, such as loss of motor skills. Some patients may develop repeated respiratory infections.

NPD-C usually affects children of school age, but the disease may strike at any time from early infancy to adulthood. Symptoms commonly found are jaundice, spleen and/or liver enlargement, difficulties with upward and downward eye movements, gait (walking) unsteadiness, clumsiness, **dystonia** (difficulty in posturing of limbs), **dysarthria** (irregular speech), learning difficulties and progressive intellectual decline, sudden loss of muscle tone which may lead to falls, **tremors** accompanying movement, and in some cases **seizures**.

Diagnosis

The diagnosis of NPD-A and B is normally clinical, helped by measuring the ASM activity in the blood (white blood cells). While this test will identify affected individuals with the two mutated genes, it is not very reliable for detecting carriers, who have only one mutated gene.

NPD-C is diagnosed by taking a small skin **biopsy**, growing the cells (fibroblasts) in the laboratory, and studying their ability to transport and store cholesterol. Cholesterol transport in the cells is tested by measuring conversion of the cholesterol from one form to another. The storage of cholesterol is assessed by staining the cells with a compound that glows under ultraviolet light. It is important that both of these tests are performed, as reliance on one or the other may lead to the diagnosis being missed in some cases. NPD-C is often incorrectly diagnosed, and misclassified as attention deficit disorder (ADD), learning disability, retardation, or delayed development.

Treatment team

The treatment team is normally composed of a nutritionist, a physical therapist and/or occupational therapist (walking and balance, motor skills and posturing), a **neurologist** (seizure medications and neurological assessments), a speech therapist, pulmonologist, a geneticist, a

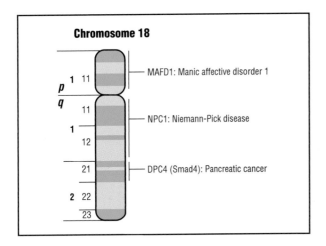

Chromosome 18

p 1 11 — MAFD1: Manic affective disorder 1

q 11

1 — NPC1: Niemann-Pick disease

12

21 — DPC4 (Smad4): Pancreatic cancer

2 22

23

Niemann-Pick disease, on chromosome 18. *(Gale Group.)*

gastroenterologist, a psychologist, a social worker, and nurses.

Treatment

No specific definitive treatment is available for patients with any NPD type, and treatment is purely supportive. For NPD-C, a healthy, low-cholesterol diet is recommended. However, research into low-cholesterol diets and cholesterol-lowering drugs do not indicate that these halt the progress of the disease or change cholesterol metabolism at the cellular level.

Recovery and rehabilitation

All types of NPD require continuous family care and medical follow-up. Long-term survival and life quality will vary from patient to patient and seem to be directly related to the nature of the disease (genetic mutation) and the medical support provided.

Clinical trials

Enzyme replacement has been tested in mice and shown to be effective for type NPD type B. It has also been used successfully in other storage diseases, such as Gaucher type I. Genzyme Corporation and Mount Sinai Medical Center have announced plans for a clinical trial using enzyme replacement therapy to begin late 2003.

A clinical trial with a drug known as Zavesca for NPD type C is underway in the United States and Europe. The drug slowed, but did not stop, the neurological decline when tested on NPD mice.

Laboratory studies of neurosteroids have recently shown encouraging results when tested on mice, but more work needs to be done before a clinical trial can be considered.

Prognosis

Patients with NPD-A commonly die during infancy. NPD-B patients may live for a few decades, but many require supplemental oxygen because of lung impairment. The life expectancy of patients with type C is variable. Some patients die in childhood while others, who appear to be less drastically affected, live into adulthood.

Special concerns

All types of NPD are autosomal recessive, which means that both parents carry one copy of the abnormal gene without having any signs of the disease. When parents are carriers, in each pregnancy, there is a 25% risk of conceiving a child who is affected with the disease and a 50% risk that the child will be a carrier.

For NPD-A and B the ASM gene has been isolated and extensively studied. DNA testing and prenatal diagnosis is currently available. Research into treatment alternatives for these types has progressed rapidly since the early 1990's. Current research focuses on bone marrow transplantation, enzyme replacement therapy, and **gene therapy**. All of these therapies have had some success against NPD-B in a laboratory environment. Unfortunately, none of the potential therapies has been effective against NPD-A.

Resources
PERIODICALS

Takahashi, T., M. Suchi, R. J. Desnick, G. Takada, and E. Schuchman. "Identification and Expression of Five Mutations in the Human Acid Sphingomyelinase Gene Causing Types A and B Niemann-Pick Disease.

Molecular Evidence for Genetic Heterogeneity in the Neuronopathic and Non-neuronopathic Forms." *The Journal of Biological Chemistry* (June 1992): 12552–12558.

Frolov, A., et al. "NPC1 and NPC2 Regulate Cellular Cholesterol Homeostasis through Generation of Low Density Lipoprotein Cholesterol-derived Oxysterols." *The Journal of Biological Chemistry* (July 2003): 25517–25525.

Choi, H. Y., et al. "Impaired ABCA1-dependent Lipid Efflux and Hypoalphalipoproteinemia in Human Niemann-Pick type C Disease." *The Journal of Biological Chemistry* (August 2003): 32569–32577.

OTHER

National Institute of Neurological Disorders and Stroke. *NINDS Niemann-Pick Disease Information Page.* <http://www.ninds.nih.gov/health_and_medical/disorders/niemann.doc.htm> (January 4, 2003).

National Tay-Sachs & Allied Diseases Association (NTSAD). *Neimann-Pick Disease.* <http://www.ntsad.org/pages/n-pick.htm> (January 4, 2004).

ORGANIZATIONS

National Niemann-Pick Disease Foundation, Inc. PO Box 49, 415 Madison Ave, Ft. Atkinson, WI 53538. (920) 563-0930 or (877) 287-3672; Fax: (920) 563-0931. nnpdf@idcnet.com. <http://www.nnpdf.org>.

Beatriz Alves Vianna
Iuri Drumond Louro

Nutritional deficiency *see*
Vitamin/nutritional deficiency

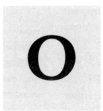

O'Sullivan-McLeod syndrome *see* **Monomelic amyotrophy**

Occipital neuralgia

Definition

Occipital neuralgia is a persistent **pain** that is caused by an injury or irritation of the occipital nerves located in the back of the head.

Description

The greater and lesser occipital nerves run from the region where the spinal column meets the neck (the suboccipital region) up to the scalp at the back of the head. Trauma to these nerves can cause a pain that originates from the lower area of the neck between the shoulder blades.

Demographics

Although statistics indicating the frequency of persons with occipital neuralgia are unknown, the condition is more frequent in females than males.

Causes and symptoms

Occipital neuralgia is caused by an injury to the greater or lesser occipital nerves, or some irritation of one or both of these nerves. The repeated contraction of the neck muscles is a potential cause. Spinal column compression, localized infection or inflammation, gout, diabetes, blood vessel inflammation, and frequent, lengthy periods of maintaining the head in a downward and forward position have also been associated with occipital neuralgia. Less frequently, the growth of a tumor can be a cause, as the tumor puts pressure on the occipital nerves.

The result of the nerve damage or irritation is pain, which is typically described as continuously aching or throbbing. Some people also have periodic jabs of pain in addition to the more constant discomfort. The level of pain can be intense, and similar to a migraine. This intense pain can cause nausea and vomiting.

The pain typically begins in the lower area of the neck and spreads upward in a "ram's horn" pattern on the side of the head. Ultimately, the entire scalp and forehead can be painful. The scalp is also often tender to the touch. Additionally, persons with occipital neuralgia may have difficulty rotating or flexing the neck, and pain may radiate to the shoulder. Pressure or pain may be felt behind the eyes, and eyes are sensitive to light, especially when **headache** is present.

Diagnosis

Diagnosis is based on the symptoms, and especially on the location of the pain. Medical history is also useful. A history of muscle tension headaches over a long period of time is a good indicator that the current pain could be a neuralgic condition such as occipital neuralgia. While many people experience a tension headache due to the contraction of neck and facial muscles, few people experience the true neuralgic pain of occipital neuralgia. Nevertheless, physical and emotional tension can be contributing factors to the condition.

Treatment team

The treatment team typically is made up of someone capable of giving a massage, and a family physician. A **neurologist** and pain specialist may also be consulted. In the rare cases that surgery is required, a neurosurgeon is also involved.

Treatment

Treatment usually consists attempting to relieve the pain. This often involves a massage to relax the muscles in the area of the occipital nerves. Bed rest may relieve acute pain. In cases in which the nerve pain is suspected of being

Key Terms

Neuralgia Pain along a nerve pathway.

Occipital nerves Two pairs of nerves that originate in the area of the second and third vertebrae of the neck, and are part of a network that innervate the neck, upper back, and head.

caused by a tumor, a more specialized examination is done using the techniques of nuclear imaging or computed tomography (**CT**). These techniques provide an image that can reveal a tumor. If present, the tumor can be removed surgically, which usually cures the condition.

In cases in which the pain is especially intense, as in a migraine type of pain, pain-relieving drugs and antidepressants can be taken. Other treatments involve the blocking of the impulses from the affected nerve by injection of compounds that block the functioning of the nerve. Steroids can also be injected at the site of the nerve to try to relieve inflammation. However, the usefulness and long-term effects of this form of steroid therapy are not clear.

In extreme cases where pain is frequent, the nerves can be severed at the point where they join the scalp. The person is pain-free, but sensation is permanently lost in the affected region of the head.

Recovery and rehabilitation

Recovery is usually complete after the bout of pain has subsided and the nerve damage has been repaired or lessened.

Clinical trials

As of April 2004, there were no **clinical trials** in the United States that are directly concerned with occipital neuralgia. However, research is being funded through agencies such as the National Institute of Neurological Disorders and Stroke to try to find new treatments for pain and nerve damage, and to uncover the biological processes that result in pain.

Prognosis

The periodic nature of mild occipital neuralgia usually does not interfere with daily life. The prognosis for persons with more severe occipital neuralgia is also good, as the pain is usually lessened or eliminated by treatment.

Resources

BOOKS

Parker, J. N., and P. M. Parker. *The Official Parent's Sourcebook on Occipital Neuralgia: A Revised and Updated Directory for the Internet Age.* San Diego: Icon Health Publications, 2003.

OTHER

Loeser, J. D. "Occipital Neuralgia." *Facial Neuralgia Resources.* April 14, 2004 (June 2, 2004). <http://www.facial-neuralgia.org/conditions/occipital.html>.

"NINDS Occipital Neuralgia Information Page." *National Institute of Neurological Disorders and Stroke.* April 12, 2004 (June 2, 2004). <http://www.ninds.nih.gov/health_and_medical/disorders/occipitalneuralgia.htm>.

ORGANIZATIONS

National Institute for Neurological Diseases and Stroke (NINDS). 6001 Executive Boulevard, Bethesda, MD 20892. (301) 496-5751 or (800) 352-9424. <http://www.ninds.nih.gov>.

National Organization for Rare Disorders. 55 Kenosia Avenue, Danbury, CT 06813-1968. (203) 744-0100 or (800) 999-6673; Fax: (203) 798-2291. orphan@rarediseases.org. <http://www.rarediseases.org>.

National Institute of Arthritis and Musculoskeletal and Skin Diseases (NIAMS). 31 Center Dr., Rm. 4C02 MSC 2350, Bethesda, MD 20892-2350. (301) 496-8190 or (877) 226-4267. NIAMSinfo@mail.nih.gov. <http://www.niams.nih.gov>.

Brian Douglas Hoyle, PhD

Occulocephalic reflex *see* **Visual disturbances; Traumatic brain injury**

Occult spinal dysraphism sequence *see* **Tethered spinal cord syndrome**

Olivopontocerebellar atrophy

Definition

Olivopontocerebellar atrophy (OPCA) is a group of disorders characterized by degeneration of three brain areas: the inferior olives, the pons, and the **cerebellum**. OPCA causes increasingly severe **ataxia** (loss of coordination) as well as other symptoms.

Description

Two distinct groups of diseases are called OPCA, leading to some confusion. Non-inherited OPCA, also called sporadic OPCA, is now considered a form of **multiple system atrophy** (MSA). Hereditary OPCA, also called inherited OPCA and familial OPCA, is caused by inheritance of a defective gene, which is recognized in some forms but not in others.

Demographics

Hereditary OPCA affects approximately 10,000 people in the United States, with males affected approximately twice as often as females. The average age of onset is 28 years.

Causes and symptoms

By definition, hereditary OPCA is caused by the inheritance of a defective gene. Several genes have been identified. The two most common are known as SCA-1 and SCA-2 (SCA stands for **spinocerebellar ataxia**). These genes cause similar, though not identical, diseases. Besides these two genes, there are at least 20 other genetic forms of the disease. For reasons that are not understood, these gene defects cause degeneration (cell death) in specific parts of the brain, leading to the symptoms of the disorder. The cerebellum is a principal center for coordination, and its degeneration leads to loss of coordination.

The most common early symptom of OPCA is ataxia, or incoordination, which may be observed in an unsteady gait or over-reaching for an object with the hand. Other common symptoms include **dysarthria** (speech difficulty), dysphagia (swallowing difficulty), nystagmus (eye tremor), and abnormal movements such as jerking, twisting, or writhing. Symptoms worsen over time.

Diagnosis

An initial diagnosis of OPCA can be made with a careful neurological examination (testing of reflexes, balance, coordination, etc.), plus a magnetic resonance image (**MRI**) of the brain to look for atrophy (loss of tissue) in the characteristic brain regions. Genetic tests exist for SCA-1 and SCA-2 forms. Many other types of tests are possible, although they are usually done only to rule out other conditions with similar symptoms or to confirm the diagnosis in uncertain cases. Because the symptoms of OPCA can be so variable, especially at the beginning of the disease, it may be difficult to obtain a definite diagnosis early on.

Treatment team

The treatment team is likely to consist of a **neurologist**, physical therapist, occupational therapist, speech/language pathologist, genetic counselor, and nursing care specialist.

Treatment

There are no treatments that reverse or delay the progression of OPCA.

Very few medications have any beneficial effect on OPCA symptoms. In some patients, Levodopa, also prescribed for **Parkinson's disease**, may initially help. Some anti-tremor medications, including propranolol, may also slightly help. **Acetazolamide** may be useful in some forms of the disease.

Treatment of OPCA is primarily directed toward reducing the danger of ataxia, and minimizing the impact of the disease on activities of daily living. Falling is the major danger early in the disease, and **assistive mobile devices** such as walkers and wheelchairs are often essential to prevent falling.

As the disease progresses, swallowing difficulties present the greatest danger. Softer foods and smaller mouthfuls are recommended. A speech-language pathologist can help devise swallowing strategies to lessen the risk of choking, and can offer advice on assisted communication as well. Late in the disease, a feeding tube may be needed to maintain adequate nutrition.

Prognosis

The life expectancy after diagnosis is approximately 15 years, although this is an average and cannot be used to predict the lifespan of any individual person.

Special concerns

Because OPCA is an inherited disease with identified genetic causes, it is reasonable to have other family members tested for the genes to determine if they, too, are at risk. This information may help family members to make personal decisions about their future, including decisions about family planning.

Resources

WEBSITES

National Ataxia Foundation. (April 19, 2004).
    <http://www.ataxia.org>.
National Organization for Rare Disorders. (April 19, 2004).
    <http://www.rarediseases.org>

Richard Robinson

▌Opsoclonus myoclonus

Definition

Opsoclonus **myoclonus** is a syndrome in which the eyes dart involuntarily (opsoclonus or dancing eyes) and muscles throughout the body jerk or twitch involuntarily (myoclonus).

Description

Opsoclonus myoclonus is a very rare syndrome that strikes previously normal infants, children, or adults, often occurring in conjunction with certain cancerous tumors, viral infections, or medication use. Onset can be very sudden and dramatic, with a quick progression.

Demographics

Most children who develop opsoclonus myoclonus are under the age of two when they are diagnosed. Boys and girls are affected equally.

Causes and symptoms

Many cases of opsoclonus myoclonus follow a bout of a viral illness such as infection with influenza, Epstein-Barr or Coxsackie B viruses, or after St. Louis encephalitis. About half of all cases are associated with a cancerous tumor; this kind of symptom that occurs due to cancer is termed a paraneoplastic syndrome. In children, the most common type of tumor that precipitates opsoclonus myoclonus is called neuroblastoma. Neuroblastoma can cause tumors in the brain, abdomen, or pelvic area. The cancerous cells develop from primitive nerve cells called neural crest cells. When opsoclonus myoclonus occurs in adults, it is usually associated with tumors in the lung, breast, thymus, lymph system, ovaries, uterus, or bladder. Rarely, opsoclonus myoclonus can occur after the use of certain medications such as intravenous phenytoin or **diazepam**, or subsequent to an overdose of the antidepressant amitriptyline.

No one knows exactly why opsoclonus myoclonus occurs. It is postulated that the presence of a viral infection or tumor may kick off an immune system response. The immune system begins trying to produce cells that will fight the invaders, either viruses or cancer cells. However, the immune cells produced may accidentally also attack areas of the brain, producing the symptoms of opsoclonus myoclonus.

Patients with opsoclonus myoclonus all have both opsoclonus and myoclonus. They experience involuntary, rapid darting movements of their eyes, as well as lightning-quick jerking of the muscles in their faces, eyelids, arms, legs, hands, heads, and trunk. Many individuals with opsoclonus myoclonus also experience weak and floppy muscles and a tremor. The movement disorder symptoms are incapacitating enough to completely interfere with sitting or standing when they are at their most severe. Difficulties eating, sleeping, and speaking also occur. Other common symptoms include mood changes, rage, irritability, nervousness, anxiety, severe drowsiness, confusion, and decreased awareness and responsiveness.

Diagnosis

Diagnosis is primarily arrived at through identification of concurrent opsoclonus and myoclonus. Laboratory testing of blood and spinal fluid may reveal the presence of

---

Key Terms

Apheresis   A procedure in which the blood is removed and filtered in order to rid it of particular cells, then returned to the patient.

Autoantibodies   Antibodies that are directed against the body itself.

Immunoadsorption   A procedure that can remove harmful antibodies from the blood.

Myoclonus   Lightning-quick involuntary jerks and twitches of muscles.

Neuroblastoma   A malignant tumor of nerve cells that strikes children.

Opsoclonus   Often called "dancing eyes," this symptom involves involuntary, quick darting movements of the eyes in all directions.

Paraneoplastic syndrome   A cluster of symptoms that occur due to the presence of cancer in the body, but that may occur at a site quite remote from the location of the cancer.

---

certain immune cells that could be responsible for attacking parts of the nervous system, such as autoantibodies. When opsoclonus myoclonus is diagnosed, a search for a causative condition such as tumor should be undertaken.

Treatment team

The treatment team will include a **neurologist** and neurosurgeon. A physical therapist, occupational therapist, and speech and language therapist may help an individual with opsoclonus myoclonus retain or regain as much functioning as possible.

Treatment

If opsoclonus myoclonus is due to the presence of a tumor, the first types of treatment will involve tumor removal and appropriate treatment of the cancer. Some adult cases of opsoclonus myoclonus resolve spontaneously, without specific treatment.

Treatment of the symptoms of opsoclonus myoclonus include clonzaepam or valproate. These may decrease the severity of both the opsoclonus and the myoclonus.

Other treatments for opsoclonus myoclonus include the administration of the pituitary hormone, called adrenocorticotropic hormone (ACTH). ACTH prompts the production of steroid hormones in the adrenal glands. When ACTH is given in high intravenous (IV) doses for about 20

---

weeks, the body produces large quantities of steroids, which can help quell any immune response that may be responsible for the opsoclonus myoclonus. Intravenous immunoglobulin treatment (IVIG), Azathioprine, and intravenous steroid treatments may also be given in an effort to suppress the immune system's response.

Two treatments that filter the blood in an effort to remove potentially damaging immune cells may also be attempted, although they are generally only able to be performed on adults. These include therapeutic apheresis and immunoadsorption. In these procedures, the patient's blood or plasma is processed to extract certain immune cells; the blood or plasma is then returned to the patient. These procedures may need to be repeated five or six times, but improvement is often rapid and may last up to two to three months.

Prognosis

The prognosis for opsoclonus myoclonus is varied. The milder the case prior to treatment, the more likely full recovery may occur. When opsoclonus myoclonus is due to a viral illness, there is a higher possibility for resolution of symptoms than when the condition results from neuroblastoma. Furthermore, although the degree of myoclonus may decrease, there are still often some residual coordination problems, difficulties with learning, behavior and/or attention, and obsessive-compulsive disorder. Children with very severe cases of opsoclonus myoclonus are likely to continue to have severe problems, and will probably never have normal intelligence or the ability to live independently.

Many children have flares of their symptoms or actual relapses of the disease when they suffer from viral illnesses, even years later. The treatments for such relapses are the same as for the initial illness.

Resources

BOOKS

Asha Das, Ramsis, K. Benjamin, and Fred H. Hochberg. "Metastatic Neoplasms and Paraneoplastic Syndromes." *Textbook of Clinical Neurology*, edited by Christopher G. Goetz. Philadelphia: W. B. Saunders Company, 2003.

Al-Lozi, Muhammad, and Alan Pestronk. "Paraneoplastic Neurologic Syndromes." *Harrison's Principles of Internal Medicine*, edited by Eugene Braunwald, et al. New York: McGraw-Hill Professional, 2001.

PERIODICALS

Dale, R. C. "Childhood Opsoclonus Myoclonus." *Lancet Neurology* 2, no. 5 (May 1, 2003): 270.

Pranzatelli, M. R. "Screening for Autoantibodies in Children with Opsoclonus-Myoclonus-Ataxia." *Pediatric Neurology* 27 no. 5 (November 1, 2002): 384–387.

Storey, Imogen, Alastair Denniston, and Sarah Denniston. "Dancing Eyes." *Hospital Medicine* 27, no. 5 (September 1, 2003): 555–556.

Yiu, V. W. "Plasmapheresis as an Effective Treatment for Opsoclonus Myoclonus Syndrome." *Pediatric Neurology* 24 no. 1 (January 1, 2001): 72–74.

ORGANIZATIONS

Opsoclonus-Myoclonus USA and International. SIU School of Medicine, 751 North Rutledge, Suite 3100, Springfield, IL 62702. (217) 545-7635; Fax: (217) 545-1903. omsusa@siumed.edu. <http://www.omsusa.org/index.htm>.

Rosalyn Carson-DeWitt, MD

Organic voice tremor

Definition

Organic voice tremor is a neurogenic voice disorder of adulthood that most often occurs as a component of essential or hereditofamilial tremor; it may occur by itself, however. Organic voice tremor must be distinguished from other conditions, which also present with voice disturbances in the early stages. These include Parkinsonism, cerebellar disease, thyrotoxicosis, and anxiety.

Description

Organic voice tremor is a disorder of voice production characterized by unsteadiness of pitch and loudness and quavering intonation. In some patients, it may result in rhythmic arrests of voicing that occur at a rate of four to six per second. Voice quality is characterized by harshness, vocal strain, abnormally low pitch, and voice stoppages. Laryngeal examination typically reveals vocal folds of normal appearance, with no evidence of aberrant innervation. The abnormal oscillations of the larynx occur as a result of vigorous up-and-down vertical movements that occurred synchronously with the oscillation of the tremor. The quavering speech quality that characterizes organic voice tremor has been thought to include extralaryngeal influences arising from **tremors** in the diaphragm, lips, and tongue (Critchley, 1949; Tomoda, et al., 1985).

The origin of organic voice tremors has not been conclusively determined, though aging and occlusive arterial disease are thought to contribute significantly to the effects. Critchley (1949) showed that essential tremor occurred in persons with confirmed lesions in the brain stem, basal ganglia (e.g., putamen and lentiform nuclei) and within neural connections joining the red nucleus, dentate nucleus, and inferior olive. Vocal tremors usually coexist with tremors in the head and limbs, but may be localized entirely

Key Terms

Dysphonia Disordered phonation or voice production.

Dystonia Abnormalities of muscle tone involving involuntary twisting or distortions of the trunk or other body parts.

Endoscopy A clinical technique using an instrument called an endoscope, used for visualization of structures within the body.

Extra-laryngeal Actions of muscles outside the larynx, but usually in its vicinity, which influence its functioning.

Extrapyramidal system Functional, rather than anatomical unit, comprised of nuclei and nerve fibers that are chiefly involved with subconscious, automatic aspects of motor coordination, but which also assist in regulation of postural and locomotor movements.

Hyperfunction Term used to describe excess effort or strain involved in producing an action.

Innervation Distribution or supply of nerves to a structure.

Neurogenic Of neurological origin.

Otolaryngologist A physician who specializes in medical and surgical treatment of disorders of the ear, nose, throat, and larynx.

Resonator As used in regard to the human speech mechanism, it is the cavity extending from the vocal folds to the lips, which selectively amplifies and modifies the energies produced during speech and voice production. It is synonymous with the term vocal tract.

Speech-language pathologist A non-physician health care provider who evaluates and treats disorders of communication and swallowing.

Thyrotoxicosis A condition caused by excess amounts of thyroid hormone.

Tremor Involuntary rhythmic movements, which may be intermittent or constant, involving an entire muscle or only a circumscribed group of muscle bundles.

---

within the larynx. Disturbed central innervation to the larynx is thought to disturb coordination between abductor and adductor groups of laryngeal muscles, which may affect the symmetry of vibration of the vocal folds, and result in excess force of approximation or abruptness of vocal fold separation during conversational speech. Symptoms may be difficult to fully appreciate in conversational speech but become quite evident in sustained vowel production (Brown and Simonson, 1963). This finding is significant for differential diagnosis of essential tremor from spasmodic dysphonia, a focal **dystonia** affecting voicing.

Demographics

Organic voice tremor is a condition that usually occurs in persons over age 50. Males and females appear to be affected equally. Specific incidence data are not available.

Causes and Symptoms

Organic voice tremor is thought to result from neural degeneration in one or more regions of the extrapyramidal system. It usually is part of a more general condition of tremor involving the head, neck, and limbs called essential tremor. For some individuals, these changes are inherited and may occur in several members of the same family,

sometimes occurring in successive generations. These persons are said to have hereditofamilial tremor. When the onset of organic voice tremor is rapid, the etiology may result from occlusive vascular disease (Brown and Simonson, 1963). When it is gradual, the etiology is likely related to progressive changes in several locations in the brain stem or basal ganglia.

Persons with organic voice tremor usually experience changes in voice slowly. In addition to changes in voice quality and reduced stability in pitch, loudness, and vocal flexibility, some patients may experience tremor in the pharynx, lips, and jaw. Some patients experience difficulties in initiating or maintaining voicing or experience sudden loss of voice during conversation. In addition to vocal tremor, some patients experience spasms in the diaphragm and expiratory musculature (Tomoda, et al.,1987), which may contribute to instability within the vocal tract and add to the quavering property of the voice.

Diagnosis

Organic voice tremor is usually made by examination of a **neurologist** and speech-language pathologist. Detailed history and medical examination is essential to determine if disruptions in voice functioning are related to other neurological conditions such as Parkinsonism, cerebellar disease, and systemic conditions such as thyrotoxicosis. Differential diagnosis needs to be made between organic voice tremor and spasmodic dysphonia, which is a focal dystonia. A complete laryngeal examination should be obtained from an otolaryngologist and include endoscopic and videostroboscopic examinations of the larynx. A battery of objective tests to assess the aerodynamic and acoustic properties of voice production should be obtained from a speech pathologist, who usually works with the otolaryngologist. In addition, neuromotor intactness of the speech mechanism (the motor speech examination), should be undertaken. In this examination attention is given to assessment of muscle strength, speed of movement, range of motion, accuracy of movement, motor steadiness, and muscle tone in the speech articulators, larynx, and resonatory systems.

Treatment Team

The treatment team for organic voice tremor consists of a neurologist, otolaryngologist, and speech-language pathologist.

Treatment

There is no cure for organic voice tremor. Medications (Sinemat or Inderal) used to treat essential tremor have not emerged as a reliable treatment modality for organic voice tremor. Koller, et al. (1985) used propranolol to treat organic voice tremor and found that voice tremor was more resistant to drug treatment than tremor in the hand. Others (Massey and Paulson, 1982; Hartman and Vishwanat, 1984; Tomoda, et al., 1987) report effective treatment of voice and hand tremors with clonazepan, and **diazepam. Botulinum Toxin** A (BOTOX) may be useful in treating some patients with organic voice tremor, in which vocal fold **spasticity** is a coexisting feature. Speech therapy may be useful in reducing laryngeal hyperfunction and in establishing improved respiratory support.

Recovery and Rehabilitation

Patients with organic voice tremor do not recover from the condition. They must learn to adapt or compensate for speech and voice deficits. Speech therapy may be useful in this regard.

Prognosis

Prognosis is very poor for clinically significant improvement of voice in those with organic voice tremor.

Resources

PERIODICALS

Ardran, G., M. Kinsbourne, and G. Rushworth. "Dysphonia due to tremor." *Journal. Neurology Neurosurgery and Psychiatry* 29 (1966): 219–223.

Aronson, A. E., and D. E. Hartman. "Adductor spasmodic dysphonia as a sign of essential (voice) tremor." *Journal of Speech and Hearing Disorders* 46 (1981): 52–58.

Aronson, A. E., J. R. Brown, E. M. Litin, and J. S. Pearson. "Spastic dysphonia. II. Comparison with essential (voice) tremor and other neurologic and psychogenic dysphonias." *Journal of Speech and Hearing Disorders* 33, no. 3 (1969): 219–231.

Brown, J. R., and J. Simonson. "Organic voice tremor: a tremor of phonation." *Neurology* 13 (1963): 520–525.

Critchley, M. "Observations on essential (hereditofamilial) tremor." *Brain* 72 (1949): 113–139.

Hartman, D. E., and B. Vishwanat. "Spastic dysphonia and essential (voice) tremor treated with primidone." *Archives of Otolaryngology* 110 (1984): 394–397.

Hachinski, V. C. "Thomsen IV Buch NH The nature of primary vocal tremor." *Canada Journal of Neurological Sciences* 2 (1975): 195–197.

Koller, W. Graner, and D. A. Mlcoch. "Essential tremor: Treatment with propanolol." *Neurology* 35 (1985): 106–108.

Tomoda, H., H. Shibasaki, Y. Kuroda, and T. Shin. "Voice tremor: Dysregulation of voluntary expiratory muscles." *Neurology* 37: 117–122.

ORGANIZATIONS

American Speech-Language and Hearing Association. 10801 Rockville Pike, Rockville, MD 20852-3279. (301) 897-5700. <http://www.asha.org>.

National Spasmodic Dysphonia Association. One East Wacker Drive, Suite 2430, Chicago, IL 60601-1905. 800-795-6732. NSDA@dysphonia.org. <http://www.dysphonia.org>.

Joel C. Kahane, PhD

Orthostatic hypotension

Definition

Orthostatic hypotension refers to a reduction of blood pressure (systolic blood pressure that occurs when the heart contracts) of at lest 20 mmHg or a diastolic pressure (pressure when the heart muscle relaxes) of at least 10 mmHg within three minutes of standing.

Description

Orthostatic hypotension is a decrease of blood pressure when standing, due to changes in the blood pressure regulation systems within the body. Normally in a healthy human there is an orthostatic pooling of venous blood in the abdomen and legs when shifting positions from the supine (lying on the back) to an erect position (standing up). This redistribution of blood flow is the result of normal physiological compensatory mechanisms built into

Key Terms

Adrenal insufficiency Problems with the adrenal glands that can be life threatening if not treated. Symptoms include sluggishness, weakness, weight loss, vomiting, darkening of the skin, and mental changes.

Amyloidosis The accumulation of amyloid deposits in various organs and tissues in the body so that normal functioning is compromised. Primary amyloidosis usually occurs as a complication of multiple myeloma. Secondary amyloidosis occurs in patients suffering from chronic infections or inflammatory diseases such as tuberculosis, rheumatoid arthritis, and Crohn's disease.

Angina pectoris Chest pain caused by an insufficient supply of oxygen and decreased blood flow to the heart muscle. Angina is frequently the first sign of coronary artery disease.

Autonomic nervous system The part of the nervous system that controls so-called involuntary functions, such as heart rate, salivary gland secretion, respiratory function, and pupil dilation.

Brain stem The stalk of the brain which connects the two cerebral hemispheres with the spinal cord. It is involved in controlling vital functions, movement, sensation, and nerves supplying the head and neck.

Claudication Cramping or pain in a leg caused by poor blood circulation. This condition is frequently caused by hardening of the arteries (atherosclerosis). Intermittent claudication occurs only at certain times, usually after exercise, and is relieved by rest.

Diuretic drugs A group of medications that increase the amount of urine produced and relieve excess fluid buildup in body tissues. Diuretics may be used in treating high blood pressure, lung disease, premenstrual syndrome, and other conditions.

Levodopa A substance used in the treatment of Parkinson's disease. Levodopa can cross the blood-brain barrier that protects the brain. Once in the brain, it is converted to dopamine and thus can replace the dopamine lost in Parkinson's disease.

Mineralocorticoid A steroid hormone, like aldosterone, that regulates the excretion of salt, potassium, and water.

Monoamine oxidase inhibitors A class of antidepressants used to treat certain types of mental depression. MAO inhibitors are especially useful in treating people whose depression is combined with other problems such as anxiety, panic attacks, phobias, or the desire to sleep too much.

Myelopathy A disorder in which the tissue of the spinal cord is diseased or damaged.

Parkinson's disease A slowly progressive disease that destroys nerve cells in the basal ganglia and thus causes loss of dopamine, a chemical that aids in transmission of nerve signals (neurotransmitter). Parkinson's is characterized by shaking in resting muscles, a stooping posture, slurred speech, muscular stiffness, and weakness.

Syncope A loss of consciousness over a short period of time, caused by a temporary lack of oxygen in the brain.

Valsalva maneuver A strain against a closed airway combined with muscle tightening, such as happens when a person holds his or her breath and tries to move a heavy object. Most people perform this maneuver several times a day without adverse consequences, but it can be dangerous for anyone with cardiovascular disease. Pilots perform this maneuver to prevent black-outs during high-performance flying.

Vasodilator Any drug that relaxes blood vessel walls.

Vertigo A feeling of dizziness together with a sensation of movement and a feeling of rotating in space.

---

body systems to prevent any adverse outcome (decrease in blood pressure, or hypotension) during positional change. Compensatory mechanisms include sympathetic nervous system activation and parasympathetic inhibition and increased heart rate and vascular resistance. Compensation responses restore cardiac output to vital organs and return blood pressure to normal. Orthostatic hypotension can occur if normal physiological mechanisms become faulty, such as inadequate cardiovascular compensation when shifting positions (i.e. change from supine to erect position), or due to excessive reduction in blood volume. Elderly persons seemed predisposed to orthostatic hypotension because of age-related changes; possible cardiovascular disease and the medications commonly taken by the elderly all predispose autonomic nervous system (ANS) functions. Additionally, hypertension present in 30% of persons over 75 years of age also predisposes a person to orthostatic hypotension, since hypertension reduces baroreflex sensitivity. Hypertension and the normal aging process (which typically causes blood vessel stiffness) decrease the sensitivity of specialized structures called baroreceptors, which function to maintain blood pressure, but initiating compensatory mechanisms such as increasing heart rate and vascular resistance. Persons affected with symptomatic orthostatic hypotension have symptoms when tilting head upward or when moving toward an erect position. Symptom severity varies among affected persons, but can include blurred vision, lightheadedness, weakness, vertigo, tremulousness and cognitive impairment. Symptoms can be relieved within one minute of lying down. Some persons have orthostatic hypertension without symptoms.

Demographics

The demographics of orthostatic hypotension are different due to variables that include the subject's position change, the specific population, and when measurements are taken. It is estimated that elderly in community living environments have prevalence rates of approximately 20% among individuals over 65 years of age and 30% in persons over 75 years of age. In frail elderly persons, the prevalence of orthostatic hypotension can be more than 50%. The disorder seems more prevalent among the elderly (especially if systolic blood pressure rises) with chronic diseases (i.e. hypertension and/or diabetes).

Causes and symptoms

Orthostatic hypotension can be caused by several different disorders that affect the entire body (systemic disorders), the **central nervous system** (CNS, consisting of the brain and spinal cord), and the autonomic nervous system (peripheral autonomic neuropathy) or as a result of taking certain medications that are commonly prescribed by clinicians. Systemic causes can include dehydration, prolonged immobility or an endocrine disorder called adrenal insufficiency. Diseases of the CNS that can cause orthostatic hypotension include MSA (multiple systems atrophy), **Parkinson's disease**, multiple strokes, brain stem lesions, myelopathy.

Medications that can cause orthostatic hypotension include Tricyclic antidepressants, antipsychotics, monoamine oxidase inhibitors, antihypertensives, diuretics, vasodilators, Levodopa, beta-blockers (heart medications), and blood pressure medications that inhibit a chemical called angiotensin (angiotensin-converting-enzyme inhibitors). Disorders that cause peripheral autonomic neuropathy include diabetes mellitus, amyloidosis, **tabes dorsalis** (late manifestations of syphilis infection), alcoholism, nutritional deficiency, pure autonomic failure or **paraneoplastic syndromes**.

The most common symptoms of orthostatic hypotension include weakness, lightheadedness, cognitive impairment, blurred vision, vertigo and tremulousness. Other symptoms that have been reported include **headache**, paracervical **pain**, lower **back pain**, syncope, palpitations, angina pectoris, unsteadiness, falling, and calf claudication.

Diagnosis

It is important that the clinician take numerous blood pressure measurements on different occasions, since blood pressure can vary (i.e. postural hypotension, another disorder causing hypotension, is often worse in the morning when rising from bed). A detailed history and physical examination is important. The clinician should focus medical evaluation on autonomic symptoms and diseases. There are bedside tests that can determine autonomic (baroreceptor) response (i.e. Valsalva maneuver). Measurements of a chemical in blood called norepinephrine while lying down and for five to 10 minutes after standing, can produce some useful information concerning deficits in autonomic nervous system functioning. Additionally, levels of another chemical in blood (called vasopressin) during upright tilting, can help to distinguish if the cause is due to ANS failure or from as a result of MSA. Pure ANS failure is characterized by increased vasopressin levels, whereas patients with MSA have no appreciable increase of vasopressin levels during head tilting.

Treatment team

Primary care practitioner (internist); or in complicated cases (severe orthostatic hypotension) a **neurologist** is consulted.

Treatment

Nonsymptomatic orthostatic hypotension is a threat for falls or syncope and could be treated by preventive measures that include avoiding warm environments and increasing one's blood pressure by squatting, stooping forward, or crossing one's leg. Additionally, persons affected with the nonsymptomatic variation should increase salt intake, sleep in the head-up position, wear waist-high compression stockings and withdraw from drugs that are known to cause orthostatic hypotension as a side effect. Treatment for symptomatic orthostatic hypotension is important since it is a manifestation of a new illness or as a result of medications. Intervention can initially be nonpharmacologic (preventive measures and adjustments) or pharmacologic therapy. Nonpharmacologic intervention includes a review of medications, since elderly patients may be taking either OTC or prescribed drugs that can induce orthostatic hypotension. Persons affected should rise slowly to the erect position after a long period of sitting or lying down. They should avoid excess heat environments (i.e. in shower or central heating systems), coughing, straining or heavy lifting since these events can precipitate episodes of orthostatic hypotension. There are certain measures that can redirect blood to increase blood pressure and reduce symptoms associated with orthostatic hypotension. These measures include squatting, sitting down, crossing legs, and stooping forward.

Pharmacological Treatment

One of the most commonly prescribed medications for treating orthostatic hypotension is fludrocortisone acetate. This chemical is a synthetic mineralocorticoid which expands circulatory volume. This drug can cause a decrease of an important body element called potassium (hypokalemia, a decrease in potassium in plasma) which is important for normal heart contraction. Elderly persons should be monitored for blood levels of potassium and cardiac status. A drug called midodrine is useful for cases of orthostatic hypotension caused by peripheral **autonomic dysfunction**, usually in conjunction with fludrocortisone. However, midodrine is not recommended in persons with coronary or peripheral arterial disease. Other medications that may be helpful include clonidine or antihypertension medications. In severe cases of ANS deficits, a combination of medications may be indicated to provide brief periods of upright posture.

Recovery and rehabilitation

The recovery is variable and is also dependent on the cause. Recovery varies according to specific health status of affected person, age complications, and comorbidities (other existing disorders).

Clinical trials

Government-sponsored research includes studies concerning treatment of orthostatic hypotension. Details can be obtained from the website: <http://www.clinical trials.gov>

Prognosis

Careful evaluation and management is important for outcome. Identifying the source is an important first step. Preventive measures and posture modification techniques and avoidance of triggers can result in significant reduction of falls, fractures, functional decline, and syncope.

Special concerns

Special attention should be given to medications that are prescribed, which may cause orthostatic hypotension as a side effect.

Resources

BOOKS

Goetz, Christopher G., et al, eds. *Textbook of Clinical Neurology*, 1st ed. Philadelphia: W.B. Saunders Company, 1999.

Marx, John A., et al eds. *Rosen's Emergency Medicine: Concepts and Clinical Practice,* 5th ed. St. Louis: Mosby, Inc., 2002.

Noble, John., et al eds. *Textbook of Primary Care Medicine,* 3rd ed. St. Louis: Mosby, Inc., 2001.

PERIODICALS

Mukai, Seiji, and Lewis A. Lipsitz. "Orthostatic Hypotension." *Clinics in Geriatric Medicine* 18:2: (May 2002).

Viramo, Petteri. "Orthostatic Hypotension and Cognotive Decline in Older People." *Journal of the American Geriatrics Society* 47:5 (May 1999).

The Consensus Committee of the American Autonomic Society and the American Academy of Neurology. "Consensus statement on the definition of orthostatic hypotension, pure autonomic failure, and multiple system atrophy." *Neurology* 46:5 (May 1996).

WEBSITES

The Family Practice Notebook.com. *Orthostatic Hypotension.* <http://www.fpnotebook.com>.

ORGANIZATIONS

American Academy of Neurology. 1080 Montreal Avenue, Saint Paul, MN 55116. 800-879-1960; Fax: (651) 695-2791. <http://www.aan.com>.

Laith Farid Gulli, MD
Alfredo Mori, MBBS

Overuse syndrome *see* **Repetitive motion disorders**

Oxazolindinediones

Definition

Oxazolindinediones are **anticonvulsants**, indicated for the treatment of absence **seizures** (sometimes called petit mal seizures) associated with **epilepsy** and other seizure disorders.

Purpose

Oxazolindinediones are thought to decrease abnormal activity and excitement within the **central nervous system** (CNS) that may trigger seizures. While oxazolindinediones is often effective in controlling petit mal seizures associated with epilepsy, there is no known cure for the disorder. If necessary, oxazolindinediones can be used in conjunction with other anti-epileptic drugs (AEDs) that prevent or control other types of seizures.

Description

In the United States, oxazolindinediones are sold under the generic name trimethadione and the brand name Tridione.

Recommended dosage

Oxazolindinediones are taken orally and are available in tablet, chewable tablet, or suspension forms. Oxazolindinediones are appropriate for pediatric and adult patients. Physicians prescribe the medication in varying total daily dosages. Typically, the total daily dosage is administered in three to four divided doses.

When beginning a course of treatment that includes oxazolindinediones, most physicians will prescribe a carefully scheduled dosing regimen. The physician will determine the proper initial dosage, and then gradually raise the patient's daily dosage over the course of several days or weeks until seizure control is achieved. Likewise, dosages are usually tapered down over time when ending treatment with oxazolindinediones.

It is important to not take a double dose of any anticonvulsant medication, including oxazolindinediones. If a daily dose is missed, it should be taken as soon as possible. However, if it is within four hours of the next scheduled dose, then the missed dose should be skipped.

Precautions

A physician should be consulted before taking oxazolindinediones with certain non-prescription medications. Patients should avoid alcohol and CNS depressants (medicines that can make one drowsy or less alert, such as antihistimines, sleep medications, and some **pain** medications) while taking oxazolindinediones or any other anticonvulsants, which can exacerbate the side effects of alcohol and other medications.

A course of treatment including oxazolindinediones may not be appropriate for persons with liver or kidney disease, anemia, eye disorders, mental illness, diabetes, high blood pressure, angina (chest pain), irregular heartbeats, or other heart problems. Periodic blood, urine, and liver function tests are advised for many patients (especially pediatric and elderly patients) using the medicine.

Persons taking oxazolindinediones should avoid prolonged exposure to sunlight and should wear protective clothing and sunscreen while outdoors. Oxazolindinediones may make skin sensitive to sunlight and prone to sunburn.

Before beginning treatment with oxazolindinediones, patients should notify their physician if they consume a large amount of alcohol, have a history of drug use, are pregnant, nursing, or plan on becoming pregnant. Anticonvulsant medications may increase the risk of some birth defects. Patients who become pregnant while taking oxazolindinediones should contact their physician.

Side effects

Patients should discuss with their physicians the risks and benefits of treatment with oxazolindinediones before taking the medication. Oxazolindinediones are usually well tolerated. However, in some patients, they may case a variety of usually mild side effects. **Dizziness**, nausea, and drowsiness are the most frequently reported side effects of anticonvulsants. Possible side effects that do not usually require medical attention, and may diminish with continued use of the medication include:

- unusual tiredness or weakness
- loss of appetite
- weight loss
- abdominal pain
- speech problems
- nausea
- diarrhea or constipation
- heartburn or indigestion
- dry mouth
- chills, joint aches, and other flu-like symptoms

If any symptoms persist or become too uncomfortable, the prescribing physician should be notified.

Other, uncommon side effects of oxazolindinediones can be serious or could indicate an allergic reaction. Patients who experience any of the following symptoms should contact a physician:

- purple spots on the skin
- jaundice (yellowing of the skin and eyes)
- bruising easily
- unusual bleeding
- dark urine, frequent urination, or burning sensation when urinating
- extreme mood or mental changes
- shakiness or unsteady walking
- severe unsteadiness or clumsiness
- excessive speech or language problems
- difficulty breathing
- chest pain
- faintness or loss of consciousness
- persistent, severe headaches
- persistent fever or pain

Interactions

Oxazolindinediones may have negative interactions with some antacids, heartburn or acid reflux prevention medications, anticoagulants, antihistamines, antidepressants, antibiotics, and monoamine oxidase inhibitors (MAOIs). Oxazolindinediones may be used in conjunction with other seizure prevention medications (anticonvulsants or anti-epileptic drugs) only if advised and monitored by a physician. Many anticonvulsants may decrease the effectiveness of oral contraceptives (birth control pills) or contraceptive injections or implants containing estrogen and progestins.

Resources

BOOKS

Devinsky, Orrin, MD. *Epilepsy: Patient and Family Guide*, 2nd ed. Philadelphia: F. A. Davis Co., 2001.

Weaver, Donald F. *Epilepsy and Seizures: Everything You Need to Know.* Toronto: Firefly Books, 2001.

OTHER

"Trimethadione." *Medline Plus.* National Library of Medicine. May 6, 2004 (May 27, 2004). <http://www.nlm.nih.gov/medlineplus/druginfo/medmaster/a601127.html>.

"Trimethdione." *Yale New Haven Health Service Drug Guide.* May 6, 2004 (May 27, 2004). <http://yale newhavenhealth.org/Library/HealthGuide/DrugGuide/topic.asp?hwid=multumd00945a1>.

ORGANIZATIONS

Epilepsy Foundation. 4351 Garden City Drive, Landover, MD 20785-7223. (800) 332-1000. <http://www.epilepsy foundation.org>.

American Epilepsy Society. 342 North Main Street, West Hartford, CT 06117-2507. <http://www.aesnet.org>.

Adrienne Wilmoth Lerner

Pain

Definition and classification

Pain is a universal human experience. The International Association for the Study of Pain (IASP) defines pain as "an unpleasant sensory and emotional experience associated with actual or potential tissue damage or described in terms of such damage." Pain may be a symptom of an underlying disease or disorder, or a disorder in its own right.

At the same time that pain is a universal experience, however, it is also a complex one. While the physical sensations involved in pain may be constant throughout history, the ways in which humans express and treat pain are shaped by their respective cultures and societies. Since the 1980s, research in the neurobiology of pain has been accompanied by studies of the psychological and sociocultural factors that influence people's experience of pain, their use of health care systems, and their compliance with various treatments for pain. As of 2003, the World Health Organization (WHO) emphasizes the importance of an interdisciplinary approach to pain treatment that takes this complexity into account.

Types of pain

Pain can be classified as either acute or chronic. Acute pain is a direct biological response to disease, inflammation, or tissue damage, and usually lasts less than one month. It may be either continuous or recurrent (e.g., sickle cell disease). Acute pain serves the long-term well-being of humans and the higher animals by alerting them to an injury or condition that needs treatment. In humans, acute pain is often accompanied by anxiety and emotional distress; however, its cause can usually be successfully diagnosed and treated. Some researchers use the term "eudynia" to refer to acute pain.

In contrast, chronic pain has no useful biological function. It can be defined broadly as pain that lasts longer than a month following the healing of a tissue injury; pain that recurs or persists over a period of three months or longer; or pain related to a tissue injury that is expected to continue or get worse. Chronic pain may be either continuous or intermittent; in either case, however, it frequently leads to weight loss, sleep disturbances, **fatigue**, and other symptoms of **depression**. According to an article in the *New York Times*, chronic pain is the most common underlying cause of suicide. Unlike acute pain, chronic pain is resistant to most medical treatments. It is sometimes called "maldynia," and is considered a disorder in its own right.

Pain that is caused by organic diseases and disorders is known as somatogenic pain. Somatogenic pain in turn can be subdivided into nociceptive pain and neuropathic pain. Nociceptive pain occurs when pain-sensitive nerve endings called nociceptors are activated or stimulated. Most nociceptors in the human body are located in the skin, joints and muscles, and the walls of internal organs. There may be as many as 1,300 nociceptors in a square inch (6.4 square centimeter) of skin. However, there are fewer nociceptors in muscle tissue and the internal organs, as they are covered and protected by the skin. Nociceptors are specialized to detect different types of painful stimuli—some are sensitive to heat or cold, while others detect pressure, toxic substances, sharp blows, or inflammation caused by infection or overuse.

In contrast to nociceptive pain, neuropathic pain results from damage to or malfunctioning of the nervous system itself. It may involve the **central nervous system** (the brain and spinal cord); the **peripheral nervous system** (the nerve trunks leading away from the spine to the limbs, plus the 12 pairs of cranial nerves on the lower surface of the brain); or both. Neuropathic pain is usually associated with an identifiable disorder such as **stroke**, diabetes, or **spinal cord injury**, and is frequently described as having a "hot" or burning quality.

Psychogenic pain is distinguished from somatogenic pain by the influence of psychological factors on the intensity of the patient's pain or degree of disability. The patient is genuinely experiencing pain—that is, he or she is not malingering—but the pain has either no organic explanation or else a weak one. Common psychogenic pain syndromes include chronic **headache** or low **back pain**; atypical facial pain; or pelvic pain of unknown origin.

Some cases of psychogenic pain belong to a group of mental disorders known as somatoform disorders. According to the *Diagnostic and Statistical Manual of Mental Disorders*, Fourth Edition (DSM-IV), somatoform disorders are defined by "the presence of physical symptoms that suggest a general medical condition," but cannot be fully explained by such a condition, by the direct effects of a drug or other substance, or by another mental disorder. The somatoform disorders include somatization disorder, characterized by chronic complaints of unexplained physical symptoms, often involving multiple sites in the body; hypochondriasis is a preoccupation with illness that persists in spite of the doctor's reassurance; and pain disorder, characterized by physical pain that is intensified by psychological factors, often becoming the focus of the patient's life and impairing his or her family relationships and ability to work.

It is important to recognize that some pain syndromes may involve more than one type of pain. For example, a cancer patient may suffer from neuropathic pain as a side effect of cancer treatment as well as nociceptive pain associated with pressure from the tumor itself on nociceptors in a blood vessel or hollow organ. In addition to the somatogenic pain, the patient may experience psychogenic pain related to the loss of physical functioning or attractiveness, coupled with anxiety about the progression or recurrence of the cancer. Other pain syndromes do not fit neatly into either somatogenic or psychogenic categories. A case in point would be certain types of chronic headache that involve the stimulation of nociceptors in the tissues of the head and neck as well as psychogenic factors related to the patient's handling of stress.

Description
How the body feels pain

A person begins to feel pain when nociceptors in the skin, muscles, or internal organs detect pressure, inflammation, a toxic substance, or another harmful stimulus. The pain message travels along peripheral nerve fibers in the form of electrical impulses until it reaches the spinal cord. At this point, the pain message is filtered by specialized nerve cells that act as gatekeepers. Depending on the cause and severity of the pain, the nerve cells in the spinal cord may either activate motor nerves, which govern the ability to move away from the painful stimulus; block out the painful message; or release chemicals that increase or lower the strength of the original pain message on its way to the brain. The part of the spinal cord that receives and "processes" the pain messages from the peripheral nerves is known as the dorsal horn.

After the pain message reaches the brain, it is relayed to an egg-shaped central structure called the thalamus, which transmits the information to three specialized areas within the brain: the somatosensory cortex, which interprets physical sensations; the limbic system, which forms a border around the brain stem and governs emotional responses to physical stimuli; and the frontal cortex, which handles thinking. The activation of these three regions explains why human perception of pain is a complex combination of sensation, emotional arousal, and conscious thought.

In addition to receiving and interpreting pain signals, the brain responds to pain by activating parts of the nervous system that send additional blood to the injured part of the body or that release natural pain-relieving chemicals, including serotonin, endorphins, and enkephalins.

Factors that affect pain perception

LOCATION AND SEVERITY OF PAIN Pain varies in intensity and quality. It may be mild, moderate, or severe. In terms of quality, it may vary from a dull ache to sharp, piercing, burning, pulsating, tingling, or throbbing sensations; for example, the pain from jabbing one's finger on a needle feels different from the pain of touching a hot iron, even though both injuries involve the same part of the body. If the pain is severe, the nerve cells in the dorsal horn transmit the pain message rapidly; if the pain is relatively mild, the pain signals are transmitted along a different set of nerve fibers at a slower rate.

The location of the pain often affects a person's emotional and cognitive response, in that pain related to the head or other vital organs is usually more disturbing than pain of equal severity in a toe or finger.

GENDER Recent research has shown that sex hormones in mammals affect the level of tolerance for pain. The male sex hormone, testosterone, appears to raise the pain threshold in experimental animals, while the female hormone, estrogen, appears to increase the animal's recognition of pain. Humans, however, are influenced by their personal histories and cultures as well as by body chemistry. Studies of adult volunteers indicate that women tend to recover from pain more quickly than men, cope more effectively with it, and are less likely to allow pain to control their lives. One explanation of this difference comes from research with a group of analgesics known as kappa-opioids, which work better in women than in men. Some researchers think that female sex hormones may increase the effectiveness of some analgesic medications, while male sex hormones may make them less effective. In addition, women appear to be less sensitive to pain when their estrogen and progesterone levels are high, as happens during pregnancy and certain phases of the menstrual cycle. It has been noted, for example, that women with irritable bowel syndrome (IBS) often experience greater pain from the disorder during their periods.

FAMILY Another factor that influences pain perception in humans is family upbringing. Some parents comfort children who are hurting, while others ignore or even punish them for crying or expressing pain. Some families allow female members to express pain but expect males to "keep a stiff upper lip." People who suffer from chronic pain as adults may be helped by recalling their family's spoken and unspoken "messages" about pain, and working to consciously change those messages.

CULTURE AND ETHNICITY In addition to the nuclear family, a person's cultural or ethnic background can shape his or her perception of pain. People who have been exposed through their education to Western explanations of and treatments for pain may seek mainstream medical treatment more readily than those who have been taught to regard hospitals as places to die. On the other hand, Western medicine has been slower than Eastern and Native American systems of healing to recognize the importance of emotions and spirituality in treating pain. The recent upsurge of interest in alternative medicine in the United States is one reflection of dissatisfaction with a one-dimensional "scientific" approach to pain.

There are also differences among various ethnic groups within Western societies regarding ways of coping with pain. One study of African American, Irish, Italian, Jewish, and Puerto Rican patients being treated for chronic facial pain found differences among the groups in the intensity of emotional reactions to the pain and the extent to which the pain was allowed to interfere with daily functioning. However, much more work on larger patient samples is needed to understand the many ways in which culture and society affect people's perception of and responses to pain.

Demographics

Acute pain, particularly in its milder forms, is a commonplace experience in the general population; most people can think of at least one occasion in the past week or month when they had a brief tension headache, felt a little muscle soreness, cut themselves while shaving, or had a similar minor injury. On the other hand, chronic pain is more widespread than is generally thought; the American Chronic Pain Association estimates that 86 million people in the United States suffer from and are partially disabled by chronic pain. Two Canadian researchers evaluating a set of 13 studies of chronic pain done in North America, Europe, and Australia reported that the prevalence of severe chronic pain in these parts of the world is about 8% in children and 11% in adults. In terms of the economic impact of chronic pain, various productivity audits of the American workforce have stated that such pain syndromes as arthritis, lower back pain, and headache cost the United States between $80 and $90 billion every year.

The demographics of chronic pain depend on the specific disorder, including:

• Chronic pelvic pain (CPP) is more common in women than in men; it is thought to affect about 14% of adult women worldwide. In the United States, CPP is most common among women of reproductive age, particularly those between the ages of 26 and 30. It appears to be more common among African Americans than among Caucasians or Asian Americans. In addition, a history of sexual abuse before age 15 is a risk factor for CPP in adult life.

• Lower back pain (LBP) is the most common chronic disability in persons younger than 45. One researcher estimates that 80% of people in the United States will experience an episode of LBP at some point in life. About 3–4% of adults are disabled temporarily each year by LBP, with another 1% of the working-age population disabled completely and permanently. While 95% of patients with LBP recover within six to 12 weeks, the back pain becomes a chronic syndrome in the remaining 5%.

• Headaches in general are very common in the adult population in North America; about 95% of women and 90% of men in the United States and Canada have had at least one headache in the past twelve months. Most of these are tension headaches. Migraine headaches are less common than tension headaches, affecting about 11% of the population in the United States and 15% in Canada. Migraines occur most frequently in adults between the ages of 25 and 55; the gender ratio is about 3 F:1 M. Cluster headaches are the least common type of chronic headaches, affecting about 0.4% of adult males in the United States and 0.08% of adult females. The gender ratio is 7.5–5 M:1 F.

• Atypical facial pain is a less-common chronic pain syndrome, affecting one or two persons per 100,000 population each year. It is almost entirely a disorder of adults. Atypical facial pain is thought to affect men and women equally, and to occur with equal frequency in all races and ethnic groups.

Evaluation of pain
Patient description and history

A doctor's first step in evaluating a patient's pain is obtaining a detailed description of the pain, including:

Adjuvant A medication or other substance given to aid another drug, such as a tranquilizer given to ease the anxiety of a cancer patient in addition to an analgesic for pain relief.

Analgesic A medication that relieves pain without causing loss of consciousness. Over-the-counter analgesics include aspirin and nonsteroidal anti-inflammatory drugs (NSAIDs).

Bursa (plural, bursae) A fluid-filled sac or pouch located in joints or other pressure points between tendons and bones. Inflammation of a bursa is known as bursitis.

Capsaicin An alkaloid derived from hot peppers that can be used as a topical anesthetic.

Dorsal horn The part of the spinal cord that receives and processes pain messages from the peripheral nervous system.

Endorphins Neuropeptides produced by the body that are released in response to stress or injury and act as natural analgesics.

Enkephalins Polypeptides that serve as neurotransmitters and short-acting pain relievers. Enkephalins also influence a person's perception of painful sensations.

Eudynia The medical term for acute pain, or pain that is a symptom of an underlying disease or disorder.

Limbic system A group of structures found in the brains of all mammals that are associated with emotions, behavior, and such body functions as appetite and temperature regulation.

Maldynia The medical term for chronic pain, or pain that has become a disease in and of itself as a result of changes in the patient's nervous system.

Malingering Knowingly pretending to be physically or mentally ill in order to get out of some unpleasant duty or responsibility, or for economic benefit.

Narcotic Another term for opioid drugs that refers to their ability to produce drowsiness as well as relieve pain.

Neurotransmitter Any of a group of chemicals that transmit nerve impulses across the gap (synapse) between two nerve cells.

Nociceptor A specialized type of nerve cell that senses pain.

Opioid Any of a number of pain-relieving drugs derived from the opium poppy or from synthetic compounds that have the same effect as natural opioids.

Pain medicine The medical specialty that deals with the study and prevention of pain, and with the evaluation, treatment, and rehabilitation of patients with acute or chronic pain.

Somatoform disorders A group of psychiatric disorders in the DSM-IV classification that are characterized by external physical symptoms or complaints related to psychological problems rather than organic illness.

Thalamus An egg-shaped structure in the brain that integrates pain sensations and other sensory impulses, and relays them to other regions of the brain.

• severity

• timing (time of day; continuous or intermittent)

• location in the body

• quality (piercing, burning, aching, etc.)

• factors that relieve the pain or make it worse (temperature or humidity; body position or level of activity; foods or medications; emotional stress, etc.)

• its relationship to mood swings, anxiety, or depression

The doctor will then take the patient's medical history, including past illnesses, injuries, and operations as well as a family history. In some cases, the doctor may need to ask about experiences of emotional, physical, or sexual abuse. The doctor will also make a list of all the medications that the patient takes on a regular basis. Other information that may help the doctor evaluate the pain includes the patient's occupation and level of functioning at work; marriage and family relationships; social contacts and hobbies; and whether the patient is involved in a lawsuit for injury or seeking workers' compensation. This information may be helpful in understanding what the patient means by "pain" as well as what may have caused the pain, particularly because many people find it easier to discuss physical pain than anxiety, anger, depression, or sexual problems.

Some doctors may give the patient a brief written pain questionnaire to fill out in the office. There are a number of different instruments of this type, some of which are designed to measure pain associated with cancer, arthritis, HIV infection, or other specific diseases. Most of these rating questionnaires ask the patient to mark their pain level on a scale from zero to 10 or zero to 100 with zero representing "no pain" and the higher number representing "worst pain imaginable" or "unbearable pain." The patient then answers a few multiple-choice questions regarding the impact of the pain on his or her employment, relationships, and overall quality of life.

Physical examination

A thorough physical examination is essential in identifying the specific disorders or injuries that are causing the pain. The most important part of pain management is removing the underlying cause(s) whenever possible, even when there is a psychological component to the pain.

Special tests

Although there are no laboratory tests or imaging studies that can demonstrate the existence of pain as such or measure its intensity directly, the doctor may order special tests to help determine the cause(s) of the pain. These studies may include one or more of the following:

- Imaging studies, usually x rays or **magnetic resonance imagings** (**MRIs**). These studies can detect abnormalities in the structure of bones or joints, and differentiate between healthy and diseased tissues.

- Neurological tests. These tests evaluate the patient's movement, gait, reflexes, coordination, balance, and sensory perception.

- Electrodiagnostic tests. These tests include **electromyography** (EMG), nerve conduction studies, and evoked potential (EP) tests. In EMG, the doctor inserts thin needles in specific muscles and observes the electrical signals that are displayed on a screen. This test helps to pinpoint which muscles and nerves are affected by pain. Nerve conduction studies are done to determine whether specific nerves have been damaged. The doctor positions two sets of electrodes on the patient's skin over the muscles in the affected area. One set of electrodes stimulates the nerves supplying that muscle by delivering a mild electrical shock; the other set records the nerve's electrical signals on a machine. EP tests measure the speed of transmission of nerve impulses to the brain by using two electrodes, one attached to the patient's arm or leg and the other to the scalp.

- Thermography. This is an imaging technique that uses infrared scanning devices to convert changes in skin temperature into electrical impulses that can be displayed as different colors on a computer monitor. Pain related to inflammation, nerve damage, or abnormalities in skin blood flow can be effectively evaluated by thermography.

- Psychological tests. Such instruments as the Minnesota Multiphasic Personality Inventory (MMPI) may be helpful in assessing hypochondriasis and other personality traits related to psychogenic pain.

Treatment

Treatment of either acute or chronic pain may involve several different approaches to therapy.

Medications

Medications to relieve pain are known as analgesics. Aspirin and other nonsteroidal anti-inflammatory drugs, or NSAIDs, are commonly used analgesics. NSAIDs include such medications as ibuprofen (Motrin, Advil), ketoprofen (Orudis), diclofenac (Voltaren, Cataflam), naproxen (Aleve, Naprosyn), and nabumetone (Relafen). These medications are effective in treating mild or moderate pain. A newer group of NSAIDs, which are sometimes called "superaspirins" because they can be given in higher doses than aspirin without causing stomach upset or bleeding, are known as COX-2 inhibitors. The COX-2 inhibitors include celecoxib (Celebrex), rofecoxib (Vioxx), and valdecoxib (Bextra).

For more severe pain, the doctor may prescribe an NSAID combined with an opioid, usually codeine or hydrocodone. Opioids, which are also called narcotics, are strong painkillers derived either from the opium poppy *Papaver somniferum* or from synthetic compounds that have similar effects. Opioids include such drugs as codeine, fentanyl (Duragesic), hydromorphone (Dilaudid), meperidine (Demerol), morphine, oxycodone (OxyContin), and propoxyphene (Darvon). They are defined as Schedule II controlled substances by the Controlled Substances Act of 1970, which means that they have a high potential for abuse in addition to legitimate medical uses. A doctor must have a special license in order to prescribe opioids. In addition to the risk of abuse, opioids cause potentially serious side effects in some patients, including cognitive impairment (more common in the elderly), disorientation, constipation, nausea, heavy sweating, and skin rashes.

If the patient's pain is severe and persistent, the doctor will give separate dosages of opioids and NSAIDs in order to minimize the risk of side effects from high doses of aspirin or acetaminophen. In addition, the doctor may prescribe opioids that are stronger than codeine—usually morphine, fentanyl, or levorphanol.

The "WHO Ladder" for the treatment of cancer pain is based on the three levels of analgesic medication. Patients with mild pain from cancer are given nonopioid medications with or without an adjuvant (helping) medication. For example, the doctor may prescribe a tranquilizer to relieve the patient's anxiety as well as the pain medication. Patients on the second "step" of the ladder are given a milder opioid and a nonopioid analgesic with or without an adjuvant drug. Patients with severe cancer pain are given stronger opioids at higher dosage levels with or without an adjuvant drug.

Acute pain following surgery is usually managed with opioid medications, most commonly morphine sulfate (Astromorph, Duramorph) or meperidine (Demerol). In some cases, NSAIDs that are available in injectable form (such as ketorolac) are also used. Patient-controlled analgesia, or PCA, allows patients to control the timing and amount of pain medication they receive. Although there are oral forms of PCA, the most common form of administration involves an infusion pump that delivers a small dose of medication through an intravenous line when the patient pushes a button. The PCA pump is pre-programmed to deliver no more than an hourly maximum amount of the drug.

Some types of chronic pain are treated by injections in specific areas of the body rather than by drugs administered by mouth or intravenously. There are three basic categories of injections for pain management:

• Joint injections. Joint injections are given to treat chronic pain associated with arthritis. The most common medications used are corticosteroids, which suppress inflammation in arthritic joints, and hyaluronic acid, which is a compound found in the joint fluid of healthy joints.

• Soft tissue injections. These are given to reduce pain in trigger points (areas of muscle that are hypersensitive to touch) and bursae, which are small pouches or sacs containing tissue fluid that cushions pressure points between tendons and bones. When a bursa becomes inflamed—a condition called bursitis—the person experiences pain in the nearby joint. Corticosteroids are the drugs most often used in soft tissue injections, although the doctor may also inject an anesthetic into a trigger point in order to relax the muscle.

• Nerve blocks. Nerve blocks are injections of anesthetic around the fibers of a nerve to prevent pain messages relayed along the nerve from reaching the brain. They may be used to relieve pain in specific parts of the body for a short period; a common example of this type of nerve block is the lidocaine injections given by dentists before drilling or extracting a tooth. Some nerve blocks are injected in or near the spinal column to control pain that affects a larger area of the body; an example is the epidural injection given to women in labor or to patients with **sciatica**. A third type of nerve block is administered to block the sympathetic nervous system as part of pain management in patients with complex chronic pain syndromes.

Medications used to treat neuropathic pain include tricyclic antidepressants, anticonvulsant medications, selective serotonin reuptake inhibitors, topical creams containing capsaicin or 5% lidocaine, and diphenhydramine (Benadryl).

Surgery

Because surgery is itself a cause of pain, few surgical treatments to relieve pain were available prior to the discovery of safe general anesthetics in the mid-nineteenth century. For most of human history, doctors were limited to procedures that could be completed within two to three minutes because the patients could not bear the pain of the operation. Ancient Egyptian doctors gave their patients wine mixed with opium, while early European doctors made their patients drunk with brandy, tied them to the benches that served as operating tables, or put pressure on a nerve or artery to numb a specific part of the body.

Modern surgeons, however, can perform a variety of procedures to relieve either acute or chronic pain, depending on its cause. These procedures include:

• removal of diseased or dead tissue to prevent infection

• removal of cancerous tissue to prevent the spread of the cancer and relieve pressure on nearby healthy organs and tissues

• correction or reconstruction of malformed or damaged bones

• insertion of artificial joints or other body parts to replace damaged structures

• organ transplantation

• insertion of pacemakers and other electrical devices that improve the functioning of damaged organs or help to control pain directly

• cutting or destroying damaged nerves to control neuropathic pain

PSYCHOTHERAPY Psychotherapy may be helpful to patients with chronic pain syndromes by exploring the connections between anger, depression, or anxiety and physical pain sensations. One type of psychotherapy that has been shown to be effective is cognitive restructuring, an approach that teaches people to "reframe" the problems in their lives—that is, to change their conscious attitudes and responses to these stressors. Some psychotherapists teach relaxation techniques, biofeedback, or other approaches to stress management as well as cognitive restructuring.

Another type of psychotherapy that is effective in treating some patients with chronic pain is hypnosis. Although there is some disagreement among researchers as to whether hypnosis works by distracting the patient's attention from painful sensations or whether it works by stimulating the release of endorphins (chemicals produced by the body that are released in response to stress or injury and act as natural analgesics), it has been approved by the American Medical Association since 1958 as a treatment for pain. Some therapists offer instruction in self-hypnosis to patients with chronic pain.

COMPLEMENTARY AND ALTERNATIVE (CAM) AP-PROACHES CAM therapies that are used in pain management include:

- **Acupuncture**. Studies funded by the National Center for Complementary and Alternative Medicine (NCCAM) since 1998 have found that acupuncture is an effective treatment for chronic pain in many patients. It is thought that acupuncture works by stimulating the release of endorphins, the body's natural painkillers.

- **Exercise**. Physical exercise stimulates the body to produce endorphins.

- Yoga. Practiced under a doctor's supervision, yoga helps to maintain flexibility and range of motion in joints and muscles. The breathing exercises that are part of a yoga practice also relax the body.

- Prayer and meditation. The act of prayer by itself helps many people to relax. In addition, prayer and meditation are ways to refocus one's attention and keep pain from becoming the center of one's life.

- Naturopathy. Naturopaths include dietary advice and nutritional therapy in their treatment, which is effective for some patients suffering from chronic pain syndromes.

- Hydrotherapy. Warm whirlpool baths ease muscular and joint pain.

- Music therapy. Music therapy may involve listening to music, making music, or both. Some researchers think that music works to relieve pain by temporarily blocking the "gates" of pain in the dorsal horn of the spinal cord, while others believe that music stimulates the release of endorphins.

Pain management

Pain management refers to a set of skills and techniques for coping with chronic pain. The goal of pain management is not complete elimination of pain; rather, the patient learns to keep the pain at a level that he or she can tolerate, and to make the most of life in spite of the pain. The American Chronic Pain Association (ACPA) lists seven coping skills that help in managing pain:

- not dwelling on physical pain symptoms

- emphasizing abilities rather than disabilities

- recognizing one's feelings about the pain and discussing them freely

- using relaxation exercises to ease the emotional tension that makes pain worse.

- doing mild stretching exercises every day (with medical approval)

- setting realistic goals for improvement and evaluating them on a weekly basis

- affirming one's basic rights: the right to make mistakes, the right to say no, and the right to ask questions

An important part of pain management is participation in a multidisciplinary pain program. Many hospitals and rehabilitation centers in the United States and Canada offer pain management programs. Ideally, the program will have its own unit apart from patient care areas. Good pain management programs offer comprehensive treatment that includes relaxation training and stress management techniques; group therapy, family therapy, personal counseling, and job retraining; physical therapy, including exercise and body mechanics; patient education regarding medications and other aspects of pain management; and aftercare or follow-up support.

The treatment team in a pain management program is usually headed by a **neurologist**, psychiatrist, or anesthesiologist with specialized training in pain management. Other members of the team include registered nurses, psychiatrists or psychologists, physical and occupational therapists, massage therapists, family therapists, and vocational counselors.

Clinical trials

As of December 2003, the National Institutes of Health (NIH) was sponsoring 35 studies related to various chronic pain conditions and the effectiveness of such treatments as acupuncture, hypnosis, yoga, COX-2 inhibitors, and several experimental drugs.

Special concerns
Pain management in special populations

Pain management in the elderly and in children poses additional challenges. Although 20% of adults over 65 take an analgesic on a regular basis, older people are more vulnerable to the drug's side effects, particularly the nausea and bleeding that sometimes results from long-term use of NSAIDs. Children require special attention because they do not have an adult's ability to describe their pain. New tools have been developed since the mid-1990s to measure pain in children and to help doctors understand their nonverbal cues.

Addiction and withdrawal

Doctors have debated the risk of opioid abuse for most of the past century. For many years, patients with severe chronic pain were not given enough of the drugs they needed to control their pain because of the fear that they would become addicted to the narcotics. In the mid-1980s, however, some experts in pain management argued that the risk of addiction was quite low, whether the patients suffered from cancer pain or from chronic pain unrelated to cancer. As a result, some synthetic narcotics—most notably oxycodone (OxyContin)—were widely prescribed and a growing number of patients became addicted to these drugs. As of 2003, researchers estimate that 3–14% of the population may have an underlying undiagnosed vulnerability to abuse these substances.

In addition to the risk of abuse, there is a risk of withdrawal symptoms and a temporary increase in pain (known as rebound pain) if opioid medications are discontinued suddenly. Withdrawal symptoms include diarrhea, runny nose and watery eyes, restlessness, insomnia, anxiety, nausea, and abdominal cramps. These symptoms are usually treated with clonidine (Catapres), an antihypertensive drug, and NSAIDs or antihistamines. The various risks of long-term use of opioids in pain management are not yet fully understood.

Resources

BOOKS

Altman, Lawrence K., MD. *Who Goes First? The Story of Self-Experimentation in Medicine.* Berkeley, CA: University of California Press, 1998.

American Psychiatric Association. *Diagnostic and Statistical Manual of Mental Disorders*, 4th edition, text revision. Washington, DC: American Psychiatric Association, 2000.

Martin, John H. *Neuroanatomy: Text and Atlas*, 3rd ed. New York: McGraw-Hill, 2003.

"Pain." *The Merck Manual of Diagnosis and Therapy*, edited by Mark H. Beers, MD, and Robert Berkow, MD. Whitehouse Station, NJ: Merck Research Laboratories, 2002.

Pelletier, Kenneth R., MD. *The Best Alternative Medicine*, Part II, "CAM Therapies for Specific Conditions: Pain." New York: Simon & Schuster, 2002.

PERIODICALS

Daitz, Ben. "In Pain Clinic, Fruit, Candy and Relief." *New York Times*, December 3, 2002.

Duenwald, Mary. "Tales from a Burn Unit: Agony, Friendship, Healing." *New York Times*, March 18, 2003.

Halsey, James H., MD. "Atypical Facial Pain." *eMedicine*, February 9, 2001 (February 24, 2004). <http://www.emedicine.com/neuro/topic25.htm>.

Harstall, Christa, and Maria Ospina. "How Prevalent Is Chronic Pain?" *Pain: Clinical Updates* 11 (June 2003): 1–4.

Lasch, Kathryn E., PhD. "Culture and Pain." *Pain: Clinical Updates* 10 (December 2002): 1–11.

Meier, Barry. "The Delicate Balance of Pain and Addiction." *New York Times*, November 25, 2003.

Singh, Manish K., MD, Elizabeth Puscheck, MD, and Jashvant Patel, MD. "Chronic Pelvic Pain." *eMedicine*, November 7, 2003 (February 24, 2004). <http://emedicine.com/med/topic2939.htm>.

Wheeler, Anthony H., MD. "Therapeutic Injections for Pain Management." *eMedicine*, October 19, 2001 (February 24, 2004). http://www.emedicine.com/neuro/topic514.htm>.

Wheeler, Anthony H., MD, James R. Stubbart, MD, and Brandi Hicks. "Pathophysiology of Chronic Back Pain." *eMedicine*, March 8, 2002 (February 24, 2004). <http://www.emedicine.com/neuro/topic516.htm>.

Yates, William R., MD. "Somatoform Disorders." *eMedicine*, November 20, 2003 (February 24, 2004). <http://www.emedicine.com/med/topic3527.htm>.

WEBSITES

<http://www.Pain.com>.

<http://www.PartnersAgainstPain.com>.

OTHER

National Institute of Neurological Disorders and Stroke (NINDS). "Pain—Hope Through Research." NIH Publication No. 01-2406. 2001.

NINDS. "Chronic Pain Information Page." Bethesda, MD: NINDS, 2001. (February 24, 2004.) <http://www.ninds.nih.gov/health_and_medical/pubs/migraineupdate.htm>.

ORGANIZATIONS

American Academy of Neurology (AAN). 1080 Montreal Avenue, Saint Paul, MN 55116. (651) 695-2717 or (800) 879-1960; Fax: (651) 695-2791. memberservices@aan.com. <http://www.aan.com>.

American Academy of Pain Medicine (AAPM). 4700 West Lake, Glenview, IL 60025. (847) 375-4731; Fax: (877) 734-8750. aapm@amctec.com. <http://www.painmed.org>.

American Chronic Pain Association. P. O. Box 850, Rocklin, CA 95677. (916) 632-3208 or (800) 533-3231. ACPA@pacbell.net. <http://www.theacpa.org>.

American Pain Foundation. 201 North Charles Street, Suite 710, Baltimore, MD 21201-4111. (888) 615-PAIN. <http://www.painfoundation.org>.

International Association for the Study of Pain (IASP) Secretariat. 909 NE 43rd Street, Suite 306, Seattle, WA 98105-6020. (206) 547-6409; Fax: (206) 547-1703. iaspdesk@juno.com. <http://www.iasp-pain.org>.

NIH Neurological Institute. P. O. Box 5801, Bethesda, MD 20824. (301) 496-5751 or (800) 352-9424. <http://www.ninds.nih.gov>.

Rebecca J. Frey, PhD

Pallidotomy

Definition

Pallidotomy is the destruction of a small portion of the brain within the globus pallidus internus, or GPi. The GPi helps control voluntary movements.

Purpose

Pallidotomy is performed to treat the symptoms of **Parkinson's disease** (PD), which results from the death of cells in a part of the brain that controls movement, called the substantia nigra. Part of the normal function of the substantia nigra is to inhibit overactivity of the GPi, which itself communicates with other portions of the brain in complex control circuits. In PD, the overactivity of the GPi is in part responsible for the slowed movements, tremor, and rigidity that are the classic symptoms of the disease. By destroying part of the GPi, some balance is restored to these movement-control circuits, allowing faster and more fluid movements.

Early on in PD, symptoms can be effectively treated with medication, especially levodopa and the dopamine agonists (drugs that act like levodopa). As the disease progresses, increasing amounts of drugs are needed to control symptoms, and the patient's response to the drugs declines. Typically, within 10 years of starting treatment, the patient will develop uncontrolled movements, called dyskinesias, in response to drug treatment. At this point, surgery is considered an option.

The GPi has two halves, which control movements on opposites sides of the body: right controls left, left controls right. Unilateral (one-sided) pallidotomy may be used if symptoms are markedly worse on one side or the other, or if the risks from bilateral (two-sided) pallidotomy are judged to be too great.

Precautions

Pallidotomy is major surgery on the brain. It may cause excessive bleeding, and care must be taken in patients susceptible to uncontrolled bleeding or who are on anticoagulant therapy.

Description

To destroy tissue in the GPi, a long needle-like probe is inserted deep into the brain, through a hole in the top of the skull. To make sure the probe reaches its target exactly, a rigid "stereotactic frame" is attached to the patient's head. This provides an immobile three-dimensional coordinate system, which can be used both to determine the precise position of the GPi and to track the probe on its way to the target.

A single "burr hole" is made in the top of the skull for a unilateral pallidotomy; two holes are made for a bilateral procedure. General anesthesia is not used for two reasons: first, the brain does not feel any **pain**; second, the patient must be awake and responsive in order to respond to the neurosurgical team as they monitor the placement of the probe. The GPi is close to the nerve that carries visual information from the eyes to the rear of the brain. Visual abnormalities during probe placement may indicate that it is too close to this region, and thus needs repositioning.

Other procedures may be used to ensure precise placement of the probe, including electrical recording and injection of a contrast dye into the spinal fluid. The electrical recording can cause some minor odd sensations, but is harmless.

When the probe is in the correct position, its tip is heated briefly. This destroys the surrounding tissue in an area about the size of a pearl. If bilateral pallidotomy is being performed, the localizing and lesioning will be repeated on the other side.

Preparation

A variety of medical tests are needed to properly locate the GPi and fit the frame. These may include computed tomography (**CT**) scans, **magnetic resonance imaging (MRI)**, and injection of dyes into the spinal fluid or ventricles (fluid-filled cavities) of the brain. The frame is attached to the head on the day of surgery, which may be somewhat painful, although the pain is lessened by local anesthetic. A mild sedative is given to ease anxiety.

Aftercare

Pallidotomy takes several hours to perform. In some medical centers, pallidotomy is performed as an outpatient procedure, and patients are sent home the same day. Most centers provide an overnight stay or longer for observation and recuperation. Movement usually improves immediately, and typically requires the reduction of medication to accommodate the improvement.

Risks

Pallidotomy carries significant risks, especially in patients who are in poor health or who are cognitively impaired. Brain hemorrhage is a possible complication, as is infection. Damage to the optic tract, which carries visual messages from the eye to the brain, is a small but significant risk, and is more significant in bilateral pallidotomy. Speech impairments may also occur, including difficulty retrieving words, and slurred speech.

All PD experts agree that risks are lowest when the surgery is performed by neurosurgeons with the most experience in the procedure. Among the best surgeons, the risk of serious morbidity or mortality (i.e., serious consequences or death) is 1–2%. Hemorrhage may occur in 2–6%, visual deficits in 0–6%, and weakness in 2–8%.

Normal results

Pallidotomy improves the patient's ability to move, especially between levodopa doses (so-called "off" periods). Studies show the surgery generally improves tremor, rigidity, and slowed movements by 25–60%. Dyskinesias typically improve by 75% or more. Improvements from unilateral pallidotomy are primarily on the side opposite the surgery. Balance does not improve, nor do "nonmotor" symptoms such as drooling, constipation, and **orthostatic hypotension** (lightheadedness on standing).

Resources

BOOKS

Jahanshahi, M., and C. D. Marsden. *Parkinson's Disease: A Self-Help Guide.* New York: Demos Medical Press, 2000.

WEBSITES

National Parkinson's Disease Foundation. <http://www.pdf.org/> (March 23, 2004).

WE MOVE. <http://www.wemove.org> (March 23, 2004).

Richard Robinson

Pantothenate kinase-associated neurodegeneration

Definition

Pantothenate kinase-associated neurodegeneration (PKAN), long known as Hallervorden-Spatz syndrome (HSS), is a very rare childhood neurodegenerative disorder that is associated with the accumulation of iron in the brain, which causes progressively worsening abnormal movements and **dementia**.

Description

In addition to its original name, Hallervorden-Spatz syndrome, pantothenate kinase-associated neurodegeneration has also been called neurodegeneration with brain iron accumulation (NBIA). The name Hallervorden-Spatz is rapidly being discontinued by those who study and treat the disease, both because the new names indicate the nature of the underlying disorder, and because Julius Hallervorden, who described the syndrome, was involved in a "selective euthanasia" program in Nazi Germany to kill retarded children.

Demographics

PKAN is so rare that there is no reliable information on its prevalence. It affects boys and girls equally. Typical age of onset is in middle childhood to early adolescence, although onset in early adulthood may occur.

Causes and symptoms

PKAN occurs due to mutation in the gene for pantothenate kinase 2 (PANK2), which is an enzyme, a type of protein that regulates a reaction inside a cell. PANK2 helps regulates the production of coenzyme A, an important intermediate in the production of energy within all cells. Mutations in the gene for PANK2 lead to loss of function of this enzyme, the consequence of which is accumulation of iron and the amino acid cysteine within

---

Key Terms

Dystonia Painful involuntary muscle cramps or spasms.

Enzyme A protein that catalyzes a biochemical reaction without changing its own structure or function.

Neurodegeneration The deterioration of nerve tissues.

---

brain cells. It is not yet known how this leads to the disease, but it is possible that cysteine interacts with iron, leading to buildup of other molecules within brain cells that puts stress on the cells and causes them to degenerate.

PKAN causes **dystonia**, a sustained posturing of lower limbs due to excessive muscle contraction. Leg dystonia leads to gait difficulties and other limitations of movement. Dystonia may also affect the upper limbs and the muscles of the face and neck. Abnormal movements may also include writhing or tremor. Ability to walk is usually lost within 15 years. **Dysarthria**, or impairment of the ability to speak, is common, and is usually accompanied by swallowing difficulty. PKAN also causes progressive dementia, or impairment of normal intellectual function, although this is more variable among patients. PKAN may also cause a degenerative eye condition, retinitis pigmentosa.

An atypical form of PKAN has similar features, but with later age of onset and more variable and less severe symptoms. Speech difficulties tend to be more common in atypical patients. Atypical patients may or may not have a recognizable gene defect.

Diagnosis

Diagnosis of PKAN begins with a neurological exam, which is followed up by a **magnetic resonance imaging (MRI)** scan to reveal a characteristic signal from the affected portions of the brain. Genetic testing may be done to look for the mutation in the PKAN gene.

Treatment team

Treatment involves a pediatric **neurologist**, a speech-language pathologist, and physical and occupational therapists.

Treatment

There is no treatment that can halt or slow the degeneration of the brain that occurs in PKAN. The recent discovery of the gene defect may lead to a better understanding of the neurodegenerative process, and thereby to better treatments.

Drug therapy for the **movement disorders** of PKAN is variably successful, and becomes less so with time. Drugs used for **Parkinson's disease** such as levodopa may be beneficial in some patients. Trihexyphenidyl may be useful. Oral antispasticity medications, including **diazepam** and dantrolene, can help reduce muscle stiffness and **spasticity**. Intrathecal baclofen has been successful in several patients. A **pallidotomy**, a type of brain surgery that destroys part of the globus pallidus internus, a structure in the brain that regulates movements, has shown some success at relieving painful dystonia and returning some function to the affected limbs.

Speech impairment may be the most severe consequence of PKAN. Assistive communication devices such as computers or letter boards offer the possibility of continued communication even as the disease worsens.

Recovery and rehabilitation
Clinical trials

PKAN is so rare there are few **clinical trials**. Some effort is underway to determine whether supplements with PANK2's normal products or related molecules may be effective.

Prognosis

The average duration of disease is 11 years. Death is usually caused by aspiration pneumonia, brought on by food inhaled into the airways.

Resources
BOOKS

The Official Patient's Sourcebook on Hallervorden-Spatz Disease: A Revised and Updated Directory for the Internet Age. San Diego: Icon Health Publications, 2002.

WEBSITES

NBIA Disorders Association. <http://www.hssa.org/> (April 27, 2004).

Richard Robinson

Papilledema *see* **Visual disturbances**

Paramyotonia congenita

Definition

Paramyotonia congenita is an inherited condition that causes stiffness and enlargement of muscles, particularly leg muscles.

Description

Paramyotonia congenita is passed on in families as an autosomal dominant trait. This means that males and females are affected equally; it also means that if one parent has the trait, the offspring have a 75% chance of also having the condition.

Demographics

Paramyotonia congenita is present from birth on. In some cases, the symptoms appear to grow more mild as the patient ages.

Causes and symptoms

Paramyotonia congenita is believed to be caused by a defect in the chloride channels of the muscles. As a result, the relaxation phase of the muscles is impaired, resulting in prolonged muscle contraction and stiffness. This "overuse" of the muscle results in the muscle becoming enlarged and bulky (called muscle hypertrophy).

Symptoms of paramyotonia congenita include stiffness and enlargement of various muscle groups, particularly those in the legs. The muscle stiffness of paramyotonia congenita is often exacerbated by cold temperatures and inactivity and relieved by warmth and **exercise**.

Diagnosis

Electromyographic (EMG) testing involves placing a needle electrode into a muscle and measuring its electrical activity. EMG testing in paramyotonia congenita may reveal differences between electrical activity in a warm muscle and electrical activity in a cooled muscle. There are a number of genetic defects that are associated with the chloride channel defect of paramyotonia congenita, some of which can be revealed through genetic testing.

Treatment team

Paramyotonia congenita is diagnosed and treated by neurologists.

Treatment

Paramyotonia congenita is usually mild enough not to require any treatment at all. If muscle stiffness is truly problematic, quinine or anticonvulsant medications (such as phenytoin) may improve functioning.

Prognosis

Paramyotonia congenita has an excellent prognosis. Although annoying, it does not cause significant disability, and the patient usually learns to make lifestyle adjustments that prevent exacerbations (for example, dressing warmly and avoiding exposure to cold).

Resources

BOOKS

Brown, Robert H., and Jerry R. Mendell. "Muscular Dystrophies and Other Muscle Diseases." In *Harrison's Principles of Internal Medicine*, edited by Eugene Braunwald, et al. NY: McGraw-Hill Professional, 2001.

Rose, Michael, and Robert C. Griggs. "Hereditary Nondegenerative Neuromuscular Disease." In *Textbook of Clinical Neurology*, edited by Christopher G. Goetz. Philadelphia: W. B. Saunders Company, 2003.

WEBSITES

National Institute of Neurological Disorders and Stroke (NINDS). *NINDS Myotonia Congenita Information Page.* November 8, 2001. <http://www.ninds.nih.gov/health_and_medical/disorders/myotoniacongenita.htm> (June 3, 2004).

Rosalyn Carson-DeWitt, MD

Paraneoplastic syndromes

Definition

Paraneoplastic syndromes (PS) are rare disorders triggered by the immune system's response to cancer cells, or by remote effects of tumor-derived factors. These syndromes are believed to occur when cancer-fighting antibodies or white blood cells, known as T-cells, mistakenly attack normal body cells. These disorders typically affect middle-aged to older people and are most common in patients with lung, ovarian, lymphatic, or breast cancer.

Description

Paraneoplastic syndromes are defined as clinical syndromes involving non-cancerous effects in the body that accompany malignant disease, and can affect any part of the nervous system from the cerebral cortex to peripheral nerves and muscles. In a broad sense, these syndromes are collections of symptoms that result from substances produced by the tumor, occurring far away from the tumor itself. When a tumor arises, the body may produce antibodies to fight it, by binding to and helping in the destruction of tumor cells. Unfortunately, in some cases, these antibodies cross-react with normal tissues and destroy them, which may stimulate the onset of PS. However, not all PS are associated with such antibodies.

Neurological symptoms generally develop over a period of days to weeks, and usually occur prior to the discovery of cancer, which can complicate diagnosis. In these cases, additional information should raise the possibility that the patient may have a hidden cancer and that neurological symptoms could be paraneoplastic. Symptoms include **fatigue**, weakness, muscular **pain** in upper arms, difficulty walking, burning, numbness or tingling sensations in the limbs (peripheral paresthesia), dry mouth, sexual function difficulty, and drooping eyelids.

Neurological signs may include **dementia** with or without brain stem signs, rapid and irregular eye movements, and ophthalmoplegia (weakness or paralysis in muscles that move the eye). Paraneoplastic syndromes involving the nervous system include: **Lambert-Eaton myasthenic syndrome** (LEMS), **stiff person syndrome** (SPS), encephalomyelitis (inflammation of the brain and spinal cord), **myasthenia gravis** (MG), cerebellar degeneration (CD), limbic and/or brain stem encephalitis, neuromyotonia, **opsoclonus myoclonus** (OM), and sensory neuropathy.

Demographics

Most paraneoplastic syndromes are rare, affecting less than 1% of persons with cancer. Exceptions include LEMS, which affects about 3% of patients with small-cell lung cancer; MG, which affects about 15% of persons with thymoma; and demyelinating **peripheral neuropathy**, which affects about 50% of patients with the rare osteosclerotic form of plasmacytoma. No race, age, or sex preference has been reported.

Causes and symptoms

Most or all paraneoplastic syndromes are activated by the body's immune system. In response to a tumor, the immune system produces an antigen that is normally expressed exclusively in the nervous system. The tumor antigen is identical to the normal antigen, but for unknown reasons the immune system identifies it as foreign and mounts an immune response.

In general (although not always), PS develops in an acute or subacute fashion, over days or weeks. Symptoms may include difficulty in walking and/or swallowing, loss of muscle tone, loss of fine motor coordination, slurred speech, memory loss, vision problems, sleep disturbances, dementia, **seizures**, sensory loss in the limbs, and vertigo. The nervous system disability is usually severe.

Diagnosis

Currently, paraneoplastic syndromes are diagnosed using two different technologies in testing blood. Blood testing with western blot using recombinant human antigens is a highly specific method; it can clearly distinguish between different paraneoplastic antibodies. Immunohistochemistry can detect paraneoplastic antibodies in blood

Key Terms

Antibodies A protein produced by the body's immune system to fight infection or harmful foreign substances.

Cytotoxic T-cells A type of white blood cells, T lymphocytes, that can kill body cells infected by viruses or transformed by cancer.

Dysarthria Problems with speaking caused by difficulty moving or coordinating the muscles needed for speech.

Nystagmus Rapid, involuntary eye movements.

Ophthalmoplegia Drooping eyelids.

serum, providing a general diagnosis, but cannot distinguish between the different PS antibodies.

The physician should search for cancer using the most sensitive technology available, including **magnetic resonance imaging (MRI)** and a fluorodeoxyglucose body **positron emission tomography (PET)** scan.

Treatment team

Due to the many manifestations of paraneoplastic syndromes, PS should be evaluated clinically by a coordinated team of doctors, including medical oncologists, surgeons, **radiation** oncologists, endocrinologists, hematologists, neurologists, and dermatologists.

Treatment

Because PS are considered to be immune-mediated disorders, two treatment approaches have been used: removal of the source of the antigen by treatment of the underlying tumor, and suppression of the immune response. For many PS, the first approach is the only effective treatment. In the LEMS and MG, plasma exchange or intravenous immune globulin is usually effective in suppressing the immune response.

Physicians often also prescribe a combination of either plasma exchange or intravenous immune globulin and immunosuppressive agents such as corticosteroids, cyclophosphamide, or tacrolimus. For most paraneoplastic syndromes, immunotherapy is not effective.

Recovery and rehabilitation

Some disorders such as the LEMS and MG respond well to immunosuppressant drugs and to treatment of the underlying tumor. The peripheral neuropathy associated with osteosclerotic myeloma generally resolves when the tumor is treated with radiotherapy. A few disorders may respond to treatment of the underlying tumor, immunosuppression, or both, or they may resolve spontaneously. In many instances, it is not clear whether the PS resolve spontaneously or in response to treatment. Disorders involving the **central nervous system**, such as encephalomyelitis associated with cancer or paraneoplastic cerebellar degeneration, usually respond poorly to treatment, although they may stabilize when the underlying tumor is treated.

Clinical trials

As of mid-2004, the numerous **clinical trials** recruiting participants for the study and treatment of paraneoplastic syndromes include:

- Interferon and Octreotide to Treat Zollinger-Ellison Syndrome and Advanced Non-B Islet Cell Cancer
- Evaluating Pancreatic Tumors in Patients with Zollinger-Ellison Syndrome
- Treatment of Zollinger-Ellison Syndrome
- The Use of Oral Omeprazole and Intravenous Pantoprazole in Patients with Hypersecretion of Gastric Acid

Updates information on these and other ongoing trials can be found at the National Institutes of Health website for clinical trials at <http://www.clinicaltrials.gov>.

Prognosis

The prognosis for persons with paraneoplastic syndromes depends on the specific type of PS, and the progression of the underlying cancer. LEMS and MG are neuromuscular junction diseases, which can recover function once the causal insult is removed, because there is no neuronal loss. Disorders such as CD are usually associated with neuronal damage, and because they evolve subacutely and treatment is often delayed, neurons die, making recovery much more difficult. Some central nervous system disorders such as OM may not involve cellular loss and, thus, patients with these disorders, like those with LEMS, have the potential for recovery.

Special concerns

It is important that caregivers for those with paraneoplastic syndromes receive adequate support. The disorder typically emerges suddenly and without warning. The neurological manifestations of PS are complex and often require 24-hour patient care. Many caregivers will require quick access to information on caring for a disabled person. This includes information on social security benefits, insurance coverage, handicapped license plates, evaluations for physical therapy; medical equipment such as hospital beds, ultra-light wheelchairs, handheld showerheads, and home healthcare and visiting nurses; and **social workers** and other support services.

Resources

BOOKS

Ruter, U., et al. *Paraneoplastic Syndromes.* Basel: S. Karger Publishing, 1998.

PERIODICALS

Robert, B. D., and P. B. Jerome. "Paraneoplastic Syndromes Involving the Nervous System." *New England Journal of Medicine* 349 (2003): 1543–1554.

Sutton, I., and J. B. Winer. "The Immunopathogenesis of Paraneoplastic Neurological Syndromes." *Clinical Science* 102 (2002): 475–486.

OTHER

"NINDS Paraneoplastic Syndromes Information Page." *National Institute of Neurological Disorders and Stroke.* May 1, 2004 (June 2, 2004). <http://www.ninds.nih.gov/health_and_medical/disorders/paraneoplastic.htm>.

Santacroce, Luigi. "Paraneoplastic Syndromes." *eMedicine.* May 1, 2004 (June 2, 2004). <http://www.emedicine.com/med/topic1747.htm>.

ORGANIZATIONS

American Autoimmune Related Diseases Association. 22100 Gratiot Avenue, Eastpointe, MI 48201-2227. (586) 776-3900 or (800) 598-4668; Fax: (586) 776-3903. aarda@aol.com. <http://www.aarda.org>.

National Cancer Institute (NCI)—National Institutes of Health. Bldg. 31, Rm. 10A31, Bethesda, MD 20892-2580. (301) 435-3848. cancermail@icicc.nci.nih.gov. <http://cancer net.nci.nih.gov>.

American Cancer Society. 1599 Clifton Road, NE, Atlanta, GA 30329-4251 or (800) ACS-2345 (227-2345). <http://www.cancer.org>.

Francisco de Paula Careta
Iuri Drumond Louro, MD, PhD

▌Parkinson's disease

Definition

Parkinson's disease (PD) is a neurodegenerative disorder that causes slowed movements, tremor, rigidity, and a wide variety of other symptoms. "Neurodegenerative" refers to the degeneration, or death, of neurons, the type of cell in the brain that is the basis for all brain activity.

Description

Parkinson's disease occurs when neurons (nerve cells) in a part of the brain called the substantia nigra degenerate, or die off. The loss of these cells disrupts the brain's normal control of movement, causing the person to experience slowed movements, stiffness or rigidity, and tremor.

Demographics

PD is one of the most common neurodegenerative diseases, second only to **Alzheimer's disease** in the number of people affected. Estimates suggest that approximately 750,000 Americans have PD. It affects older people much more than younger, and indeed, old age is the single greatest risk factor for PD. The average age at diagnosis is 62. Onset before age 40 is extremely rare. Men are slightly more likely to be affected than women.

Causes and symptoms

In the vast majority of cases, the cause of PD is unknown. Besides old age, there are several well-recognized risk factors. These include exposure to pesticides or herbicides, rural living, and drinking well water. Because of this, it is assumed that some type of environmental pollutant, either a pesticide or something associated with its use, is involved in causing PD. Other known risk factors include welding and exposure to manganese, further strengthening the case for an environmental toxin.

There is also evidence that genes play an important role in determining the risk of PD. PD can run in families, affecting members of the family at a much higher rate than expected by chance alone. Among identical twins, the situation is complex: if one twin develops the disease early, the other is more likely to as well; but if one twin has typical late-onset PD, the other is no more likely to develop the disease than would be expected by chance.

Several genes have been identified that cause PD in some people, but the number of people affected by these genes is quite small. Therefore, the interest of these genes is more in what they can reveal about the disease process than in providing the solution to the mystery of what causes PD in most people. Two of the genetic mutations identified involve a protein called alpha-synuclein, whose normal function is unknown. It is believed that the mutations prevent the normal breakdown of alpha-synuclein, leading it to accumulate in the neuron, where it then goes on to damage the cell. Another gene mutation that causes PD affects a protein called parkin, which normally helps break down proteins. It is believed that the loss of parkin causes build-up of proteins (though not of alpha-synuclein), again leading to damage. Researchers believe that environmental toxins may also cause similar problems, and it now seems likely that problems in protein breakdown are a significant step leading to PD, whether of genetic or environmental causation. Finally, a combination of genetic and environmental factors is likely to be important in most cases. For instance, a person with a genetically weaker ability to dispose of proteins, who was also exposed to pesticides, might develop PD, whereas a person with different genes but the same exposure might not.

Whatever the ultimate cause, people with PD share the same pathology, or disease process, in their brains. The symptoms of PD arise when cells in the substantia nigra (SN) degenerate. The SN is located at the base of the brain, near the top of the spinal column. Neurons of the SN receive messages from, and send messages to, several other portions of the brain, all of which are involved in the control of movement. By interacting with these other regions, the SN helps to ensure that movements will be smooth, fluid, and controlled.

SN cells communicate with other cells by releasing the chemical dopamine. Dopamine released by SN cells stimulates cells in other brain regions to act. As SN cells die, they release less dopamine, and the receiving cells are not stimulated as much. This leads to the disordered movement of PD. The SN is also involved in regulating numerous other types of brain behaviors, and late-stage PD is marked by a wide variety of symptoms that probably reflect loss of this regulation.

The earliest symptoms of PD, and the most widely recognized, are tremor, slowed movements (bradykinesia), and stiffness or rigidity. Symptoms often begin on one side of the body, and progress over time to involve both sides. The tremor of PD is a rest tremor—the shaking occurs when the patient is not trying to use the limb, and diminishes when the limb is in use. Bradykinesia and stiffness, along with loss of some balance reflexes, can combine to cause postural instability, and increase the likelihood of falling down.

Other symptoms of PD include:

- **orthostatic hypotension**, or loss of blood pressure upon standing, which can cause **dizziness** and fainting
- painful foot cramps
- micrographia, or reduced size of handwriting
- reduced voice volume
- reduced facial expression
- excessive sweating
- constipation
- decreased ability to smell
- male impotence
- drooling
- sleep disturbance
- **depression**
- anxiety
- panic attacks
- late-stage **dementia**

Diagnosis

Parkinson's disease is diagnosed by a careful neurological examination, testing movements, coordination, reflexes, and other aspects of function. If the physician suspects PD, the patient will usually be referred to a **neurologist** for definitive diagnosis. Unilateral (one-sided) tremor, slowed movements, and muscle stiffness are generally enough to confirm the diagnosis; two of the three are usually considered definitive. Several specialized tests may be used, including imaging of the brain with **magnetic resonance imaging (MRI)** or **positron emission tomography (PET)**. These are not essential to diagnosis in most cases, but may help to confirm the diagnosis in difficult cases and to distinguish PD from similar diseases such as **progressive supranuclear palsy**, **corticobasal degeneration**, or **multiple system atrophy**. Clues that the disease is one of these, rather than PD, include early or rapidly progressing dementia, loss of coordination, or early and prominent orthostatic hypotension (lightheadedness upon standing).

Certain medications can cause a PD-like syndrome, and it is important to rule these out. These drugs include certain antipsychotic medications (haloperidol) and antivomiting drugs (metoclopramide).

Treatment team

Treatment of PD is headed by a neurologist, who may be either a general neurologist or a **movement disorders** specialist. The movement disorders specialist is most likely to be aware of the most current trends in treatment. Since PD therapy continues to undergo rapid advances, it may be an advantage to see a specialist when possible. Other team members may include a speech/language pathologist for addressing voice and **swallowing disorders**, a geriatric medicine specialist to coordinate other medical and social issues, a **neuropsychologist** for expertise on cognitive aspects of PD and its treatment, and a neurosurgeon.

Treatment

There are no treatments that have been proven to slow the course of PD, although research published in 2003 suggested that coenzyme Q10 may offer a slight benefit in this regard. The study has not been replicated, and its authors noted it would be premature to recommend treatment with this very expensive supplement. Additional claims have been made that two medications used to treat PD symptoms—selegiline and dopamine agonists—may have

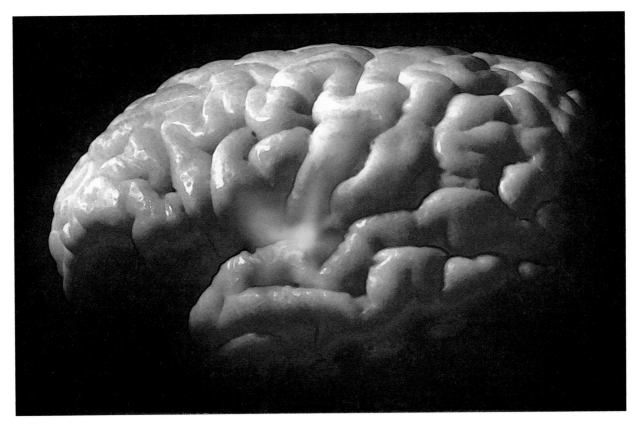

The highlight indicates the area of the brain affected by Parkinson disease. *(David Gifford / Photo Researchers, Inc.)*

some disease-slowing effects. These claims are not widely accepted.

The treatment of the symptoms of PD is complex for several reasons. First, PD is a progressive disease, getting worse over time, so that the medications and doses that work well early in the disease are insufficient later on. Second, the most effective drugs have long-term side effects that are troubling and difficult to control. Third, there are a lot of different treatment options, and finding the right combination can be time consuming. Fourth, the PD patient is likely being treated for other conditions associated with advancing age, and these conditions or their treatment may interfere with treatment of PD. Finally, a major treatment option for late-stage PD is surgery, but the risks of surgery are significant, and determining when and what kind of surgery to perform is a complicated decision.

Once the diagnosis of PD has been made, a central question is when to begin treatment. Treatment is typically not started right away (unless the patient elects to use coenzyme Q10), but instead is delayed until symptoms begin to interfere with his or her ability to work or engage in activities of daily living. This may be a year or even more after diagnosis.

Drug treatment

The next question is what drug to begin with. The most powerful treatment for the symptoms of PD is levodopa, which is taken into the brain and substitutes for the dopamine no longer being made by the substantia nigra. Similar in effect are the dopamine agonists, which mimic the effect of dopamine on the cells that normally receive dopamine from the SN. Three other medications also commonly used in PD, whose effects are not nearly as strong as either levodopa or the dopamine agonists, are **anticholinergics**, selegiline, and **amantadine**. These are often prescribed early on, when symptoms are not severe, saving the more powerful medications for later on.

Anticholinergics include benztropine and trihexyphenidyl. The loss of SN activity means that another brain system that controls movement, the cholinergic system, is relatively overactive. Anticholinergics dampen the activity of this system, restoring some balance to the control of movement. Anticholinergics are usually well tolerated in younger patients, but their side effects can be a significant barrier to their use in the elderly. Side effects include sedation, confusion, hallucinations, **delirium**, dry mouth, constipation, and urinary retention.

Selegiline inhibits the action of monoamine oxidase B, an enzyme in the brain that breaks down dopamine. Thus, selegiline prolongs the activity of dopamine in the brain. It can cause insomnia and hallucinations, as well as orthostatic hypotension. It may also interact with certain types of antidepressants, and for this reason, selegiline may be discontinued when beginning treatment for depression. In the early 1990s, selegiline was examined for its potential for neuroprotection, or disease slowing. The results of that trial were inconclusive; selegiline had such a significant and long-lasting symptomatic benefit that it was difficult to examine its disease-slowing effects independently.

Amantadine improves PD symptoms through an unknown mechanism. It is beneficial for each of the major movement symptoms of PD, although its effects are not strong. It also can lessen dyskinesias, which are unwanted movements that develop late in PD due to treatment. Amantadine can cause orthostatic hypotension and confusion.

Most drugs have side effects, and drugs for PD are no exception. The most effective drugs for PD, levodopa and the dopamine agonists, cause a set of side effects called "dopaminergic" side effects, indicating they derive from mimicking the action of dopamine. Dopaminergic side effects include nausea and vomiting, orthostatic hypotension, excessive sleepiness, hallucinations, and dyskinesias (in more advanced patients). Nausea, vomiting, and orthostatic hypotension tend to lessen with use, and do not pose long-term problems for most patients. Excessive sleepiness is a problem for many patients. Dyskinesias are an unavoidable effect of dopaminergic treatments, although dopamine agonists tend to cause less of it than levodopa. Dyskinesias tend to appear after three or more years of successful treatment, and become worse over time. Episodes of dyskinesias can be lessened by reducing the dose of the dopaminergic drug, but may lose symptomatic benefit. Adjusting drugs to minimize dyskinesias while maintaining good symptom control is a central challenge of managing PD.

Levodopa is the most effective treatment for PD symptoms, and is the drug used most often at the beginning of disease in elderly patients, because it is less likely to cause hallucinations than dopamine agonists. It is given in a pill that also contains another medication, called carbidopa, which inhibits an enzyme that would act on dopamine in the bloodstream, thus allowing more of it to reach the brain. In order for levodopa to be taken up by the gut and to pass from the bloodstream to the brain, a carrier that also moves amino acids from food must transport the drug. For this reason, doctors typically suggest that patients avoid taking levodopa with or right after a protein-rich meal. Levodopa may also be given with another medication, called a COMT inhibitor, which further prevents its breakdown in the bloodstream. A new pill combines levodopa, carbidopa, and a COMT inhibitor.

Dopamine agonists are almost as effective as levodopa for combating PD symptoms, and have the advantage that their use does not lead to dyskinesias as frequently as levodopa does. For this reason, many movement disorder specialists begin their patients on a dopamine agonist rather than levodopa. This is especially true for younger patients, who can anticipate more years of dopaminergic therapy, and a higher likelihood of developing dyskinesias as a result. There are four major dopamine agonists available in the United States: pergolide, pramipexole, bromocriptine, and ropinirole. Each is taken as a pill, and can be taken alone or in combination with levodopa or other medications. Some patients respond better to one than another, and inadequate relief from one does not mean the same should be expected from another. The U.S. Food and Drug Administration was expected to approve a fifth dopamine agonist, called apomorphine, by mid-2004. Unlike the others, it is injected, and provides very rapid, short-term symptomatic relief when a dose of levodopa wears off.

Excessive sleepiness is a potentially dangerous side effect for all the dopaminergic drugs (levodopa and the dopamine agonists). This can take the form of predictable, peak-dose sleepiness, or general increase in sleepiness during the day, or a sudden, unpredictable "attack" of sleepiness and falling asleep. The latter can be dangerous if it occurs while driving or performing another activity requiring full awareness. Patients are cautioned to be aware of changes in sleepiness especially after changing a medication, and to avoid driving whenever possible if excessive sleepiness does become a side effect issue.

Complications of advanced disease

After several years of successful treatment, most patients begin to develop one or more motor complications. These often begin with "wearing off," a reduction in the duration of effect of a given dose of levodopa, which initially can be countered by dosing more frequently. Another complication is "on-off," in which the symptomatic benefit of a given dose suddenly switches off and the patient becomes rigid, with tremor and slowed movements emerging. When this occurs at home, the patient will typically just take another dose of medication, and wait for it to begin to work. It is more of a problem when it occurs while the patient is out and about, and frequent on-off episodes may make the patient reluctant to leave the home. Apomorphine injection may be useful in this situation, since it works very rapidly (approximately seven minutes), and can therefore be used as a "rescue" for sudden off periods. Dyskinesias are a third motor complication. Dyskinesias are uncontrolled writhing movements that typically occur at the peak of effect of a levodopa dose. In some cases for some patients, dyskinesias are mild enough that they are not problematic. In other cases, they interfere with function, and attempting to reduce them becomes an important treatment issue. While drug adjustments can have some effect, as the disease progresses it becomes more and more difficult to maintain adequate symptom control while avoiding dyskinesias. At this stage, the patient may consider surgery for treatment of PD symptoms.

Other complications arise in advanced PD, especially in "non-motor" symptoms, those that do not affect movement. Low voice volume may be amenable to speech therapy treatment, with one of the most effective programs being **Lee Silverman voice treatment**, which focuses on conscious attempts to increase volume. Orthostatic hypotension may be treatable with increased salt intake, compression stockings, and medication. Drooling may become an issue in later-stage disease; there are both drug treatments and non-drug therapies available to reduce this problem. Constipation is a significant problem for many advanced PD patients, and can be treated with standard measures such as increasing the fiber in the diet and bulking laxatives.

Panic attacks and anxiety are common in PD. These can be addressed both through helping the patient understand that this is a feature of the disease, and through antianxiety medication. Depression affects many PD patients, and can worsen other aspects of the disease. It usually responds well to antidepressant medications. Dementia (loss of memory and impairment of other thinking functions) occurs more frequently in PD patients than in the population at large. Treatment is similar to that in non-PD patients, although some medications cannot be used because they have undesirable side effects for PD patients. Psychosis-hallucinations, paranoia, nightmares, and delusions may be a response to dopaminergic medications. If these side effects cannot be controlled through modification of treatments, an antipsychotic drug may be useful.

Surgery

Brain surgery is a treatment option in late-stage PD. The best candidate is the individual who continues to respond to levodopa, but whose treatment is complicated by unacceptable dyskinesias even after medication adjustment. Dementia or other significant health-related conditions may make the patient unsuitable for the rigors of surgery. The patient is usually evaluated by the neurologist, a neuropsychologist, and a neurosurgeon before deciding whether surgery is the right option.

There are two types of surgery for PD. An "ablative" lesion destroys a small portion of the brain, and in so doing, restores the balance of neural activity within the movement control circuits of the brain; ablation means to destroy or remove. The second option is **deep brain stimulation** (DBS), which accomplishes the same thing by implanting an electrode in the target brain region; electrical pulses shut the region down. Ablative lesions are simpler and less prone to long-term complications, but they are not adjustable after the lesion has been made. DBS is more complex, expensive, and time consuming, and carries a significant risk for infection or equipment malfunction, but it can be adjusted to more precisely target the brain region, thereby enhancing the surgical effect.

Three brain regions are targeted in PD surgery. Ablation of the thalamus (thalamotomy) is primarily effective in controlling tremor, and is not widely performed anymore since other, more effective targets are available. The globus pallidus internus (GPi) can either be ablated (**pallidotomy**) or stimulated (GPi DBS), which is effective for all the major motor symptoms of PD (tremor, bradykinesia, rigidity), and can improve them by 25–60%. It is also effective for reducing dyskinesias by up to 90%. The subthalamic nucleus can be stimulated in STN DBS, and is highly effective for all the major motor symptoms and dyskinesias, to a somewhat greater extent than GPi DBS. An additional advantage of STN DBS is that it is safer to do on both sides of the brain (left and right, termed bilateral) than GPi DBS. Therefore, if the patient is affected by disabling symptoms on both sides, as is often the case in advanced PD, bilateral STN DBS may be a better choice.

Clinical trials

Parkinson's disease is the subject of intense research, and there are usually several large and important **clinical trials** going on at any time. Trials may focus on slowing the disease, determining the best drug treatment, or refining surgical methods and targets.

Two experimental forms of surgery have been the subject of recent clinical trials. The first is the implantation of cells into the substantia nigra to replace the lost dopamine-producing cells. The implanted cells come from fetal tissue. Fetal-tissue transplants have led to success, but also to uncontrolled dyskinesias in some patients. For this reason, such trials on are on hold until a better understanding of this problem is discovered and methods are developed to avoid it.

The second form of surgery delivers a growth factor to the substantia nigra via an implanted pump and tube.

The growth factor, called GDNF, has been shown to slow cell death in experimental systems. A small group of patients undergoing this surgery has improved, although these results are quite preliminary.

Prognosis

PD is a progressive disease, and the loss of brain tissue in the SN is inevitable. PD patients tend to live almost as long as age-matched individuals without PD, although with an increasing level of disability. Loss of motor control can lead to an increased risk for falls, and swallowing difficulty can cause choking or aspiration (inhaling) of food. Aspiration pneumonia is a common cause of death in late-stage PD patients.

Resources

BOOKS

Cram, David L. *Understanding Parkinson's Disease: A Self-Help Guide.* Milford, CT: LPC, 1999.

Hauser, Robert, and Theresa Zesiewicz. *Parkinson's Disease: Questions and Answers*, 2nd edition. Coral Springs, FL: Merit Publishing International, 1997.

Jahanshahi, Marjan, and C. David Marsden. *Parkinson's Disease: A Self-Help Guide.* San Diego: Demos Medical Publishing, 2000.

WEBSITES

WE MOVE. <http://www.wemove.org> (April 27, 2004).

Parkinson's Disease Foundation. <http://www.pdf.org> (April 27, 2004).

Richard Robinson

Paroxysmal hemicrania

Definition

Paroxysmal hemicrania (PH) is a rare form of **headache**. Paroxysmal hemicrania usually begins in adulthood, and affected persons experience severe throbbing, claw-like, or boring **pain**. The pain is usually on one side of the face, near or in the eye, temple, and occasionally reaching to the back of the neck. Red and tearing eyes, a drooping or swollen eyelid on the affected side of the face, and nasal congestion may accompany this pain. Persons experiencing the headache pain of paroxysmal hemicrania may also feel dull pain, soreness, or tenderness between attacks.

Description

Paroxysmal hemicrania syndromes have two forms: chronic, in which persons experience attacks on a daily basis for a year or more, and episodic, in which the headaches do not occur for months or years. Episodic paroxysmal hemicrania is four times more common than the chronic form.

Chronic paroxysmal hemicrania (CPH), also known as Sjaastad syndrome, is a primary headache disorder first described by the Norwegian **neurologist** Ottar Sjaastad in 1974. In 1976, Sjaastad proposed the term chronic paroxysmal hemicrania after observing two patients, who had daily, solitary, severe headache pain that remained on one side of the head. The main feature of chronic paroxysmal hemicrania is frequent attacks of strictly one-sided severe pain localized in or around the eye or temple regions, lasting from 2–45 minutes in duration, and occurring 2–40 times per day.

Attacks of chronic paroxysmal hemicrania do not occur in recognizable time patterns. Episodic paroxysmal hemicrania (EPH), a more rare form of the disorder, is characterized by bouts of frequent, daily attacks with the same clinical features of CPH, but separated by relatively long periods without headache. Most episodic headaches in paroxysmal hemicrania occur at night or other recognizable time patterns.

Demographics

In the United States, CPH is a rare syndrome, but the number of diagnosed cases is increasing. The prevalence of CPH is not known, but it occurs more often than cluster headaches, a disorder of that can sometimes be confused with CPH. Internationally, many cases of CPH have been described throughout the world, in different races and different countries.

Chronic paroxysmal hemicrania affects more women than men. In the past, because of female preponderance, CPH was considered a disease exclusive to women. However, CPH has been reported in increasing numbers of men. A study conducted in 1979 reported a female-to-male ratio of 7:1, but a review of 84 patients in 1989 reported a female-to-male ratio of 2.3:1. Chronic paroxysmal hemicrania can occur at any age, and the mean age of onset is 34 years.

Episodic paroxysmal hemicrania occurs in both sexes, with a slight female preponderance (1.3:1). The age of onset is variable; studies show EPH onset is 12–51 years.

Causes and symptoms

No definite cause of paroxysmal hemicrania is known. Persons who experience these headaches usually do not have additional neurological disorders, with the exception of **trigeminal neuralgia**, which has been observed in a small number of persons also having paroxysmal hemicrania. History of head or neck trauma is reported in about 20% of persons with paroxysmal hemicrania, but these findings are similar to cluster headache or migraine headaches. Occasionally, attacks may be provoked mechanically by bending or rotating the head and by applying external pressure against the back of the neck. There is no inheritable pattern or familial disposition known for paroxysmal hemicrania, and affected individuals do not have a higher incidence of other types of headaches, such as CH or migraine, than the general population.

Headache is the main symptom of both types of paroxysmal hemicrania. Chronic PH involves headaches that are one-sided, severe, affecting the eye or temple area, and lasting two to 45 minutes, occurring more than five times per day. Episodic paroxysmal hemicrania involves attacks of severe pain in the eye or temple area that last about one to 30 minutes, with a frequency of three or more events per day, and clear intervals between bouts of attacks that may last from months to years.

Both chronic and episodic paroxysmal hemicrania involve symptoms such as nasal congestion on the affected side, rhinorrhea (runny nose), and swelling of the eyelid on the affected side with tearing. Sweating, both on the forehead and generalized over the body, is also common.

Diagnosis

The diagnosis of paroxysmal hemicrania is based on a person's history and clinical symptoms. There are conditions involving underlying lesions in the brain (such as tumors or arteriovenous malformation) that can lead to symptoms similar to the headaches of paroxysmal hemicrania. Because of this, various tests of the brain are recommended to exclude structural abnormalities.

Laboratory studies such as routine blood tests can help identify metabolic and other causes of headache and facial pain. Imaging studies including computed tomography (**CT**) scan, or preferably **magnetic resonance imaging (MRI)** of the brain may be needed to rule out structural disorders of the eye, ear, nose, neck, skull, and brain.

Testing the effectiveness of the drug indomethiacin may also be a useful tool in the assessment of one-sided headaches. The response to indomethacin is part of the criteria for a diagnosis of paroxysmal hemicrania. During two different periods, the drug is administered intramuscularly, and patterns of headache pain are evaluated. In paroxysmal hemicranias, indomethiacin relieves pain, prevents recurring pain, and/or decreases the frequency of pain. As the effects of indomethacin clear the body, the pain returns in its usual form and pattern.

Treatment team

A neurologist is the primary consultant for PH treatment. An ophthalmologist is also important to evaluate any eye disorders such as glaucoma.

Key Terms

Cluster headache A painful recurring headache associated with the release of histamine from cells.

Migraine A severe recurring vascular headache; occurs more frequently in women than men.

Trigeminal neuralgia A condition resulting from a disorder of the trigeminal nerve resulting in severe facial pain.

Treatment

The nonsteroidal anti-inflammatory drug (NSAID) indomethacin often provides complete relief from symptoms. Other less effective NSAIDs, calcium-channel blocking drugs (such as verapamil), and corticosteroids may be used to treat the disorder. Patients with both PH and trigeminal neuralgia (a condition of the fifth cranial nerve that causes sudden, severe pain typically felt on one side of the jaw or cheek) should receive separate treatment for each disorder.

Recovery and rehabilitation

When headaches are severe enough or frequent enough to interfere with a person's daily activities such as work, family life, and home responsibilities, a specially trained physical therapist can provide a variety of treatment and education services to manage or reduce headaches, including:

- exercises (stretching, strengthening, and aerobic conditioning)
- safe sleep, standing, and sitting postures
- performing daily activities safely
- relaxation

Clinical trials

As of mid-2004, there were no ongoing **clinical trials** specific to the study or treatment of paroxysmal hemicrania. The National Institute for Neurological Disorders and Stroke (NINDS), however, carries out multifaceted research on headaches and their causes.

Prognosis

Many patients experience complete relief or near-complete relief of symptoms following medical treatment for paroxysmal hemicrania. PH headaches may occur throughout life, but have also been known to go into remission or stop spontaneously.

Special concerns

Chronic paroxysmal hemicrania headaches have been reported to improve during pregnancy; however, they often recur after delivery. In some persons, menstruation lessens the headaches, while in others, headaches are worse during menstruation. Birth control pills do not seem to influence the frequency of attacks, and the effects of menopause on paroxysmal hemicrania are unknown.

Resources

BOOKS

Paulino, Joel, and Ceabert J. Griffith. *The Headache Sourcebook*. New York: McGraw-Hill/Contemporary Books, 2001.

PERIODICALS

Antonaci, F. "Chronic Paroxysmal Hemicrania and Hemicrania Continua. Parenteral Indomethacin: The 'Indotest.'" *Headache* 38, no. 2 (February 1998): 122–128.

Trucco, M., F. Maggioni, R. Badino, and G. Zanchin. "Chronic Paroxysmal Hemicrania, Hemicrania Continua and SUNCT Syndrome in Association with Other Pathologies: A Review." *Cephalalgia* 24 (2004): 173–184.

OTHER

"NINDS Paroxysmal Hemicrania Information Page." *National Institute of Neurological Disorders and Stroke*. May 8, 2004 (June 2, 2004). <http://www.ninds.nih.gov/health_and_medical/disorders/paroxysmal_hemicrania.htm>.

ORGANIZATIONS

American Council for Headache Education. 19 Mantua Road, Mt. Royal, NJ 08061. (856)423-0258 or (800) 255-ACHE (255-2243); Fax: (856) 423-0082. achehq@talley.com. <http://www.achenet.org>.

National Headache Foundation. 820 N. Orleans, Suite 217, Chicago, IL 60610-3132. (773) 388-6399 or (888) NHF-5552 (643-5552); Fax: (773) 525-7357. info@headaches.org. <http://www.headaches.org>.

Greiciane Gaburro Paneto
Iuri Drumond Louro, MD, PhD

Parsonage-Turner syndrome

Definition

Parsonage-Turner syndrome (PTS) is a rare syndrome of unknown cause, affecting mainly the lower motor neurons of the brachial plexus. The brachial plexus is a group of nerves that conduct signals from the spine to the shoulder, arm, and hand. PTS is usually characterized by the sudden onset of severe one-sided shoulder **pain**, followed by paralysis of the shoulder and lack of muscle control in the arm, wrist, or hand several days later. The syndrome can vary greatly in presentation and nerve involvement.

Description

PTS, also known as brachial plexus neuritis or neuralgic amyotrophy, is a common condition characterized by inflammation of a network of nerves that control and supply (innervate) the muscles of the chest, shoulders, and arms. Individuals with the condition first experience severe pain across the shoulder and upper arm. Within a few hours or days, weakness, wasting (atrophy), and paralysis may affect the muscles of the shoulder. Although individuals with the condition may experience paralysis of the affected areas for months or, in some cases, years, recovery is usually eventually complete.

Local pain around the shoulder girdle is the prevalent symptom of Parsonage-Turner syndrome. It is usually sudden and often severe, often awakening persons during the night. The pain worsens progressively for up to two days. Described as a constant, severe ache associated with tenderness of the muscles, the pain is not affected by coughing. However, it is accentuated by arm movements and muscular pressure, but almost unaltered by movements of the neck. The pain is commonly distributed across the back of the scapula (shoulder blade) and the tip of the shoulder. Pain often radiates down the outer side of the arm and up along the neck, and seldom spreads down as far as the outer side of the forearm, below the elbow. There is no exact correlation between the localization of the pain and the distribution of the subsequent muscle paralysis.

However, in general, pain radiating below the elbow is associated with involvement of the biceps or triceps, and **radiation** into the neck involves the sternocleidomastoid and trapezius muscles. Usually the severe pain lasts from a few hours to three weeks and then disappears rather suddenly; at the same time, muscular wasting and weakness are occurring. A less severe pain may persist considerably longer.

As the pain subsides, paralysis of some muscles of the shoulder girdle, and often of the arm, develops. Usually, muscle weakness appears suddenly, but sometimes gradually increases over two or three days, or up to one week in rare cases. The paralysis involves limpness and rapid wasting of the affected muscles. Tendon reflexes might be affected, depending on the severity and extent of muscular paralysis and wasting. Weakened reflexes are frequently encountered, and fasciculations (fine **tremors**) occasionally occur.

Demographics

In the United States, the incidence is approximately 1.64 cases per 100,000 people per year. Internationally, PTS has been described in many countries around the

Key Terms

Atrophy   Degeneration or wasting of tissues.

Brachial plexus   A group of nerves that exit the cervical (neck) and upper thoracic (chest) spinal column to provide muscle control to the shoulder, arms, and hands.

Scapula   The bone also known as the shoulder blade.

Trapezius   Muscle of the upper back that rotates the shoulder blade, raises the shoulder, and flexes the arm.

Triceps   Muscle of the back of the upper arm, primarily responsible for extending the elbow.

world, although specific rates of incidence have not been reported. There is a male predominance in PTS with a male-to-female ratio ranging from 2:1–4:1. Individuals as young as three months or as old as 74 years can be affected with PTS; however, the prevalence is highest in young to middle-aged adults. When a child develops Parsonage-Turner syndrome, hereditary PTS should be considered.

Causes and symptoms

The exact cause of PTS is unknown, but the condition has been linked to many previous events or illnesses such as:

- viral infection (particularly of the upper respiratory tract)
- bacterial infection (e.g., pneumonia, diphtheria, typhoid)
- parasitic infestation
- surgery
- trauma (not related to shoulder)
- vaccinations (e.g., influenza, tetanus, diphtheria, tetanus toxoids, pertussis, smallpox, swine flu)
- childbirth
- miscellaneous medical investigative procedures (e.g., lumbar puncture, administration of radiologic dye)
- systemic illness (e.g., polyarteritis nodosa, lymphoma, systemic **lupus** erythematosus, **temporal arteritis**, Ehlers-Danlos syndrome)

In addition to these possible causes, a rare hereditary form of PTS has been localized to a defect on chromosome 17, and should be considered a distinct disorder. This form of the disorder occurs in a younger age group, affects males and females equally (autosomal-dominant inheritance), and is characterized by recurrent attacks that often cause pain on both sides of the body.

Acute pain in the shoulder girdle or arm is almost always the first symptom. Shortly thereafter, muscle weakness and wasting in the shoulder girdle and arm occur. The pain, which may be extraordinarily severe for a short time, eventually abates.

Diagnosis

PTS is a clinical syndrome, and therefore diagnosis is made by exclusion. Other disorders of the upper extremity or cervical spine have to be excluded, including abnormalities of the rotator cuff, acute calcific tendinitis, adhesive capsulitis, cervical **radiculopathy**, peripheral **nerve compression**, acute **poliomyelitis**, and **amyotrophic lateral sclerosis** (ALS). PTS may sometimes be confused with peripheral nerve compression or traction injury of the brachial plexus. Affected persons, however, do not experience the acute intense pain associated with PTS, and the loss of strength occurs simultaneously with the sensory changes.

In PTS, x rays of the cervical spine and shoulder show normal findings compatible with the patient's age. Nerve conduction studies and **electromyography** (EMG) are helpful in localizing the lesion. Three to four weeks after the onset of pain, EMG studies show changes consistent with PTS. Arthrography or ultrasound may be useful to rule out a tear of the rotator cuff. **MRI** may reveal muscles changes associated with PTS.

Treatment team

A specialist in neuromuscular disease may be consulted to confirm diagnosis and evaluate any potentially underlying causes. An orthopedic surgeon is important when nerve grafting or tendon transfer is necessary. Physical and occupational therapists may be asked to provide a comprehensive rehabilitation program.

Treatment

No specific treatment has yet been proved efficient in PTS. In the early stages, pain may require treatment. Common analgesic drugs are usually sufficient. Usually, steroidal medications do not relieve the pain or improve muscle function in PTS. Rest is recommended, and immobilization of the affected upper extremity may be helpful in relieving the pain and in preventing stretching of the affected muscles.

As pain subsides, physical therapy is recommended. Passive range of motion exercises of the shoulder and elbow are suggested to maintain full range of motion.

Surgical stabilization of the scapula to the thorax, or tendon transfers have been performed with benefit in persons with PTS who experience continuing pain and muscle weakness.

Recovery and rehabilitation

Physical therapy should focus on the maintenance of full range of motion (ROM) in the shoulder and other affected joints. Passive range of motion (PROM) and active range of motion (AROM) exercises should begin as soon as the pain has been controlled adequately, followed by regional conditioning of the affected areas. Strengthening of the rotator cuff muscles and scapular stabilization may be indicated. Passive modalities (e.g., heat, cold, transcutaneous electrical nerve stimulation) may be useful as adjunct pain relievers.

Another type of rehabilitation therapy in PTS is occupational therapy. Functional conditioning of the upper extremity may be helpful. Assistive devices and orthotics (such as splints or devices for grasping and reaching) may be used, depending on the particular disabilities present.

Clinical trials

As of mid-2004, there were no ongoing **clinical trials** specific for PTS.

Prognosis

The overall prognosis for persons with PTS is good, as recovery of strength and sensation usually begins spontaneously as early as one month after the onset of symptoms. Almost 75% of persons with PTS experience complete recovery within two years. However, the period of time for complete recovery is variable, ranging from six months to five years. It seems that the delay in recovering strength depends on the severity and duration of pain, weakness, or both. Furthermore, patients with involvement of upper trunk lesions have the most rapid recovery. Although not very common, relapse might occur within a few months to several years after full recovery. In general, complete restoration of normal strength and function usually occurs within five years.

Resources

BOOKS

Liverson, Jay Allan. *Peripheral Neurology: Case Studies.* Oxford, UK: Oxford University Press, 2000.

PERIODICALS

Parsonage, M. J., and J. W. Aldren Turner. "Neuralgic Amyotrophy. The Shoulder-Girdle Syndrome." *Lancet* 1948, I: 973–1,978.

Simon, J. P. A., and G. Fabry. "Parsonage-Turner Syndrome after Total-Hip Arthroplasty." *The Journal of Arthroplasty* 16 (2001): 518–520.

OTHER

"Parsonage-Turner Syndrome." *Yale New Haven Health.* May 6, 2004 (June 2, 2004). <http://yalenewhaven health.org/library/healthguide/IllnessConditions/topic.asp?hwid=nord726>.

ORGANIZATIONS

American Autoimmune Related Diseases Association. 22100 Gratiot Avenue, Eastpointe, MI 48021. (586) 776-3900. aarda@aarda.org. <http://www.aarda.org/>.

NIH/National Arthritis and Musculoskeletal and Skin Diseases Information Clearinghouse. 1 AMS Circle, Bethesda, MD 20892-3675. (301) 495-4484 or (877) 226-4267. niamsinfo@mail.nih.gov. <http://www.niams.nih.gov>.

Greiciane Gaburro Paneto
Iuri Drumond Louro

Pellegra *see* **Vitamin/nutritional deficiency**

Pemoline *see* **Central nervous system stimulants**

Perineural cysts

Definition

Perineural cysts (also called Tarlov cysts) are abnormal fluid-filled sacs located in the sacrum, the base of the spine.

Description

Perineural cysts appear to be dilated or ballooned areas of the sheaths that cover nerve roots exiting from the sacral area of the spine. The spaces or cysts created by the dilated sheaths are directly connected to the subarachnoid area of the spinal column, the area through which cerebrospinal fluid flows. Many people have perineural cysts but no symptoms at all; in fact, the majority of people with these cysts are completely unaware of their existence. However, when conditions cause these perineural cysts to fill with cerebrospinal fluid and expand in size, they can begin to compress important neighboring nerve fibers, resulting in a variety of symptoms, including **pain**, weakness, and abnormal sensation.

Demographics

More women than men develop perineural cysts.

Causes and symptoms

A variety of conditions that can increase the flow of cerebrospinal fluid may cause perineural cysts to expand in size, creating symptoms. Such conditions include traumatic injury, shock, or certain forms of exertion (such as heavy lifting) or **exercise**. Prolonged sitting or standing may cause cysts to fill and retain fluid. Other research suggests that herpes simplex virus can cause the body chemistry to become more alkaline, which predisposes the

Key Terms

Cerebrospinal fluid   A fluid that bathes the brain and the spinal cord.

Cyst   A fluid-filled sac.

Sacrum   An area in the lower back, below the lumbar region.

Subarachnoid   The space underneath the layer of meningeal membrane called the arachnoid.

cerebrospinal fluid to fill the perineural cysts, thus prompting the advent of symptoms.

The symptoms of expanding perineural cysts occur due to compression of nerve roots that exit from the sacral area. Symptoms may include **back pain** and **sciatica**, a syndrome of symptoms that occur due to compression or inflammation of the sciatic nerve. Sciatica results in burning, tingling, numbness, stinging, or electric shock sensations in the lower back, buttocks, thigh, and down the leg to below the knee. Severe sciatica may also result in weakness of the leg or foot. Other more severe symptoms of perineural cysts include loss of bladder control and problems with sexual functioning.

Diagnosis

Because most perineural cysts don't cause symptoms, most perineural cysts are never diagnosed. When symptoms do develop that are suggestive of perineural cysts, **MRI** will usually demonstrate their presence, and CT myelography (a test in which dye is injected into the spine) may demonstrate the cerebrospinal fluid flow between the spinal subarachnoid area and the cyst.

Treatment team

Neurologists and neurosurgeons usually treat individuals with perineural cysts. A urologist may be called in to consult with individuals whose cysts are interfering with bladder or sexual functioning.

Treatment

Although using a needle to drain fluid from perineural cysts can temporarily relieve their accompanying symptoms, eventually the cysts will refill with cerebrospinal fluid and the symptoms will recur. Similarly, steroid injections can provide short-term pain relief. Pain may also be temporarily controlled by injecting the cysts with fibrin glue (a substance produced from blood chemicals involved in the clotting mechanism). Using diet or dietary

supplements to decrease the body's alkalinity may prevent perineural cysts from filling with more fluid. Medications used to treat chronic nerve-related pain (such as **anticonvulsants** and antidepressants) may be helpful.

When pain is intractable despite a variety of interventions, or when weakness or other neurological symptoms become severe, surgery to remove the cysts may be necessary. This is the only permanent treatment for perineural cysts; once removed, they very rarely recur.

Prognosis

Most individuals with perineural cysts have no symptoms whatsoever. Those who do have symptoms run a risk of neurological damage if the cysts continue to compress nerve structures over time. Individuals who undergo neurosurgery to remove the cysts usually have an excellent outcome, with no cyst recurrence.

Resources

BOOKS

Braunwald, Eugene, et al., eds. *Harrison's Principles of Internal Medicine.* NY: McGraw-Hill Professional, 2001.

Goetz, Christopher G., ed. *Textbook of Clinical Neurology.* Philadelphia: W. B. Saunders Company, 2003.

Goldman, Lee, et al., eds. *Cecil Textbook of Internal Medicine.* Philadelphia: W. B. Saunders Company, 2000.

PERIODICALS

Acosta, Frank L., et al. "Diagnosis and Management of Sacral Tarlov cysts." *Neurosurgical Focus* 15, no. 2 (August 2003). Available online at <http://www.aans.org/education/journal/neurosurgical/aug03/15-2-15.pdf> (June 3, 2004).

Voyadzis, J. M., et al. "Tarlov cysts: a study of 10 cases with review of the literature." *Journal of Neurosurgery* 95 (July 2001): 25–32.

WEBSITES

National Institute of Neurological Disorders and Stroke (NINDS). *NINDS Tarlov Cysts Information Page.* July 10, 2003. <http://www.ninds.nih.gov/health_and_medical/disorders/tarlov_cysts.htm> (June 3, 2004).

Tarlov Cyst Support Group. <http://www.tarlovcyst.net/> (June 3, 2004).

Rosalyn Carson-DeWitt, MD

Periodic paralysis

Periodic **paralysis** (PP) is the name for several rare, inherited muscle disorders marked by temporary weakness, especially following rest, sleep, or exercise.

Description

Periodic paralysis disorders are genetic disorders that affect muscle strength. There are two major forms, hypokalemic and hyperkalemic, each caused by defects in different genes.

In hypokalemic PP, the level of potassium in the blood falls in the early stages of a paralytic attack, while in hyperkalemic PP, it rises slightly or is normal. (The root of both words, "kali," refers to potassium.) Hyperkalemic PP is also called potassium-sensitive PP.

Causes and symptoms

Both forms of PP are caused by inheritance of defective genes. Both genes are dominant, meaning that only one copy of the defective gene is needed for a person to develop the disease. A parent with the gene has a 50% chance of passing it along to each offspring, and the likelihood of passing it on is unaffected by the results of previous pregnancies.

The gene for hypokalemic PP is present equally in both sexes, but leads to noticeable symptoms more often in men than in women. The normal gene is responsible for a muscle protein controlling the flow of calcium during muscle contraction.

The gene for hyperkalemic PP affects virtually all who inherit it, with no difference in male-vs.-female expression. The normal gene is responsible for a muscle protein controlling the flow of sodium during muscle contraction.

The attacks of weakness in hypokalemic PP usually begin in late childhood or early adolescence and often become less frequent during middle age. The majority of patients develop symptoms before age 16. Since they begin in the school years, the symptoms of hypokalemic PP are often first seen during physical education classes or after-school sports, and may be mistaken for laziness, or lack of interest on the part of the child.

Attacks are most commonly brought on by:

• strenuous **exercise** followed by a short period of rest

• large meals, especially ones rich in carbohydrates or salt

• emotional **stress**

• alcohol use

• infection

• **pregnancy**

The weakness from a particular attack may last from several hours to as long as several days, and may be localized to a particular limb, or might involve the entire body.

The attacks of weakness of hyperkalemic PP usually begin in infancy or early childhood, and may also become

---

---

less severe later in life. As in the hypokalemic form, attacks are brought on by stress, pregnancy, and exercise followed by rest. In contrast, though, hyperkalemic attacks are not associated with a heavy meal but rather with missing a meal, with high potassium intake, or use of glucocorticoid drugs such as prednisone. (**Glucocorticoids** are a group of steroids that regulate metabolism and affect muscle tone.)

Weakness usually lasts less than three hours, and often persists for only several minutes. The attacks are usually less severe, but more frequent, than those of the hypokalemic form. Weakness usually progresses from the lower limbs to the upper, and may involve the facial muscles as well.

Diagnosis

Diagnosis of either form of PP begins with a careful medical history and a complete physical and neurological exam. A family medical history may reveal other affected relatives. Blood and urine tests done at the onset of an attack show whether there are elevated or depressed levels of potassium. Electrical tests of muscle and a muscle **biopsy** show characteristic changes.

Challenge tests, to aid in diagnosis, differ for the two forms. In hypokalemic PP, an attack of weakness can be brought on by administration of glucose and insulin, with exercise if necessary. An attack of hyperkalemic PP can be induced with administration of potassium after exercise during **fasting**. These tests are potentially hazardous and require careful monitoring.

Genetic tests are available at some research centers and are usually recommended for patients with a known family history. However, the number of different possible mutations leading to each form is too great to allow a single comprehensive test for either form, thus limiting the usefulness of **genetic testing**.

Treatment

Severe respiratory weakness from hypokalemic PP may require intensive care to ensure adequate ventilation. Potassium chloride may be given by mouth or intravenously to normalize blood levels.

Attacks requiring treatment are much less common in hyperkalemic PP. Glucose and insulin may be prescribed. Eating carbohydrates may also relieve attacks.

Prognosis

Most patients learn to prevent their attacks well enough that no significant deterioration in the quality of life occurs. Strenuous exercise must be avoided, however. Attacks often lessen in severity and frequency during middle age. Frequent or severe attacks increase the likelihood of permanent residual weakness, a risk in both forms of periodic paralysis.

Prevention

There is no way to prevent the occurrence of either disease in a person with the gene for the disease. The likelihood of an attack of either form of PP may be lessened by avoiding the triggers (the events or combinations of circumstances which cause an attack) for each.

Hypokalemic PP attacks may be prevented with use of **acetazolamide** (or another carbonic anhydrase inhibitor drug) or a diuretic to help retain potassium in the bloodstream. These attacks may also be prevented by avoiding such triggers as salty food, large meals, a high-carbohydrate diet, and strenuous exercise.

Attacks of hyperkalemic PP may be prevented with frequent small meals high in carbohydrates, and the avoidance of foods high in potassium such as orange juice or bananas. Acetazolamide or thiazide (a diuretic) may be prescribed.

Resources

BOOKS

Harrison's Principles of Internal Medicine. Anthony S. Fauci, et al., eds. New York: McGraw-Hill, 1997.

Greenberg, David A., et al. *Clinical Neurology.* 2nd ed. Norwalk, CT: Appleton & Lange, 1993.

ORGANIZATIONS

Muscular Dystrophy Association. 3300 East Sunrise Drive, Tucson, AZ 85718. (800) 572-1717. <http://www.mdausa.org>.

The Periodic Paralysis Association. 5225 Canyon Crest Drive #71-351, Riverside, CA 92507. (909) 781-4401. <http://www.periodicparalysis.org>.

Richard Robinson

▌ Peripheral nervous system

Definition

The peripheral nervous system (PNS) consists of all parts of the nervous system, except the brain and spinal cord, which are the components of the **central nervous system** (CNS). The peripheral nervous system connects the central nervous system to the remainder of the body, and is the conduit through which neural signals are transmitted to and from the central nervous system. Within the peripheral nervous system, sensory neurons transmit impulses to the CNS from sensory receptors. A system of motor neurons transmit neural signals from the CNS to effectors (glands, organs, and muscles).

Description

The peripheral nervous system is composed of nerve fibers that provide the cellular pathways for the various signals on which the proper operation of the nervous system relies. There are two types of neurons operating in the PNS. The first is the sensory neurons that run from the myriad of sensory receptors throughout the body. Sensory receptors provide the connection between the stimulus such as heat, cold, and **pain** and the CNS. As well, the PNS also consists of motor neurons. These neurons connect the CNS to various muscles and glands throughout the body. These muscles and glands are also known as effectors, meaning they are the places where the responses to the stimuli are translated into action.

The peripheral nervous system is subdivided into two subsystems: the sensory-somatic nervous system and the autonomic nervous system.

The sensory-somatic nervous system

The sensory-somatic nervous system is the sensory gateway between the environment outside of the body and the central nervous system. Responses tend to be conscious.

The sensory nervous system comprises 12 pairs of cranial nerves and 31 pairs of spinal nerves. Some pairs are exclusively sensory neurons such as the pairs involved in smell, vision, hearing, and balance. Other pairs are strictly made up of motor neurons, such as those involved in the movement of the eyeballs, swallowing, and movement of the head and shoulders. Still other pairs consist of a sensory and a motor neuron working in tandem such as those involved in taste and other aspects of swallowing. All of the spinal neuron pairs are mixed: they contain both sensory and motor neurons. This allows the spinal neurons to properly function as the conduit of transmission of the signals of the stimuli and the subsequent response.

The autonomic nervous system

The autonomic nervous system (ANS) consists of three subsystems: the sympathetic nervous system, the parasympathetic nervous system, and the enteric nervous system. The ANS regulates the activities of cardiac muscle, smooth muscle, endocrine glands, and exocrine glands. The ANS functions involuntarily (i.e., reflexively)

Key Terms

Central nervous system (CNS) Composed of the brain and spinal cord.

Peripheral nervous system (PNS) All parts of the nervous system, except the brain and spinal cord.

in an automatic manner without conscious control. Accordingly, the ANS is the mediator of visceral reflex arcs.

In contrast to the somatic nervous system that always acts to excite muscle groups, the autonomic nervous systems can act to excite or inhibit innervated tissue. The autonomic nervous system achieves this ability to excite or inhibit activity via a dual innervation of target tissues and organs. Most target organs and tissues are innervated by neural fibers from both the parasympathetic and sympathetic systems. The systems can act to stimulate organs and tissues in opposite ways (antagonistically). For example, parasympathetic stimulation acts to decrease heart rate. In contrast, sympathetic stimulation results in increased heart rate. The systems can also act in concert to stimulate activity (e.g., both increase the production of saliva by salivary glands, but parasympathetic stimulation results in watery as opposed to viscous or thick saliva). The ANS achieves this control via two divisions of the ANS, the sympathetic nervous system and the parasympathetic nervous system.

The autonomic nervous system also differs from the somatic nervous system in the types of tissue innervated and controlled. The somatic nervous system regulates skeletal muscle tissue, while the ANS services smooth muscle, cardiac muscle, and glandular tissue.

Although the sympathetic systems share a number of common features (i.e., both contain myelinated preganglionic nerve fibers that usually connect with unmyelinated postganglionic fibers via a cluster of neural cells termed ganglia), the classification of the parasympathetic and the sympathetic systems of the ANS is based both on anatomical and physiological differences between the two subdivisions.

The sympathetic nervous system

The nerve fibers of the sympathetic system innervate smooth muscle, cardiac muscle, and glandular tissue. In general, stimulation via sympathetic fibers increases activity and metabolic rate. Accordingly, sympathetic system stimulation is a critical component of the fight or flight response.

The cell bodies of sympathetic fibers traveling toward the ganglia (preganglionic fibers) are located in the thoracic and lumbar spinal nerves. These thoraco-lumbar fibers then travel only a short distance within the spinal nerve (composed of an independent mixture of fiber types) before leaving the nerve as myelinated white fibers that synapse with the sympathetic ganglia that lie close to the side of the vertebral column. The sympathetic ganglia lie in chains that line both the right and left sides of the vertebral column, from the cervical to the sacral region. Portions of the sympathetic preganglionic fibers do not travel to the vertebral ganglionic chains, but travel instead to specialized cervical or abdominal ganglia. Other variations are also possible. For example, preganglionic fibers can synapse directly with cells in the adrenal medulla.

In contrast to the parasympathetic system, the preganglionic fibers of the sympathetic nervous system are usually short, and the sympathetic postganglionic fibers are long fibers that must travel to the target tissue. The sympathetic postganglionic fibers usually travel back to the spinal nerve via unmyelineted or gray rami before continuing to the target effector organs.

With regard to specific target organs and tissues, sympathetic stimulation of the pupil dilates the pupil. The dilation allows more light to enter the eye and acts to increase acuity in depth and peripheral perception.

Sympathetic stimulation acts to increase heart rate and increase the force of atrial and ventricular contractions. Sympathetic stimulation also increases the conduction velocity of cardiac muscle fibers. Sympathetic stimulation also causes a dilation of systemic arterial blood vessels, resulting in greater oxygen delivery.

Sympathetic stimulation of the lungs and smooth muscle surrounding the bronchi results in bronchial muscle relaxation. The relaxation allows the bronchi to expand to their full volumetric capacity and thereby allow greater volumes of air passage during respiration. The increased availability of oxygen and increased venting of carbon dioxide are necessary to sustain vigorous muscular activity. Sympathetic stimulation can also result in increased activity by glands that control bronchial secretions.

Sympathetic stimulation of the liver increases glycogenolysis and lipolysis to make energy more available to metabolic processes. Constriction of gastrointestinal sphincters (smooth muscle valves or constrictions) and a general decrease in gastrointestinal motility assure that blood and oxygen needed for more urgent needs (such as fight or flight) are not wasted on digestive system processes that can be deferred for short periods. The fight or flight response is a physical response; a strong stimulus or emergency causes the release of a chemical called noradrenaline (also called norepinephrine) that alternately stimulates or inhibits the functioning of a myriad of glands and muscles. Examples include the acceleration of the heartbeat, raising of blood pressure, shrinkage of the pupils of the eyes, and the redirection of blood away from the skin to muscles, brain, and the heart.

Sympathetic stimulation results in renin secretion by the kidneys and causes a relaxation of the bladder. Accompanied by a constriction of the bladder sphincter, sympathetic stimulation tends to decrease urination and promote fluid retention.

Acetylcholine is the neurotransmitter most often found in the sympathetic preganglionic synapse. Although there are exceptions (e.g., sweat glands utilize acetylcholine), epinephrine (noradrenaline) is the most common neurotransmitter found in postganglionic synapses.

The parasympathetic nervous system

Parasympathetic fibers innervate smooth muscle, cardiac muscle, and glandular tissue. In general, stimulation via parasympathetic fibers slows activity and results in a lowering of metabolic rate and a concordant conservation of energy. Accordingly, the parasympathetic nervous subsystem operates to return the body to its normal levels of function following the sudden alteration by the sympathetic nervous subsystem; the so-called "rest and digest" state. Examples include the restoration of resting heartbeat, blood pressure, pupil diameter, and flow of blood to the skin.

The preganglionic fibers of the parasympathetic system derive from the neural cell bodies of the motor nuclei of the occulomotor (cranial nerve: III), facial (VII), glossopharyngeal (IX), and vagal (X) cranial nerves. There are also contributions from cells in the sacral segments of the spinal cord. These cranio-sacral fibers generally travel to a ganglion that is located near or within the target tissue. Because of the proximity of the ganglia to the target tissue or organ, the postganglionic fibers are much shorter.

Parasympathetic stimulation of the pupil from fibers derived from the occulomotor (cranial nerve: III), facial (VII), and glossopharyngeal (IX) nerves constricts or narrows the pupil. This reflexive action is an important safeguard against bright light that could otherwise damage the retina. Parasympathetic stimulation also results in increased lacrimal gland secretions (tears) that protect, moisten, and clean the eye.

The vagus nerve (cranial nerve: X) carries fibers to the heart, lungs, stomach, upper intestine, and ureter. Fibers derived from the sacrum innervate reproductive organs, portions of the colon, bladder, and rectum.

With regard to specific target organs and tissues, parasympathetic stimulation acts to decrease heart rate and decrease the force of contraction. Parasympathetic stimulation also reduces the conduction velocity of cardiac muscle fibers.

Parasympathetic stimulation of the lungs and smooth muscle surrounding the bronchi results in bronchial constriction or tightening. Parasympathetic stimulation can also result in increased activity by glands that control bronchial secretions.

Parasympathetic stimulation usually causes a dilation of arterial blood vessels, increased glycogen synthesis within the liver, a relaxation of gastrointestinal sphincters (smooth muscle valves or constrictions), and a general increase in gastrointestinal motility (the contractions of the intestines that help food move through the system).

Parasympathetic stimulation results in a contracting spasm of the bladder. Accompanied by a relaxation of the sphincter, parasympathetic stimulation tends to promote urination.

The chemical most commonly found in both pre- and postganglionic synapses in the parasympathetic system is the neurotransmitter acetylcholine.

The enteric nervous system

The enteric nervous system is made up of nerve fibers that supply the viscera of the body: the gastrointestinal tract, pancreas, and gallbladder.

Regulation of the autonomic nervous system

The involuntary ANS is controlled in the hypothalamus, while the somatic system is regulated by other regions of the brain (cortex). In contrast, the somatic nervous system may control motor functions by neural pathways that contain only a single axon that innervates an effector (i.e., target) muscle. The ANS is comprised of pathways that must contain at least two axons separated by a ganglia that lies in the path between the axons.

ANS reflex arcs are stimulated by input from sensory or visceral receptors. The signals are processed in the hypothalamus (or regions of the spinal cord) and target effector control is then regulated via myelinated preganglionic neurons (cranial and spinal nerves that also contain somatic nervous system neurons). Ultimately, the preganglionic neurons terminate in a neural ganglion. Direct effector control is then regulated via unmyelinated postganglionic neurons.

The principal **neurotransmitters** in ANS synapses are acetylcholine and norepinephrine.

General PNS disorders

General PNS disorders include loss of sensation or hyperesthesia (abnormal or pathological sensitivity). Sensations such as prickling or tingling without observable stimulus (paresthesia) or burning sensations are also abnormal.

Stabbing or throbbing pains are often due to neuralgia (e.g., **trigeminal neuralgia**, also known as tic douloureux). Neuritis (an inflammation of the nerve) can be caused by a number of factors, including trauma, infection (both bacterial and viral), or chemical injury.

Resources

BOOKS

Goldman, Cecil. *Textbook of Medicine*, 21st ed. New York: W. B. Saunders Co., 2000.

Guyton & Hall. *Textbook of Medical Physiology*, 10th ed. New York: W. B. Saunders Company, 2000.

Tortora, G. J., and S. R. Grabowski. *Principles of Anatomy and Physiology*, 9th ed. New York: John Wiley and Sons Inc., 2000.

Brian Douglas Hoyle, PhD
Paul Arthur

Peripheral neuropathy

Definition

Peripheral neuropathy is a condition involving the nerves of the peripheral portion of the nervous system. Neurobiologists describe the **peripheral nervous system** as any part of that system found in the arms or legs. The nerves that traverse the arms and legs occur in fibrous groups identified from the vascular system by their whitish color. These nerve tracts, or bundles of similar type nerve cell fibers, exit the brain and spinal cord from the intervertebral spaces in the spinal column to the rest of the body. The majority of the peripheral nerves are responsible for sensations such as touch, **pain**, and temperature. There is a greater concentration of particular types of nerve cells located in both the hands and feet. This concentration is a result of the need for sensory integration with the numerous small muscles and intricacy of movement in these regions of the body.

When certain traumatic conditions exist in the peripheral nerves, some people experience a highly uncomfortable condition in which they describe sensations as burning, tingling, shooting pain, overall persistent pain, and a wide variety of additional discomforting sensations. When this condition this persistent, it is called peripheral neuropathy. Peripheral neuropathy is also known as somatic neuropathy or distal sensory polyneuropathy.

This disorder is primarily recorded in persons with diabetes, compromised immune systems, or those who have suffered some sort of injury to these nerves. The traumas can range from overexposure to certain chemical toxins, penetration injury, fractures, staying in one position too long, severe impact, or even prolonged compression, as in the wearing of inappropriate footwear. Athletes who use their feet in sports such as tennis, basketball, soccer, or any running **exercise** are at moderate-to-severe risk. Among those with diabetes and HIV the risk is highest. As a result of high computer usage, the incidence of **carpal tunnel syndrome**, a type of peripheral neuropathy, is rising.

Many researchers assume the condition itself is caused by the loss of myelin (a waxy type substance) along the axon of the nerve cell. The role of myelin will be discussed later in the description of the nerves themselves. As a result of this loss of myelin, patients describe a variety of symptoms such as those previously described. A variety of initial complaint descriptions like aching, throbbing, the feeling of cold such as frostbite or even heat sensation so severe some patients compare it to "walking on a bed of coals," are the first clues to the possibility of advancing neuropathy.

Because the initial symptoms are similar to many other disorders, doctors are sometimes hesitant to diagnose peripheral neuropathy until the disease has reached a more advanced stage. By that time rehabilitation and treatment may take longer and be less effective.

Description

Many persons with peripheral neuropathy in the legs experience an inability to walk properly. The incidence of injuries from falling increase, and affected persons may eventually develop a shuffling-type gait. In the hands, many people with this disorder must wear a brace or some sort of support. They lack their previous dexterity and fingers become numb. Manual tasks become difficult or almost impossible.

This disease may affect the nerves in several ways. If a single nerve is involved, the condition is called mononeuropathy. This condition is considered rare as it is unusual to find a condition in which only a single nerve maybe involved. Trauma is likely to involve multiple neurons and toxins or diabetes will most likely produce a global reaction.

Another condition likely to exist is one in which two or more nerves in separate areas of the body are affected. This case is described as multiple mononeuropathy. While this is still a less frequent scenario it is more common that the disease will occur in the same areas of either side of the body. This situation is more common when the cause is systemic rather than a physical injury.

Most often many nerves in the same vicinity are simultaneously involved, which is known as polyneuropathy. This is the most common expression of the disorder. Damage to nerve fibers may eventually result in loss of

Key Terms

Diabetic neuropathy A complication of diabetes mellitus in which the peripheral nerves are affected. Diabetic neuropathy is primarily due to metabolic imbalance and secondarily to nerve compression.

Mononeuropathy Neuropathy affecting a single nerve.

Multiple mononeuropathy Neuropathy affecting several individual nerve trunks.

Myelin A covering composed of fatty substances that forms a protective sheath around nerves and speeds the transmission of impulses along nerve cells.

Neuropathy Disease or disorder of the peripheral nerves.

Polyneuropathy Peripheral neuropathy affecting multiple nerves.

Schwann cell The cell that wraps around a nerve fiber to form a protective myelin sheath.

motor function or a reduction in proprioceptive or sensation types of responses. This type of neuropathy causes the greatest distress among patients. Treatment is difficult and often the nerve damage is irreversible. A halt to the advancement of the disease is one of the most promising types of relief a patient can expect.

Demographics

Statistics on the occurrence of this disorder are not always reliable. Because peripheral neuropathy can accompany a great number of other disorders, many cases go undiagnosed. Carpal tunnel syndrome, which is on the increase, is just one form of peripheral neuropathy and affects millions of people worldwide. There is evidence that some forms of this disease are inherited. Those neuropathies that are inherited are called either sensorimotor neuropathies or sensory neuropathies.

Race has not been found as a contributing factor in the onset of peripheral neuropathy. In fact, the only risk factors aside from inheritance are those that result from traumas, reaction to toxic substances, and malnutrition. While malnutrition has been erroneously paired with certain social demographics this does not necessarily mean that those who suffer from inadequate nutritional intake are more susceptible. Trauma and associated diseases, such as diabetes and HIV, are the major factors associated with this neuropathy. The occurrence of peripheral neuropathy is about 2,400 cases per 100,000 population

(2.4%). However with continued aging the rates increase to about 8,000 per 100,000 people (8%).

Causes and symptoms

One of the more prevalent and reasonable descriptions of how the disease is caused lies in the declining myelination of the actual nerve cells and fibers. In order to illustrate this condition, a discussion of one of the more common and most often discussed type of nerve cell will aid in the understanding of this type of neuropathy. The motor neuron, which is responsible for the initiation of movement, is a large nerve cell with a body and a long extension called the axon. The cell terminates at the end of the axon into a branched formation from which **neurotransmitters** are released to stimulate other motor neurons. The axon is the region of the cell along which electrical signals are passed. These electrical impulses are generated in the cell body and travel at high speeds to the ends of the neuron. The branched ends, called the synaptic end bulbs release acetylcholine which, in turn, activates the next cell body to produce an electrical signal and on down the fiber of a new nerve cell in the tract.

A waxy lipid is generated inside a specialized cell, the Schwann cell, that wraps around the axon of the nerve cell. Many Schwann cells grow along the axon and act as a kind of insulation for the nerve cell. The Schwann cells assure that the electric charge goes where the **central nervous system** (CNS) intends it to go. In diseases such as **multiple sclerosis**, the degeneration and death of these Schwann cells cause CNS electrical signals to go in random directions, preventing the muscles from responding properly.

It is assumed that in peripheral neuropathy the same sort of condition may occur. Whether due to trauma or a reaction to toxins, the myelin appears to start disappearing in many nerve cells and the otherwise contained electrical signals spread throughout the affected region. In turn, the neighboring neurons receive an overstimulation of random impulses and movement is impaired.

Muscle weakness is one of the first symptoms of peripheral neuropathy and is maximized soon after the beginning of the disease or about three to four weeks after onset. Sensory nerve cells, especially those that transmit pain are overstimulated and can cause severe aching and shooting pains, including the feeling of extreme cold or heat. Misdirected signals can cause cramping in advanced stages.

Diagnosis

Once a physician suspects a patient may be affected with from peripheral neuropathy, the diagnosis can be confirmed by a series of tests. An EMG (a recording of electrical activity in the muscles) allows the physician to see how much of a small electrical current passing through a suspected nerve region is lost due to damage in the nerves. The difference in electrical charge from its origin to its endpoint provides a measure of potential damage.

Nerve conduction tests are performed by having a machine determine the speed at which a nerve impulse passes through a nerve region. The slower the passage, the greater the neuropathy. This may relate to the loss of myelin around the nerve axons and fibers or actual physical damage. Nerve biopsies are performed in the more serious conditions. The **biopsy** will permit the physician to see the actual condition of the nerve and rule out other causes for the pain the patient experiences.

Finally, a simple blood test can be administered. Toxins that may damage nerves are screened for. Vitamin levels are observed since nutrition may be a causative factor. Vitamin B6 has been demonstrated in some studies to be toxic for some patients with peripheral neuropathy. A diabetic condition is examined for presence or absence or degree of severity.

For persons with HIV, certain drugs such as didanosine (ddI, Videx), zalcitabine (ddC, Hivid), and stavudine (d4T, Zerit) are common culprits in the occurrence of peripheral neuropathy. Not everyone taking these drugs will acquire peripheral neuropathy, but those with the disease appear to have had a damaging response to these chemicals. Additionally, in some cases, alcohol consumption may be a contributing factor.

Treatment team

The family physician and a **neurologist** are the traditional specialists in recognizing and treating peripheral neuropathy. Alternative therapists include nutritionists and acupuncturists, who also have found a place among those seeking treatment for peripheral neuropathy. One thing agreed upon is that peripheral neuropathy is often treatable. Better results occur with those patients who receive an early diagnosis and are younger, although physical therapists working with patients in all stages of the disease have reported improvement over time.

Treatment

A variety of treatments are available to patients with peripheral neuropathy. Some report a significant degree of improvement after taking higher doses of vitamin B12. Physical therapies and exercise influence the nerves to respond to correct stimuli and decrease the loss of myelin. Treatment is aimed at two goals. The first is to try and alleviate or eliminate the cause of the underlying disease. The second is to relieve its symptoms. Painkillers are often prescribed (including morphine) for the most severe cases. Prosthetic devices can be used when muscle weakness has reduced a person's ability to walk.

Managing diabetes is extremely important in those patients who have developed peripheral neuropathy as a symptom of the disease. Good nutrition, exercise, and avoiding alcohol are highly recommended. Those with HIV may experiment with alternate therapies and, again, focus on good nutrition and exercise.

Recovery and rehabilitation

The recovery from peripheral neuropathy varies. Those who are diagnosed early stand a better chance of a full recovery than those who are diagnosed after the disease has progressed over a long period. While not all cases are reversible, many patients have made a full recovery with proper treatment. For many, a halt in the progression of the disease is highly possible and often achieved. No quick cures have been found, however, and those who do improve do so after a great deal of work and commitment to recovery.

One of the aspects of the disease not often discussed is the emotional and psychological impact this disease has on its sufferers. Many find the constant pain an unbearable condition and are left to live a life dependent on painkilling drugs. Others are distraught at the loss of movement and weakness that accompany the disorder. For these patients, there are support groups and websites devoted to the sharing of ideas and promising new therapies. Relatives and friends can be very supportive in recognizing that this is a real and diagnosable disease with proven treatments. Peripheral neuropathy is not an imaginary condition and it is not only possible to find cessation from advancing symptoms, but a partial if not total recovery.

Clinical trials

Many **clinical trials** are underway to search for treatments and prevention methods for peripheral neuropathy. A clinical trial is a research study designed to test or target a specific aspect of a research topic. They are designed to ask and attempt to answer very specific questions about the causation and new therapies for medical or other research types of questions. Many new vaccines or new ways of using known treatments for a specific pathology have been discovered in clinical trials. They are often the source of new drug therapies or alternate types of treatment. Often, the criteria for entering a clinical trial is very specific, but the results can prove to be enormously helpful.

Some of the current clinical trials for peripheral neuropathy include the following: The University of Chicago is undertaking two separate clinical trials for the study of a particular drug's effectiveness in relieving the pain of diabetic peripheral neuropathy, as well as slowing the rate of progression. Washington University of St. Louis School of

Medicine is sponsoring a trial to study treatments for those with peripheral neuropathy resulting from HIV infection. Information on these studies and other ongoing clinical trials can be found at the National Institutes of Health website for clinical trials at <http://www.clinicaltrials.gov>.

Prognosis

Prognosis varies for persons with peripheral neuropathy. Quick identification and diagnosis is critical to beginning therapies in the early phases of the disease. Age is also a contributing factor, as younger persons fare better than older patients when they follow a multi-disciplinary approach to the disease. However, most patients can find a degree of relief from symptoms and the advancement of the disease.

Special concerns

While there are many cases in which peripheral neuropathy is unavoidable, most podiatrists recommend good foot hygiene. Recommendations include using appropriate and supportive footwear. Support measures such as arch and wrist braces may help in prevention of some types of peripheral neuropathy. If a person finds that one of the conditions of their employment is repetitive motion of the hand, as in typing, newer more ergonomic types of keyboards may reduce pressure on the nerves associated with carpal tunnel syndrome.

Resources

BOOKS

Golovchinsky, Vladimir. *Double-Crush Syndrome.* Hingham, MA: Kluwer Academic Publishers, 2000.

Senneff, John A. *Numb Toes and Aching Soles: Coping with Peripheral Neuropathy.* San Antonio, TX: Medpress, 1999.

Stewart, John D. and M. M. Stewart. *Focal Peripheral Neuropathies,* 3rd ed. New York: Lippincott Williams & Wilkins Publishers, 2000.

OTHER

National Institute of Diabetes and Digestive and Kidney Diseases. "Diabetic Neuropathies: The Nerve Damage of Diabetes." January 4, 2004 (June 1, 2004). <http://diabetes.niddk.nih.gov/>.

"Nerve and Muscle Disease; Peripheral Neuropathy." *The Cleveland Clinic Neurosciences Center.* May 15, 2004 (June 1, 2004). <http://www.clevelandclinic.org/neuroscience/treat/nerve/neuropathies.htm>.

"NINDS Peripheral Neuropathy Information Page." *National Institute of Neurological Disorders and Stroke.* May 15, 2004 (June 1, 2004). <http://www.ninds.nih.gov/health_and_medical/disorders/peripheralneuropathy_doc.htm>.

"Peripheral Neuropathy." *AIDS Education Global Information System.* May 15, 2004 (June 1, 2004). <http://www.aegis.com/topics/oi/oi-neuropathy.html>.

ORGANIZATIONS

National Institute of Neurological Disorders and Stroke (NINDS). P.O. Box 5801, Bethesda, MD 20824. (800) 352-9424. <http://www.ninds.nih.gov>.

The Neuropathy Association. 60 E. 42nd Street, Suite 942, New York, NY 10165-0999. (212) 692-0662. info@neuropathy.org. <http://www.neuropathy.org>.

Brook Ellen Hall, PhD

Periventricular leukomalacia

Definition

Periventricular leukomalacia is a brain condition affecting fetuses and newborns in which there is softening, dysfunction, and death of the white matter of the brain.

Description

The brain is composed of outer gray matter and inner white matter. The gray matter is responsible for processing information involved in muscle control, sensory perception, emotion, and memory. The white matter is responsible for transmitting information throughout the brain, to the spinal cord, and outside of the brain to the muscles. The ventricles are four cavities within the brain, all of which are interconnected with each other and with the central spinal canal, and through which the cerebrospinal fluid circulates. "Periventricular" refers to the white matter that surrounds the ventricles. "Leukomalacia" means softening of the white tissue. When the white matter softens, the brain tissue begins to die.

Demographics

Periventricular leukomalacia strikes fetuses and newborns, particularly those who have undergone some kind of oxygen deprivation, such as may occur due to complications of prematurity. Some 4–26% of all premature infants in neonatal intensive care units have evidence of periventricular leukomalacia. As many as 76% of premature infants who die of complications of prematurity have evidence of periventricular leukomalacia on autopsy.

The risk of a baby developing periventricular leukomalacia is higher in those babies with smaller birth weights, who are twins, who are born at less than 32 weeks and require mechanical ventilation, and/or who are born of mothers who have abused cocaine. The following conditions also increase a baby's likelihood of developing periventricular leukomalacia:

- low blood pressure
- increased acidity of the blood

Key Terms

Cerebral palsy A group of symptoms, including difficulty with muscle control and coordination and sometimes mental retardation, that occur after oxygen deprivation in the early newborn period.

Cyst A fluid-filled sac.

Intraventricular hemorrhage Bleeding into the brain, specifically into the ventricles.

Ischemia Abnormally low flow of blood to an organ or tissue of the body, resulting in oxygen deprivation of that organ or tissue.

Leukomalacia Softening of the brain's white matter.

Periventricular Located around the brain's ventricles.

Hypoxemia Abnormally low blood oxygen.

Hypoxia Abnormally low oxygen reaching the body's organs and tissues.

Ventricles Four cavities within the brain, all of which are interconnected with each other and with the central spinal canal, and through which the cerebrospinal fluid circulates.

- high blood pressure
- low blood carbon dioxide
- abnormalities of the placenta

Causes and symptoms

Premature babies are at high risk of a variety of complications, including low blood oxygen (hypoxemia), decreased delivery of oxygen to the body's tissues (**hypoxia**), and/or decreased flow of oxygen-rich blood to the body's tissues (ischemia). All of these complications can result in oxygen deprivation of the susceptible newborn brain tissue, and potentially in subsequent brain damage. Without a constant flow of enough oxygen and nutrients, the oxygen-starved brain tissue will begin to soften and die. Additionally, premature infants have a very high risk of bleeding into the brain (intraventricular hemorrhage). When this occurs, the area around the brain hemorrhage is particularly susceptible to periventricular leukomalacia.

Other risk factors for periventricular leukomalacia include early rupture of the amniotic membranes (the birth sac) prior to delivery of the baby, and infections within the mother's uterus during pregnancy and/or labor and delivery of the baby.

Symptoms of periventricular leukomalacia include tight, contracted, spastic leg muscles, delayed motor development, delayed intellectual development, problems with coordination, impaired vision and hearing, and **seizures**. More than 60% of all babies who have periventricular leukomalacia will actually develop **cerebral palsy**, particularly if the periventricular leukomalacia has been accompanied by intraventricular hemorrhage. Cerebral palsy is a constellation of symptoms that occur due to significant oxygen deprivation of the brain tissue, resulting in lifelong difficulties with coordination between the brain and muscles, and sometimes accompanied by **mental retardation**.

Diagnosis

Periventricular leukomalacia can be diagnosed through cranial ultrasound, which allows the brain to be examined using ultrasound techniques through the soft spots, or fontanelles, in the baby's skull. When a baby has periventricular leukomalacia, the ultrasound exam will reveal cysts (fluid-filled compartments) or empty cavities within the brain tissue. **Magnetic resonance imaging (MRI)** scans of the brain may also reveal the characteristic abnormalities of periventricular leukomalacia.

Treatment team

Most premature babies are treated by a perinatologist (a specialist in the care of premature infants). A pediatric **neurologist** may be consulted if a baby is suspected of having periventricular leukomalacia or intraventricular bleeding.

Treatment

There is no cure for periventricular leukomalacia. Efforts, instead, are made to help affected children reach their full potential through a variety of modalities throughout childhood.

Recovery and rehabilitation

The rehabilitation team will depend on the extent of a child's physical and intellectual challenges. Physical therapy, occupational therapy, speech and language therapy, and a specialized educational setting may all be necessary.

Prognosis

The prognosis for babies with periventricular leukomalacia is quite variable, and is dependent on the other complications of prematurity that a baby may face. Deficits may range from mild to devastating disability or even death.

Special concerns

Some studies have suggested that the risk of periventricular leukomalacia is decreased by the administration of steroids to women in premature labor. Other preventive measures include any steps that may decrease the likelihood of intraventricular hemorrhage, such as careful labor management and monitoring, and care in an experienced neonatal intensive care unit.

Resources

BOOKS

DeGirolami, Umberto, Douglas C. Anthony, and Matthew P. Frosch. "The Central Nervous System." In *Robbins Pathologic Basis of Disease*, edited by Richard E. Behrman, et al. Philadelphia: W.B. Saunders Company, 1999.

Stoll, Barbara J., and Robert M. Kliegman. "Nervous System Disorders." In *Nelson Textbook of Pediatrics*, edited by Richard E. Behrman, et al. Philadelphia: W.B. Saunders Company, 2004.

PERIODICALS

Okumara, A. "Abnormal Sharp Transients on Electroencephalograms in Preterm Infants with Periventricular Leukomalacia." *Journal of Pediatrics* 143, no. 1 (July 1, 2003): 26–30.

Sofue, A. "Sharp Wave in Preterm Infants with Periventricular Leukomalacia." *Pediatric Neurology* 29, no. 3 (September 1, 2003): 214–217.

WEBSITES

National Institute of Neurological Disorders and Stroke (NINDS). *Periventricular Leukomalacia Fact Sheet.* (May 23, 2004). <http://www.ninds.nih.gov/health_and_medical/disorders/periventricular_leukomalacia.htm>.

Rosalyn Carson-DeWitt, MD

PET scan *see* **Positron emission tomography (PET)**

Phantom limb

Definition

Phantom limb is the term for abnormal sensations perceived from a previously amputated limb. The abnormal sensations may be painful or nonpainful in nature. It is presumed to be due to central and **peripheral nervous system** reorganization as a response to injury. Phantom limb **pain** is often considered to be a form of neuropathic pain, a group of pain syndromes associated with damage to nerves.

Description

Phantom limb syndrome was first described by Ambroise Pare in 1552. Pare, a French surgeon, noticed this phenomenon in soldiers who felt pain in their amputated limbs. Mitchell coined the term "phantom limb" in 1871. Phantom limb syndrome can be subdivided into phantom limb sensation and phantom limb pain. Stump or residual limb pain refers to pain that may persist at the residual site of amputation and may be grouped under phantom limb syndrome as well.

The onset of pain after amputation usually occurs within days to weeks, although it may be delayed months or years. Pain may last for years, and tends to be intermittent rather than constant. Pain may last up to 10–14 hours a day and can vary in severity from mild to debilitating The abnormal "phantom" sensations and pain are usually located in the distal parts of the missing limb. Pain and tingling may be felt in the fingers and hand, and in the lower limbs, in the toes and the feet.

Demographics

The incidence of phantom limb pain is estimated in 50–80% of all amputees. Phantom limb sensation is more frequent and occurs in all amputees at some point. There is no known association with age, gender, or which limb is amputated. Studies have shown a decreased incidence of phantom limb syndrome in those born without limbs versus actual amputees.

Causes and symptoms

The exact etiology of phantom limb pain is unknown. Phantom limb is thought to be secondary to the brain plasticity and reorganization. The human brain has an enormous capacity to alter its connections and function in response to everyday learning or to the setting of injury. These processes of reorganization may occur in retained nerves in the amputated limbs, the spinal cord, or various parts of the brain, including the thalamus and the cerebral cortex. Although phantom pain is presumably a result of a response to amputation injury, phantom limb pain may occur in nonamputees with spinal cord damage causing loss of sensation. This suggests that the phantom limb phenomenon may be a result of damage to pathways responsible for painful sensation in general. Research studies in primates and patients with limb amputation have shown that after amputation, the area of the brain that is responsible for processing the sensations from the missing limb are taken over by areas neighboring the missing limb.

Patients may feel a variety of sensations emanating from the absent limb. The limb may feel completely intact despite its absence. Nonpainful sensations may include changes in temperature, itching, tingling, shock-like sensations, or perceived motion of the phantom limb. The limb may feel as if it is retracting into the stump in a phenomenon called telescoping. Painful sensations include burning, throbbing, or stabbing in nature. Touching the remaining stump may elicit sensations from the phantom. The quality of the pain may change over time and may not remain constant. Patients may also feel pain from the retained stump itself. Stump pain is often associated with phantom limb sensations and may be related in etiology.

Diagnosis

The diagnosis of phantom limb is a clinical one. A history of previous limb amputation and the subsequent symptoms of abnormal sensations from the missing limb are key to the diagnosis. Spinal cord damage affecting pathways mediating sensation may also be associated with phantom limb. There are no imaging or clinical tests useful in diagnosing phantom limb.

Treatment team

The treatment team for phantom limb pain may involve the participation of neurologists, pain specialists, physical therapists, neurosurgeons, or rehabilitation specialists. Neurologists and pain specialists may help in prescribing medications to treat the phantom limb pain. Physical therapists may help to facilitate and maintain mobility. Neurosurgeons may perform surgery to place electrical nerve stimulators in the spinal cord or lesion procedures to help treat the pain.

Treatment

There are few controlled clinical studies on phantom limb treatment, and therefore no consensus on the best treatment. Treatment is directed towards the management of painful symptoms. Nonpainful symptoms rarely require treatment. Treatment for phantom limb pain involves the use of medications, nonmedical, electrical, and surgical therapy.

Medical treatment of phantom limb pain involves agents typically used for neuropathic pain. Medications such as **anticonvulsants**, muscle relaxants, and antidepressants may be tried. Opiate medications have also been used. Ketamine, an anesthetic agent, or calcitonin has been shown to be effective in some clinical studies.

Various electrical and nonmedical treatments may be tried. Trancutaneous electrical nerve stimulation (TENS) and biofeedback may be used. Massage, ultrasound, and **acupuncture** modalities may be tried as well. Training patients to discriminate sensory signals in the stump appears to be helpful in reducing pain. In research studies, allowing individuals to see a reflection of the normal, intact limb moving in the position of the amputated limb helped alleviate symptoms of phantom limb pain.

Surgical treatments for phantom limb pain are limited in benefit. Lesions of various pain centers in the spinal cord and brain can be performed, and may provide short-term relief on most occasions.

Recovery and rehabilitation

Prospective studies of phantom pain show that in two years, many amputees will experience a reduction of symptoms. Physical and occupational therapists may help in the treatment of phantom limb pain by maintaining range of motion and mobility.

Clinical trials

There are ongoing **clinical trials** conducted by the National Institutes of Neurological Disorders and Stroke (NINDS) studying touch perception in patients with upper limb amputation.

Prognosis

The prognosis for phantom limb varies from individual to individual. Medical treatment shows the most benefit in treating symptoms. Some studies show that in a two-year period, many amputees will experience a reduction or disappearance of their phantom limb pain. The results of the studies are somewhat limited due to the heterogeneity of the populations studied.

Special concerns

Phantom limb may have a chronic course and may lead to feelings of **depression** or anxiety. These feelings may require treatment by a psychiatrist. Patients with phantom limb should continue to be active and participate in community and social activities. There are various support groups for amputees.

Resources
BOOKS

Ramachandran, V. S., and Sandra Blakeslee. *Phantoms in the Brain: Probing the Mysteries of the Human Mind.* New York: William Morrow, 1998.

"Phantom Pain." Chapter 16. In *Practical Management of Pain*, 3rd edition, edited by P. Prithvi Raj. St. Louis, MO: Mosby 2000.

PERIODICALS

Flor, H. "Phantom-limb Pain: Characteristics, Causes, and Treatment." *Lancet Neurology* 1 (2002): 190–195.

Hill, A. "Phantom Limb Pain: A Review of the Literature on Attributes and Potential Mechanisms." *Journal of Pain and Symptom Management* 17 (February 1999): 125–142.

Nikolajsen, L., and T. S. Jensen. "Phantom Limb Pain." *British Journal of Anaesthesia* 87 (2001): 107–116.

Pharmacotherapy

OTHER

National Institutes of Neurological Disorders and Stroke (NINDS). *Pain: Hope Through Research.* NIH Publication No. 01-2406. Bethesda, MD: NINDS, 2001.

ORGANIZATIONS

American Chronic Pain Association. P.O. Box 850, Rocklin, CA 95677-0850. (916) 632-0922 or (800) 533-3231; Fax: (916) 632-3208. ACPA@pacbell.net. <http://www.theacpa.org>.

American Pain Foundation. 201 North Charles Street, Suite 710, Baltimore, MD 21201. (410) 783-7292 or (888) 615-7246; Fax: (410) 385-1832. info@painfoundation.org. <http://www.painfoundation.org>.

The Pain Relief Foundation. Clinical Sciences Centre, University Hospital Aintree, Lower Lane, Liverpool, L9 7AL, UK. 0151.529.5820; Fax: 0151.529.5821. pri@liv.ac.uk. <http://www.painrelieffoundation.org.uk/index.html>.

Peter T. Lin, MD

Pharmacotherapy

Definition

Pharmacotherapy is the use of medicine in the treatment of diseases, conditions, and symptoms.

Description

History of pharmacotherapy

Pharmacotherapy is not a contemporary science. The use of drugs to treat illness is a practice that has been accepted for thousands of years. A famous example is Hippocrates, who is generally credited with revolutionizing medicine in ancient Greece by using beneficial drugs to heal illness. Traditionally, plants have been the source of medicinal drugs, but modern day medicine in the United States mostly utilizes synthesized or purified bioactive compounds, rather than an entire sample of plant matter. The advantage to this method of pharmacotherapy is that the dose of medicine rendered is standardized and pure, rather than an unknown drug dosage administered in addition to a wide variety of other chemicals present in the plant. Modern pharmacotherapy is the most common course of treatment for illness in the United States.

Pharmacokinetics and pharmacodynamics

Pharmacokinetics is the study of the concentration of a drug and its metabolites in the body over time. A drug that remains in the body for a longer time period will require lower subsequent doses to maintain a specific concentration. How quickly a drug clears from the body is a function of its absorption, bioavailability, distribution, metabolism, and excretion properties.

The absorption of a drug is the rate at which it leaves its site of administration. The bioavailability of a drug describes the extent to which it is available at the site of action in a bioactive metabolic form. A drug absorbed from the stomach and intestine passes through the liver before reaching the systemic circulation. If the liver biotransforms the drug extensively into an inactive form, its availability in bioactive form would be greatly reduced before it reaches its site of action. This is known as the first pass effect. Sometimes the liver biotransforms an inactive drug into an active form.

Which parts of the body drugs distribute to affects the length of time the drugs remain in the body. Fat-soluble drugs may deposit in fat reservoirs and remain in the body longer than drugs that are not fat-soluble. Drugs are metabolized within cells, often into inactive forms. The rate at which a drug is excreted from the body also affects its pharmacokinetics. Pharmacokinetic information about a drug allows the determination of an optimal dosage regimen and form of administration that will produce a specified drug concentration in the body for a desired period of time.

While pharmacokinetics is the study of drug concentration versus time, pharmacodynamics is the study of drug effect versus concentration, or what effect a drug has on the body. Pharmacodynamics measures a quantifiable drug-induced change in a biochemical or physiological parameter. Pharmacodynamics is the study of the mechanism of action of a drug. Medicinal drugs have targets to reach at the site of action. These targets are usually a specific type of drug receptor. Drug and drug receptor interactions can be measured. Complex pharmacodynamic equations combine with measurable pharmacokinetic values to determine the overall effect of a drug on the body over time.

Pharmacogenetics and pharmacogenomics

Pharmacogenetics is the study of the extent to which genetic differences influence the response of an individual to a medication. This science is still at an early stage in its development, but its importance is well understood. While drug treatment remains the cornerstone of modern medicine, in some cases it has adverse side effects or no effect at all. Adverse drug reactions are a leading cause of disease and death. It has been known for some time that genetic variation often causes these unanticipated situations.

While pharmacogenetics is the term used to describe the relationship between a genetically determined variability and the metabolism of drugs, pharmacogenomics is a separate and much more recent term that expands the concept. Pharmacogenomics includes the identification of

Key Terms

Biotransformation The conversion of a compound from one form to another by the action of enzymes in the body of an organism.

Genome The entire collection of genes of an individual.

Genotype The structure of DNA that determines the expression of a trait. Genotype is the genetic constitution of an organism, as distinguished from its physical appearance or phenotype.

all genetic variations that influence the efficacy and toxicity of drugs, describing the junction of pharmaceutical science with knowledge of genes. Pharmacogenomics is the application of the concept of genetic variation to the whole genome. Pharmacogenomics takes the concept of pharmacogenetics to the level of tailoring drug prescriptions to individual genotypes. There is an emerging trend towards defining both terms as pharmacogenomics.

There are many worrisome issues associated with modern pharmacotherapy that necessitate the study of pharmacogenomics. The optimal dose for many drugs is known to vary among individuals. The daily dose for the drug propranolol varies 40-fold and the dose for warfarin can vary by 20-fold between individuals. Also, the same drug does not always work in every patient. Thirty percent of schizophrenics do not respond to antipsychotic treatment. A major concern is adverse drug reactions. In the United States, adverse effects are a major cause of death. Research has demonstrated that gene polymorphisms influence drug effectiveness and toxicity, leading to these inconsistencies in patient response, affecting all fields of pharmacotherapy. Some drugs are known to produce potentially fatal side reactions at therapeutically effective doses. The current accepted method of addressing this situation involves determining the correct concentration of the drug for the patient so that therapy can be ceased before potentially irreversible damage. At best this is complicated, time-consuming, and expensive. It is also potentially dangerous for the patient.

The goal of pharmacogenomics is to maximize beneficial drug responses while minimizing adverse effects for individuals. In the future, pharmacogenomics may hold the promise of personalized drugs. However, genetic variation is not solely responsible for variable drug response. Other factors such as health, diet, and drug combinations are all very relevant.

Pharmacoepidemiology and pharmacoeconomics

Epidemiology is the study of the distribution and determinants of disease in large populations. Epidemiology has a precise and strict methodology for the study of disease. Pharmacoepidemiology is the application of epidemiology to the study of the effects of drugs in large numbers of people. The discipline of pharmacoepidemiology maintains a close watch on the therapeutic drugs commonly used in society. If the drug monitoring and reviewing process is not implemented, potential adverse effects of drugs and their misuse could have seriously deleterious effects on the population.

Pharmacoepidemiological studies performed on a population seek to address many different issues. Studies are performed to identify and quantify adverse drug effects, including delayed adverse effects. This is where most research in pharmacoepidemiology has focused. Analyses evaluate the efficiency and toxicity of drugs in specific patient groups such as pregnant and lactating women. Studies are performed on unanticipated side effects of drugs, along with anticipated side effects to monitor their severity. Research is done on the expected beneficial effects of drugs to verify their efficacy. Also, unanticipated beneficial effects of some drugs are examined. Factors that may affect drug therapy are studied to draw correlations between them and effects on pharmacotherapy. Such factors include sudden changes in drug regimen, age, sex, diet, patient compliance, other diseases, concurrent recreational drug usage, and genetics.

Pharmacoepidemiology can be used in conjunction with pharmacogenomics to examine how genetic patterns present in a population may affect a society's use of a specific therapeutic, or the need for gene-specific pharmacogenomic studies in a population. Studies are performed to examine a few candidate genes where genetic variability has been shown to have biological consequences. Subsequent research attempts to correlate phenotypic markers with genetic characteristics by association studies, involving the analysis of either a specific drug response as a continuous trait or of separate groups (drug responders versus drug non-responders). These genetic association studies are complex and depend on the frequency of the trait, frequency of the genetic variation within the population, the number of contributing genes, and the relative risk associated with the genetic variation. Reviews of drug utilization are generally done on overuse of drugs or use of costly drugs. Expensive drugs may be reviewed in a cost-benefit analysis involving pharmacoeconomics.

Pharmacoeconomics has a close relationship to the discipline of pharmacoepidemiology. Analysis of cost effectiveness, cost benefit, and cost utility are incorporated in pharmacoepidemiological research. A related topic of controversy is the validity of using economic analysis of pharmaceuticals as a proxy for prescribing medication, or a reason for prescribing one medication over another. The influence of pharmacoeconomic data on the choice of medication prescribed may be considerable. A general concern is whether a physician has the best interest of the patient in mind or of economics when choosing a medication. While the two concerns are not necessarily in contradiction, they sometimes may be. These topics are also being explored in prescribing research.

Resources

BOOKS

Goodman Gilman, Alfred, Joel G. Hardman, Lee E. Limbird, Perry B. Molinoff, and Raymond W. Ruddon, eds. *Goodman & Gilman's The Pharmacological Basis of Therapeutics.* New York: McGraw-Hill Health Professions Division, 1996.

Thomas, Clayton L., ed. *Taber's Cyclopedic Medical Dictionary.* Philadelphia: F. A. Davis Company, 1993.

WEBSITES

Pharmacogenetics and Pharmacogenomics Knowledge Base. <http://pharmgkb.org/index.jsp> (May 23, 2004).

Maria Basile, PhD

Phenobarbital

Definition

Phenobarbital is a barbiturate, a drug that has sedative and hypnotic effects. The drug is classed as a **central nervous system** agent and subclassed as an anticonvulsant (antiseizure).

Purpose

Phenobarbital is used to control the **seizures** that occur in **epilepsy**, and can relieve anxiety. For short-term use, phenobarbital can help those with insomnia fall asleep.

Description

Phenobarbital is available in tablet or capsule form, and as a liquid. All three forms are taken orally one to three times each day with or without food. When taken once a day, the drug is typically taken near bedtime.

Recommended dosage

The dosage is prescribed by a physician. Typically, the total daily dose ranges 30–120 mg. For treatment of seizures, the dosage can be 60–200 mg daily. The daily dosage for children is typically 3–6 mg per 2.2 lb (1 kg) of body weight.

Key Terms

Anticonvulsant drugs Drugs used to prevent convulsions or seizures. They often are prescribed in the treatment of epilepsy.

Hypnotics A class of drugs that are used as a sedatives and sleep aids.

Sedative A medication that has a calming effect and may be used to treat nervousness or restlessness. Sometimes used as a synonym for hypnotic.

Dosages should not be exceeded. It is also important to adhere to the proper timetable for use of the medication. Use of the drug should not be discontinued without consulting a physician.

Precautions

Phenobarbital is potentially habit forming if taken over an extended period of time. When being prescribed to overcome insomnia, the drug should not be used for a period longer than two weeks. Furthermore, phenobarbital should not be taken in a dose that exceeds the prescribed amount. Ingestion of more than the recommended dosage can result in unsteadiness, slurred speech, and confusion. More serious results of overdose include unconsciousness and breathing difficulty.

Long-term use can lead to tolerance, making it necessary to take increased amounts of the drug to achieve the desired effect. This poses a risk of habitual use; however, it should be noted that people with seizure disorders seldom have problems with phenobarbital dependence. Nevertheless, with chemical dependency, symptoms of withdrawal from phenobarbital begin eight to 12 hours after the last dose, and progress in severity. Initial symptoms may include anxiousness, insomnia, and irritability. Twitching and **tremors** in the hands and fingers precludes increasing weakness, **dizziness**, nausea, and vomiting. Symptoms can sometimes become severe or life-threatening, with seizures, **delirium**, or coma.

While there is evidence of risk to a fetus, the benefits of phenobarbital for a pregnant woman can sometimes warrant its use. This must be determined by a physician.

Side effects

Common side effects include drowsiness, **headache**, dizziness, **depression**, stomachache, and vomiting. More severe side effects include nightmares, constipation, and **pain** in muscles and joints. Side effects that require immediate medical attention occur rarely, and include seizures, profuse nosebleeds, fever, breathing or swallowing difficulties, and a severe skin rash.

Interactions

Phenobarbital can interact with a number of prescription and nonprescription medications including acetaminophen, anticoagulants such as warfarin, chloramphenicol, monoamine oxidase inhibitors (MAOIs), antidepressants, asthma medicine, cold medicine, anti-allergy medicine, sedatives, steroids, tranquilizers, and vitamins. Interactions with these medications can increase the drowsiness caused by phenobarbital. Decreased efficiency of anticoagulants can increase the risk of bleeding. Phenobarbital can also react with oral contraceptives, which can decrease the effectiveness of the birth control medication.

Resources

PERIODICALS
Beghi, E. "Overview of Studies to Prevent Posttraumatic Epilepsy." *Epilepsia* (2003; Suppl): 21–26.

Galindo, PA., et al. "Anticonvulsant Drug Hypersensitivity." *Journal of Investigative Allergological and Clinical Immunology* (December 2002): 299–304.

Kokwaro, GO., et al. "Pharmacokinetics and Clinical Effect of Phenobarbital in Children with Severe Falciparum Malaria and Convulsions." *British Journal of Clinical Pharmacology* (October 2003): 453–457.

Pennell, P. B. "Antiepileptic Drug Pharmacokinetics during Pregnancy and Lactation." *Neurology* (September 2003): S35–42.

OTHER
U.S. National Library of Medicine. *Drug Information: Phenobarbital.* MEDLINEplus Health Information. December 28, 2003 (May 23, 2004). <http://www.nlm.nih.gov/medlineplus/print/druginfo/medmaster/a682007.html>.

ORGANIZATIONS
The Epilepsy Foundation. 4351 Garden City Drive, Landover, MD 20785-7223. (800) 332-1000. <http://www.epilepsy foundation.org/>.

Brian Douglas Hoyle, PhD

Phytanic acid storage disease *see* **Refsum disease**

Pick disease

Definition

Pick disease is a rare neurodegenerative disorder that affects pre-senile adults. It is characterized by atrophy of the tissues in the frontal and temporal lobes of the brain and by the presence of aggregated tau protein that accumulates in Pick bodies in the neurons of the affected regions. Named for the German physician who studied patients who with the disease, Pick disease is grouped together with other non-Alzheimer's dementias, under the category of frontotemporal **dementia** (FTD), which is now the preferred term for Pick disease. FTD is classified by the *Diagnostic and Statistical Manual of Mental disorders*, Fourth Edition (DSM-IV) as a Dementia Due to Other General Medical Conditions.

Description

The disease is named after the German physician, Arnold Pick, but it was not named by him. German psychiatrist and pathologist Alois Alzheimer named the illness in 1923 following post-mortem examinations of Pick's patients. One of these patients was a 71-year old man who died following progressive mental deterioration. His autopsy revealed atrophy of the frontal cortex. This feature is seen nearly universally among patients with FTD. The disease is also referred to as frontotemporal lobar degeneration, progressive **aphasia** and semantic dementia.

The disease may be inherited through mutations associated with chromosomes 17, 9 and 3, or develop sporadically.

Demographics

Alzheimer's disease and other non-Alzheimer's dementias are much more common than FTD. The average age of onset is 54 years, and most cases arise between the ages of 40 and 60. Few diagnoses are made in individuals older than 75 years of age, but FTD has been diagnosed in people as young as 20.

At autopsy, 8–10% of all cases of pre-senile dementia meet the diagnostic criteria for FTD disease, although some estimates put the incidence of the disease in the United States at as much as 15% of individuals with dementia. Epidemiological studies have estimated that FTD affects as few as one in 100,000 people. The familial incidence of FTD disease may be higher in Europe; a Dutch study indicated a prevalence of 28 per 100,000 individuals. The incidence increases with age, affecting 10.7 per 100,000 in the 50–60-year age range and 28 per 100,000 in the 60–70-year age range. FTDs account for about 3% of dementias. One-fifth to one-half of individuals diagnosed with FTD has a first-degree relative that has also been diagnosed with dementia.

Discrepancies in neuropathological diagnosis have led some groups to suspect that its incidence is much greater than previously indicated. There is some suggestion that as imaging techniques improve the disease is becoming more frequently recognized in younger patients.

Causes and Symptoms

The molecular cause of Pick disease are a series of mutations linked to chromosomes 17, 9 and 3. One of these mutations is located on the long arm of chromosome 17 (17q35) at the locus known to hold the gene for the tau protein, and accounts for between 9–14% of all FTDs. This gene has also been implicated in Alzheimer's disease. Mutations on chromosomes 9 and 3 have not yet been identified. The gene encodes a scaffold protein that maintains the shape of brain neurons by stabilizing cellular microtubules. Mutations to the tau protein cause it to form clumps and limit its ability to assemble microtubules. The aggregates that form in the neurons of the affected regions of the brain are called Pick bodies. As in Alzheimer's disease, the tau protein is hyperphoshorylated in FTD.

The brain regions most severely affected by the tau mutation are the frontal and temporal lobes. These parts of the brain control reasoning and judgment, behavior and speech. In addition to the accumulation of tau protein, these regions atrophy over the course of the disease.

The clinical features of frontotemporal dementia includes changes in the patient's behavior, and may include additional emotional, neurological and language symptoms. Patients show poor reasoning, judgment and mental flexibility, but memory may not be affected.

Initially, patients become disinhibited and restless, and lose the ability to control their actions or to chose socially acceptable behavior. As the condition progresses, repetitive and ritualistic behaviors, such as hand rubbing or clapping, develop. Hyperoral behaviors are often associated with this phase, and may include overeating, hoarding or fixations on specific foods.

Later, apathy, uncaring and unsympathetic attitudes, and mood changes may develop. The patient may also develop language difficulties, including aphasia and reduced reading and writing comprehension, **dysarthria** and echolalia. Most patients with FTD eventually become mute.

Some patients with FTD will develop ALS, also known as Lou Gehrig's disease, parkinsonian, or psychiatric symptoms.

Diagnosis

Frontotemporal dementia is commonly misdiagnosed as Alzheimer's disease, because of the similarity in their clinical courses. However, FTD should be suspected if Alzheimer's-like symptoms are present in patients of a pre-senile age. Patients show early declines in social conduct, emotional expression and insight. Conversely, perception, spatial skills, memory generally remain intact or well preserved. The following behavioral disorders, altered speech and language, and physical signs also support FTD diagnosis.

The diagnostic criteria for FTD were reviewed and updated at a consensus conference in 1998. The criteria comprising the clinical profile are divided into two groups: core diagnostic features, which must be present, and supportive diagnostic features, which are present in many patients with FTD. Changes to character and altered social conduct are prominent features of the disease and prevalent at all stages.

Core Diagnostic Features

- insidious onset and gradual progression
- early decline in social conduct
- early impaired regulation of personal conduct
- early emotional blunting
- early loss of insight

Supportive Diagnostic Features

- altered behavior: decline in hygiene, mental rigidity, hyperorality and dietary changes, stereotyped behavior
- speech and language: less spontaneous and limited speech, sterotypy, echoalia, mutism
- physical signs: primitive reflexes, incontinence, rigidity and tremor, low blood pressure, frontal or anterior temporal abnormality

Neuropsychological tests reveal a lack of verbal fluency, ability to abstract and limited executive function. Because of the clinical similarities between FTD and Alzheimer's disease, it is difficult not to misdiagnose FTD as Alzheimer's disease. However, one study found that a word fluency test may be the best method of differentiating FTD from Alzheimer's disease.

Neuroimaging studies, such as **CT scans**, will generally show atrophy and reduced blood flow to the frontal and anterior temporal lobes, but will not be conclusive in all cases. Several studies suggest that functional imaging with single photon emission CT or **positron emission tomography** may be better at identifying FTD in its early stages, showing decreased blood flow to the frontal and temporal lobes. Electroencephalograms (EEG) may show non-specific changes in electrical activity, but are usually normal.

Like Alzheimer's disease, a diagnosis of FTD can be confirmed with autopsy. Gross inspection reveals significant atrophy of the cortex and the white matter of the

Key Terms

Alzheimer's disease A progressive, neurodegenerative disease characterized by loss of function and death of nerve cells in several areas of the brain, leading to loss of mental functions such as memory and learning. Formerly called pre-senile dementia.

Analgesics A class of pain-relieving medicines, including aspirin and Tylenol.

Anticholinergic drugs Drugs that block the action of the neurotransmitter acetylcholine. They are used to lessen muscle spasms in the intestines, lungs, bladder, and eye muscles.

Aphasia The loss of the ability to speak, or to understand written or spoken language. A person who cannot speak or understand language is said to be aphasic.

Cytoplasm The substance within a cell including the organelles and the fluid surrounding the nucleus.

Dementia Loss of memory and other higher functions, such as thinking or speech, lasting six months or more.

Dysarthria Slurred speech.

Echolalia Involuntary echoing of the last word, phrase, or sentence spoken by someone else.

Electroencephalogram A record of the tiny electrical impulses produced by the brain's activity picked up by electrodes placed on the scalp. By measuring characteristic wave patterns, the EEG can help diagnose certain conditions of the brain.

Hydrocephalus An abnormal accumulation of cerebrospinal fluid within the brain. This accumulation can be harmful by pressing on brain structures, and damaging them.

Hypothyroidism A disorder in which the thyroid gland produces too little thyroid hormone causing a decrease in the rate of metabolism with associated effects on the reproductive system. Symptoms include fatigue, difficulty swallowing, mood swings, hoarse voice, sensitivity to cold, forgetfulness, and dry/coarse skin and hair.

Microtubules Slender, elongated, anatomical channels.

Parkinson's disease A slowly progressive disease that destroys nerve cells in the basal ganglia and thus causes loss of dopamine, a chemical that aids in transmission of nerve signals (neurotransmitter). Parkinson's is characterized by shaking in resting muscles, a stooping posture, slurred speech, muscular stiffness, and weakness.

---

frontal and anterior temporal lobes. Neuronal inclusions called "Pick bodies" are characteristic of the disease, but not always present or necessary for diagnosis. Pick bodies are cytoplasmic silver-staining masses made up of 10-to 20-nm filaments. Other investigators have further classified the pathology into three distinct subsets.

• FTD Type A: lobar atrophy with swollen poorly staining neurons and Pick bodies

• FTD Type B: lobar atrophy with swollen poorly staining neurons, but no Pick bodies

• FTD Type C: lobar atrophy, lacking swollen poorly staining neurons and Pick bodies

Differential Diagnosis

FTD is rare and other diseases, such as **hydrocephalus**, tumors, hypothyroidism, vascular dementia, and vitamin B12 deficiency should be ruled out. However, an accurate and rapid diagnosis saves well-intentioned but futile attempts to treat for other conditions such as **depression** or mania.

Treatment

There is no known treatment for frontotemporal dementia and no way to slow the progression of the disease. Treatment focuses on patient care, symptom management, monitoring symptom progression and providing assistance with daily activities and personal care.

During the early stages of the disease speech therapy, occupational therapy, and behavior modification may improve day-to-day functioning and improve autonomy. Disorders that contribute to confusion, such as heart failure, **hypoxia**, thyroid disorders, and infections should be treated appropriately.

Some medications, such as **anticholinergics**, analgesics, cimetidine, **central nervous system** depressants, and lidocaine may heighten confusion and non-essential ones should be discontinued. In addition, it is inadvisable to prescribe drugs used to treat Alzheimer's disease, as many may increase agitation and aggressivity.

As the disease progresses, a patient's capacity to care for himself will decline and he will become more dependent on caregivers. Around the clock care may be required in the most advanced stages or the disease; family members should consider hiring an in-home caregiver or consider institutional care to meet the patient's needs.

Clinical trials

As of early 2004, two NIH sponsored **clinical trials** were recruiting patients with frontotemporal dementia. Both were operating out of the National Institute of Neurological disorders and Stroke (NINDS) in Bethesda, MD. The Memory and Aging Center at the University of California, San Francisco is also conducting several diagnostic and genetic studies of FTD. Contact information is listed under resources, below.

Prognosis

Patients with frontotemporal dementia have a poor prognosis. The disease is much more aggressive than Alzheimer's disease. Total disability occurs early after diagnosis. Most patients die within two to 10 years after diagnosis, with median survival at three years from diagnosis and six years after symptom inception. Death is usually due to infection or from body system failure.

Resources

BOOKS

Goldman, L., and J. C. Bennett, eds. *Cecil Textbook of Medicine*, 21st ed. W. B. Saunders Company, 2000.

PERIODICALS

Coleman, L. W., K. B. Digre, G. M. Stephenson, et al. "Autopsy-Proven, Sporadic Pick Disease With Onset at Age 25 Years." *Archives of Neurology* 59 (May 2002): 856–859.

Hodges, J. R., R. Davies, J. Xuereb, et al. "Survival in frontotemporal dementia." *Neurology* 61 (2003): 349-354.

Gydesen, S., J. M. Brown, A. Brun, et al. "Chromosome 3 linked frontotemporal dementia (FTD-3)." *Neurology* 59 (2002): 1585-1594.

Munoz, D. G., D. W. Dickson, C. Bergeron, et al. "The Neuropathology and Biochemistry of Frontotemporal Dementia." *American Neurological Association* (June 23, 2003).

ORGANIZATIONS

The National Institute of Neurological Disorders and Stroke (NINDS). 9000 Rockville Pike, Bethesda, MD 20892. (800) 411-1222. prpl@mail.cc.nih.gov.

UCSF Memory and Aging Center. 350 Parnassus Avenue, Suite 706, San Francisco, CA 94143-1207. (415) 476-6880; Fax: (415) 476-4800. <http://memory.ucsf.edu>.

Pick's Disease Support Group. <http://www.pdsg.org.uk/>.

The Association for Frontotemporal Dementias. <http://www.ftd-picks.org>.

Hannah M. Hoag, MSc

Pinched nerve

Definition

A pinched nerve is a general term that describes an injury to a nerve or group of nerves. The damage may include compression, constriction or stretching. Nerves that pass near or through bones or other rigid tissues are most susceptible to pinching. Pinched nerves result in numbness, **pain**, burning and tingling sensations radiating out from the affected area.

Description

Pinched nerves can be grouped into two types depending on where they occur in the body. Pinched nerves can occur within or in the vicinity of the vertebral column. For example, herniation of vertebral discs causes pain along the pathway of the nerve that is affected. Similarly, stenosis, or narrowing, of the vertebral column puts pressure on nerves traveling through the vertebrae. Another group of pinched nerves are referred to as nerve entrapment syndromes and they affect peripheral nerves, most commonly in the arms.

At least 80% of all herniated discs occur in people between the ages of 30 and 50. Between these ages, the tough outer core of the vertebral discs weakens and the soft gel-like inner core, which is under pressure, can more easily squeeze through weakened areas. After age 50, the inner core begins to harden, making herniation of discs less common. The amount of pain and discomfort resulting from a herniated disc varies depending on which disk has herniated and the amount of rupture. One of the most common problems associated with herniated discs is **sciatica**.

Nerve entrapment syndromes refer to a particular type of pinched nerve, in which peripheral nerves are chronically compressed resulting in pain or loss of function in an extremity. The most common nerve entrapment syndromes affect the median, ulnar and radial nerves of the arms. Nerve entrapment syndromes are extremely common, accounting for about 10–20% of all cases seen in neurosurgical practices. The most common entrapment syndrome is **carpal tunnel syndrome**. Cubital tunnel syndrome of the ulnar nerve, which runs down the arm and through the elbow, also occurs frequently.

Causes and symptoms

A nerve can be thought of as a wire encased in insulation that carries electrical information from one part of the body to another part. When the insulation or the wire itself becomes damaged the electrical signal does not move along the nerve efficiently or, in severe cases, the signal is not transmitted at all. The brain interprets this faulty transmission as pain, numbness or burning. Several different types of damage can occur to nerve cells that cause a disruption in the transfer of electrical signal. Compression or pressure on a nerve in one area will result in symptoms such as numbness or tingling in the region from which the nerve should be sending signals. The myelin sheath, which covers the nerve and is analogous to the insulation covering an electrical wire, can be damaged by scarring, in effect causing a short circuit of the nerve. Scar tissue hinders movement of a nerve in its tissue bed as the body moves and compromises the ability of the nerve to function properly, either by stressing the nerve fibers themselves or by impairing the blood supply to the nerve cell. Nerves can also be pulled or stretched, which constricts the nerve fibers. This is called a traction of the nerve and results in a decreased electrical flow through the nerve. The brain interprets the slow electrical signal as numbness, pain, or tingling.

Pinched Nerves in the Spine

Herniated discs are the most common reason for a pinched nerve along the vertebrae. This condition occurs when the gel-like core of a vertebral disc (nucleus puposus) ruptures through the tougher outer section (annulus) of the disc. The extrusion puts pressure on the adjacent nerve root causing it to function improperly. The discs that most often suffer from herniation are those in the cervical spine and the lumbar spine because they are the most flexible.

Lumbar disc herniations usually occur between lumbar segments 4 and 5, which cause pain in the L5 nerve, or between lumbar segment 5 and sacral segment 1, which cause pain on the S1 nerve. Pinching of the L5 nerve causes weakness in the big toe and ankle and pain on the top of the foot that may extend up to the buttocks. Pinching of the S1 nerve causes weakness in the ankle and numbness and pain in the sole and side of the foot. If the sciatic nerve, which runs from lumbar segment 3 down the vertebral column, is pinched by a herniation, the resulting condition is known as sciatica and it can cause pain, burning or tingling in the buttocks and leg. Lumbar disc herniations often heal on their own and conservative treatments are used to provide some relief from symptoms and to aid healing. Such treatments include physical therapy, chiropractic manipulations, non-steroidal anti-inflammatory drugs, oral steroids and, in some cases, an injection of a steroid such as cortisone. In more severe

cases, surgery to remove the pressure of the disc from the nerve is warranted. This is most often performed using microsurgical techniques.

Cervical disc herniations occur less frequently than lumbar disc herniations because there is less force in the cervical spine and less disc material between vertebrae. When nerve roots exiting the cervical spine are pinched, they can cause a **radiculopathy**, or a pain in the arm. Rarely, the nerves between the first and second or second and third cervical segments can be pinched. These nerves are sensory nerves and can cause chronic headaches. Usually cervical disc herniations heal on their own and conservative treatments are used to relieve symptoms and pain. These treatments include rest, non-steroidal anti-inflammatory drugs, physical therapy, chiropractic treatments and manual traction. Epidural injections of cortisone may also help relieve pain. Surgical techniques can also be used to remove the herniated disc from impinging on nerves.

Stenosis, or narrowing, of the spinal canal can cause a pinching of the spinal cord. This occurs commonly with age and may cause weakening of muscles or loss of coordination. Often symptoms develop slowly and worsen over a long period of time. Usually treatment for this condition requires surgery to relieve pressure on the spinal canal.

Nerve Entrapment Syndromes

Most nerve entrapment syndromes are caused by injury to the nerve as it travels between a canal consisting of bone or ligament. One side of the canal is able to move so that the injury is aggravated by repetitive rubbing or slapping against the edges of the canal. Rest and splinting are therefore effective treatments for entrapment syndromes. Symptoms of entrapment syndromes usually proceed from pain and numbness to weakness and muscle atrophy.

The most common nerve entrapment syndrome is **carpal tunnel syndrome** (CTS), with a reported occurrence between 1–10% of the population. Statistics indicate that nearly half of a million surgeries for CTS are performed yearly. It occurs most often in people who perform repetitive motions with their hands, such as bankers, computer operators, secretaries, grocery store workers and bank tellers.

The carpal tunnel is in the wrist of the hand. It is bound on the palm side by the transverse carpal tunnel ligament which attaches to the four carpal tunnel bones that extend around the back of the wrist. The inside of the carpal tunnel houses ten flexor tendons, which are used to bend fingers, as well as the median nerve and the ulnar nerve. The median nerve, which is aggravated in CTS, is between the transverse carpal tunnel ligament and the flexor tendons. When the hand moves, the flexor tendons may glide back and forth through the carpal tunnel up to .75 in (2 cm) in either direction. These tendons are covered in a substance called tenosynovium that allows them to move easily. When the tendons move rapidly, the tenosynovium may heat up and expand, putting pressure on the median nerve. This pressure results in pain and tingling in the thumb, index finger, middle finger and along the thumb side of the fourth finger. Symptoms may also include a dull, aching pain in the wrist, extending up to the elbow. Most people suffering from CTS find that the pain worsens at night and they will awaken with numbness in the middle fingers and thumb. Both bending the wrist and extending the wrist cause increased pain. Given time, CTS may continue to aggravate the median nerve, resulting in scar tissue that only enhances the syndrome.

CTS is usually treated with conservative treatments including rest and splinting of the wrist, especially at night. Using non-steriodal anti-inflammatory medications may relieve some of the swelling in the carpal tunnel. Injections of cortisone into the carpal tunnel are also effective at relieving swelling. Surgery can also be used in severe cases to relieve pressure on the median nerve.

Ulnar nerve entrapment syndrome occurs when the ulnar nerve is injured. The ulnar nerve extends down the arm and into the hand, enervating the ring finger and the little finger. In the elbow, it passes through a tunnel called the cubital tunnel. Most ulnar nerve entrapments occur in the cubital tunnel, although some can occur at the wrist. Most commonly, trauma to the elbow or repetitive bending of the elbow puts pressure on the ulnar nerve that damages the myelin sheath insulating and protecting the nerve.

Symptoms include tenderness on the inside of the elbow, numbness in the hand especially the ring and little fingers and decreased coordination and strength in the hand. Conservative treatments for ulnar nerve entrapment include rest and splinting of the elbow and corticosteroids to reduce pain. In severe cases, surgery to move the ulnar nerve from behind the elbow to the front of the elbow relieves the pressure on the nerve.

Suprascapular nerve entrapment is a rare type of entrapment syndrome that most often occurs in athletes. The major symptom is a dull pain near the shoulder blade, which can progress to weakness and muscle atrophy. The pain is not localized, but does not extend to the neck or arm.

Tarsal tunnel syndrome is another uncommon type of nerve entrapment syndrome that causes burning, tingling and pain in the plantar surface of the foot. Bending of the ankle worsens the pain and there is a weakening of muscles in the big toe.

Resources

BOOKS

Beers, Mark H., ed. *Merk Manual of Medical Information.* Merk Research Laboratories, 2003.

Fried, Scott M. *Light at the End of the Carpal Tunnel: A Guide to Understanding and Relief from the Pain of Nerve Problems.* Healing Books, 1998.

Tierney, Lawrence M., Stephen J. McPhee, and Maxine A. Papadakis, eds. *Current Medical Diagnosis and Treatment.* McGraw-Hill, 2003.

OTHER

Hochschuler, Stephen H. "What You Need to Know about Sciatica." *SpineHealth.com.* (September 22, 2003). <http://www.spine-health.com/topics/cd/d_sciatica/sc01.html>.

Luskin, Brandon. "Pinched Nerve—What Is It?" *SpineUniverse.com.* (November 24, 2003). <http://www.spineuniverse.com/displayarticle.php/article232.html>.

National Institute of Neurological Disorders and Stroke. *Pinched Nerve Information Page.* (July 1, 2001). <http://www.ninds.nih.gov/health_and_medical/disorders/pinchednerve.htm>.

Pang, Dachling, and Kamran Sahrakar. "Nerve Entrapment Syndromes." *Emedicine.* (October 4, 2001). <http://www.emedicine.com/med/topic2909.htm>.

Ullrich Jr., Peter F. "Cervical Disc Herniation." *SpineHealth.com.* (July 2001). <http://www.spine-health.com/topics/cd/overview/cervical/cerv01.html>.

Ullrich Jr., Peter F. "Lumbar Disc Herniation." *SpineHealth.com.* (March 15, 2001). <http://www.spine-health.com/topics/cd/overview/lumbar/young/lum01.html>.

"Ulnar Nerve Entrapment." *American Academy of Orthopaedic Surgeons.* (November 2000). <http://www.orthoinfo.org/fact/thr_report.cfm?Thread_ID=143&topcategory=Arm>.

ORGANIZATIONS

National Rehabilitation Information Center (NARIC). 4200 Forbes Boulevard Suite 202, Lanham, MD 20706-4829.

Key Terms

Corticosteroids A group of hormones produced naturally by the adrenal gland or manufactured synthetically. They are often used to treat inflammation. Examples include cortisone and prednisone.

Histamine · A substance released by immune system cells in response to the presence of an allergen. It stimulates widening of blood vessels and increased porousness of blood vessel walls so that fluid and protein leak out from the blood into the surrounding tissue, causing localized inflammation of the tissue.

Prostaglandins A group of hormonelike molecules that exert local effects on a variety of processes including fluid balance, blood flow, and gastrointestinal function. They may be responsible for the production of some types of pain and inflammation.

Sacroiliac joint The joint between the triangular bone below the spine (sacrum) and the hip bone (ilium).

Serotonin A widely distributed neurotransmitter that is found in blood platelets, the lining of the digestive tract, and the brain, and that works in combination with norepinephrine. It causes very powerful contractions of smooth muscle and is associated with mood, attention, emotions, and sleep. Low levels of serotonin are associated with depression.

---

(301) 562-2400 or (800) 346-2742; Fax: (301) 5 62-2401. naricinfo@heitechservices.com. <http:// www.naric.com>.

Juli M. Berwald, PhD

Piriformis syndrome

Definition

Piriformis syndrome is a neuromuscular disorder caused by the compression or irritation of the sciatic nerve by the piriformis muscle. It is usually the result of a traumatic injury to the buttocks or hip region. The piriformis muscle is a long, narrow, pyramid-shaped muscle, located deep in the buttocks, that runs from the base of the spine to the top of the femur. Sciatic irritation causes nagging aches, **pain**, tingling and numbness in the area extending from the buttocks to the tibia.

Description

Piriformis syndrome is a frequent cause of low **back pain**. Yoeman first described it in 1928, although the term itself wasn't introduced until 1947, when Robinson correctly identified **sciatica** as a symptom, not a disease. Diagnosis of the condition remains controversial among physicians because its definition and pathophysiology lack consensus.

The condition is caused by the irritation or compression of the proximal sciatic nerve by the piriformis muscle, which at the sacral vertebrae, runs through the sciatic notch and inserts at the greater trochanter of the femur. The piriformis muscle is used to help rotate the leg outwards.

It is particularly common among skiers, tennis players, long-distance bikers, and truck drivers. In addition, in as much as 20% of the population, the sciatic nerve passes through the piriformis muscle, contributing to the development of the condition.

Demographics

Due to discrepancies in diagnosis, the incidence of piriformis syndrome ranges from very rare to being responsible for approximately 6% of sciatica cases. Women may be affected more frequently than men, with some reports suggesting a six-fold incidence among females. Some reports find that it is most commonly diagnosed in patients between 30 and 40 years old.

Causes and Symptoms

There is little consensus over the cause of piriformis syndrome. The syndrome is attributed to mechanical or chemical irritation of the sciatic nerve. Approximately 50% of patients have a history of buttocks, lower back or hip injury, although it is frequently diagnosed in people who sit for long periods of time, presumably because the position leads to compression of the sciatic nerve.

The release of chemical mediators, such as serotonin, prostaglandin E, bradykinin, and histamine, into the region surrounding the sciatic nerve during inflammation contributes to irritation.

Piriformis syndrome is characterized by chronic nagging pain, tingling or numbness starting at the buttocks and extending along the length of the thigh, sometimes descending to the calf. It may worsen with sitting, or with lower limb movement.

Diagnosis

Piriformis syndrome is primarily a diagnosis of exclusion, aimed at identifying the piriformis muscle as the primary cause of the pain. Diagnoses should be made through a physical examination, and a complete neurologic examination.

Several maneuvers that contract or stretch the piriformis muscle can be performed. Freiberg's maneuver—an inward rotation of the thigh—stretches the piriformis muscle. In sitting patients, Pace's maneuver will elicit pain with the abduction of the affected leg. In Beatty's maneuver, the patient lies on a table on his non-affected leg, and the knee of the affected leg is bent knee and placed on the table. Raising the knee several inches off the table causes pain in the buttocks, and indicates piriformis syndrome

Imaging studies of the lower spine can exclude disc protrusion or degeneration, or osteoarthritis, hip and joint disease, and other spinal causes. Nerve conduction studies show delayed F waves and H reflexes.

Treatment Team

The structure of the treatment team will vary on the severity of the condition and on the success of initial interventions. Generally the treatment team is composed of a physiotherapist and a massage therapist. In advanced cases that do not respond to mechanical or pharmacological therapy, surgery may be recommended.

Treatment

Treatment for piriformis syndrome includes avoiding activities that aggravate the condition, such as running and bicycling. Patients who experience pain while sitting for long periods of time, should stand frequently, or raise the painful area from the seat.

Physiotherapy aimed at relaxing tight piriformis muscles, hip external rotators and adductors, strengthen hip abductors, or that increase the mobility of the sacroiliac joint can be beneficial. Home stretching routines can also be designed for the patient. Ultrasound has been effective for some patients.

Pharmacotherapy, including non-steroidal anti-inflammatory drugs, analgesics and muscle relaxants may help. An injection of corticosteroid into the piriformis muscle, close to the sciatic nerve, can also ease pain and reduce swelling. In severe cases, surgical resection of the piriformis muscle can be performed.

Prognosis

When piriformis syndrome is diagnosed and treated early, prognosis is good.

Special Concerns

Other causes of sciatica must be ruled out. A rapid and accurate diagnosis of piriformis syndrome can localize the cause of the pain, and can prevent sentencing a patient to long-term chronic pain management.

Resources

BOOKS

DeLee, J. C. and D. Drez Jr. *DeLee & Drez's Orthopaedic Sports Medicine, Principles and Practice,* 2nd ed. Philadelphia: Saunders, 2003.

PERIODICALS

Papadopoulos, E. C. and Khan, S. N. "Piriformis syndrome and low back pain: a new classification and review of the literature." *Orthopedic Clinics of North America* 35 (January 2004).

OTHER

"Piriformis Syndrome," Section 5, Chapter 62. In *The Merck Manual of Diagnosis and Therapy.* <http://www.merck.com>.

ORGANIZATIONS

National Rehabilitation Information Center (NARIC). 4200 Forbes Boulevard, Suite 202. Lanham, MD 20706-4829. (301) 562-2400 or (800) 346-2472; Fax: (301) 562-2401. naricinfo@heitechservices.com. <http://www.naric.com>.

National Organization of Rare Disorders (NORD). P.O. Box 1968 (55 Kenosia Avenue), Danbury, CT 06813-1968. (203) 744-0100 or (800) 999-NORD (6673); Fax: (203) 789-2291. orphan@rarediseases.org. <http://www.rarediseases.org>.

Hannah M. Hoag, MSc

Plexopathies

Definition

Plexopathies are a form of **peripheral neuropathy** (i.e., a form of damage to peripheral nerves).

Common plexopathies include brachial plexopathy affecting the upper thorax (chest and upper back), arm, and shoulder region, cervical plexopathy affecting the neck and head, and lumbosacral plexopathy affecting the lower back and legs.

Description

A branching network of nerves in which individual nerve fibers can pass from one peripheral nerve to another is termed a nerve plexus. Within the **peripheral nervous system**, there are several such plexi (e.g., the cervical plexus, brachial plexus, lumbar plexus, sacral plexus, etc.) that are often associated with neuropathy and **pain**. These neuropathies are termed plexopathies.

Neural plexi

Neural plexi are branching and interwoven connections among peripheral nerves that allow a redistribution of nerve fibers among the peripheral nerves. As nerves are traced through the peripheral nervous system, they divide into branches that then communicate with branches of nearby nerves. Because peripheral nerves are composed of aggregates or collections of individual nerve fibers, individual fibers are able to pass through the branching connections (e.g., the individual nerve fiber that controls a specific muscle in a distant appendage) to then continue their course within a new peripheral nerve. Although the branching between nerves can be complex, in most cases the nerve fibers pass intact without branching and individual fibers remain separate and distinct.

For example, the brachial plexus is a neural plexus (a grouping and branching of nerves) located deep in the neck, shoulder, and maxilla region that is responsible for the proper innervation and control of the muscles of the shoulder, upper chest, and arms (upper limbs). Because of the complexities of branching nerve roots, trunks, and cords of the brachial plexus, injuries to the brachial plexus region often cause loss or impairments of function at distant muscle groups.

Injury to the median nerve of the brachial plexus can cause a loss of flexion of the fingers. This loss of flexion results in a loss of the critical ability to oppose the thumb with individual fingers. Median nerve impairment can also result in a loss of range of motion of the arm. Individuals who sustain median nerve injury causing loss of index finger flexion may develop an index finger that "points" or remains extended. Because the median nerve ultimately passes through the carpal tunnel of the wrist, injuries or inflammation of the wrist (e.g., **carpal tunnel syndrome**) can result in pain and loss of feeling far away from the wrist itself.

Diverse symptoms

Pain, numbness, tingling, and weakness in the area of the affected neural plexus (including the lumbar, sacral, which is also known as the combined lumbsacral plexi, cervical, brachial, etc.), or in the distal appendage or area of the service by nerve fibers traversing through a particular plexus are symptoms of a potential plexopathy. Trauma, disease, or disorder can result in a plexopathy.

Depending on the source of the damage, treatment for plexopathies can include direct surgical correction, medication to relieve pain, and/or physical therapy.

Plexopathies are often initially diagnosed by a careful evaluation of the patient's history and symptoms, but electromyographic examination and nerve conduction studies are often the most accurate means to localize and determine the exact nature and site of the plexopathy.

Key Terms

Peripheral neuropathy (PN)   Damage to nerves in the peripheral nervous system (nerves other than the brain or spinal cord).

Symptoms related to plexopathies can be mild or severe, from diffuse irritation to intense and intractable pain as sometime experienced by cancer patients. In cancer patients, the source of pain may be direct damage to the nerves caused by tumor invasion or by damage to adjacent tissue (such as by **radiation** therapy, called a radiation plexopathy).

Damage to the cervical plexus caused by trauma or head and neck tumors often results in pain or a complaint of "aching discomfort" in the neck and head. Cervical plexopathy may be caused by trauma or by head and neck tumors. Brachial plexopathy is commonly related to breast cancer, lung cancer, lymphoma, or metastatic tumor. Similarly, tumors in the pelvis and abdomen may result in plexopathies and pain in the lumar, sacral (lumbosacral) plexi with pain experienced in the abdomen and upper regions of the leg. Specific plexopathy in the sacral region may result in pain in the perineal and perirectal regions.

In many plexopathies, diagnosis can be delayed or made complex by the fact that initial complaints of pain or discomfort may precede (sometimes by weeks, months, or years) the onset of other symptoms of disorder.

Resources

BOOKS

Goetz, C. G., et al. *Textbook of Clinical Neurology.* Philadelphia: W. B. Saunders Company, 1999.

Goldman, Cecil. *Textbook of Medicine*, 21st ed. New York: W. B. Saunders Co., 2000.

WEBSITES

"Physical Medicine and Rehabilitation—Plexopathy Articles." *eMedicine.com.* May 9, 2004 (May 27, 2004). <http://www.emedicine.com/pmr/PLEXOPATHY.htm>.

Paul Arthur

Poliomyelitis

Definition

Poliomyelitis is an infectious disease that is caused by a subgroup of viruses. The hallmark of the disease is the rapid development of paralysis. Poliomyelitis is also commonly called polio. Once a cause of widespread public health measures to control epidemics, polio is now on the brink of eradication.

Description

The term poliomyelitis comes from the Greek words *polio*, meaning gray, and *myelon*, referring to the spinal cord. The term is accurate, as an important consequence of the disease is the involvement of the spinal cord with resulting paralysis.

Poliomyelitis was first described in 1789, although it likely dates back many centuries prior to that time. Outbreaks occurred in Europe and the United States beginning in the early nineteenth century. For the next hundred years, outbreaks became a regular summer and fall event in northern regions. As time passed, the number of cases and people crippled by the infection rose. By 1952, more than 21,000 people in the United States were paralyzed after a bout of poliomyelitis.

The manufacture and widespread use of several vaccines beginning in the 1950s drastically reduced the number of cases of poliomyelitis. In the United States, the last reported case of polio acquired from a wild-type (original form of a naturally occurring) virus was in 1979.

Demographics

Humans are the only known carriers of the polio virus. Poliomyelitis most commonly affects children under the age of five. Several generations ago, the disease was much more common than it is now. Even in the 1950s, poliomyelitis was global in its occurrence. Many children in underdeveloped and developed countries, including the United States, were susceptible. With the successful development of vaccines and the implementation of global vaccination campaigns, the infection has been drastically reduced. As of 2004, only isolated pockets of disease remain. These hot spots include areas in Africa, India, and the eastern Mediterranean.

Males and females are equally susceptible to polio. Irreversible paralysis, usually in the legs, occurs in about one of every 200 polio infections.

Causes and symptoms

Poliomyelitis originates with a viral infection. Poliovirus is a member of a group of viruses designated as enteroviruses. The viruses contain ribonucleic acid (RNA) as their genetic material. More specifically, the various polioviruses belong in a group (or family) called Picornaviridae.

There are three types of poliovirus that are related to each other based on their recognition by the body's immune system. This sort of a relationship is called a serotype. The three poliovirus serotypes are P1, P2, and P3. Even though they are closely related immunologically, developing immunity to one serotype is no guarantee of protection from infection from the other two serotypes. Thus, vaccines are geared towards producing an immune response that will be protective against all three serotypes.

Enteroviruses can be found in the gastrointestinal tract and are not often dissolved by the acidic conditions. Thus, poliovirus can be swallowed and remain intact, capable of causing an infection. As the virus particles lodge at the back of the throat in the pharynx, or are swallowed and end up in the intestinal tract, the viruses can begin to multiply. Like all viruses, the multiplication requires a host cell, in this case, cells lining the throat and intestines.

Shortly after the virus enters a person, viral particles can be recovered from the throat and from feces. About one week later, the virus is not usually detectable in the throat. However, virus can continue to be excreted in the feces for several more weeks. During this time, symptoms of the disease do not develop. Thus, the virus can be unknowingly passed to others via the oral or fecal-to-oral route. This transmission is a common method of transfer of a variety of viral and bacterial infections in settings like daycare centers.

Subsequently, the poliovirus invades lymph tissue. From there, the virus can enter the bloodstream and infect cells of the **central nervous system**. This typically takes from six to 20 days after infection. Multiplication of the virus inside motor neurons in environments like the brain destroys the host cells and causes paralysis. The appearance of paralysis is rapid.

Up to 95% of polio infections do not produce any symptoms or damage. However, these individuals can still excrete the virus in their feces, and so are capable of infecting others. For every 200 people who escape the effects of poliomyelitis, about one person becomes paralyzed.

Approximately 4–8% of polio infections are minor, and consist of fairly nonspecific symptoms, including sore throat and fever, nausea, vomiting, abdominal **pain**, or constipation. Recovery is complete in about a week. Indeed, a person may not know the difference between this brush with polio and the flu. This condition is known as abortive poliomyelitis. There is no involvement of the central nervous system.

In 1–2% of infections, a condition called nonparalytic aseptic meningitis is produced. Nonspecific symptoms characterize this condition, followed several days later by stiffness in the neck, back, and/or legs. The symptoms last from 2–10 days. Recovery is complete.

Less than 1% of those who are infected with the poliovirus develop what is termed flaccid paralysis. Paralysis appears anywhere from one to 10 days after symptoms

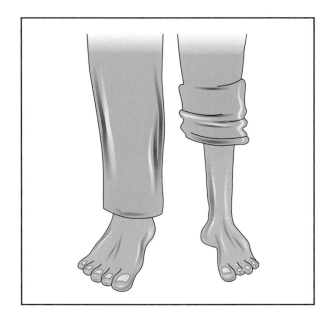

Diagram showing the difference between a healthy leg and foot and those deformed by polio. *(Illustration by Electronic Illustrators Group.)*

that include loss of reflexes, severe muscle aches, and muscle spasms in the arms, legs, or back. In children, the initial symptoms can begin to fade before paralysis appears.

Over the next few days, the paralysis becomes worse. For many people, muscle strength eventually returns. However, for those who still have weak muscles and/or paralysis a year later, the changes are likely permanent.

Types of paralytic poliomyelitis

There are three types of paralysis that can develop in poliomyelitis. The first is called spinal polio. This is the most common form of polio-related paralysis, and accounted for nearly 80% of all polio-related paralysis from 1969 to 1979. This type produces the classical image of a person whose legs have been paralyzed. The second type is known as bulbar polio. This type accounts for about 2% of known cases. Stiffness and paralysis typically occurs in the neck and head. The third type of polio-related paralysis is called bulbospinal polio. A combination of the previous two conditions, it accounts for nearly 20% of paralysis.

Postpolio syndrome

In almost half of those who contract polio in childhood, muscle pain and weakness reappears three or four decades later. Postpolio syndrome does not appear to be caused by a recurrence of the viral infection, as no virus can be detected in the feces. Rather, it may result from motor neurons damaged in the initial bout of polio that fail to operate properly decades later. The reason for the failure is not known.

Diagnosis

The diagnosis of poliomyelitis is based on the recovery of the virus from the throat or feces of a person. It is possible to isolate the virus from the cerebrospinal fluid, but this is uncommon. When the virus is recovered, specialized testing can be done to determine if the virus is wild type (that is, it has been acquired from the environment), or whether it is a vaccine type (polio vaccines utilize intact, but weakened viruses).

Another means of diagnosis relies on the detection of antibodies that have been produced by the virus. Since antibodies are produced as a part of the vaccination process, physicians focus on the increasing levels of antibodies over a short time as evidence that the body is battling an active viral infection.

Still another diagnostic test detects increased number of white blood cells and protein in the cerebrospinal fluid. This is a more general response to infections. Other conditions can present similar symptoms, and need to be ruled out when diagnosing poliomyelitis. These include **Guillain-Barré syndrome**, meningitis, and encephalitis.

Treatment team

The treatment team ideally consists of the family physician, **neurologist**, infectious disease specialist, physical therapists, occupational therapists, specialty nurses, and family members. In field conditions in developing countries, the treatment team may consist of a physician and direct caregivers only. World health agencies rapidly mobilize to provide care and vaccinations in order to contain isolated outbreaks in developing countries.

Treatment

Prevention is the watchword for poliomyelitis, and prevention consists of vaccination. There are two polio vaccines available; inactivated (Salk) poliovirus vaccine, and oral poliovirus vaccine.

The inactivated vaccine was devised by American physician Jonas Salk (1914–1995) in the 1950s. The vaccine contains all three serotypes of the poliovirus. The viruses, which are inactivated and incapable of causing an infection, are grown in a type of monkey kidney cell. When injected, the viruses stimulate an immune response that is protective. Initially, vaccine impurity was the cause of illness and death in some people who received the Salk vaccine. Refinement of the vaccine preparation eliminated these unwanted effects. Still, in the 1990s, a controversy arose regarding the vaccine as a suggested source of acquired immunodeficiency syndrome (**AIDS**), based on the known presence of the AIDS virus in monkey tissue cells. However, scrupulously conducted examinations ruled out this suggestion.

Key Terms

Disease eradication A status whereby no further cases of a diseases occur anywhere, and continued control measures are unnecessary.

Flaccid paralysis Loss of muscle tone resulting from injury or disease of the nerves that innervate the muscles.

Wild-type virus A virus occurring naturally in the environment or a population in its original form.

The oral vaccine was developed by Polish-born American physician Albert Sabin (1906–1993) in the late 1950s and was licensed for use in 1963. This vaccine has largely replaced the injected Salk vaccine. The vaccine also contains live, but weakened (attenuated) poliovirus.

A series of vaccinations given at two, four, six to 18 months, and four to six years produces a lifelong immunity to the three poliovirus serotypes. In regions where poliomyelitis is actively occurring, even a single dose of vaccine can provide adequate protection from infection during the outbreak.

In 2002, a new formulation of polio vaccine was approved for use in the United States. In addition to the polioviruses, the vaccine also bestows immunity to the virus that causes hepatitis B.

Recovery and rehabilitation

There is no cure for poliomyelitis. Some people can partially recover from paralysis, while the condition is irreversible in others. Physical and occupational therapies can be helpful in providing strengthening exercises and assistive devices for walking, but these are seldom available in remote areas of developing countries where polio outbreaks still occur.

Prognosis

Among those who are paralyzed by the viral infection, 5–10% overall die due to the paralysis of muscles used for breathing. For every 100 people who become paralyzed by the viral infection, two to five children and 15–30% of adults will die from polio.

Special concerns

Vaccination can produce reactions ranging from a transient and minor skin irritation and allergic reaction to some components of the oral vaccine to paralysis. The latter, termed vaccine-associated paralytic polio, is very rare. The condition is associated more with the injectable vaccine than with the vaccine given orally. Nonetheless,

adults can be affected. From 1980–1998, 152 adults in the United States developed some degree of paralysis from polio vaccination.

The decision by Nigeria to suspend its vaccination program in 2001 contributed to a rise in the number of polio cases in the African country. Nigeria has since reinstated the vaccination program. The Nigerian experience points out that continued vigilance is necessary to keep poliomyelitis under control.

Since the widespread availability of vaccines, the number of cases of poliomyelitis worldwide has decreased by over 99% since 1988. That year, the estimated number of cases was more than 350,000. As of April 2003, the number of cases was reduced to 1,919. The dramatic reduction in the disease is attributed to a multinational worldwide vaccination effort that began in 1988. The program was spearheaded by organizations such as the World Health Organization.

The effort intensified during the first half of 2004, with the urgent distribution of polio vaccine to 250 million children in the world's remaining hotspots. As of April 2004, the number of polio cases worldwide caused by a wild-type virus was reduced to 89. World health officials aim to interrupt the transmission of all wild-type polio virus by the year 2005.

Resources

BOOKS

Bruno, Richard L. *The Polio Paradox: Understanding and Treating "Post-Polio Syndrome" and Chronic Fatigue.* New York: Warner Books, 2003.

Oshinsky, David, *Polio: An American Story.* New York: Oxford University Press, 2004.

Salgado, Sebastio, and Kofi Annan. *The End of Polio: A Global Effort to End a Disease.* Boston: Bulfinch, 2003.

PERIODICALS

Centers for Disease Control and Prevention. "Progress toward global eradication of poliomyelitis." *Morbidity and Mortality Weekly Report* (July 2003): 366–369.

OTHER

Dowdle, Walter, et al. "Preventing Polio from Becoming a Reemerging Disease." Panel Summary from the 2000 Emerging Infectious Diseases Conference in Atlanta, Georgia. *CDC.* April 23, 2004 (June 2, 2004). <http://www.cdc.gov/ncidod/eid/vol7no3_supp/dowdle.htm>.

World Health Organization. "Poliomyelitis." April 14, 2004 (June 2, 2004). <http://www.who.int/mediacentre/factsheets/fs114/en/>.

ORGANIZATIONS

World Health Organization. Avenue Appia 20, Geneva, Switzerland. + 41 22 791 2111; Fax: + 41 22 791 3111. info@who.int. <http://www.who.int>.

Brian Douglas Hoyle, PhD

Polymyositis

Definition

Polymyositis (PM) is an inflammatory muscle disease with an unknown cause. The disease has a gradual onset and generally begins in the second decade of life and, thus, it rarely affects persons under the age of 18. It causes muscles to exhibit varying degrees of decreased strength, usually affecting those muscles that are closest to the trunk of the body. Trouble with swallowing (dysphagia) may occur with polymyositis.

Description

In polymyositis, muscles exhibit varying degrees of weakness, evolving gradually over weeks to months. It is known that PM begins when white blood cells, the immune cells of inflammation, spontaneously invade muscles, and is thus termed an autoimmune disease. In PM, muscle fibers are found to be in varying stages of necrosis (tissue death) and regeneration. The muscles affected are typically those closest to the trunk or torso, resulting in weakness that can be severe. Eventually, patients have difficulty rising from a sitting position, climbing stairs, lifting objects, or reaching overhead. In some cases, distal muscles (those not close to the trunk of the body) may also be affected later in the course of the disease. Polymyositis is a chronic illness with periods of increased symptoms, called flares or relapses, and decreased symptoms, known as remissions.

Polymyositis mimics many other muscle disorders and remains a diagnosis of exclusion. It should be viewed as a syndrome of diverse causes that occurs separately or in association with other autoimmune disorders or viral infections. A similar **inflammatory myopathy** is often associated with skin rash and is referred to as **dermatomyositis**.

Demographics

Polymyositis in the United States is most common among African Americans. The disorder is most prevalent in women in a male/female ratio of 1:2. In the United States, its incidence is one per 100,000 persons per year; internationally, a lower incidence among the Japanese has been observed. The age of onset is normally above the second decade of life and it is rare or nonexistent for persons under the age of 20.

Causes and symptoms

To date, no cause of polymyositis has been isolated by scientific researchers. While the initial inciting agent remains unknown, possibilities include infection with certain viruses or muscle trauma. There are many infectious agents that are thought to trigger the disease, mainly Coxsackie virus B1, HIV, human T-lymphotropic virus 1 (HTLV-1), hepatitis B and C, influenza, echovirus, and adenovirus. Certain drugs are also thought to be potential triggers, including D-penicillamine, hydralazine, procainamide, and phenytoin.

There are indicators of heredity (genetic) susceptibility that can be found in some patients, mainly the HLA (human leukocyte antigen) genes, which are responsible for encoding some proteins that can activate the immune system.

The muscle weakness affecting mainly the proximal (closest to the trunk of the body) muscles is the first sign of PM. The onset can be gradual or rapid, but normally progresses over weeks or months. This results in varying degrees of loss of muscle strength and atrophy (tissue degeneration). The loss of strength can be noticed as difficulty getting up from chairs, climbing stairs, or lifting above the shoulders. Trouble with swallowing (dysphagia) and weakness lifting the head from the pillow may occur. Occasionally, the muscles ache at rest or with use, and are tender to the touch (occurs in about 25% patients). Persons with polymyositis can also feel **fatigue**, a general feeling of discomfort, and have weight loss, and/or low-grade fever. Heart and lung involvement can lead to irregular heart rhythm and shortness of breath.

Diagnosis

Persons with polymyositis generally seek initial medical help due to weakness. A physician typically reviews the condition of other body systems, including the skin, heart, lungs, and joints. Blood tests are helpful to reveal abnormal high levels of muscle enzymes in the serum of PM patients, mainly creatinine phosphokinase (CPK) and aldolase. In PM, muscle damage causes the muscular cells to break open and spill their content into the bloodstream. Since most of CPK and aldolase exist in muscles, an increase in the amount of these enzymes in the blood indicates that muscle damage has occurred, or is occurring. Blood tests can also point to active inflammation.

The muscle **biopsy** is one of the best ways to diagnose myositis and other muscle disorders. A muscle biopsy is used to confirm the presence of muscle inflammation typical only of polymyositis. This is a surgical procedure whereby muscle tissue is removed for analysis by a pathologist, a specialist in examining tissue under a microscope. Muscles often used for biopsy include the quadriceps muscle of the front of the thigh, the biceps muscle of the arm, and the deltoid muscle of the shoulder. The results can show conditions such as inflammation, or swelling, of the muscle, damage to the muscle, and loss of muscle mass, or atrophy.

Imaging of the muscles using radiology tests such as **magnetic resonance imaging (MRI)** can show areas of inflammation of muscle, swelling, or scarring. This sometimes can be used to determine muscle biopsy sites. MRIs show signal intensity abnormalities of muscle due to inflammation.

Another test, an electromyogram (EMG), is used to measure the activity of muscles and to provide clues to the cause of muscle weakness or paralysis, muscle problems such as muscle twitching, numbness, tingling, or **pain**, and nerve damage or injury. EMG is useful in the diagnosis of PM and to exclude other nerve-muscle diseases. Although EMG and MRI imaging are helpful in many cases, the diagnosis of PM is definite when a patient has subacute elevated levels of serum creatine kinase and characteristic findings on muscle biopsy.

Treatment team

A **neurologist** or rheumatologist is the primary consultant for PM, with allied health care areas that include, but are not limited to, physical therapy.

Treatment

In PM, high-dose corticosteroids constitute the first line of treatment, and are effective in more than 70% of patients. Alternatives include immunosuppressant medications, notably azathioprine, methotrexate, and intravenous immunoglobulins (IVIg).

Recovery and rehabilitation

Before the era of corticosteroids, PM was a particularly severe disease with a spontaneous survival rate of less than 40%. Polymyositis in adults now has a relatively favorable prognosis, with a five-year survival rate of around 90%. Only 30–50% of persons with polymyositis

achieve complete recovery; the majority of patients have persistent functional problems. However, patients can ultimately do well, especially with early medical treatment of disease and early recognition of disease flares. The disease frequently becomes inactive, and rehabilitation of atrophied (withered) muscles becomes a long-term project.

Clinical trials

The National Institute of Environmental Health Sciences (NIEHS) is recruiting patients for a study entitled "Myositis in Children." The aim of the study is to learn more about the immune system changes and medical problems associated with myositis. The National Institute of Arthritis and Musculoskeletal and Skin Diseases (NIAMS) is examining whether infliximab (Remicade[r]) is safe for treatment of PM. Updated information is available at The National Institutes of Health website for **clinical trials** at <http://www.clinicaltrials.gov>.

Prognosis

The prognosis for PM and the response to therapy vary from very good to satisfactory. Most patients respond well to treatment, although residual weakness is common. Osteoporosis, a common complication of chronic corticosteroid therapy, may be significant. For African Americans, older people, females, people with interstitial lung disease and associated malignancies, those who delay treatment, and those with trouble swallowing or heart involvement, the prognosis is much less favorable.

Special concerns

Exercise is generally beneficial, and helps to get the most out of diseased muscles. Falls and injuries, however, can cause substantial disability. People with PM, therefore, have the difficult task of undertaking regular exercise within their capability, but avoiding injury through accident. Because weakened muscles cannot carry an excess load, keeping to an ideal weight is critical. Although this may seem obvious, weight control is more difficult when exercise is limited.

A well-balanced diet is helpful. Patients with severe inflammation of the muscles may need extra protein. Feeding should be avoided prior to bedtime in patients with trouble swallowing.

Resources

BOOKS

Staff. *The Official Patient's Sourcebook on Polymyositis: A Revised and Updated Directory for the Internet Age.* San Diego: Icon Health International, 2004.

PERIODICALS

Mastaglia, F. L., M. J. Garllep, B. A. Phillips, and P. J. Zilko. "Inflammatory Myopathies: Clinical, Diagnostic and

Therapeutic Aspects." *Muscle & Nerve* (April 2003): 407–425.

OTHER

"NINDS Polymyositis Information Page." *National Institute of Neurological Disorders and Stroke.* May 2, 2004 (June 2, 2004). <http://www.ninds.nih.gov/health_and_medical/disorders/polymyos_doc.htm>.

"Myositis." *Medline Plus.* May 1, 2004 (June 2, 2004). <http://www.nlm.nih.gov/medlineplus/myositis.html>.

ORGANIZATIONS

Myositis Association of America. 755 Cantrell Ave., Suite C, Harrisonburg, VA 22801. (540) 433-7686; Fax: (540) 432-0206. maa@myositis.org. <http://www.myositis.org>.

Marcos do Carmo Oyama
Iuri Drumond Louro, MD, PhD

Pompe disease

Definition

Pompe disease is a genetically inherited disorder that results in the progressive deterioration of muscle function. The disorder was first described by the Dutch pathologist J.C. Pompe in 1932. Pompe disease is an autosomal recessive disorder, which means that both unaffected parents are carriers and there is a 25% risk of having an affected offspring. Pompe disease is caused by mutations in a gene that encodes an enzyme (a protein that speeds up chemical reactions) called acid alpha-glucosidase. This enzyme is required for breaking down stored sugars in the body.

Description

Pompe disease is also known as glycogen storage disease, type II. Glucose molecules make up sugar, and glucose is stored in the body as glycogen. In this form of the disease, glycogen accumulates in discreet structures in the cell called the lysosomes. Other types of Pompe disease involve the failure to break down glycogen, leading to accumulation in the interior of the cell (not the lysosomal organelles). Glycogen storage diseases collectively, therefore, are all progressive neuromuscular diseases that result from defects in the breakdown or storage of glycogen.

Pompe disease can be categorized into three distinct forms that are determined by the age of onset: the infantile, juvenile, and the adult-onset form. In general, the earlier the onset, the more severe the clinical features of the disease are manifested. Muscle deterioration is the hallmark of Pompe disease. Muscle wasting is progressive, meaning that eventually, patients will lose their ability (or in affected infants, fail to develop an ability) to walk, or perform activities that require sustained motion.

Demographics

In the United States, it is estimated that approximately 1 out of 40,000 individuals is affected with Pompe disease. This estimation is based on population frequencies from a variety of races, but independent of sex or age of onset. Although the frequency has been reported to be less (1 in 50,000) in some Asian populations, including Taiwanese and Southern Chinese, it is felt that most populations share a similar gene frequency found in populations in the United States. As this is an autosomal recessive disorder, males and females are equally affected. Although there are gene mutations that are found in different populations, these gene mutations (otherwise known as an individuals' genotype) do not correlate with the observable clinical feathers (phenotype).

Causes and symptoms

Acid alpha-glucosidase is an enzyme found in discrete organelles within the cell called the lysosomes. Lysosomes are important for storage and release of various molecules that serve as building blocks for the cell or as a source of energy. Lysosomes transport enzymes, like acid alpha-glucosidase, to break down glycogen by breaking down or hydrolyzing specific bonds between sugar molecules. Unlike other types of glycogen storage diseases, Pompe disease patients do not have a condition with low blood sugar (hypoglycemia) or have impairments in energy production. Acid alpha-glucosidase is not the predominant enzyme required to break down glycogen, although it does play a role. Regardless, a deficiency of this enzyme results in an accumulation of glycogen. Toxicity of the accumulated glycogen results in injury to the cells and with enough damage, injury of the entire organ.

Genetic mutations in the acid alpha-glucosidase gene can produce several effects: normal amounts of enzyme can be produced, but with decreased function; or, mutations can also result in a decreased amount of enzyme produced with no defects in function; finally, specific mutations can result in the absence of proper amino acid sequences that are used to produce the acid alpha glucosidase protein.

INFANTILE POMPE DISEASE Infantile Pompe disease typically becomes apparent before the child reaches six months of age. It is particularly progressive, and characterized by rapid muscle deterioration. Failure to reach milestones such as rolling over, sitting up, or standing is typical. Progressive muscular involvement can include tissues that are part of the skeletal system, the cardiac system, and the respiratory system. The cause of death is

Key Terms

Autosomal recessive disorder A genetic disorder that is inherited from parents that are both carriers, but do not have the disorder. Parents with an affected recessive gene have a 25% chance of passing on the disorder to their offspring with each pregnancy.

Glycogen The principle form of carbohydrate energy (glucose) stored within the muscles and liver.

Myopathy Abnormal muscle weakness.

usually due to respiratory and/or heart failure. The heart usually becomes enlarged (cardiomegaly) and becomes dysfunctional, a condition called cardiomyopathy. Cardiomegaly accompanies thickening of the left ventricle of the heart followed by obstruction of blood outflow. Skeletal muscle involvement leads to floppiness and muscle weakness (**myopathy**). Breathing can also become labored due to respiratory muscle injury. This cellular injury will eventually compromise the ability of the respiratory system to function.

JUVENILE POMPE DISEASE Unlike the infant form, children with the juvenile form of Pompe disease usually develop symtomatology after six months of age, but before the age of 20. They may initially complain about muscle weakness and experience failure to progress in terms of motor development, even though intelligence is normal. These patients usually do not have cardiac involvement, and this becomes less likely the older the patient is at the time that clinical manifestations occur. Skeletal and respiratory system failure can eventually lead to death in these patients.

ADULT-ONSET POMPE DISEASE In this form, the course of the disease is less rapid and can develop in persons from 20–60 years old. Patients typically find it difficult to go up a flight of stairs or experience **exercise** intolerance. There is an absence of cardiac abnormality involvement in this type of the disease, and therefore, these patients usually die of complications related to respiratory system dysfunction.

Diagnosis

As there are many disorders that can cause muscle weakness, it is important that laboratory tests, in combination with a physical evaluation, be performed to diagnose Pompe disease. Creatinine kinase, an enzyme involved in muscle function, is also a biomarker for muscle degradation and can be measured in patients' skin cells or other tissues. People with Pompe disease have elevated CK levels, often up to 10 times greater than normal. The test for enzyme activity can also be performed using skin cells or blood cells by a clinical biochemical geneticist. An echocardiogram can help establish the level of heart involvement by testing whether the functions of the heart are normal.

Treatment

There is no cure for Pompe disease. Treatment, therefore, serves only to help minimize the symptoms. The clinical course is typically not affected by drugs that are used to treat the respiratory or cardiac defects. A high protein diet may be helpful and has led to significant improvements in respiratory function in some cases. Ibuprofen has been shown to be effective at relieving muscle aches.

It should be noted that enzyme replacement therapy has been described in Pompe disease recently with some dramatic effects in very small numbers of patients. Although it is still investigational, it may become more available in the future.

Recovery and rehabilitation

As there is no cure for Pompe disease and it is often rapid in its progression, emphasis is placed upon maintaining function for as long as possible, rather than recovery. Occupational therapy can be helpful with positioning devices and strategies for accomplishing daily tasks. Physical therapists can assist with exercises to help maintain maximum possible range of motion and purposeful muscle movement. Speech therapists often provide assistance in feeding strategies for infants affected with Pompe disease.

In the early onset form, it is important and challenging for parents to consider the special needs of babies affected with Pompe disease. This adjustment is often difficult for parents, not only in terms of logistical considerations, but also with the realization that their children will have significant limitations. Parents often utilize community support groups or other counseling to help with these experiences. The late onset form has different emotional and physical issues, as the affected person must cope with progressive lack of mobility and independent function.

Clinical trials

There are several promising ongoing **clinical trials** for the treatment of Pompe disease. In one study, the safety and effectiveness of a recombinant human acid alpha-glucosidase enzyme is being used as a potential enzyme replacement therapy. This recombinant form allows scientist to make a lot of protein, in this case the enzyme that is defective in Pompe disease, and deliver it to patients. Patients diagnosed with infantile-onset Pompe disease who are less than or equal to six months old (or severely affected) are being studied. (Contact information: Duke University Medical Center, Durham, North Carolina, 27710, Stephanie DeArmey (919) 681-1946, Dearm001@mc.duke.edu; Priya Kishnani, M.D., Principal Investigator.) Other treatment studies are also being invested.

Prognosis

As heart and respiratory muscles quickly weaken, babies affected with Pompe disease usually die within the first year of life. The juvenile form of the disease has a slower progression, with a fatal outcome usually occurring between 20–30 years old. The cause of death is usually respiratory failure. Although the adult form can be fatal, it is likely that these patients will live for several decades following a diagnosis.

Special concerns

Because Pompe disease is a genetic disorder and unaffected carrier parents have a 25% chance of having another affected fetus with each pregnancy, the appropriate genetic counseling is recommended. It should be conveyed to patients and parents that being affected with the disease means that there is a possible risk for other family members to have or pass on the disorder. Prenatal diagnosis is also an option for an expecting mother that wants to know the child's genotype in order to make reproductive decisions.

Resources

PERIODICALS

Bakker, H. D., M. C. Loonen, J. B. de Klerk, A. J. Reuser, and A. T. van der Ploeg. "The natural course of infantile Pompe's disease: 20 original cases compared with 133 cases from the literature." *Pediatrics* 112, no. 2 (August 2003): 332–40.

OTHER

Association for Glycogen Storage Disease (UK). *The Pompe Disease Page.* <http://www.pompe.org.uk/> (March 30, 2004).

Johns Hopkins University, OMIM—Online Mendelian Inheritance in Man. *Glycogen Storage Disease II.* <http://www.ncbi.nlm.nih.gov/entrez/dispomim.cgi?id=232300> (March 30, 2004).

National Institute of Neurological Disorders and Stroke. *NINDS Pompe Disease Information Page.* <http://www.ninds.nih.gov/health_and_medical/disorders/pompe.htm> (March 30, 2004).

ORGANIZATIONS

Acid Maltase Deficiency Association (AMDA). P.O. Box 700248, San Antonio, TX 78270. 210-494-6144; Fax: 210-490-7161. tianrama@aol.com. <http://www.amda-pompe.org>.

Association for Glycogen Storage Disease. P.O. Box 896, Durant, IA 52747. 563-785-6038; Fax: 563-785-6038. maryc@agsdus.org. <http://www.agsdus.org>.

Muscular Dystrophy Association. 3300 East Sunrise Drive, Tucson, AZ 85718-3208. (520) 529-2000 or (800) 572-1717; Fax: (520) 529-5300. mda@mdausa.org. <http://www.mdausa.org/>.

Bryan Richard Cobb, PhD

Porencephaly

Definition

Porencephaly is a rare condition in which fluid-filled hollows or cavities develop on the surface of the brain. These cavities usually form at sites where damage has been caused by infection, loss of blood flow, or **stroke** during brain development, but may also be genetic in origin. Equivalent terms are cerebral porosis, perencephaly, porencephalia, and (no longer in favor) polyporencephaly. The prefix "por" comes from the Latin *porus,* for hole or cavity.

Description

In porencephaly, large dimples, craters, or clefts develop on the surface of the brain. These cavities or cysts are filled with fluid and lined with smooth tissue. They are usually caused by injuries to the fetal or newborn brain before full development of the convolutions or gyri (singular gyrus) on the surface of the cerebrum, especially by infection, ischemia (reduction of blood flow through a vessel), infarction (blockage of blood flow through a vessel), or stroke (bleeding in the brain). The cerebral gyri develop abnormally around a porencephaly cavity, both anatomically and microscopically, and may take on a radiating pattern. Areas of abnormally small gyri (polymicrogyria) may develop on areas of the cerebrum not directly adjacent to a porencephalic cavity.

Porencephaly cavities sometimes develop symmetrically, that is, with a cavity on one side of the brain being matched by a similar cavity on the other side. When a pair of symmetric cavities are very large, they may leave only a thin arch of cerebral cortex running front to back over the top of the brain like a basket handle, a condition termed basket brain. In the most extreme cases, virtually the entire cerebrum may be replaced by fluid, a condition termed **hydranencephaly**.

Demographics

Porencephaly is rare, and its exact incidence is unknown. A 1984 study from the University of Colorado found in a study of 18,000 patients with seizure disorder

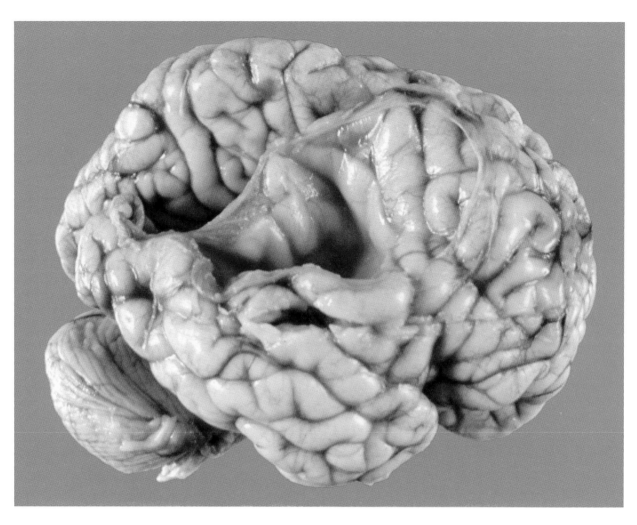

Cavities in a hemisphere of a brain affected with porencephaly. *(Custom Medical Stock Photo. All Rights Reserved.)*

or retarded neural development that 11 had porencephaly, a rate of 1:1650 in that abnormal population.

Causes and symptoms

Any agent or event that causes localized tissue death in the brain during development can cause porencephaly. The body walls off the injured area with a barrier of smooth tissue (encysts it), and eventually the dead tissue is cleared away and replaced with cerebrospinal fluid. One infectious agent that can cause porencephaly is cytomegalovirus, which can also cause **microcephaly** (small brain). Ischemic brain necrosis, the death of a portion of the brain due to restriction of blood flow through a specific vessel, most often the middle cerebral artery, can also cause porencephaly. Rarely, porencephaly can be caused by a mechanical injury such as accidental penetration of the skull by an amniocentesis needle.

Because porencephaly usually follows from a disruption during development rather than from a genetic defect, it falls into a class of cerebral defects in between primary malformations (those occurring without any specific injury or trigger, and usually genetic in origin) and secondary malformations (those resulting from injury, infection, or some other external cause). The question of whether a given case of porencephaly is primary (genetic) or secondary is important because geneticists wish to provide accurate counseling to prospective parents with family histories of porencephaly. If a familial case of porencephaly is due to infection or injury, there is probably no increased genetic risk for future generations. If, on the other hand, a familial case of porencephaly is due to heritable genetic abnormalities affecting clotting factors, for instance, there may be increased risk for a fetus affected in future pregnancies. Research by the National Institute of Neurological Disorders and Stroke, an arm of the National Institutes of Health, commenced in 2000 to determine if acquired and/or genetic abnormal coagulation factors in the blood are associated with porencephaly, stroke, and **cerebral palsy**.

The symptoms of porencephaly are varied, and depend on the severity of the defects in each individual case. Persons with porencephaly may suffer early death, **epilepsy**, moderate or severe **mental retardation**, blindness, epilepsy, rigidity, and paralysis.

Diagnosis

Imaging technologies such as ultrasound, x-ray computerized tomography, and **magnetic resonance imaging** (**MRI**) can diagnose porencephaly before or after birth. Ultrasound is preferred for fetal imaging, both because it is cheaper than MRI or computed tomography (**CT**) **scan** and, in most cases, just as informative; and because of lingering concerns that magnetic resonance imaging might, by some unknown mechanism, be capable of disrupting the normal formation of organs. (X rays are not used because fetuses are known to be extremely vulnerable to ionizing radiation.) An initial diagnosis can sometimes be made by shining a light through the newborn's skull.

Treatment team

As with other severe congenital defects of the brain, the membership of a porencephaly patient's treatment team will depend on the severity and exact nature of the damage. A pediatric **neurologist** and physical therapist will probably be involved, at minimum.

Treatment

Treatment is addressed to alleviating symptoms, not to curing the underlying problem, as there is no treatment to induce the brain to grow missing sections of the cerebrum. Treatment includes physical therapy for rigidity, **spasticity**, or movement difficulties; medication to prevent **seizures**; and, if necessary, the installation of a shunt or drain to remove excess cerebrospinal fluid from the inside of the skull.

Clinical trials

As of early 2004, the National Institute of Neurological Disorders and Stroke was sponsoring research entitled "Study of Abnormal Blood Clotting in Children with Stroke." More information can be found by contacting the National Institute of Neurological Disorders and Stroke (NINDS), 9000 Rockville Pike, Bethesda, Maryland, 20892, Patient Recruitment and Public Liaison Office, telephone: (800) 411–1222, email: prpl@mail.cc.nih.gov.

Prognosis

Most persons with porencephaly die before reaching adulthood. Each individual's prognosis will depend on the location and severity of the lesions on their cerebrum.

Resources

BOOKS

Graham, David I. and Peter L. Lantos. *Greenfield's Neuropathology*, 6th edition. Bath, UK: Arnold, 1997.

OTHER

National Institute of Neurological Disorders and Stroke. *NINDS Porencephaly Information Page.* <http://www.ninds.nih.gov/health_and_medical/disorders/porencephaly.htm> (April 7, 2004).

ORGANIZATIONS

National Organization for Rare Disorders. 55 Kenosia Avenue, Danbury, CT 06813-1968. (203) 744-0100 or (800) 999-6673; Fax: (203) 798-2291. orphan@rarediseases.org. <http://www.rarediseases.org>.

March of Dimes Birth Defects Foundation. 1275 Mamaroneck Avenue, White Plains, NY 10605, USA. (914) 428-7100 or 888-MODIMES (663-4637); Fax: (914) 428-8203. askus@marchofdimes.com. <http://www.marchofdimes.com>.

Larry Gilman, PhD

Positron emission tomography (PET)

Definition

Positron emission tomography (PET) is a noninvasive scanning technique that utilizes small amounts of radioactive positrons (positively charged particles) to visualize body function and metabolism.

Description

PET is the fastest growing nuclear medicine tool in terms of increasing acceptance and applications. It is useful in the diagnosis, staging, and treatment of cancer because it provides information that cannot be obtained by other techniques such as computed tomography (**CT**) and **magnetic resonance imaging (MRI)**.

PET scans are performed at medical centers equipped with a small cyclotron. Smaller cyclotrons and increasing availability of certain radiopharmaceuticals are making PET a more widely used imaging modality.

Physicians first used PET to obtain information about brain function, and to study brain activity in various neurological diseases and disorders including **stroke**, **epilepsy**, **Alzheimer's disease**, **Parkinson's disease**, and Huntington's disease; and in psychiatric disorders such as **schizophrenia**, **depression**, obsessive-compulsive disorder, **attention deficit hyperactivity disorder** (ADHD), and **Tourette syndrome**. PET is now used to evaluate patients for these cancers: head and neck, lymphoma, melanoma, lung, colorectal, breast, and esophageal. PET also is used to evaluate heart muscle function in patients with coronary artery disease or cardiomyopathy.

Procedure

PET involves injecting a patient with a radiopharmaceutical similar to glucose. An hour after injection of this tracer, a PET scan creates an image of a specific metabolic function by measuring the concentration and distribution of the tracer throughout the body.

When it enters the body, the tracer courses through the bloodstream to the target organ, where it emits positrons. The positively charged positrons collide with negatively charged electrons, producing gamma rays. The gamma rays are detected by photomultiplier-scintillator combinations positioned on opposite sides of the patient. These signals are processed by the computer and images are generated.

PET provides an advantage over CT and MRI because it can determine if a lesion is malignant. The two other modalities provide images of anatomical structures, but often cannot provide a determination of malignancy. CT and MRI show structure, while PET shows function. PET has been used in combination with CT and MRI to identify abnormalities with more precision and indicate areas of most active metabolism. This additional information allows for more accurate evaluation of cancer treatment and management.

Resources

BOOKS

Bares, R., and G. Lucignani. *Clinical PET.* Kluwer Academic Publishers, 1996.

Gulyas, Balazs, and Hans Muller-Gartner. *Positron Emission Tomography: A Critical Assessment of Recent Trends.* Kluwer Academic Publishers, 1996.

Kevles, Bettyann Holtzmann. *Medical Imaging in the Twentieth Century.* Rutgers University Press, 1996.

PERIODICALS

"Brain Imaging and Psychiatry: Part 1." *Harvard Mental Health Letter* 13 (Jan. 1997): 1.

"Brain Imaging and Psychiatry: Part 2." *Harvard Mental Health Letter* 13 (February 1997): 1403.

Goerres, G. "Position Emission Tomography and PET CT of the Head and Neck: FDG Uptake in Normal Anatomy, in Benign Lesions, and Changes Resulting from Treatment." *American Journal of Roentgenology* (November 2002): 1337.

Kostakoglu, L. "Clinical Role of FDG PET in Evaluation of Cancer Patients." *Radiographics* (March-April 2003): 315.

Shreve, P. "Pitfalls in Oncologic Diagnosis with FDG PET Imaging: Physiologic and Benign Variants." *Radiographics* 62 (January/February 1999).

"Studies Argue for Wider Use of PET for Cancer Patients." *Cancer Weekly Plus* 15 (December 1997): 9.

OTHER

Di Carli, M. F. "Positron Emission Tomography (PET)." *1st Virtual Congress of Cardiology* October 4, 1999. <http://www.fac.org>.

Madden Yee, Kate. "Start-up Enters Breast Imaging Arena with Scintimammography, PET Offerings." *Radiology News* March 14, 2001. <http://www.auntminnie.com>.

"Nycomed Amersham and the Medical Research Council: Major Collaboration in World Leading Imaging Technology." *Medical Research Center* 2001. <http://www.mrc.ac.uk/whats_new/press_releases/PR_2001/mrc_02_01.html>.

Dan Harvey
Lee A. Shratter, MD
Rosalyn Carson-DeWitt, MD

Post-polio syndrome

Definition

Post-polio syndrome is a slowly progressing weakness that affects polio survivors decades after their initial bout with the disease.

Description

In order to understand post-polio syndrome, it's important to understand polio infection in general. Although people of any age can become infected with poliovirus, it tends to infect young children in particular. About 1% of all people who become infected with poliovirus will actually become ill. Initial symptoms include fever, nausea,

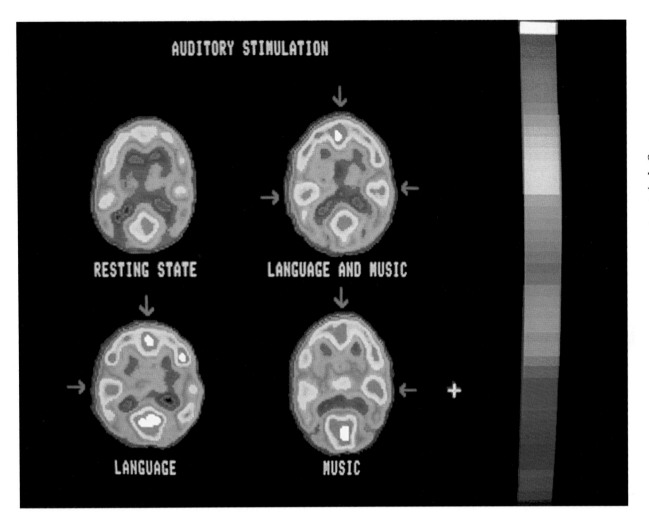

Results of a brain stimulation test made with positron emission tomography. *(© Roger Ressmeyer/Corbis. Reproduced by permission.)*

Key Terms

Electron   One of the small particles that make up an atom. An electron has the same mass and amount of charge as a positron, but the electron has a negative charge.

Gamma ray   A high-energy photon emitted by radioactive substances.

Half-life   The time required for half of the atoms in a radioactive substance to disintegrate.

Photon   A light particle.

Positron   One of the small particles that make up an atom. A positron has the same mass and amount of charge as an electron, but the positron has a positive charge.

and vomiting, followed by several symptom-free days. Some individuals then recover completely. Others go on to develop new symptoms, including severe head, back, and neck **pain**. These symptoms signal that the virus is invading the nervous system, causing inflammation, injury, and destruction of motor nerves (the nerves that are necessary for muscle movement). As motor nerves are destroyed, the muscles cannot receive messages from the brain. Without input from the brain, muscle tone becomes weak and floppy, and paralysis sets in. Over time, the muscle becomes atrophic (shrunken in size). Paralysis is usually asymmetric; that is, it affects only one side of the body. The paralyzed limbs retain their ability to feel. When the muscles of respiration are affected, the patient may need to be put on a mechanical ventilator.

It only takes a few days for the weakness and/or paralysis to progress to its maximum level of severity. Recovery continues for about six months, during which time the remaining unaffected motor nerves begin sprouting new branches to the muscles, in an attempt to compensate for the nerves that were completely destroyed. During this phase, the patient will regain some degree of functioning. After six months have passed, whatever disability remains will usually be permanent.

Post-polio syndrome occurs some decades after the original infection with polio. Initially, the subtly gradual progressive muscle weakness is barely noticed by the patient, but over time the decrement becomes increasingly obvious. In general, the more severe the original polio infection, the more severe the disability from post-polio syndrome.

Demographics

Only 1% of all people infected with poliovirus actually develop full-fledged polio. About 25-50% of polio survivors will eventually be affected with post-polio syndrome.

Causes and symptoms

Attempts to completely delineate the process by which post-polio syndrome develops have not been totally successful. A number of working theories have been developed.

- The newer nerve sprouts that grew in order to compensate for lost motor units overtax the rest of the nerve, and over time the nerve begins to fail.

- Injured nerves that regained function end up failing after years of overuse attempting to compensate for lost motor units.

- Remaining particles of the poliovirus may precipitate a chemical response in the immune system that accidentally destroys the body's own nerves.

- Spinal cord changes in polio survivors may adversely affect nerves over time.

Symptoms of post-polio syndrome include severe **fatigue**; decreased energy; gradually progressive muscle weakness and muscle atrophy; involuntary muscle twitching (fasciculation); muscle, joint and **back pain**; difficulty breathing and swallowing; and problems with sleep. The most severe muscle problems seem to occur in those muscles that were already affected by the initial bout of polio, although muscles that were not originally affected may also develop some new degree of weakness.

Diagnosis

Diagnosis should be suspected in any polio survivor experiencing new muscle weakness.

Four criteria are required to diagnose post-polio syndrome in a patient with gradually increasing muscle weakness:

Key Terms

Atrophy   Wasting or shrinking of a body part, such as a muscle.

Motor nerve   A nerve that is involved in muscle movement.

Polio   A disease caused by the poliovirus that can result in muscle weakness and/or paralysis.

Poliovirus   The virus responsible for the disease called polio.

Sphincter   A band of muscle that encircles an opening in the body, allowing the opening to open and close (anal sphincter, esophageal sphincter).

- known history of poliovirus infection with residual muscle weakness

- history of recovery of some degree of muscle function, with a period of stability lasting at least 15 years

- at least one limb demonstrating residual muscle atrophy, weakness, lack of normal reflex, and continued normal sensation

- normal function of sphincter muscles (the muscles around the anus and the lower part of the esophagus)

Treatment team

The treatment team will depend in part on the specific symptoms encountered. In general, once diagnosed, the patient will benefit from work with a physical therapist, occupational therapist, and speech and language therapist. Specialists in arthritis, orthopedics, rehabilitation, and pulmonology may also be helpful.

Treatment

There is no cure for post-polio syndrome. Efforts are primarily directed at retaining mobility and improving patient comfort. Anti-inflammatory medications can help relieve muscle and joint pain by decreasing inflammation. Braces, wheelchairs, or motorized scooters may help very compromised patients retain some independence and mobility. Respiratory and sleep problems may interact with each other to create considerable distress. They may be relieved by the use of supplemental oxygen and/or breathing devices to help keep the airway open while sleeping.

Recovery and rehabilitation

The physical therapist should design a thoughtful **exercise** program to maintain and increase flexibility, although it is important not to overtax already weakened muscles and nerves. Occupational therapy can help the individual learn methods to compensate for muscle weakness, and still retain independence in the activities of daily living. Speech and language therapists can be helpful for swallowing problems.

Clinical trials

A **clinical trial** through the National Institute of Neurological Disorders and Stroke is studying whether the drug **modafinil** might be helpful in treating the relentless fatigue of post-polio syndrome.

Prognosis

Because the increase in muscle weakness is so gradual, post-polio syndrome is generally thought to have a good prognosis, rarely causing significantly more severe impairment and disability. In a few rare cases, however, progressive weakening of the muscles of respiration can result in death.

Resources

BOOKS

Modlin, John F. "Poliovirus." In *Principles and Practice of Infectious Diseases,* edited by Gerald L. Mandell. London: Churchill Livingstone, Inc., 2000.

Nath, Avindra, and Joseph R. Berger. "Poliomyelitis." In *Cecil Textbook of Medicine,* edited by Lee Goldman. Philadelphia: W.B. Saunders Company, 2003.

Roos, Karen L. "Viral Infections." In *Textbook of Clinical Neurology,* edited by Christopher G. Goetz. Philadelphia: W.B. Saunders Company, 2003.

WEBSITES

National Institute of Neurological Disorders and Stroke (NINDS). *Post-polio Syndrome Fact Sheet.* Bethesda, MD: NINDS, 2003.

ORGANIZATIONS

National Institute of Neurological Disorders and Stroke (NINDS). 9000 Rockville Pike, Bethesda, Maryland 20892. 800-411-1222. prpl@mail.cc.nih.gov. <http://clinicaltrials.gov/ct/show/NCT00067496?order=1>.

Rosalyn Carson-DeWitt, MD

Postinfectious encephalomyelitis *see* **Acute disseminated encephalomyelitis**

Postural hypotension *see* **Orthostatic hypotension**

Prednisone *see* **Glucocorticoids**

Primary lateral sclerosis

Definition

Primary lateral sclerosis (PLS) is a rare disease that causes progressive weakness in voluntary muscles such as in the legs, hands, and tongue. PLS is one of the diseases, along with **amyotrophic lateral sclerosis** (or Lou Gehrig's disease), that are grouped together as **motor neuron diseases**.

Description

Motor neuron diseases like primary lateral sclerosis develop because the nerve cells that normally control the movement of voluntary muscles degenerate and die. The disease is typically detected in middle age, after age 50. The symptoms of the disorder become progressively worse, with muscles typically affected in the following order: legs and feet, main part of the body (the trunk), arms and hands, and face. PLS is not fatal, and people with the disorder can usually maintain mobility with the use of canes or other assistance.

Demographics

Primary lateral sclerosis predominates in those over 50 years of age, although people in their mid-30s can be affected. PLS is rare in younger people, although one case of a 20-year-old has been reported. It is estimated that only about 500 people in the United States have the disease. Due to its historically rare occurrence, it is not yet possible to know if the disease is more prevalent in males or females. The incidence of PLS is uncertain. ALS is known to affect two to three people per 100,000. Tentative estimates of the occurrence of PLS are on the order of one person in 10 million, which would make it only about 0.5 percent as prevalent as the already rare ALS.

Causes and symptoms

The cause of the disease is the progressive degeneration and death of the nerves (neurons) that control the movement of voluntary muscles. There is no evidence of a genetic basis for the disease. Some other process determines the nerve cell death. PLS affects a part of the neuron called the cell body (or soma). Specifically, it is the cell bodies of upper motor neurons that are affected. Upper motor neurons are located in the brain. Their loss affects the transmission of a signal to other neurons that eventually control the muscle activity. This specificity distinguishes PLS from ALS. ALS, the most common motor neuron disease, affects both the upper neurons and lower motor neurons located in the spinal cord.

PLS is characterized by weakness of voluntary muscles. Typically, the disease is first noticed as a weakening

Key Terms

Gait Manner in which a person walks.

Motor neuron disease A neuromuscular disease, usually progressive, that causes degeneration of motor neuron cells and loss or diminishment of voluntary muscle control.

of the legs, hands, or tongue. Other symptoms include difficulty in maintaining balance and clumsiness, sudden muscle spasms, foot dragging, and difficulty in speaking. The neuron death does not affect regions of the brain that control intellect and behavior.

The muscle weakness becomes progressively worse. For some people, this process can stretch over decades. For others, the progression is much faster. While PLS is related to Lou Gehrig's disease, in PLS there is no degeneration of the spinal motor neurons or the wasting away of muscle mass than occurs in ALS.

Diagnosis

Diagnosis is based on the observance of the muscle weakness and the progressive worsening of the weakness. The diagnosis can be delayed because the disease is mistaken for ALS.

Treatment team

Treatment of PLS involves the family physician, a **neurologist**, and others such as physical therapists. The prolonged nature of the disease means that the energy and commitment of the patient and treatment team must be maintained for a long periods of time, usually decades.

Treatment

The treatment aims to reduce the discomfort and inconvenience of the disease. There is currently no cure for PLS. Medications such as baclofen, **diazepam**, and **gabapentin** have shown effectiveness in reducing muscle spasms in many patients with PLS.

Recovery and rehabilitation

As primary lateral sclerosis is a slowly progressive disorder, emphasis is placed upon maintaining maximum function rather than recovery. Physical therapists can assist with stretching and strengthening exercises to help maintain range of motion and decrease muscle **fatigue** and spasms. Physical therapists are often involved in assessing gait (manner of walking) and balance, and help select the proper type and size of cane or other device to assist with mobility.

Clinical trials

As of April 2004, one clinical trial was recruiting patients in North America. People between the ages of 40 and 75 were sought in the trial, which seeks to relate measurements of voluntary muscle activity to brain activity. The intention is to better understand the areas of the brain that are involved with PLS. Updated information on the trial can be found at the National Institutes for Health website on **clinical trials** at <www.clinicaltrials.gov>. Aside from the clinical trial, research studies are being funded that seek to develop techniques to diagnose, treat, prevent, and hopefully someday to cure motor neuron diseases.

Prognosis

Because PLS can be a slowly progressing disease, the outlook for a normal life span is good. While life can be greatly changed, a person is still usually able to walk, albeit with the assistance of a cane or other device.

Resources

BOOKS

Parker J. N., and P. M. Parker. *The Official Parent's Sourcebook on Primary Lateral Sclerosis: A Revised and Updated Directory for the Internet Age.* San Diego, Icon Health Publications, 2002.

OTHER

"NINDS Primary Lateral Sclerosis Information Page." *National Institute of Neurological Disorders and Stroke.* <http://www.ninds.nih.gov/health_and_medical/disorders/primary_lateral_sclerosis.htm> (April 12, 2004).

ORGANIZATIONS

National Institute for Neurological Diseases and Stroke (NINDS). 6001 Executive Boulevard, Bethesda, MD 20892. (301) 496-5751 or (800) 352-9424. <http://www.ninds.nih.gov>.

ALS Association (ALSA). 27001 Agoura Road, Suite 150, Calabasas Hills, CA 91301-5104. (818) 880-9007 or (800) 782-4747; Fax: (818) 880-9006. info@alsa-national.org. <http://www.alsa.org>.

Primary Lateral Sclerosis Newsletter. 101 Pinta Court, Los Gatos, CA 95032. (408) 356-8227. 73112.611@compuserve.com.

Brian Douglas Hoyle, PhD

Primidone

Definition

Primidone belongs to the class of medications known as **anticonvulsants**. It is indicated for the control of **seizures** in the treatment of **epilepsy** and other seizure disorders. Primidome may be prescribed alone or as part of a combination of medications for preventing seizures.

Key Terms

Barbiturate A class of drugs including phenobarbital that have sedative properties and depress respiratory rate, blood pressure, and nervous system activity.

Epilepsy A disorder associated with disturbed electrical discharges in the central nervous system that cause seizures.

Seizure A convulsion, or uncontrolled discharge of nerve cells that may spread to other cells throughout the brain.

Purpose

Primidone is thought to decrease abnormal activity within the brain that may trigger seizures. While primidone controls some types of seizures associated with epilepsy (grand mal, psychomotor, and focal seizures) there is no known cure for the disorder. Additionally, primidone has shown promise in alleviating some forms of essential **tremors**, but is not approved in the United States for this use.

Description

In the United States, primidone is also sold under the names Myidone and Mysoline. Although the precise mechanism by which primidone exerts its therapeutic effects is unknown, it is thought to help slow and control nerve impulses in the brain. The active metabolites of primidone are **phenobarbital** and phenylmethylmalonamide (PEMA), both barbiturate-type compounds with anticonvulsant and sedative properties. Primidone is supplied in chewable tablets (in Canada), tablets to be swallowed whole, and in suspension (syrup) forms for oral administration.

Recommended dosage

Primidone is available in 50 milligram (mg) and 250 mg tablets, and is prescribed by physicians in varying dosages. The usual initial dose for adults, teenagers, and children over eight years of age is 100 mg or 125 mg per day. Dosages are gradually increased until arriving at the lowest possible dosage that results in control of seizures. Children under eight years of age typically take an initial daily dose of 50 mg. The maximum daily dose for anyone taking primidone usually is not greater than 2000 mg.

The prescribing physician will schedule a patient's daily dosages, gradually increasing them over the course of several weeks. Primidone may not exert its full therapeutic effect during the initial dose-increasing period.

Primidone should be taken at approximately the same time every night. If a daily dose is missed, it should be taken as soon as possible. However, if it is almost time for the next dose, the missed dose should be skipped. Double doses of primidone should not be taken.

A patient should consult their physician before they stop taking primidone. Suddenly discontinuing this medicine may cause seizures to return or occur more frequently. When ending treatment including primidone, physicians typically direct patients to taper their daily dosages gradually.

Precautions

A physician should be consulted before taking primidone with non-prescription medications. Patients should avoid alcohol and CNS depressants (medicines that can make one drowsy or less alert, such as antihistimines, sleep medications, and some **pain** medications) while taking primidone because it can exacerbate their side effects. Primidone may not be suitable for persons with a history of porphyria, asthma or other chronic lung diseases, liver disease, kidney disease, mental illness, high blood presure, angina (chest pain), irregular heartbeats, or other heart problems. Patients should notify their physician if they consume a large amount of alcohol, have a history of drug use, are pregnant, or plan to become pregnant.

Anticonvulsant medications, namely phentoyn and phenobarbital, have been shown to cause birth defects. Physicians usually advise women of childbearing age to use effective birth control while taking this medication. Patients who become pregnant while taking primidone should contact their physician immediately.

Side effects

Patients and their physicians should weigh the risks and benefits of primidone before beginning treatment. Most patients tolerate primidone well, but may experience a variety of mild side effects. If any symptoms persist or become too uncomfortable, consult the prescribing physician. The following common side effects usually do not require medical attention and may lessen after taking primidone for several weeks:

- dizziness, unsteadiness, or clumsiness
- nausea or vomiting
- decreased sexual desire or ability
- loss of appetite
- mood or mental changes
- tremors

Other, less common side effects of primidone may be serious. Contact a physician immediately if any of the following symptoms occur:

- rash or bluish patches on the skin

- unusual excitement or restlessness (especially in children, seniors, or patients taking high dosages)
- double vision
- uncontrolled back-and-forth or rolling eye movements
- speech or language problems
- chest pain
- irregular heartbeat
- faintness or loss of consciousness
- persistent, severe headaches
- persistent fever or pain.

Interactions

Primidone may have negative interactions with adrenocorticoids (cortisone-like medications), antibiotics, antidepressants, anticoagulants, antihistimines, asthma medications, barbituates, and monoamine oxidase inhibitors (MAOIs). Primidone should be used in conjunction with other seizure prevention medications, especially valproic acid, only if advised and closely monitored by a physician. Primidone may decrease the effectiveness of oral contraceptives (birth control pills) that contain estrogen.

Resources

BOOKS

Devinsky, Orrin. *Epilepsy: Patient and Family Guide,* 2nd. ed. Philadelphia: F. A. Davis Co., 2001.

Weaver, Donald F. *Epilepsy and Seizures: Everything You Need to Know.* Toronto: Firefly Books, 2001.

OTHER

"Primidone (systemic)." *Thompson Micromedex.* <http://health.yahoo.com/health/drug/202479/> (April 4, 2004).

"Primidone (systemic)." *Medline Plus.* National Library of Medicine. <http://www.nlm.nih.gov/medlineplus/druginfo/uspdi/202479.html> (April 4, 2004).

ORGANIZATIONS

American Epilepsy Society. 342 North Main Street, West Hartford, CT 06117-2507. <http://www.aesnet.org>.

Epilepsy Foundation, 4351 Garden City Drive, Landover, MD 20785-7223. (800) 332-1000. <http://www.epilepsyfoundation.org>.

Adrienne Wilmoth Lerner

▌Prion diseases

Definition

Prion diseases are also called transmissible spongiform encephalopathies (TSEs) because of the sponge-like holes they leave in infected brains. The infectious agents in prion diseases are prions, or proteinaceous infectious particles, that can reproduce themselves. Prions have the ability to transform normal, benign protein molecules into infectious, deadly ones by altering their structure. These deadly proteins initiate a sequence of events in which many benign proteins are transformed into new deadly ones upon contact. Prions are distinct from all other infectious materials in that they do not contain any genetic material. There are multiple prion diseases, including bovine spongiform **encephalopathy** (BSE), or "mad cow disease." Some prion diseases are hereditary, and involve a mutation in the gene that encodes for the prion protein. Prion diseases are transmissible within a species and between compatible species.

Description

Research on prion diseases was founded by Dr. Stanley Prusiner, a **neurologist** at the University of California San Francisco. He spent two decades working on the revolutionary topic of self-reproducing prions. At the time, many other scientists regarded their existence as a preposterous idea. Despite being shunned by the scientific community, Dr. Prusiner was able to prove that prions were truly infectious proteins that could cause brain disease in people and animals. The Nobel Prize for Medicine or Physiology was awarded to Dr. Prusiner in 1997 for discovering this new type of disease-causing agents that contain no DNA.

Prion diseases are transmissible between hosts of a single species and different, compatible species. The term "spongiform" in TSE comes from the spongy appearance of the damaged brain tissue. Some examples of infectious prion diseases include scrapie in sheep and goats, **kuru** in cannibalistic humans of Papua New Guinea, and BSE, or mad cow disease, which is transmitted to humans through infected beef products. Prion diseases can also be transmitted through injections of infected material from a compatible organism. Because of the ability of prions to cross many species barriers, all organisms that carry prion diseases are potential vectors for human infection.

Prion diseases can also be hereditary, as seen in some cases of **Creutzfeldt-Jakob disease** (CJD), fatal familial insomnia (FFI), and **Gerstmann-Straussler-Scheinker disease** (GSS). Hereditary prion diseases occur when the PRNP gene that encodes for the normal human PrP^C protein, found on the surface of neurons, is mutated so that the prion PrP^{Sc} protein (Sc for scrapie) is formed. The PrP^{Sc} protein has a different conformational structure than the normal protein and is the infectious agent. PrP^{Sc} proteins can convert similar PrP^C proteins upon contact into more infectious agents, thereby reproducing themselves. Prion diseases are inherited when at least one copy of the mutated PRNP gene is present. Nervous tissue from patients with hereditary prion diseases is also infectious.

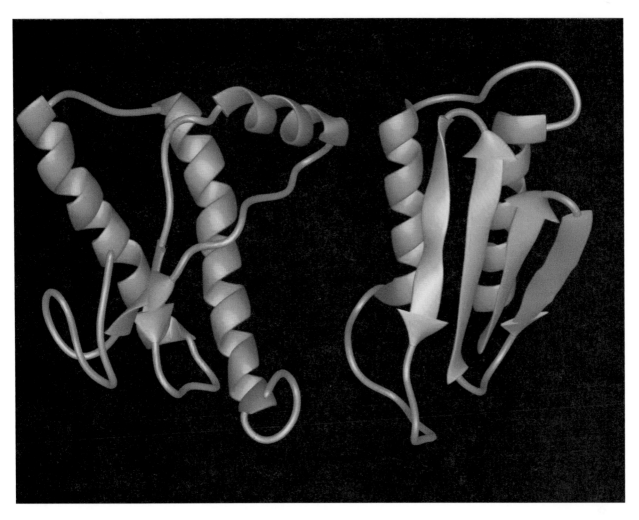

A computer-generated illustration showing, on the left, a human prion protein in its normal shape at the molecular level, and, on the right, a disease-causing, abnormally shaped prion protein. The blue arrow indicates beta strands, the green spiral shapes are alpha helices, and the yellow strands depict the chain connecting the regions. *(AP/Wide World. Reproduced by permission.)*

A third category of prion disease is sporadic. CJD and FFI sometimes occur in people with no known history of the disease in their family and with no known exposure to infectious materials. The cause of disease in these cases is unknown. Patients with sporadic prion diseases may have a susceptibility polymorphism in their PRNP gene, and may have spontaneous mutations forming prion proteins.

Demographics

Sporadic CJD, with no recognizable pattern of transmission, has an incidence of about one case per million people per year worldwide, making up 85% of total CJD cases, and 80% of all prion disease cases. In the United States, there are approximately 200 sporadic CJD cases per year. Approximately 15% of CJD cases are inherited and associated with a different prion type than that of sporadic CJD. Inherited CJD may show up in geographic clusters. A 60- to 100-fold increase in CJD is seen in Libya- or Slovakia-born Israelis due to a PRNP gene mutation rather than transmission or environmental factors. Other communities genetically at increased risk are found in some areas of Chile. CJD cases caused by accidental transmission routes such as surgical instruments and transplants are extremely rare and make up less than 1% of total cases. In the United States, the CJD cases are almost always in patients older than 30 years of age. In the United States, patients under 30 dying of CJD are less than one case per 100 million people per year, whereas in the United Kingdom, patients dying of a variant CJD (vCJD) in this age group make up over 50% of the CJD cases.

GSS is rarer than CJD, striking one person in every 10 million people. These figures are likely to be underestimated since prion diseases may be misdiagnosed as other neurological disorders. Kuru occurs in approximately 1%

of the indigenous New Guinea population it is associated with. Kuru is found mostly in children older than five years and adult females under 40 years of age.

BSE has been transmitted to humans primarily in the United Kingdom, causing vCJD. An epidemic of mad cow disease began in the United Kingdom in 1985 when cattle feed was contaminated with brain tissue from scrapie-infected sheep. More than 170,000 cattle were infected before the disease was brought under control. Cattle feed containing sheep matter was banned in 1988. In 1989, slaughter techniques that allow nervous tissue to be included in beef intended for human consumption were banned. The mad cow disease epidemic of the United Kingdom reached its peak in 1992, but then declined quickly. More than one million cattle may have been infected with BSE in the United Kingdom. However, as of December 2003, only 143 cases of vCJD have been reported in the United Kingdom, out of 153 cases worldwide. The percentage of BSE cases in cattle reported outside of the United Kingdom is steadily increasing as surveillance increases and disease rates rise. The BSE epidemic in the United Kingdom may have peaked, and may now be in decline. How much of the population has vCJD in the incubation phase is yet to be determined.

To prevent the spread of BSE to the United States, severe restrictions were placed on the importation of ruminants and ruminant products from Europe. In 1997, the U.S. Department of Agriculture (USDA) also implemented a ban on the use of ruminant tissue in ruminant feed. In 2002, the CDC reported a case of vCJD in the United States in a 22-year-old patient who was born and grew up in the United Kingdom. Mad cow disease made its first appearance in cattle of the United States in December 2003, when the USDA announced a possible diagnosis in a cow from Washington State. This diagnosis was confirmed within the month at a laboratory in the United Kingdom. The cow was believed to be imported from Canada in the year 2001 and had been slaughtered for human consumption. The USDA recalled all beef slaughtered at the same slaughter plant on the same date as the infected cow.

Causes and symptoms

Ingested prions are absorbed through Peyer's patches of the small intestine, lumps of lymphoid tissue that readily allow the passage of gut antigens straight through them. Peyer's patches are a part of the mucosal-associated lymphoid tissue that presents microorganisms to the immune system and would normally facilitate a protective immune response. Prions do not activate any immune response. Prions passed through Peyer's patches travel to various sites in the lymph system, such as nodes and the spleen. Because many lymph sites are innervated, prions gain access to the nervous system, make their way to the spinal cord, and eventually the brain.

Prions are not killed by high doses of ultraviolet **radiation** as are bacteria and viruses. Prions are also resistant to high temperatures, strong degradative enzymes, and chemicals. Because of these properties, prions are resistant to many methods of sterilization and to protective, degradative enzymes in the human brain. The plaques formed in the brain by prion proteins are amyloid deposits similar to those seen in **Alzheimer's disease**. Most brain cells contain enzymes that degrade these aggregations. Prions are resistant to these enzymes. The plaques continue to grow and cause damage to the brain, usually along with the formation of large vacuoles that give the brain a spongiform appearance. Brain damage manifests itself in a loss of coordination, paralysis, **dementia**, and wasting, followed by death. Pneumonia also frequently occurs in patients with prion diseases. All prion diseases are inevitably fatal; there are no known cures.

Prion diseases can be inherited in an autosomal dominant matter. This means if one parent carries the mutation on their PRNP gene, each offspring has a 50% chance of inheriting the mutation. In this manner, patients with a prion disease have inherited at least one copy of a mutated PRNP gene on human chromosome 20. There are a variety of mutations in the gene that cause resultant mutated proteins to be expressed, with each type of mutation resulting in a different prion strain, and a different inherited prion disease. Strains show very different and reproducible patterns of brain degeneration. Extracts of autopsied brain tissue from infected patients have been used for research on prion diseases. It has been demonstrated that only animals whose PRNP gene is similar enough to humans can be infected with human prions. Similarly humans can only be infected by prions from animals whose PRNP gene ultimately encodes for a prion protein that is similar to humans. Prions transform their normal cellular counterparts into other prions only between prion-compatible species. Infectious prion diseases are transmitted through consumption of infected materials or through injection of ground-up infected tissues. Prion diseases are not contagious in the traditional sense. Individuals who live with patients with prion diseases are at no increased risk. While casual contact does not transmit the disease, brain tissue and cerebrospinal fluid from patients with prion diseases should be avoided.

Inherited prion diseases

GERSTMANN-STRAUSSLER-SCHEINKER DISEASE Caused by the GSS prion, this disease was first described in 1928. GSS is associated with variations in at least one PRNP gene sequence at positions 102 and 117. It is also highly associated with a polymorphism on both gene copies at position 129 on the human PRNP gene. GSS typically occurs between the ages of 35 and 55. It is characterized by progressive cerebellar **ataxia** and associated motor complications, following a time course of 2–10 years before death. Dementia with GSS is less common than with CJD, except in very late stages of disease following a long time course. GSS is almost always inherited, but has been known to occur sporadically as well.

CREUTZFELDT-JAKOB DISEASE Caused by the CJD prion, this disease is associated with variations in the PRNP gene at positions 178 and 200, along with an insertion of extra DNA in the familial form. CJD was first described in the 1920s as a progressive dementia, following a course of one year, ending in death. CJD presents with a variety of motor disturbances, including twitching. CJD typically occurs between the ages of 50 and 75. While CJD is an inherited disease, the majority of CJD occurs sporadically. Other CJD cases are due to accidental exposure to infected material.

FATAL FAMILIAL INSOMNIA Caused by the FFI prion, FFI is a rare disorder first described in 1986. It is caused by inherited mutations in the PRNP gene at position 178 and a polymorphism at position 129. FFI typically occurs between the ages of 40 and 60, and is characterized by progressive sleep disturbance classified as untreatable insomnia, ataxia (motor dysfunction), and dysautonomia (sensory dysfunction). The disease course is 7–18 months, followed by death. Postmortem studies associate this prion disease with severe selective atrophy of the thalamus, a brain region controlling sleep and wakefulness. Sporadic FFI has been reported without the characteristic gene mutation.

ALPERS SYNDROME Alpers syndrome is the term used to describe prion diseases in infants.

Infectious prion diseases

SCRAPIE Caused by the scrapie prion, scrapie is the first prion disease ever studied. Scrapie was first described in sheep and goats more than 200 years ago. It is transmitted through feed contaminated with nervous tissue. It can also be transmitted through pasture infected with placental tissue from infected sheep. The term "scrapie" comes from the behavior of infected sheep that rub up against the fences of their pens to remain upright despite severe ataxia, a loss of muscular coordination due to brain damage. Autopsies of infected animals reveal spongiform encephalopathy. In 1943, scrapie was demonstrated as transmissible when a contaminated vaccine infected healthy sheep.

KURU Decades after scrapie was first discovered, a similar disorder was described in humans called kuru.

Kuru was characterized in 1950 as a progressive cerebellar ataxia associated with a shivering tremor, with a disease course of three to nine months, followed by death. The word *kuru* comes from the Fore language and means 'tremor.' Caused by the kuru prion, kuru primarily occurred in the Fore highland people of southern New Guinea, whose cultural practice used to involve ritualistic ingestion of the brain tissue of recently deceased family members. The brain tissue was ground into a pale gray soup, heated, and consumed. Statistically, women of the Fore tribe were more likely than men to develop kuru, due to their greater involvement in the preparation of the brain tissue. Infection in the female population was probably via both ingestion and through minor skin abrasions. Clinically, kuru resembles CJD. Since this practice has stopped, the disease has ceased to occur.

BOVINE SPONGIFORM ENCEPHALOPATHY Humans consuming infected beef are susceptible to the BSE prion strain. Strain typing shows one major strain. BSE is especially insidious in that it is compatible with and transmissible to a wide variety of species. While food items containing blood or nervous tissue are potential vectors for human infection, milk and milk products from cows are not believed to pose any risk for transmitting the BSE prion to humans (see also vCJD).

ACQUIRED CREUTZFELDT-JAKOB DISEASE While CJD is an inherited disease it can also be acquired through iatrogenic transmission, which is accidental exposure to CJD prion-contaminated material through a medical procedure using tainted human matter or surgical instruments. Recipients of corneal transplants and of grafts of dura mater (brain-associated connective tissue) have been infected with CJD. Because prions are resistant to many sterilization procedures and to degradation, surgical instruments used in brain surgery have infected new patients two years after being sterilized. More than 100 people have been infected with CJD through injections of human growth hormones prepared from pools of pituitary glands that included materials from humans with CJD. At present, growth hormones are prepared through recombinant DNA technology and surgical instruments used on potentially infected patients have new sterilization guidelines, so the transmission of CJD via these routes has ceased to occur. The National Center for Infectious Diseases has not found any iatrogenic CJD cases linked to contact with pathogens from surfaces like floors or countertops.

VARIANT CREUTZFELDT-JAKOB DISEASE (VCJD) Variant CJD appeared in 1996 during the mad cow disease epidemic in the United Kingdom. The specific strain found in these patients indicates that they have been infected with prions from contaminated beef, the BSE prion. However, victims of vCJD are homozygous for a polymorphism on the PRNP gene at position 129. Patients with

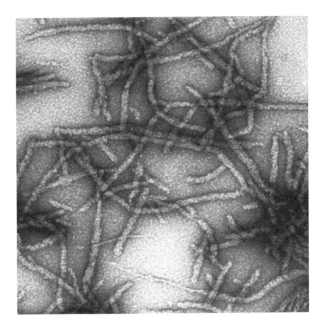

Close-up of prion structure. Amyloid fibrils form when the protein alters. *(© CNRS/Corbis Sygma. Reproduced by permission.)*

vCJD may develop the disease at an unusually early age with the current median age of 29 years at death. However, the incubation time period before the onset of symptoms may be as long as 40 years. The vCJD affects people between 15 and 60 years of age. The clinical symptoms associated with vCJD differ from those seen with CJD, including psychiatric or sensory symptoms early in the course of the disease, delayed onset of neurological abnormalities that follow a pattern identifiable as but different from CJD, and a duration of illness of at least six months, followed by death. As of January 2004, evidence indicates there has never been a case of vCJD transmitted through direct contact of one person to another.

MISCELLANEOUS INFECTIOUS PRION DISEASES Cats and mink are susceptible to species-specific forms of TSE. In many mid-western states of the United States, some elk and mule deer carry a form of TSE called chronic wasting disease (CWD). CWD prions may possibly be transmissible to humans consuming venison the same way as mad cow disease can be transmitted through contaminated beef.

Diagnosis

There is currently no single diagnostic test for any prion disease. Physicians initially rule out other treatable forms of dementia such as classical encephalitis. Standard diagnostic tests include a spinal tap to exclude other diseases and an electroencephalogram (EEG) to record the patient's brain wave pattern. **CT scans** and **magnetic resonance imaging (MRI)** scans can rule out the possibility of **stroke** and reveal characteristic patterns of brain degeneration associated with various types of prion diseases.

Diagnosis classically relied on clinical symptoms, transmissibility, and postmortem neuropathology. With these diagnosis criteria, many cases of prion diseases may have been misdiagnosed as other neurodegenerative disorders. However, modern diagnosis is also dependent on detection of prion proteins, and identification of mutations in the PRNP gene. A genetic sequence analysis can be performed for a number of different mutations associated with familial CJD. The types of mutations present determine which symptoms will be most prominent. However, the presence of these mutations on the PRNP gene does not necessarily result in CJD. Most CJD patients contain a specific protein in their cerebrospinal fluid and an abnormal EEG brain wave pattern, diagnostic for CJD. However, confirmation requires neuropathological testing of brain tissue obtained through brain **biopsy** or autopsy. Brain biopsies are usually performed only when required to exclude another, treatable condition.

A diagnosis of prion disease is confirmed through examination of the brain tissue. Visible postmortem characteristics of the brain include noninflammatory lesions, vacuoles, amyloid protein deposits forming plaques that follow prion type-specific patterns, and measurable biochemical changes. While dramatic alterations in the brain's appearance are primarily the case, more subtle and noncharacteristic changes have also been reported. Some forms of prion disease with shorter durations only create plaques in a small percentage of patients.

Clinical signs of prion disease in sheep and cattle include cerebellar ataxia (loss of muscle coordination), polydipsia (excessive drinking), and an itching syndrome that, along with the lack of coordination, causes the animals to rub up against fences. However, animals are not diagnosed with prion disease until brain autopsy reveals neuropathology similar to that seen in humans.

Treatment team

Primary-care physicians may notice symptoms of a neurological disorder in a patient and refer them to a neurologist, specialists in brain disorders. They would act as the treatment team for patients with prion diseases.

Oversight of the BSE Action Plan in the United States is done by the Department of Health and Human Services (DHHS). Under this plan, surveillance for human disease is the responsibility of the Centers for Disease Control and Prevention (CDC). Protection against this disease is the responsibility of the Food and Drug Administration (FDA). Research is primarily the responsibility of the National Institutes of Health (NIH).

Treatment

There is no known effective treatment to arrest or cure prion diseases. Treatment focuses on alleviating the patient's symptoms, increasing their comfort, and palliative care. Treatment may include medications to control **pain** and motor disorders, catheters to collect urine, intravenous fluids to maintain hydration, and frequently repositioning the patient to avoid bedsores.

Possible future treatments developed may include chemicals that bind to and stabilize PrP^C, agents destabilizing the PrP^{SC} protein, or agents that interfere with the intereaction between PrP^C and PrP^{SC}.

Recovery and rehabilitation

There is no recovery or rehabilitation for prion diseases.

Clinical trials

As of January 2004, no **clinical trials** on prion diseases have taken place. In September 2001, the government announced an agenda of the design and implementation of clinical trials on CJD. The trials were originally planned after a vCJD patient received an unproven treatment in California and seemed to be improving. The treatment was with the anti-malaria drug quinacrine, which blocks the formation of prion plaques in mouse cell culture but has undetermined effects in humans with prion diseases. Sadly, the patient died in December 2001. While planned clinical trials will focus on quinacrine, as of January 2004 they are still being designed. Other patients have taken this treatment outside of clinical trials and the results suggest possible limited benefit along with damaging side effects. Another unproven treatment is pentosan polysulphate, which also has dangerous side effects. The first patient to receive this treatment showed some improvement in the condition. As of October 2003, four other patients have been granted permission for its use.

Prognosis

Prions bring about slow degeneration of the **central nervous system**, inevitably leading to death. A very long time period passes between a patient's infection and the initial appearance of clinical symptoms, an incubation process that may take up to 40 years in humans. However, once the symptoms appear, the patient generally dies within a few months with rapid, progressive symptoms. At this time, prion diseases are fatal diseases.

Special concerns

Highly effective public health control procedures have been implemented in Europe to prevent potential BSE-infected tissue from entering the human food chain.

Key Terms

Electroencephalogram   A recording of the electrical signals produced by the brain.

Polymorphism   A difference in DNA sequence among individuals; genetic variation.

The current risk of becoming infected with vCJD from eating beef and beef products in the United Kingdom is very small, at a rate of one case per 10 billion servings. Other countries have equal or lesser rates of risk. To reduce the risk of being infected with vCJD from food while traveling to geographical areas associated with risk, travelers who do not wish to avoid eating beef entirely may reduce their risk by selecting beef products in solid pieces, as opposed to ground beef tissue.

As of January 2004, there is no evidence that blood or blood products have transmitted TSEs to humans. However, to reduce the theoretical risk of transmission from blood products to humans, those individuals who have lived cumulatively for five or more years in Europe since the year 1980 to the present have been deferred by the FDA from donating blood or blood products. Individuals living specifically in the United Kingdom for three months or more from 1980 to 1996 are also deferred. Variant CJD (vCJD) is more likely to be transmitted through blood than classical CJD.

The CDC has established a National Prion Disease Pathology Surveillance Center (NPDPSC) that provides free, high-tech diagnostic services to physicians in the United States. Relatives of CJD patients who wish to assist research have their physician send brain tissue, blood, cerebrospinal fluid, and urine samples to the center.

Prion research has been done in yeast, a convenient organism easily used in scientific study. Yeast can be infected with prions, begin forming their own prion proteins, and pass the infection on to further generations of yeast. It has been noted that yeast can be "cured" of their prion disease by increasing the activity of chaperone proteins, which help maintain the normal conformational structure of the PrP^C protein and keep it from being converted to prion conformation.

Resources

BOOKS

Cann, Alan J. *Principles of Molecular Virology.* New York: Academic Press, 2001.

Rhodes, Richard. *Deadly Feasts: The Prion Controversy and the Public's Health.* New York: Touchstone, 1998.

PERIODICALS

Horwich, A. L., and J. S. Weissmann. "Deadly Conformations—Protein Misfolding in Prion Disease." *Cell* 89 (1997): 499–510.

Mastrianni, J. A., M. T. Curtis, et al. "Prion Disease (PrP-A117V) Presenting with Ataxia Instead of Dementia." *Neurology* 45, no. 11 (1995): 2042–2050.

OTHER

Biosafety in Biomedical and Microbiological Laboratories. *The Prion Diseases.* BMBL Section VII-D Table 1, National Institutes of Health.

Centers for Disease Control and Prevention. *Bovine Spongiform Encephalopathy Detected in Canada.* Articles (2003).

Centers for Disease Control and Prevention. *BSE and CJD Information and Resources.* Bovine Spongiform Encephalopathy Main Index (2003).

Centers for Disease Control and Prevention. "Creutzfeldt-Jakob Disease Associated with Cadaveric Dura Mater Grafts." *Morbidity and Mortality Weekly Report* (1997) 46(45): 1066–9.

Centers for Disease Control and Prevention. *Fact Sheet: New Variant Creutzfeldt-Jakob Disease.* Articles (2003).

Centers for Disease Control and Prevention. *Preliminary Investigation Suggests BSE-Infected Cow in Washington State Was Likely Imported from Canada.* Articles (2003).

Centers for Disease Control and Prevention. *Questions and Answers Regarding Bovine Spongiform Encephalopathy (BSE) and Creutzfeldt-Jakob Disease (CJD).* Articles (2003).

Centers for Disease Control and Prevention. *Questions and Answers Regarding Bovine Spongiform Encephalopathy in Canada.* Articles (2003).

Centers for Disease Control and Prevention. *Questions and Answers Regarding Creutzfeldt-Jakob Disease Infection-Control Practices.* Articles (2003).

Centers for Disease Control and Prevention. *Update 2002: Bovine Spongiform Encephalopathy and Variant Creutzfeldt-Jakob Disease.* Articles (2002).

Creutzfeldt-Jakob Disease Foundation Inc. *Creutzfeldt-Jakob Disease.* CJD Info.

Creutzfeldt-Jakob Disease Voice. *Creutzfeldt-Jakob Disease Fact Sheet.* CJD Info.

FDA Press Office. *FDA Prohibits Mammalian Protein in Sheep and Cattle Feed.* FDA Talk Paper (1997).

Heaphy, S. *Prions and BSE.* University of Leicester, UK: BSE Risk Assessment (2004).

Kimball, John W., PhD. *Kimball's Biology.* 2003 (March 23, 2004). Online textbook <http://biology-pages.info>.

Meikle, James. *Anger at Two-year Delay in CJD Drug Tests.* The Guardian UK (2003).

Sander, David M., PhD. *Prion Diseases.* Virology Course 335 (1999), Tulane University.

Schonberger, Lawrence, and Ermias Belay. *Bovine Spongiform Encephalopathy and Variant Creutzfeldt-Jakob Disease.* Centers for Disease Control and Prevention Travelers' Health Information (2003-2004).

UCSF Today *Two Old Drugs May Help Fight Prion Disease.* University of California San Francisco.

Veneman, Ann M. *Statement Regarding Canada's Announcement of BSE Investigation.* USDA Statement No. 0166.03 (2003).

ORGANIZATIONS

Centers for Disease Control and Prevention. 1600 Clifton Road, Atlanta, GA 30333. (404) 639-3534 or (800) 311-3435. <http://www.cdc.gov>.

CJD Foundation, Inc. P.O. Box 5313, Akron, OH 44334, (330) 665-5590 or (800) 659-1991; Fax: (330) 668-2474. crjakob@aol.com. <http://www.cjdfoundation.org>.

National Organization for Rare Disorders. 55 Kenosia Avenue, P.O. Box 1968, Danbury, CT 06813. (203) 744-0100 or (800) 999-6673; Fax: (203) 798-2211. orphan@rarediseases.org. <http://www.rarediseases.org>.

National Prion Disease Pathology Surveillance Center. Case Western Reserve University 2085 Adelbert Road, Room 418, Cleveland, OH 44106. (216) 368-0587; Fax: (216) 368-4090. cjdsurv@cwru.edu. <http://www.cjdsurv.com>.

National Institutes of Health. 9000 Rockville Pike, Bethesda, MD 20892. (301) 496-4000. nihinfo@od.nih.gov. <http://www.nih.gov>.

Office International des Epizooties. 12, rue de Prony, Paris, France 75017. 33-(0)1 44 15 18 88; Fax: 33-(0)1 42 67 09 87. oie@oie.int. <http://www.oie.int>.

Patient Advocate Foundation. 700 Thimble Shoals Blvd, Suite 200, Newport News, VA 23606. (757) 873-8999 or (800) 532-5274. help@patientadvocate.org. <http://www.patientadvocate.org>.

United States Food and Drug Administration. 5600 Fishers Lane, Rockville, MD 20857. (888) 463-6332. <http://www.fda.org>.

Maria Basile, PhD

Progressive locomotor ataxia *see* **Tabes dorsalis**

Progressive sclerosing poliodystrophy *see* **Alpers' disease**

Progressive multifocal leukoencephalopathy

Definition

Progressive multifocal leukoencephalopathy is a rare, fatal disease of the white matter of the brain that almost solely strikes individuals who already have weakened immune systems.

Description

In progressive multifocal leukoencephalopathy, myelin (the substance that wraps around nerve fibers, providing insulation and speeding nerve transmission) is progressively destroyed. Although the disease is caused by a very prevalent virus (called JC virus), it only develops in individuals who are immunocompromised (have weakened immune systems).

Multiple areas of the brain are affected by the demyelination associated with progressive multifocal leukoencephalopathy. Additionally, other abnormalities and bizarre cells take up residence within the brain, causing destruction of normal brain tissue and impairing normal function.

Demographics

The causative virus in progressive multifocal leukoencephalopathy, JC virus, is extremely common. It is thought to be present in upwards of 85% of all children before the age of nine, and probably is present in an even greater percentage of adults. However, the JC virus does not actually cause any symptoms or disease, except in individuals who have severely compromised immune systems. About 62.2% of all progressive multifocal leukoencephalopathy cases occur in individuals with lymphatic cancers (lymphoproliferative disease, such as Hodgkin's disease and other lymphomas); 6.5% occur in individuals with cancer of bone marrow cells (myeloproliferative disease or leukemias); 2.2% occur in individuals with carcinomatous disease (cancers that affect the lining of tissues or organs of the body); and 10% occur in individuals with any of a number of acquired immunodeficiency states (such as systemic lupus erthematosus, sarcoidosis, and organ transplant survivors). Among patients with Acquired Immunodeficiency Syndrome (AIDS), about 10% of patients develop progressive multifocal leukoencephalopathy. Only 5.6% of all cases of progressive multifocal leukoencephalopathy occur in individuals with no other underlying source of immunocompromise.

Causes and symptoms

Although much is left to be defined about the mechanism whereby progressive multifocal leukoencephalopathy affects an individual, researchers believe that the JC virus resides in the kidneys of most individuals. In normal, nonimmunocompromised individuals, the virus stays within the kidneys, doing no harm. In immunocompromised individuals, the virus is reactivated, travels through the circulatory system to the brain, and selectively destroys myelinated nerve cells.

Patients with progressive multifocal leukoencephalopathy experience a range of symptoms that grow

Progressive multifocal leukoencephalopathy

Key Terms

Immunocompromise A condition in which the immune system is weak and ineffective.

Myelin An insulating layer of fats around nerve fibers that allows nerve impulses to travel more quickly.

gradually worse over time, including **headache** and difficulties with speech, thinking, walking, weakness, vision problems (even blindness), memory problems, confusion, slowness of movement, paralysis of half of the body, and **seizures**. Eventually, patients lapse into a coma and die, usually within just months of the onset of their initial symptoms.

Diagnosis

Diagnosis is usually suggested by a patient's characteristic symptoms of progressive multifocal leukoencephalopathy, in combination with evidence of white matter destruction visualized on **CT** or **MRI** scanning of the brain. Specialized tests on cerebrospinal fluid (called polymerase chain reactions) may demonstrate the presence of JC virus DNA. However, only brain **biopsy** can result in an absolutely definitive diagnosis.

Treatment team

Patients with progressive multifocal leukoencephalopathy are usually seen by neurologists, as well as by hematologist/oncologists for patients with lymphoma or leukemia, infectious disease specialists for patients with AIDS, and a rheumatologist for individuals with specific autoimmune disease.

Treatment

There are no treatments available to cure progressive multifocal leukoencephalopathy. Some degree of slowing of the relentless progression of the disease has been noted in certain patients treated with the AIDS drug AZT.

Prognosis

Progressive multifocal leukoencephalopathy is uniformly fatal, usually within one to four months of the initial symptoms. A few patients have had brief remissions in the disease progression, and have lived for several years beyond diagnosis.

Resources

BOOKS

Berger, Joseph R., and Avindra Nath. "Progressive Multifocal Leukoencephalopathy." In *Cecil Textbook of Internal*

Medicine, edited by Lee Goldman, et al. Philadelphia: W. B. Saunders Company, 2000.

Roos, Karen L. "Viral Infections." In *Textbook of Clinical Neurology*, edited by Christopher G. Goetz. Philadelphia: W. B. Saunders Company, 2003.

Tyler, Kenneth L. "Viral Meningitis and Encephalitis." In *Harrison's Principles of Internal Medicine*, edited by Eugene Braunwald, et al. NY: McGraw-Hill Professional, 2001.

PERIODICALS

Pruitt, A. A. "Nervous System Infections in Patients with Cancer." *Neurol Clin* 21, no. 1 (February 1, 2003): 193–219

WEBSITES

National Institute of Neurological Disorders and Stroke (NINDS). *NINDS Progressive Multifocal Leukoencephalopathy Information Page.* May 29, 2002. (June 4, 2004). <http://www.ninds.nih.gov/health_and_medical/disorders/pml_doc.htm>.

Rosalyn Carson-DeWitt, MD

Progressive supranuclear palsy

Definition

Progressive supranuclear palsy (PSP) is a rare degenerative disorder that causes serious and permanent deficits in movement and cognitive function.

Description

Progressive supranuclear palsy is also known as Steele-Richardson-Olszewski syndrome, reflecting the names of persons who discovered the syndrome. PSP is a neurodegenerative disease (symptoms worsen with time) first described as a distinct disorder in 1964. Characteristics of PSP include slow movement and stiffness, which are also seen similarly in **Parkinson's Disease** (PD). Persons affected by PSP tend to have more postural imbalance with falls than patients with PD. Additionally tremor is usually absent in PSP patients, while those with PD have tremor. PSP is an uncommon disorder and initially it may be difficult to clinically distinguish between PSP and PD. PSP usually begins to produce symptoms in the sixth decade (50–59 years of age) of life and the disorder progressively worsens more quickly than PD. Patients with PSP typically become disabled within five to ten years after diagnosis (PD has a slower progression and typically persons can become disabled 20 years after onset). PSP is the most common Parkinson-like or Parkinson-plus disease.

Demographics

The estimated prevalence (number of existing cases) among persons older than 55 years is approximately seven per 100,000 persons. Studies indicate that there may be a slightly higher male prevalence (1.53), than female prevalence (1.23) per 100,000. In Perth, Australia, the incidence (number of new cases) is estimated at three to four per million cases. The incidence rate for ages 50-99 is 5.3 per 100,000. The peak incidence (the peak age range for new cases) is in the early sixties. PSP is not thought to be genetically transmitted in families, but there are some reported cases of inherited transmission. Survey research (using a questionnaire) in 1996 revealed that patients with PSP were less likely than controls to have completed 12 years of education, which suggests that education level is a marker for direct risk factors which can include chemical exposure or nutritional problems. In 1999 a high prevalence of PSP was found in Guadeloupe (French West Indies) which is related to ingestion of certain teas that are forms of custard apple (called "soursop" and "sweetsop").

Causes and symptoms

The cause of degeneration of nerve cells is unknown. Patients affected with PSP have a gradual and progressive damage to cells in the midbrain, which eventually leads to atrophy (shrinkage and loss of normal cell architecture). Patients have neuronal loss and neurofibrillary tangles in the **diencephalon**, brain stem and basal ganglia. Several theories have been proposed as potential causes. Initially, the main causes of PSP was thought to be due to a virus (possibly related to the influenza virus) or to a slow acting toxin (i.e. "MPTP", a drug of abuse contaminant, herbal Caribbean teas, Cycad nut poisoning in Guam).

However, recent genetic research as of 1999 suggests PSP may be a genetic disorder transmitted with autosomal recessive transmission. The gene implicated with the condition is called the tau gene. Analysis of the tau gene using molecular biology techniques indicate that the tau gene in PSP is different from genes observed in **Alzheimer disease** patients. Studies indicate that the tau gene in PSP is similar to the gene in another disease (Cortico basal degeneration). These genetic studies indicate that some nerve cells may be partially controlled by genetic susceptibility and also related to other environmental stressors/triggers such as viruses and/or toxins.

The symptoms of PSP are insidious and typically there is a prolonged phase of **headaches, dizziness, fatigue**, arthralgias and **depression**. The most common symptoms include postural instability and falls (seen in 63% of patients) and dyarthria (a symptom expressed in 35% of patients). Other important symptoms include bradykinesia and visual disturbance (diplopia, burning eyes, blurred vision and sensitivity to light) in 13% of affected PSP patients. The front neck muscles or back neck muscles may be affected. The rigidity of the spine is characterized by a stiff extended spine. PSP patients also exhibit eye movement paralysis. The eye lids may be held wide open with eye movement paralysis resulting in a facial expression that can be described as "staring," "astonished," or "puzzled."

Eye movement difficulties usually begin with difficulty looking up or down. There may be difficulty looking right or left. These eye abnormalities may cause difficulty during driving and reading. There is no treatment for eye movement abnormalities. Patients with PSP do not have eye muscle or eye nerve problems; the problem originates in the brain stem area.

Diagnosis

Lab tests and neuroimaging can be performed to eliminate other possible causes. One specific high resolution neuroimaging study called **PET** (**positron emission tomography**) scan can provide information about blood flow and oxygen supply to the brain. PET scan analysis has revealed a decrease in blood flow and oxygen metabolism in areas of the brain thought to degenerate in PSP patients (i.e. caudate, putamen and thalamus). Sleep patterns in PSP affected patients are often abnormal and demonstrated increased awakenings, diminished total sleep time, and progressive loss of REM sleep. Patients can also develop REM sleep behavior disorder consisting of abnormal motor activity with vivid dreams during REM sleep.

Autopsy results after examination of brain tissue reveals neuronal loss and neurofibrillary tangles and gliosis in the reticular formation and ocular (eye) motor nuclei, as well as neuronal pathology in the midbrain. **MRI** neuroimaging studies can detect abnormal patterns in affected areas within the brain.

Treatment team

As the disease progresses, specialists are required as part of the treatment team. Consultation with rehabilitation medicine specialist may help with walking stability and safety. A speech therapist may modify diet if swallowing is impaired. Consultation with an eye specialist (ophthalmologist) may be indicated for the treatment of eye problems.

Treatment

There is no effective therapy for PSP. Mediation generally has little or short term effects. Treatment is supportive (palliative) until the person dies. Supportive treatment can include speech therapy, walkers, antidepressants, artificial tears (to avoid drying of eyes from excess exposure) and caregiver support. Only few persons

---

Key Terms

Basl ganglia   Brain structure at the base of the cerebral hemispheres involved in controlling movement.

Bradykinesia   Extremely slow movement.

Brain stem   The stalk of the brain which connects the two cerebral hemispheres with the spinal cord. It is involved in controlling vital functions, movement, sensation, and nerves supplying the head and neck.

Diencephalon   A part of the brain that binds the mesencephalon to the cerebral hemispheres, it includes the thalmus and the hypothalmus.

Diplopia   A term used to describe double vision.

Dysarthria   Slurred speech.

Neurofibrillary tangles   Abnormal structures, composed of twisted masses of protein fibers within nerve cells, found in the brains of persons with Alzheimer's disease.

---

demonstrate benefit with medication that increases the **neurotransmitters** dopamine (dopaminergic) or acetylcholine (cholinergic drugs). A well balanced diet is recommended and gastrostomy (a surgical procedure to redirect bowels to pass through an opening in the stomach) is performed when feeding becomes problematic due to dysphagia (difficulty swallowing), or risk of bronchoaspiration (food lodging in the lungs due to abnormal swallowing) is possible.

Recovery and rehabilitation

PSP is a chronic and progressive disorder which means that symptoms worsen with the passing of time. Close follow-up care is advisable, and during visits it is necessary to provide family with direction and education. If the patient opts for experimental treatment protocols, it is mandatory to inform all concerned about potential side effects. Physical therapy involvement can help to maximize safety at home and provide instruction in the use of walking aids (i.e. wheelchair, walker).

Clinical trials

The National Institute of Neurological Disorders and Stroke (NINDS) are currently sponsoring research concerning diagnosis, treatment and causes of PSP. Additionally, studies concerning Parkinson's and Alzheimer's disease are being performed since a better understanding of related diseases may provide valuable information concerning PSP.

Prognosis

In most patients the disease is fatal within six to 10 years. Complications of PSP are related to abnormal balance, immobility (a late feature of PSP) and decreased cognition. Falls may cause patients to injure bones. Late onset immobility can cause infectious complications (pneumonia, urinary tract infection, or sepsis).

Special concerns

A well balanced diet is recommended and physical therapy may help with walking problems and falls which are the two major causes of disability. Educational concerns are important and should be directed to the patient, family members and caregivers. Education includes an understanding of the natural history of PSP and should include information concerning prognosis, complications, supportive therapy. Patients and families may benefit from PSP support group involvement.

Resources

BOOKS

Goetz, Christopher G., et al., eds. *Textbook of Clinical Neurology,* 1st ed. Philadelphia: W. B. Saunders Company, 1999.

Goldman, Lee, et al. *Cecil's Textbook of Medicine,* 21st ed. Philadelphia: W. B. Saunders Company, 2000.

PERIODICALS

Litvan, Irene. "Diagnosis and Mangement of Progressive Supranuclear Palsy." *Seminars in Neurology* 21 (2001).

WEBSITES

Hain, Timothy C. *Progressive Supranuclear Palsy.* <http://neuronwu.edu/meded/MOVEMENT/psp2.htm>.

Progrssive Supranuclear Palsy. <http://healthlink.mcw.edu/article.922569615.html>.

Progressive Supranuclear Palsy. <http://health.allrefer.com>.

Progressive Supranuclear Palsy Fact Sheet. <http://www.ninds.nih.gov/health_and_medical/pubs/psp.htm>.

Progressive Supranuclear Palsy. <http://www.cmdg.org>.

ORGANIZATIONS

Society for Progressive Supranuclear Palsy, Woodholme Medical Building. 1838 Greene Tree Road, #515, Baltimore, MD 21208. (410) 486-3330 or 800-457-4777; Fax: (410) 486-4383. spsp@psp.org. <http://www.psp.org>.

The PSP Association, The Old Rectory, Wappenham, Towcester, Northants NN12 8SQ, United Kingdom. 011-44-1327-860299; Fax: 011-44-1327-861007. psp.eur@virgin.net. <http://www.pspeur.org>.

Laith Farid Gulli, MD
Nicole Mallory, MS, PA-C

Pseudobulbar palsy

Definition

Pseudobulbar palsy refers to a group of symptoms—including difficulty with chewing, swallowing, and speech, as well as inappropriate emotional outbursts—that accompany a variety of nervous system disorders.

Description

Pseudobulbar palsy refers to a cluster of symptoms that can affect individuals suffering from a number of nervous system conditions, such as **amyotrophic lateral sclerosis**, **Parkinson's disease**, **stroke**, **multiple sclerosis**, or brain damage due to overly rapid correction of low blood sodium levels.

Causes and symptoms

Pseudobulbar palsy occurs when nervous system conditions cause degeneration of certain motor nuclei (nerve clusters responsible for movement) that exit the brain stem.

Patients with pseudobulbar palsy have progressive difficulty with activities that require the use of muscles in the head and neck that are controlled by particular cranial nerves. The first noticeable symptom is often slurred speech. Over time, speech, chewing, and swallowing become progressively more difficult, eventually becoming impossible. Sudden emotional outbursts, in which the patient spontaneously and without cause begins to laugh or cry, are also a characteristic of pseudobulbar palsy.

Diagnosis

Diagnosis is usually made by noting the symptom cluster characteristic of pseudobulbar palsy. Diagnostic tests will be run to determine what underlying neurological disorder has led to the development of pseudobulbar palsy. In particular, neuroimaging (**CT** and **MRI** scans) can be used to diagnose many of the conditions that prompt the development of pseudobulbar palsy.

Treatment team

Neurologists usually care for patients with the kinds of conditions that include the symptoms of pseudobulbar palsy.

Treatment

There are no cures for pseudobulbar palsy; the symptoms usually progress over the course of several years, leading to complete disability. Some medications may improve the emotional symptoms associated with pseudobulbar palsy; these include levodopa, **amantadine**, amitriptyline, and fluoxetine.

Prognosis

The prognosis for pseudobulbar palsy is quite poor. When the symptoms progress to disability, there is a high risk of choking and aspiration (breathing food or liquids into the lungs), which can lead to severe pneumonia and death. The conditions with which pseudobulbar palsy is associated also have a high risk of progression to death.

Resources

BOOKS

Friedman, Joseph. "Mood, Emotion, and Thought." In *Textbook of Clinical Neurology*, edited by Christopher G. Goetz. Philadelphia: W. B. Saunders Company, 2003.

Murray, T. Jock, and William Pryse-Phillips. "Amyotrophic Lateral Sclerosis." In *Noble: Textbook of Primary Care Medicine*, edited by John Noble, et al. St. Louis: W. B. Saunders Company, 2001.

Rosalyn Carson-DeWitt, MD

Pseudotumor cerebri

Definition

Pseudotumor cerebri is a chronic elevation of intracranial pressure that causes papilloedema and possibly blindness, which occurs in the absence of a mass lesion in the brain.

Description

Pseudotumor cerebri primarily affects obese women of childbearing age, and its cause is not known. The disorder is possibly the result of an abnormality in venous blood outflow from the brain, or from an abnormality in cerebrospinal fluid (CSF) flow. The increase in intracranial pressure can result in **headache**, visual impairment, **pain**, and hearing problems.

Demographics

Three significant studies concerning pseudotumor cerebri have been conducted in Iowa and Louisiana, the Mayo Clinic in Rochester, Minnesota, and Benghazi, Libya. The incidence of pseudotumor cerebri increases in women between 14 and 44 years of age, who are obese. In the Iowa and Louisiana study, the incidence was 19.3 per 100,000 in women who were 20% over ideal weight. In the Mayo Clinic study, the annual incidence number of new cases between 1976 and 1990 was found to be approximately eight per 100,000 for obese women 15–44 years old. In the Benghazi study (from 1982–1989), the annual incidence was 21 per 100,000 obese women 15–44 years old. No evidence of any racial or ethnic predilection exists.

Key Terms

Cerebrospinal fluid A colorless and clear fluid that contains glucose and proteins that bathe and nourish the brain and spinal cord.

Recombinant human growth hormone A synthetic form of growth hormone that can be given to a patient to help skeletal growth.

Papilloedema Edema or swelling in the optic disk (a portion of the optic nerve that collects nerves from the light sensitive layer of the eye, also called the retina).

Intraocular Inside the eye.

Causes and symptoms

The cause of pseudotumor cerebri is unknown, but it is thought to result from a faulty mechanism in CSF or venous flow from the brain. Certain risk factors have been associated with the disorder that include female gender, menstrual irregularity, obesity, recent weight gain, endocrine (hormone) disorders such as hypothyroidism (underactive thyroid disorder), or medication taken such as cimetidine (anti-ulcer), corticosteroids, lithium (used to treat bipolar disorder), tetracycline, sulfa antibiotics, recombinant human growth hormone, oral contraceptives, and vitamin A intake in infants.

Patients can have symptoms such as headache, ringing sounds in the ears, double vision (diplopia), or pain in the arms. Additionally, patients may have **back pain**, neck pain, or stiffness and arthralgias in the shoulder, knee, and wrist. Patients usually develop papilloedema, which can causes visual obscurations (dimming), progressive loss of peripheral vision, blurring, and sudden visual loss (resulting from intraocular hemorrhage).

Diagnosis

Neuroimaging studies are the best diagnostic tools, especially brain **magnetic resonance imaging (MRI)** scans. **MRI** scans provide good images that can reveal other possible disease states that cause increased intracranial pressure. General and special blood tests are typically ordered. CSF studies are also indicated and are usually done by inserting a needle into the lumbar region of the spine to withdraw a fluid sample. CSF studies are done to detect an infection within the **central nervous system**; the sample is used for tumor tests.

Treatment team

Management of pseudotumor cerebri requires a lumbar puncture that is performed by a **neurologist** or

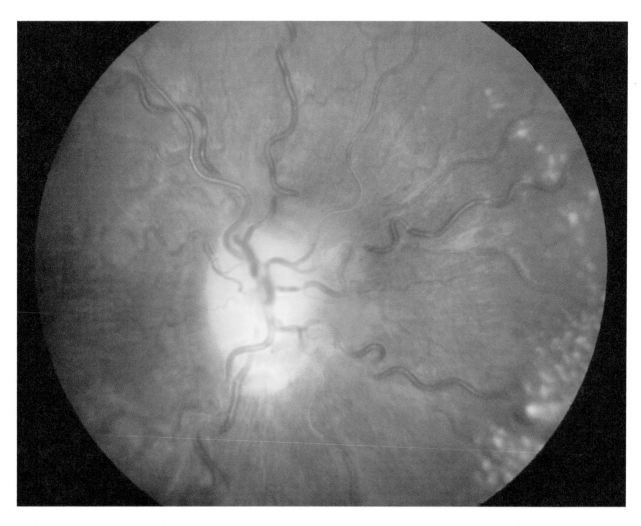

Retinal photograph showing the effects of a pseudotumor cerebri. *(Phototake, Inc. All rights reserved.)*

internist. Visual problems may be monitored by a neuro-ophthalmologist. Neurosurgical consultations are necessary if treatment does not arrest or reverse the condition quickly, within hours to days.

Treatment

Patients who do not develop visual loss are often treated with a drug called **acetazolamide** (a carbonic anhydrase inhibitor) that lowers intracranial pressure. In persons who present with more severe symptoms such as early loss of vision, a short treatment course with high-dose corticosteroids (prednisone) is recommended. Tapering down from the initial corticosteroid dose is individualized and based on the improvement of symptoms. If new visual loss is noted despite treatment, emergency surgical intervention may be indicated. A procedure called a lumboperitoneal shunt is the method of choice utilized for prompt reduction of intracranial hypertension; this is a surgical redirection of fluid flow in the brain, which creates an outflow of fluid from the brain that decreases intracranial pressure.

Recovery and rehabilitation

A formal weight loss and **exercise** program is required once the diagnosis is established. Admission to the hospital is uncommon, but some patients may be admitted for a short stay for intravenous fluid hydration and pain management in cases of intractable headache. Admission to the hospital is also indicated if the patient is a surgical candidate due to severe visual loss. Patients require education concerning blindness and weight reduction. Programs designed to lose weight should include an exercise program and psychological consultations. Many patients do not successfully lose enough weight and may require drastic treatment approaches such as gastric resection or stapling.

Clinical trials

The National Institute of Health is conducting a trial concerning the role of thrombosis inside blood vessels and the development of pseudotumor cerebri.

Prognosis

Typically, persons affected with pseudotumor cerebri can develop blindness, which is the only severe and permanent complication of this disorder. The blindness, which progressively worsens, is due to papilloedema.

Special concerns

Diligent treatment is required since eye deficits in one or both eyes can have a very quick onset and can be disabling. The disorder is not statistically correlated with weight gain during pregnancy; however, both pregnancy and pseudotumor cerebri are linked to weight gain and female gender (within childbearing age).

Resources

BOOKS

Marx, John A., et al (eds). *Rosen's Emergency Medicine: Concepts and Clinical Practice*, 5th ed. St. Louis: Mosby, Inc., 2002.

Noble, John., et al (eds). *Textbook of Primary Care Medicine*, 3rd ed. St. Louis: Mosby, Inc., 2001.

WEBSITES

Health Topics A-Z. (May 23, 2004.) <http://www.medhelp.org>.

ORGANIZATIONS

Pseudotumor Cerebri Support Network. 8247 Riverside Drive, Powell, OH 43065. (614) 895-8814. <http://www.pseudo tumorcerebri.com>.

Laith Farid Gulli, MD
Robert Ramirez, DO
Nicole Mallory, MS, PA-C

Pyridostigmine *see* **Cholinergic stimulants**

R

Radiation

Definition

Radiation and radioisotopes are extensively used medications to allow physicians to image internal structures and processes *in vivo* (in the living body) with a minimum of invasion to the patient. Higher doses of radiation are also used as means to kill cancerous cells.

Radiation is actually a term that includes a variety of different physical phenomena. However, in essence, all these phenomena can be divided into two classes: phenomena connected with nuclear radioactive processes are one class, the so-called radioactive radiation (RR); electromagnetic radiation (EMR) may be considered as the second class.

Both classes of radiation are used in diagnoses and treatment of neurological disorders.

Description

There are three kinds of radiation useful to medical personnel: alpha, beta, and gamma radiation. Alpha radiation is a flow of alpha particles, beta radiation is a flow of electrons, and gamma radiation is electromagnetic radiation.

Radioisotopes, containing unstable combinations of protons and neutrons, are created by neutron activation. This involves the capture of a neutron by the nucleus of an atom, resulting in an excess of neutrons (neutron rich). Proton-rich radioisotopes are manufactured in cyclotrons. During radioactive decay, the nucleus of a radioisotope seeks energetic stability by emitting particles (alpha, beta, or positron) and photons (including gamma rays).

Radiation—produced by radioisotopes—allows accurate imaging of internal organs and structures. Radioactive tracers are formed from the bonding of short-lived radioisotopes with chemical compounds that, when in the body, allow the targeting of specific body regions or physiologic processes. Emitted gamma rays (photons) can be detected by gamma cameras and computer

enhancement of the resulting images and allows quick and relatively noninvasive (compared to surgery) assessments of trauma or physiological impairments.

Because the density of tissues is unequal, x rays (a high frequency and energetic form of electromagnetic radiation) pass through tissues in an unequal manner. The beam passed through the body layer is recorded on special film to produce an image of internal structures. However, conventional x rays produce only a two-dimensional picture of the body structure under investigation.

Tomography (from the Greek *tomos*, meaning "to slice") is a method developed to allow the detailed construction of images of the target object. Initially using the x rays to scan layers of the area in question, with computer assisted tomography a computer then analyzes data of all layers to construct a 3D image of the object.

Computed tomography (also known as CT, **CT scan**) and computerized axial tomography (CAT) scans use x rays to produce images of anatomical structures.

Single proton (or photon) emission computed tomography (SPECT) produces three-dimensional images of an organ or body system. SPECT detects the presence and course of a radioactive substance that is injected, ingested, or inhaled. In neurology, a SPECT scan can allow physicians to examine and observe the **cerebral circulation**. SPECT produces images of the target region by detecting the presence and location of a radioactive isotope. The photon emissions of the radioactive compound containing the isotope can be detected in a manner that is similar to the detection of x rays in computed tomography (CT). At the end of the SPECT scan, the stored information can be integrated to produce a computer-generated composite image.

Positron emission tomography (PET) scans utilize isotopes produced in a cyclotron. Positron-emitting radionuclides are injected and allowed to accumulate in the target tissue or organ. As the radionuclide decays, it emits a positron that collides with nearby electrons to result in the emission of two identifiable gamma photons. **PET**

scans use rings of detectors that surround the patient to track the movements and concentrations of radioactive tracers. PET scans have attracted the interest of physicians because of their potential use in research into metabolic changes associated with mental diseases such as **schizophrenia** and **depression**. PET scans are used in the diagnosis and characterizations of certain cancers and heart disease, as well as clinical studies of the brain. PET uses radio-labeled tracers, including deoxyglucose, which is chemically similar to glucose and is used to assess metabolic rate in tissues and to image tumors, and dopa, within the brain.

Electromagnetic radiation

In contrast to imaging produced through the emission and collection of nuclear radiation (e.g., x rays, CT scans), **magnetic resonance imaging (MRI)** scanners rely on the emission and detection of electromagnetic radiation.

Electromagnetic radiation results from oscillations of components of electric and magnetic fields. In the simplest cases, these oscillations occur with definite frequency (the unit of frequency measurement is 1 Hertz (Hz), which is one oscillation per second). Arising in some point (under the action of the radiation source), electromagnetic radiation travels with the velocity that is equal to the velocity of the light, and this velocity is equal for all frequencies. Another quantity, wavelength, is often used for the description of electromagnetic radiation (this quantity is similar to the distance between two neighbor crests of waves spreading on a water surface, which appear after dropping a stone on the surface). Because the product of the wavelength and frequency must equal the velocity of light, the greater the wave frequency, the less its wavelength.

MRI scanners rely on the principles of atomic nuclear-spin resonance. Using strong magnetic fields and radio waves, MRIs collect and correlate deflections caused by atoms into images. MRIs allow physicians to see internal structures with great detail and also allow earlier and more accurate diagnosis of disorders.

MRI technology was developed from nuclear magnetic resonance (NMR) technology. Groups of nuclei brought into resonance, that is, nuclei absorbing and emitting photons of similar electromagnetic radiation such as

radio waves, make subtle yet distinguishable changes when the resonance is forced to change by altering the energy of impacting photons. The speed and extent of the resonance changes permit a non-destructive (because of the use of low-energy photons) determination of anatomical structures.

MRI images do not utilize potentially harmful ionizing radiation generated by three-dimensional x-ray CT scans, but rely on the atomic properties (nuclear resonance) of protons in tissues when they are scanned with radio frequency radiation. The protons in the tissues, which resonate at slightly different frequencies, produce a signal that a computer uses to tell one tissue from another. MRI provides detailed three-dimensional soft tissue images.

These methods are used successfully for brain investigations.

Radiation therapy (radiotherapy)

Radiotherapy requires the use of radioisotopes and higher doses of radiation that are used diagnostically to treat some cancers (including brain cancer) and other medical conditions that require destruction of harmful cells.

Radiation therapy is delivered via external radiation or via internal radiation therapy (the implantation/injection of radioactive substances).

Cancer, tumors, and other rapidly dividing cells are usually sensitive to damage by radiation. The goal of radiation therapy is to deliver the minimally sufficient dosage to kill cancerous cells or to keep them from dividing. Cancer cells divide and grow at rates more rapid than normal cells and so are particularly susceptible to radiation. Accordingly, some cancerous growths can be restricted or eliminated by radioisotope irradiation. The most common forms of external radiation therapy use gamma and x rays. During the last half of the twentieth century, the radioisotope cobalt-60 was the frequently used source of radiation used in such treatments. More modern methods of irradiation include the production of x rays from linear accelerators.

Iodine-131, phosphorus-32 are commonly used in radiotherapy. More radical uses of radioisotopes include the use of boron-10 to specifically attack tumor cells. Boron-10 concentrates in tumor cells and is then subjected to neutron beams that result in highly energetic alpha particles that are lethal to the tumor tissue.

Precautions

Radiation therapy is not without risk to healthy tissue and to persons on the health care team, and precautions (shielding and limiting exposure) are taken to minimize exposure to other areas of the patient's body and to personnel on the treatment team.

Therapeutic radiologists, radiation oncologists, and a number of technical specialists use radiation and other methods to treat patients who have cancer or other tumors.

Care is taken in the selection of the appropriate radioactive isotope. Ideally, the radioactive compound loses its radioactive potency rapidly (this is expressed as the half-life of a compound). For example, gamma-emitting compounds used in SPECT scans can have a half-life of just a few hours. This is beneficial for the patients, as it limits the contact time with the potentially damaging radioisotope.

The selection of radioisotopes for medical use is governed by several important considerations involving dosage and half-life. Radioisotopes must be administered in sufficient dosages so that emitted radiation is present in sufficient quantity to be measured. Ideally the radioisotope has a short enough half-life that, at the delivered dosage, there is insignificant residual radiation following the desired length of exposure.

New areas of radiation therapy that may prove more effective in treating brain tumors (and other forms of cancers) include three-dimensional conformal radiation therapy (a process where multiple beans are shaped to match the contour of the tumor) and stereotactic radiosurgery (used to irradiate certain brain tumors and obstructions of the cerebral circulation). Gamma knives use focused beams (with the patient often wearing a special helmet to help focus the beams), while cyberknifes use hundreds of precise pinpoint beams emanating from a source of irradiation that moves around the patient's head.

Resources

BOOKS

Saha, Gopal B. *Fundamentals of Nuclear Pharmacy.* New York: Springer-Verlag, 1999.

WEBSITES

Society of Nuclear Medicine. "What Is Nuclear Medicine?" May 12, 2004 (May 27, 2004). <http://www.snm.org/nuclear/index.html>.

Alexander Ioffe

Radiculopathy

Definition

Radiculopathy refers to disease of the spinal nerve roots (from the Latin *radix* for root). Radiculopathy produces **pain**, numbness, or weakness radiating from the spine.

Description

At the joints between the vertebrae, sensory nerves (nerves conducting sensory information toward the **central nervous system**) and motor nerves (nerves conducting commands to muscles away from the central nervous system) connect to the spinal cord. Each spinal nerve divides or fans out just before merging with the spinal cord. These smaller, separate nerve bundles are termed the roots of the nerve because they are reminiscent of the way the roots of a plant divide in the ground.

Damage to the spinal nerve roots can lead to pain, numbness, weakness, and paresthesia (abnormal sensations in the absence of stimuli) in the limbs or trunk. Pain may be felt in a region corresponding to a dermatome, an area of skin innervated by the sensory fibers of a given spinal nerve or a dynatome, an area in which pain is felt when a given spinal nerve is irritated. Dynatomes and dermatomes may overlap, but do not necessarily coincide.

Radiculopathies are categorized according to which part of the spinal cord is affected. Thus, there are cervical (neck), thoracic (middle back), and lumbar (lower back) radiculopathies. Lumbar radiculopathy is also known a **sciatica**. Radiculopathies may be further categorized by what vertebrae they are associated with. For example, radiculopathy of the nerve roots at the level of the seventh cervical vertebra is termed C7 radiculopathy; at the level of the fifth cervical vertebra, C5 radiculopathy; at the level of the first thoracic vertebra, T1 radiculopathy; and so on.

Radiculopathy is to be distinguished from myelopathy, which involves pathological changes in or functional problems with the spinal cord itself rather than the nerve roots. Sometimes, radiculopathy is also distinguished from radiculitis, the latter being defined as irritation (hence the "itis" suffix) of a nerve root that causes pain in the dermatome or dynatome corresponding to that nerve. Radiculopathy, on the other hand, denotes spinal nerve dysfunction (not just irritation) presenting with pain, altered reflex, weakness, and nerve-conduction abnormalities. Pain may not be present with radiculopathy, but is always present with radiculitis.

Demographics

Millions of persons experience some form of radiculopathy at some point in their lives. Because many of the causes of radiculopathy are long-term diseases (e.g., ankylosing spondylosis, diabetes) or diseases that tend to affect the elderly (e.g., arthritis), radiculopathy occurs more often in the middle-aged and elderly than in the young. However, injuries due to sports, heavy lifting, or bad posture affect the young as well. Cervical **disc herniation** with radiculopathy (mostly involving the C4 to C5 levels) affects 5.5 per 100,000 adults every year, with the highest risk being for adults 35 to 55 years year old.

Key Terms

Dermatome An area of skin that receive sensations through a single nerve root.

Dynatome An area in which pain is felt when a given spinal nerve is irritated.

Motor nerves Nerves conducting commands to muscles away from the central nervous system.

Sensory nerves Nerves conducting sensory information toward the central nervous system.

Causes and symptoms

Radiculopathy can be caused by any disease or injury process that compresses or otherwise injures the spinal nerve roots. Violent blows or falls, cancer, some infections such as flu and **Lyme disease**, diseases that lead to degeneration of the vertebrae and/or intervertrebral discs (osteoarthritis), slipped or herniated discs, scoliosis, and other factors can cause radiculopathy. For example, extreme backward bending of the neck can trigger cervical radiculopathy. This has given rise to a recently-recognized category of radiculopathy termed "salon sink radiculopathy," so-called because salon patrons are asked to tip their heads sharply backward into sinks for shampooing. Spondylosis (immobilization and growing-together of one or more vertebral joints, often due to osteoarthritis) can deform the structures of bone, cartilage, and ligament through which spinal nerves must pass, leading to cervical and lumbar radiculopathy. Thoracic and lumbar radiculopathies are a common result of diabetes, which can impair blood flow to the spinal nerve roots.

Diagnosis

Radiculopathy is a possible diagnosis when numbness, pain, weakness, or paresthesia of the extremities or torso are reported by a patient, especially in a dermatomal pattern. However, these symptoms can also be caused by **nerve compression** remote from the spine, and the physician must rule out this possibility before ruling in favor of radiculopathy. Electrodiagnostic studies can help distinguish radiculopathy from other diagnoses. These techniques include current perception threshold testing, which tests patient ability to sense alternating electric currents at several frequencies; electromyographic nerve conduction tests; and testing of sensory evoked potentials (changes in brain waves in response to sensory stimuli).

When radiculopathy is diagnosed, the location of the affected nerve roots and, ultimately, the cause of their dysfunction must be determined. Diagnosticians look at the precise features of radicular symptoms in order to determine the spinal level of the affected root or roots. For example, radiculopathy at the C7 level (the nerve root most often affected by herniated cervical disc) is characterized by weak triceps and wrist extensor muscles and a numb middle finger. Radiculopathy at the L3 (third lumbar disc) level is characterized by decreased patellar (kneecap) reflex, loss of sensation and/or pain in the anterior (forward) part of the thigh, and weakness in quadriceps muscle; and so on.

X ray or **MRI** may be used to confirm the diagnosis. A herniated disc, for example, will be revealed by imaging. A herniated disc is one that has partly popped or bulged out from between the vertebra above and below it. This may place pressure on the nerve roots and on the spinal cord itself.

In persons with spinal cancer or other progressive disorders, the appearance of radiculopathy may be an important sign that pressure is beginning to be exerted by the tumor or some other changing structure. This may signal that it is time for surgical intervention.

Treatment team

Diagnosis of radiculopathy will usually involve a **neurologist**. An orthopedist will usually be involved as well. Other specialists will be required depending on the cause of the radiculopathy (e.g., oncologist, if cancer is present). Treatment will usually call for a physical therapist. An orthopedic surgeon would perform any necessary surgery.

Treatment

Treatment for radiculopathy varies with the nature and severity of the disease process or injury that has caused the disorder. Conservative (non-surgical) treatment is often attempted first. This consists primarily of rest, **exercise**, and medication. Patient-specific exercises are prescribed by a physical therapist for the targeted strengthening of muscles and other supporting tissues to relieve pressure on affected spinal nerve roots. Weight loss may be advised to decrease stress on the spine. Medications may include oral opioids (e.g., morphine) or other analgesic (anti-pain) medications. In severe cases, injection of an opioid by an external or implanted pump directly into the affected area may be prescribed. Epidural corticosteroid injections, selective nerve root block, and epidural lysis (destruction) of adhesions are also used to treat radiculopathy. A soft neck collar may be prescribed for persons with cervical radiculopathy.

When conservative treatment fails, surgery may be necessary. The primary purpose of surgery is to take pressure off of affected nerve roots or the blood vessels that serve them and to stabilize spinal structure, but surgery may also sever nerves in order to relieve severe pain. Fusion of vertebrae (i.e., removal of the flexible intervertebral disc and joining of the adjacent vertebrae so that they grow into a single bone) was for many decades a common treatment for intractable radiculopathy, but as of 2003, a novel implant, the Bryan disc, was under study by the US Food and Drug Administration. The Bryan disc is a flexible disc or ring of titanium and Teflon that is used to replace the intervertebral disc in patients with degenerative disc disease. Two versions of the disc, one cervical (for the neck) and the other lumbar (for the lower back) were under development. Early reports from surgeons were positive. The advantage of such an implant over fusion is that the patient does not lose flexibility in that part of their spine.

Recovery and rehabilitation

Exercise is key to the treatment of both conservative and surgical treatment of radiculopathy. It may even be curative in some cases. It is also an important aspect of recovery from surgery. Exercise is done as directed by a physical therapist.

Clinical trials

As of mid-2004, a clinical trial sponsored by the National Institute of Dental and Craniofacial Research was recruiting participants. The goal of this clinical trial was to evaluate the effectiveness of two drugs (i.e., nortriptyline and MS Contin, a type of morphine) in treating lumbar radiculopathy, also known as sciatica. This was a phase II clinical trial, meaning that it involved a medium-size group (100–300 participants) to evaluate effectiveness and side effects of the treatment. Persons interested in participating should contact the Patient Recruitment and Public Liaison Office at telephone (800) 411-1222, or e-mail at: prpl@mail.cc.nih.gov.

Prognosis

Prognosis varies with the underlying process causing the radiculopathy. For sports injuries, at one extreme, the prognosis is excellent; for degenerative disc disorders, even surgery may not completely or permanently resolve the problem. However, new surgical techniques are improving this picture.

Resources

PERIODICALS

Kilcline, Bradford A. "Acute Low Back Pain: Guidelines for Treating Common and Uncommon Syndromes." *Consultant* (October 1, 2002).

Lauerman, William C. "When Back Surgery Fails: What's the Next Step?" *Journal of Musculoskeletal Medicine* (June 1, 1999).

Lenrow, David A. "Chronic Neck Pain: Mapping Out Diagnosis and Management; Part 1: Step-by-step Algorithms Can Show the Way to Effective Treatment." *Journal of Musculoskeletal Medicine* (June 1, 2002).

"Neck Problems Tied to Salon Sinks." *Daily News* (Los Angeles) (October 6, 1999).

OTHER

"Cervical Radiculopathy." *Neuroland.* http://neuroland.com/spine/c_radi.htm (April 29, 2004).

Skelton, Alta, "Lumbar radiculopathy." <http://www.spineuniverse.com/displayarticle.php/article1469.html> (April 29, 2004).

ORGANIZATIONS

National Institute for Neurological Diseases and Stroke (NINDS). 6001 Executive Boulevard, Bethesda, MD 20892. (301) 496-5751 or (800) 352-9424. <http://www.ninds.nih.gov>.

Larry Gilman, PhD

Ramsay-Hunt syndrome type II

Definition

Ramsay-Hunt syndrome type II is a very rare, progressive neurological disorder that causes **epilepsy**, tremor, mental impairment, and eventually death.

Description

Ramsay-Hunt syndrome type II begins in adulthood. It is a relentlessly progressive degenerative disease that culminates in death, characterized by Parkinson-like **tremors**, and muscle jerks (**myoclonus**).

Demographics

The average age of onset is about 30 years of age.

Causes and symptoms

Some cases seem to be caused by abnormalities of the mitochondria within the cell. Mitochondria are the cells' power stations. They are organelles within each cell that are responsible for producing energy.

Some cases of Ramsay-Hunt syndrome type II appear to be inherited in an autosomal dominant fashion, meaning that a child who has one parent with the abnormal gene has a 50:50 chance of inheriting the disorder. Other cases appear to be inherited in an autosomal recessive fashion, meaning that individuals who develop the disease have inherited defective genes from both parents.

Key Terms

Mitochondria The organelles within each cell that are responsible for the production of energy.

Myoclonus Involuntary jerking or twitching of muscles.

Ramsay-Hunt syndrome type II begins as an intention tremor in the limbs, particularly the arms. An intention tremor is an involuntary shaking or trembling that occurs when an individual is attempting a purposeful movement; the tremor is not manifested when the individual is at rest. The intention tremor generally occurs in just one limb. Over time, the entire muscular system is affected. In addition to the tremor, individuals with Ramsay-Hunt syndrome type II experience sudden twitching or contraction of muscle groups, called myoclonus. Some individuals experience progressive hearing impairment. As the disease progresses, the individual experiences decreased muscle tone, increasing weakness, disturbances of fine motor control, difficulty walking, epilepsy, and (in some cases) mental deterioration. The disease usually progresses over the course of about 10 years, ultimately resulting in the death of the patient.

Diagnosis

An electroencephalogram (EEG) may reveal certain abnormalities of the electrical patterns in the brain. Muscle **biopsy** may or may not reveal mitochondrial abnormalities.

Treatment team

Ramsay-Hunt syndrome type II is usually diagnosed and treated by a **neurologist**. In an effort to maintain functioning as long as possible, other treatment members may include physical therapists, occupational therapists, and speech and language therapists.

Treatment

There is no cure for Ramsay-Hunt syndrome type II. **Seizures** may respond to antiseizure medications such as **phenobarbital**, clonazepam, or valproic acid. The involuntary muscle jerking (myoclonus) may decrease with such medication as valproic acid; **benzodiazepines** such as clonazepam; L-tryptophan; 5-hydroxytryptophan with carbidopa; or piracetam.

Prognosis

Ramsay-Hunt syndrome type II generally progresses to death within about 10 years of the onset of symptoms.

Resources

BOOKS

Foldvary-Schaefer, Nancy, and Elaine Wyllie. "Epilepsy." In *Textbook of Clinical Neurology*, edited by Christopher G. Goetz. Philadelphia: W.B. Saunders Company, 2003.

PERIODICALS

Sacquegna, T. "Normal Muscle Mitochondrial Function in Ramsay-Hunt Syndrome." *Italian Journal of Neurological Science* 10 (1) (1 February 1989): 73–75.

Tassinari, C. A. "Dyssenergia Cerebellaris Myoclonica (Ramsay-Hunt Syndrome): A Condition Unrelated to Mitochondrial Encephalomyopathies." *Journal of Neurology, Neurosurgery, and Psychiatry* 52 (2) (1 February 1989): 262–265.

WEBSITES

National Institute of Neurological Disorders and Stroke (NINDS). *Ramsay-Hunt Syndrome Type II Fact Sheet.* (May 23, 2004.) <http://www.ninds.nih.gov/health_and_medical/disorders/ramsey2.htm>.

ORGANIZATIONS

National Ataxia Foundation. 2600 Fernbrook Lane, Suite 119, Minneapolis, MN 55447-4752. (763) 553-0020; Fax: (763) 553-0167. naf@ataxia.org. <http://www.ataxia.org>.

WE MOVE. 204 West 84th Street, New York, NY 10024. (212) 875-8389 or (800) 437-MOV2. wemove@wemove.org. <http://www.wemove.org>.

Rosalyn Carson-DeWitt, MD

Rasmussen's encephalitis

Definition

Rasmussen's encephalitis, also termed Rasmussen's syndrome, is a rare degenerative brain disease that initially affects only one side of the brain. It first manifests in childhood with the onset of epileptic **seizures**. Later, it progresses to paralysis of one side of the body (hemiparesis), blindness in one eye (**hemianopsia**), and loss of mental function. The seizures in Rasmussen's encephalitis usually resist therapy with anticonvulsant drugs, but respond well to hemispherectomy, the surgical removal of the entire affected side of the brain.

Description

Rasmussen's encephalitis usually appears in children, but may also strike in adulthood. It initially affects only one side (hemisphere) of the brain. The disease causes uncontrollable seizures and other symptoms that become progressively worse. The affected hemisphere shows changes characteristic of chronic inflammation, including long-term atrophy or shrinkage, hence, the term encephalitis (inflammation of the brain). Unless the affected hemisphere is removed, the disorder eventually spreads to the brain's other hemisphere.

Demographics

Rasmussen's encephalitis is very rare; between 1958, when the syndrome was first identified, and 2000, barely 100 cases were identified. The medical literature does not describe a higher incidence of this disease in either gender or in any particular racial group or geographical area.

Causes and symptoms

For many years, the cause of Rasmussen's encephalitis was a mystery. It seemed to resemble a viral infection, but despite much research, no organism could be consistently found in the brains of those who had suffered from the disorder. Finally, in the early 1990s, it was discovered that Rasmussen's encephalitis is an autoimmune disease, that is, a disorder in which the body is attacked by its own immune system.

Specifically, the body responds to one of the glutamate receptors, GluR3, as if it were an invading organism. Glutamate is a neurotransmitter, or one of the chemicals that neurons use to signal to each other. A receptor is a complex molecule embedded in the cell membrane of a neuron that detects the presence of a specific neurotransmitter and responds by causing some change in the neuron itself, such as admitting a flow of sodium, potassium, or calcium ions into the cell. There are at least 20 distinct receptors for glutamate in the brain, one of which is denoted GluR3. In Rasmussen's encephalitis, the body (for reasons still unknown) produces anti-GluR3 antibodies. Attracted by these antibodies, groupings of special immune system proteins, termed complement, gather on neurons in the affected parts of the brain, eventually forming "membrane attack complexes" that damage the neurons. It is not known why this autoimmune response attacks only one side of the brain at first, but it was hypothesized that a breach in the blood-brain barrier in one part of the brain might allow initial access of antibodies to neurons. The arrival of lymphocytes in the affected area, with consequent swelling of tissues, may then cause further damage to the blood-brain barrier and allow more anti-GluR3 antibodies access to the neurons. Finally, it remains possible that infection by cytomegalovirus may play a role in triggering the autoimmune processes of Rasmussen's encephalitis. Cytomegalovirus DNA has been detected in the brains of some patients.

The first symptom of Rasmussen's encephalitis is seizures, usually beginning suddenly before the age of 10. Loss of control over voluntary movements, loss of speech ability (**aphasia**), hemiparesis (weakness on one side of the body), **dementia**, **mental retardation**, and eventually, death, will follow if untreated.

Diagnosis

Rasmussen's encephalitis is diagnosed by the sudden onset of epileptic seizures in childhood, gradual worsening of seizures, gradual intellectual deterioration, the onset of hemiparesis and other one-sided symptoms, and the elimination of other possible causes for these symptoms.

Treatment

Early in the progress of Rasmussen's encephalitis, anticonvulsant drugs may help control seizures. Use of the anti-cytomegalovirus drug ganciclovir early in the syndrome produces improvement in some patients. Also, some patients have shown dramatic positive response to removal of anti-GluR3 antibodies from the blood by a process known as plasmapheresis. Currently, researchers are studying the hypothesis that drugs to prevent the formation of membrane-attack complexes might slow or halt the progression of Rasmussen's encephalitis as well as of other neurodegenerative diseases. However, the treatment of choice remained hemispherectomy, surgical removal of the affected half of the brain.

Remarkably, children may show little or no change in personality and no loss of intelligence or memory after having half their brain removed. Some children are irritable, withdrawn, or depressed immediately after surgery, but these symptoms are not permanent. So flexible is brain development that a child with a hemispherectomy may become fluent in one or more languages even if the left side of the brain, where the speech centers are usually located, is removed. Blindness or vision loss in one eye usually results from hemispherectomy, but normal hearing in both ears may be recovered. The older the patient is when the surgery is performed, however, the more likely they are to suffer permanent sensory, speech, and motor losses.

Recovery and rehabilitation

Rehabilitation begins immediately after hemispherectomy with passive range-of-motion exercises. Physical, occupational, and speech therapists are required. For children of school age, **neuropsychological testing** can help determine what academic setting or grade level is best. Children with hemispherectomies are often able to participate in school at the level appropriate for their age.

Prognosis

The prognosis for children below the age of 10 who are treated early in the course of the syndrome is good. This group can often achieve normal psychosocial and intellectual functioning. Without hemispherectomy, however, persons with Rasmussen's encephalitis eventually suffer near-continuous seizures, mental retardation, and death.

Resources

BOOKS

Graham, David I., and Peter L. Lantos. *Greenfield's Neuropathology*, 6th edition. Bath, UK: Arnold, 1997.

PERIODICALS

Cleaver, Hannah. "Girl Left with Half a Brain Is Fluent in Two Languages." *Daily Telegraph* (London, England), May 23, 2002.

Duke University. "Mild Injury May Render Brain Cells Vulnerable to Immune System Attack." *Ascribe Higher Education News Service* October 23, 2002.

Lilly, Donna J. "Functional Hemispherectomy: Radical Treatment for Rasmussen's Encephalitis." *Journal of Neuroscience Nursing* April 1, 2000.

Mercadante, Marcos T. "Genetics of Childhood Disorders: XXX. Autoimmune Disorders, Part 3: Myasthenia Gravis and Rasmussen's Encephalitis." *Journal of the American Academy of Child and Adolescent Psychiatry* (September 1, 2001).

Zuckerberg, Aaron. "Why Would You Remove Half a Brain? The Outcome of 58 Children after Hemispherectomy–The Johns Hopkins Experience: 1968–1996." *Pediatrics* (August 1, 1997).

OTHER

"NINDS Rasmussen's Encephalitis Information Page." *National Institute of Neurological Disorders and Stroke.* March 30, 2004 (June 2, 2004). <http://www.ninds.nih.gov/health_and_medical/disorders/rasmussn_doc.htm>.

ORGANIZATIONS

National Organization for Rare Disorders (NORD). P.O. Box 1968 (55 Kenosia Avenue), Danbury, CT 06813-1968. (203) 744-0100 or (800) 999-NORD; Fax: (203) 798-2291. orphan@rarediseases.org. <http://www.rarediseases.org>.

Larry Gilman, PhD

Reflex sympathetic dystrophy

Definition

Reflex sympathetic dystrophy is the feeling of **pain** associated with evidence of minor nerve injury.

Description

Historically reflex sympathetic dystrophy (RSD) was noticed during the Civil War in patients who suffered **pain** following gunshot **wounds** that affected the median nerve (a major nerve in the arm). In 1867 the condition was called causalgia from the Greek term meaning "burning pain." Causalgia refers to pain associated with major nerve injury. The exact causes of RSD are still unclear. Patients usually develop a triad of phases. In the first phase, pain and sympathetic activity is increased. Patients will typically present with swelling (**edema**), stiffness, pain, increased vascularity (increasing warmth), hyperhydrosis, and x-ray changes demonstrating loss of **minerals** in bone (demineralization). The second phase develops three to nine months later, It is characterized by increased stiffness and changes in the extremity that include a decrease in warmth and atrophy of the skin and muscles. The late phase commencing several months to years later presents with a pale, cold, painful, and atrophic extremity. Patients at this stage will also have **osteoporosis**.

It has been thought that each phase relates to a specific nerve defect that involves nerve tracts from the periphery spinal cord to the brain. Both sexes are affected, but the number of new cases is higher in women, adolescents, and young adults. RDS has been associated with other terms such as Sudeck's atrophy, post-traumatic osteoporosis, causalgia, shoulder-hand syndrome, and reflex neuromuscular dystrophy.

Causes and symptoms

The exact causes of RSD at present is not clearly understood. There are several theories such as sympathetic overflow (overactivity), abnormal circuitry in nerve impulses through the sympathetic system, and as a post-operative complication for both elective and traumatic

Key Terms

Atrophy Abnormal changes in a cell that lead to loss of cell structure and function.

Osteoporosis Reduction in the quantity of bone.

surgical procedures. Patients typically develop pain, swelling, temperature, color changes, and skin and muscle wasting.

Diagnosis

The diagnosis is simple and confirmed by a local anesthetic block along sympathetic nerve paths in the hand or foot, depending on whether an arm or leg is affected. A test called the **erythrocyte sedimentation rate** (ESR) can be performed to rule out diseases with similar presentation and arising from other causes.

Treatment

The preferred method to treat RSD includes sympathetic block and physical therapy. Pain is improved in motion of the affected limb improves. Patients may also require tranquilizers and mild **analgesics**. Patients who received repeated blocks should consider surgical symathectomy (removal of the nerves causing pain).

Prognosis

The prognosis for treatment during phase one is favorable. As the disease progresses undetected into phase two or three the prognosis for recovery is poor.

Resources

BOOKS

Canale, S., et al. *Campbell's Operative Orthopaedics,* 9th ed. Mosby, Inc., 1998.

Goetz, Christopher G., et al., eds. *Textbook of Clinical Neurology,* 1st ed. W. B. Saunders Company, 1999.

Rockwood, Charles A., David P. Green, et al. *Fractures in Adults,* 4th ed. Lippincott-Raven Publishers, 1996.

Ruddy, Shaun, et al., eds. *Kelly's Textbook of Rheumatology,* 6th ed. W. B. Saunders Company, 2001.

OTHER

Reflex Sympathetic Dystrophy Syndrome Association of America. <http://www.rsds.org/fact.html>.

Laith Farid Gulli, MD
Robert Ramirez, BS

Refsum disease

Definition

Refsum disease is one of several inherited disorders that are collectively called leukodystrophies. Refsum disease results from defects in the formation of the myelin sheath, a fat covering that protects the nerves in the brain and spinal cord.

Description

Refsum disease has also been called Refsum-Thiébaut disease and Refsum-Thiébaut-Klenk-Kahlke disease since Drs. W. Kahlke, E. Klenk, M.F. Thiébaut, and Sigvald Bernhard Refsum all contributed to the identification and clinical characterization of the disorder. The Norwegian **neurologist**, Sigvald Refsum first described the disorder in 1946.

Refsum disease is a rare genetic disorder that affects the ability of the body to breakdown fats, a process called fatty acid oxidation. As a result, a metabolite called phytanic acid accumulates in the blood as well as other tissues. Phytanic acid is not produced by the human body but is obtained from meat, dairy, and fish products. Phytanic acid is a branched chain fatty acid. The accumulation of this compound in the blood was detected by the German scientist Klenk and Kahlke around 1963. Phytanic acid can also be produced through the breakdown of a substance that is found in green leafy vegetables called phytol.

Refsum disease is inherited as an autosomal recessive disorder, which means that two unaffected carrier parents have a 25% chance of having an affected child in every pregnancy. Other less commonly used synonyms for Refsum syndrome include: **ataxia** hereditaria hemeralopia polyneuritiformis, hemeralopia heredotaxia polyneuritiformis, hereditary motor sensory neuropathy type IV, heredopathia atactica poluneuritiformis, and phytanic acid storage syndrome.

Demographics

Refsum disease is an extremely rare disorder that affects males and females with equal frequency. It has been observed in Norwegian populations as well as others.

Causes and symptoms

One of the earliest symptoms in Refsum disease that the patients develop is night blindness. The age of onset of all clinical manifestations tends to occur during childhood and usually develop before 50 years of age. It is a progressive disorder characterized by periods of subtle worsening and often appears to be in remission.

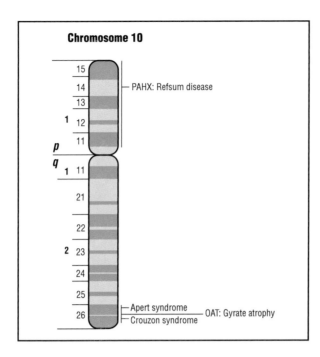

Chromosome 10

15
14 — PAHX: Refsum disease
13
1 12
11
p
q 1 11
21
22
2 23
24
25
26 — Apert syndrome — OAT: Gyrate atrophy
Crouzon syndrome

Refsum disease, on chromosome 10. *(Gale Group.)*

Key Terms

Autosomal recessive disorder A genetic disorder that is inherited from parents that are both carriers, but do not have the disorder. Parents with an affected recessive gene have a 25% chance of passing on the disorder to their offspring with each pregnancy.

Leukodystrophy A genetically determined progressive disorder that affects the brain, spinal cord, and peripheral nerves.

Myelin A fat-like substance that forms a protective sheath around nerve fibers.

People with Refsum disease typically experience progressive hearing loss due to nerve damage that occurs early during development. They can develop a progressive degeneration of the eye leading to blindness due to an atypical form of retinitis pigmentosa, a degenerative condition associated with night blindness and pigment changes in the retina. The visual loss involves progressive constriction of the visual fields and these patients can develop nystagmus (an involuntary oscillation of the eyeball) as well as cataracts.

Cerebellar ataxia (brain-damage-related loss of motor coordination) can also occur with Refsum disease, leading

to an unsteady gait. They can have syndactyly of the fingers, where two fingers appear fused due to a failure to separate during embryo formation. The neurological damage appears to be localized toward the head and trunk of the body (rather than the limbs). A fetus with Refsum disease often develops heart disease and can also be born with skeletal abnormalities in bone formation. It is also common for people with Refsum disease to lose their sense of smell. Finally, changes in the skin can also occur with Refsum disease.

Refsum was the first genetic disorder identified to be caused by defects in lipid (fat) metabolism. It is currently felt to be caused by mutations in a gene (PAHX) that encodes a protein called phyanoly-CoA hydroxylase and is important for metabolizing phytanic acid.

Diagnosis

The diagnosis for Refsum disease is made based on the development of clinical manifestations and biochemical analysis detecting elevated phytanic acid in the blood.

Treatment team

There are several specialists that are helpful in the diagnosis, treatment, and long-term care of patients with Refsum disease. A neurologist is helpful initially in diagnosing the disorder, as well as providing the appropriate follow-up studies and treatment regimen. A genetic counselor is helpful in explaining the recurrence risks to the family, especially if they are considering reproductive implications.

Treatment

Dietary treatment involving the restriction of foods that contain phytanic acid began in Norway in 1966 by Professor Lorentz Eldjarn, the Head of the Central Laboratory and Institute for Clinical Biochemistry at the Oslo University Hospital, Rikshospitalet. This treatment continues today. Additionally, plasmapheresis or the removing of plasma from the patient's blood may also be helpful and necessary.

Recovery and rehabilitation

Recovery with treatment is often possible for many of the symptoms, although treating patients with Refsum disease cannot reverse damage to the eyesight and hearing.

Clinical trials

The National Institute for Neurological Diseases and Stroke and the National Institutes of Health supports research to help increase understanding and awareness or Refsum disease, as well as to find new prevention, treatments, or a cure for this disorder. One study, which is aimed at determining the effectiveness of an oral bile acid therapy regimen is currently recruiting patients with the infantile form of Refsum disease. (Contact information: Kenneth Setchell, Study Chair, Children's Hospital Medical Center, Cincinnati OH; (513) 636-4548).

Prognosis

The prognosis for Refsum disease is highly variable. Without treatment, the prognosis is poor. In patients who are treated appropriately, many neurological symptoms and ichthyosis (scaly, dry skin) generally disappear.

Resources

BOOKS

Iocn Health Publications. *The Official Parent's Sourcebook on Refsum Disease: A Revised and Updated Directory for the Internet Age.* San Diego: Icon Group International, 2002.

PERIODICALS

Richterich, R., P. van Mechelen, and E. Rossi. "Refsum's disease (heredopathia atactica polyneuritiformis): An inborn error of lipid metabolism with storage of 3,7,11,15-tetramethylhexadecanoic acid." *Am J Med* 39: 230–41.

OTHER

"NINDS Refsum Disease Information Page." National Institute of Neurological Disorders and Stroke. (March 10, 2004). <http://www.ninds.nih.gov/health_and_medical/disorders/refsum_doc.htm>.

ORGANIZATIONS

National Organization for Rare Disorders (NORD). P.O. Box 1968 (55 Kenosia Avenue), Danbury, CT 06813-1968. (203) 744-0100 or (800) 999-NORD (6673); Fax: (203) 798-2291. orphan@rarediseases.org. <http://www.rarediseases.org>.

National Tay-Sachs and Allied Diseases Association. 2001 Beacon Street Suite 204, Brighton, MA 02135. (617) 277-4463 or (800) 90-NTSAD (906-8723; Fax: (617) 277-0134. info@ntsad.org. <http://www.ntsad.org>.

Bryan Richard Cobb, PhD

Repetitive stress injuries *see* **Repetitive motion disorders**

Repetitive motion disorders

Definition

Repetitive motion disorders are a group of syndromes caused by injuries to muscles, tendons, nerves, or blood vessels from repeated or sustained exertions of different body parts. Most of these disorders involve the hands,

arms, or neck and shoulder area. Other names for repetitive motion disorders include repetitive trauma disorders, repetitive strain injuries (RSIs), overuse syndrome, work-related disorders, and regional musculoskeletal disorders.

Description

Repetitive motion disorders are characterized by **pain**, loss of strength and coordination, numbness or tingling, and sometimes redness or swelling in the affected area. The symptoms come on gradually, and are usually relieved temporarily by resting or avoiding the use of the affected body part. Repetitive motion disorders are commonly thought of as work related, but they can occur as a result of academic, leisure-time, or household activities as well.

Demographics

The demographics of repetitive motion disorders vary according to the specific syndrome. As of 2004, about 50% of all industrial injuries in the United States and Canada are attributed to overuse disorders. Professional athletes, dancers, and musicians experience one of these disorders at a much higher percentage at some point in their careers. The Institute of Medicine's 2001 study, Musculoskeletal Disorders and the Workplace, reported that nearly a million American workers were treated in 1999 for work-related pain or impaired function in the arms, hands, or back. Other experts estimate that overuse injuries cost the United States economy between $27 million and $45 million every year.

Race is not known to be a factor in repetitive motion disorders. Gender has a significant effect on the demographics of some disorders, but it is not clear whether the higher incidence of some disorders in women reflects different occupational choices for men and women, or whether it reflects biological differences. For example, de Quervain's syndrome is a common overuse disorder in women involved with childcare, because repeated lifting and carrying of small children places severe strains on the wrist joint. On the other hand, some researchers think that the greater frequency of this disorder in women is related to the effects of female sex hormones on connective tissue, as women's ligaments are slightly looser during pregnancy and at certain points in the menstrual cycle.

Some repetitive motion disorders appear to be age related. **Carpal tunnel syndrome** is more common in middle-aged than in younger women, and trigger finger is most common in people aged 55–60. It is not yet known whether the widespread use of computers in the workplace will change the age distribution of repetitive motion disorders as present workers grow older.

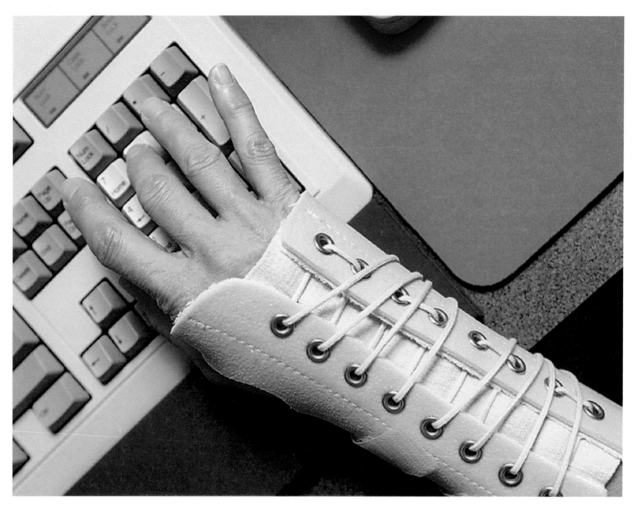

The Industrial Revolution led to increased job specialization, which meant that more and more workers were employed doing one task repeatedly rather than many different tasks. Office work is a case in point. *(© Photo Reasearchers. Reproduced by permission.)*

Causes and symptoms

SOFT TISSUE DAMAGE Repetitive motion disorders are the end result of a combination of factors. One basic cause of repetitive motion disorders, however, is microtraumas, which are tiny damages to or tears in soft tissue that occur from routine stresses on the body or repeated use of specific muscles and joints. When microtraumas are not healed during sleep or daily rest periods, they accumulate over time, causing tissue damage, inflammation, and the activation of pain receptors in peripheral nerves.

NERVE COMPRESSION Some repetitive motion disorders are associated with entrapment neuropathies, which are functional disorders of the **peripheral nervous system**. In an entrapment neuropathy, a nerve is damaged by compression as it passes through a bony or fibrous tunnel. Carpal tunnel syndrome, de Quervain's syndrome, ulnar nerve syndrome, and **thoracic outlet syndrome** are examples of entrapment neuropathies.

Compression damages peripheral nerves by limiting their blood supply. Even slight pressures on a nerve can limit the flow of blood through the smaller blood vessels surrounding the nerve. As the pressure increases, transmission of nerve impulses is affected and the patient's sensation and coordination are affected, with further increases in **nerve compression** producing greater distortion of sensation and range of motion.

TECHNOLOGICAL AND SOCIAL FACTORS Economic and social factors that have affected people's occupations and leisure-time activities over the past two centuries have contributed to the increase in repetitive motion disorders. The Industrial Revolution led to increased job specialization, which meant that more and more workers were employed doing one task repeatedly rather than many different tasks. In addition, industrialization brought about the invention of complex tools and machinery that affect the tissues and organs of the human body in many ways.

The high levels of psychological and emotional tension in modern life also contribute to repetitive stress injuries by increasing the physical stresses on muscles and joints.

INDIVIDUAL RISK FACTORS Risk factors that are associated with repetitive stress injuries include the following:

- Awkward or incorrect body postures. Each joint in the body has a position within its range of motion in which it is least likely to become injured. This position is called the neutral position. Any deviation from the neutral position puts increased strain on body tissues. Inadequate work space, using athletic or job-related equipment that is not proportioned to one's height, or improper technique are common reasons for RSIs related to body posture.

- Use of excessive force to perform a task. Pounding on piano keys or hammering harder than is necessary to drive nails are examples of this risk factor.

- Extended periods of static work. This type of work requires muscular effort, but no movement takes place. Instead, the muscles contract, preventing blood from reaching tissues to nourish the cells and carry away waste products. Over time, the muscle tissue loses its ability to repair microtraumas. Examples of static work include sitting at a desk for hours on end or holding the arms over the head while painting a ceiling.

- Activities that require repetitive movements. Assembly-line work and word processing are examples of job-related repetitive motion. In addition, such leisure-time activities as knitting, embroidery, gardening, model construction, golf or tennis, etc. can have the same long-term effects on the body as work-related activities.

- Mechanical injury. Tools with poorly designed handles that cut into the skin or concentrate pressure on a small area of the hand often contribute to overuse disorders.

- Vibration. There are two types of vibration that can cause damage to the body. One type is segmental vibration, which occurs when the source of the vibration affects only the part of the body in direct contact with it. An example of segmental vibration is a dentist's use of a high-speed drill. Overexposure of the hands to segmental vibration can eventually damage the fingers, leading to Raynaud's phenomenon. The second type is whole-body vibration, which occurs when the vibrations are transmitted throughout the body. Long-distance truckers and jackhammer operators often develop back injuries as the result of long-term whole-body vibration.

- Temperature extremes. Cold temperatures decrease blood flow in the extremities, while high temperatures lead to dehydration and rapid **fatigue**. In both cases, blood circulation is either decreased or redirected, thus slowing down the process of normal tissue recovery.

- Psychological stress. People who are worried, afraid, or angry often carry their tension in their neck, back, or shoulder muscles. This tension reduces blood circulation in the affected tissues, thus interfering with tissue recovery. In addition, emotional stress has been shown to influence people's perception of physical pain; workers who are unhappy in their jobs, for example, are more likely to seek treatment for work-related disorders.

- Structural abnormalities. These abnormalities include congenital deformities in bones and muscles, changes in the shape of a bone from healed breaks or fractures, bone spurs, and tumors. Overdevelopment of certain muscle groups from athletic workouts may result in entrapment neuropathies in the shoulder area.

- Other systemic conditions or diseases. People with such disorders as rheumatoid arthritis (RA), joint infections, hypothyroidism, or diabetes are at increased risk of developing repetitive motion disorders. Pregnancy is a risk factor for overuse disorders affecting the hands because of the increased amount of fluid in the joints of the wrists and fingers.

Symptoms

The symptoms of repetitive motion disorders include the following:

- Pain. The pain of an RSI is typically felt as an aching sensation that gets worse if the affected joint(s) or limb is moved or used. The pain may be severe enough to wake the patient at night.

- Paresthesias. Paresthesia refers to an abnormal sensation of pricking, tingling, burning, or "insects crawling beneath the skin" in the absence of an external stimulus.

- Numbness, coldness, or loss of sensation occur in the affected area.

- Clumsiness, weakness, or loss of coordination result.

- Impaired range of motion or locking of a joint occur.

- Popping, clicking, or crackling sounds in a joint are experienced.

- Swelling or redness in the affected area are observed.

Diagnosis
History and physical examination

The diagnosis of a repetitive motion disorder begins with taking the patient's history, including occupational history. The doctor will ask about the specific symptoms in the affected part, particularly if the patient suffers from rheumatoid arthritis, diabetes, or other general conditions as well as overuse of the joint or limb.

The next step is physical examination of the affected area. The doctor will typically palpate (feel) or press on

Key Terms

Alexander technique   A form of movement therapy that emphasizes correct posture and the proper positioning of the head with regard to the spine.

de Quervain's syndrome   Inflammation of the tendons contained within the wrist, associated with aching pain in the wrist and thumb. Named for the Swiss surgeon who first described it in 1895, the syndrome is sometimes called washerwoman's sprain because it is commonly caused by overuse of the wrist.

Entrapment neuropathy   A disorder of the peripheral nervous system in which a nerve is damaged by compression as it passes through a bony or fibrous passage or canal. Many repetitive motion disorders are associated with entrapment neuropathies.

Ergonomics   The branch of science that deals with human work and the efficient use of energy, including anatomical, physiological, biomechanical, and psychosocial factors.

Median nerve   The nerve that supplies the forearm, wrist area, and many of the joints of the hand.

Neuropathy   Any diseased condition of the nervous system.

Paresthesia   The medical term for an abnormal touch sensation, usually tingling, burning, or prickling, that develops in the absence of an external stimulus. Paresthesias are a common symptom of repetitive motion disorders.

Peripheral nervous system   The part of the human nervous system outside the brain and spinal cord.

Raynaud's phenomenon   A disorder characterized by episodic attacks of loss of circulation in the fingers or toes. Most cases of Raynaud's are not work-related; however, the disorder occasionally develops in workers who operate vibrating tools as part of their job, and is sometimes called vibration-induced white finger.

Transcutaneous electrical nerve stimulation (TENS)   A form of treatment for chronic pain that involves the use of a patient-controlled device for transmitting mild electrical impulses through the skin over the injured area.

Trigger finger   An overuse disorder of the hand in which one or more fingers tend to lock or "trigger" when the patient tries to extend the finger.

Ulnar nerve   The nerve that supplies some of the forearm muscles, the elbow joint, and many of the short muscles of the hand.

---

the sore area to determine whether there is swelling as well as pain. He or she will then perform a series of maneuvers to evaluate the range of motion in the affected joint(s), listen for crackles or other sounds when the joint is moved, and test for weakness or instability in the limb or joint. There are simple physical tests for specific repetitive motion disorders. For example, the Finkelstein test is used to evaluate a patient for de Quervain's syndrome. The patient is asked to fold the thumb across the palm of the affected hand and then bend the fingers over the thumb. A person with de Quervain's will experience sharp pain when the doctor moves the hand sideways in the direction of the elbow. Tinel's test is used to diagnose carpal tunnel syndrome. The doctor gently taps with a rubber hammer along the inside of the wrist above the median nerve to see whether the patient experiences paresthesias.

Laboratory tests

Laboratory tests of blood or tissue fluid are not ordinarily ordered unless the doctor suspects an infection or wishes to rule out diabetes, anemia, or thyroid imbalance.

Imaging studies

Imaging studies may be ordered to rule out other conditions that may be causing the patient's symptoms or to identify areas of nerve compression. When surgery is being planned, x rays may be helpful in identifying stress fractures, damage to cartilage, or other abnormalities in bones and joints. **Magnetic resonance imaging (MRI)** can be used to identify injuries to tendons, ligaments, and muscles as well as areas of nerve entrapment.

Electrodiagnostic studies

The most common electrodiagnostic tests used to evaluate repetitive motion disorders are **electromyography** (EMG) and nerve conduction studies (NCS). In EMG, the doctor inserts thin needles in specific muscles and observes the electrical signals that are displayed on a screen. This test helps to pinpoint which muscles and nerves are affected by pain. Nerve conduction studies are done to determine whether specific nerves have been damaged. The doctor positions two sets of electrodes on the patient's skin over the muscles in the affected area. One set of electrodes stimulates the nerves supplying that muscle by delivering a mild electrical shock; the other set records the nerve's electrical signals on a machine.

Treatment team

A mild repetitive motion disorder may be treated by a primary care physician. If conservative treatment is ineffective, the patient may be referred to an orthopedic surgeon or neurosurgeon for further evaluation and surgical treatment. Patients whose disorders are related to job dissatisfaction, or who have had to give up their occupation or favorite activity because of their disorder, may benefit from psychotherapy.

Physical therapists and occupational therapists are an important part of the treatment team, advising patients about proper use of the injured body part and developing a home **exercise** program. Some patients benefit from having their workplace and equipment evaluated by the occupational therapist or an ergonomics expert. Professional athletes, dancers, or musicians usually consult an expert in their specific field for evaluation of faulty posture or technique.

Treatment

Conservative treatment

Conservative treatment for overuse injuries typically includes:

- Resting the affected part. Complete rest should last no longer than two to three days, however. What is known as "relative rest" is better for the patient because it maintains range of motion in the affected part, prevents loss of muscle strength, and lowers the risk of "sick behavior." Sick behavior refers to using an injury or illness to gain attention or care and concern from others.

- Applying ice packs or gentle heat.

- Oral medications. These may include mild pain relievers (usually NSAIDs); amitriptyline or another tricyclic antidepressant; or vitamin B6.

- Injections. Corticosteroids may be injected into joints to lower inflammation and swelling. In some cases, local anesthetics may also be given by injection.

- Splinting. Splints are most commonly used to treat overuse injuries of the hand or wrist; they can be custom-molded by an occupational therapist.

- Ergonomic corrections in the home or workplace. These may include changing the height of chairs or computer keyboards; scheduling frequent breaks from computer work or musical practice; correcting one's posture; and similar measures.

- Transcutaneous electrical nerve stimulation (TENS). TENS involves the use of a patient-controlled portable device that sends mild electrical impulses through injured tissues via electrodes placed over the skin. It is reported to relieve pain in 75–80% of patients treated for repetitive motion disorders.

Surgery

Repetitive motion disorders are treated with surgery only when conservative measures fail to relieve the patient's pain after a trial of six to 12 weeks. The most common surgical procedures performed for these disorders include nerve decompression, tendon release, and repair of loose or torn ligaments.

Complementary and alternative (CAM) treatments

CAM treatments that have been shown to be effective in treating repetitive motion disorders include:

- **Acupuncture**. Studies funded by the National Center for Complementary and Alternative Medicine (NCCAM) since 1998 have found that acupuncture is an effective treatment for pain related to repetitive motion disorders.

- Sports massage, Swedish massage, and shiatsu.

- Yoga and tai chi. The gentle stretching in these forms of exercise helps to improve blood circulation and maintain range of motion without tissue damage.

- Alexander technique. The Alexander technique is an approach to body movement that emphasizes correct posture, particularly the proper position of the head with respect to the spine. It is often recommended for dancers, musicians, and computer users.

- Hydrotherapy. Warm whirlpool baths improve circulation and relieve pain in injured joints and soft tissue.

Recovery and rehabilitation

Recovery from a repeated motion disorder may take only a few days of rest or modified activity, or it may take several months when surgery is required.

Rehabilitation is tailored to the individual patient and the specific disorder involved. Rehabilitation programs for repetitive motion disorders focus on recovering strength in the injured body part, maintaining or improving range of motion, and learning ways to lower the risk of re-injuring the affected part. Professional musicians, dancers, and athletes require highly specialized rehabilitation programs.

Clinical trials

As of early 2004, there were four **clinical trials** related to repetitive motion disorders sponsored by the National Institutes of Health (NIH) that are recruiting subjects. One is a comparison of amitriptyline (an antidepressant medication) and acupuncture as treatments for CTS. A second study will evaluate the effectiveness of a protective brace in preventing overuse disorders associated with hand-held power tools. The third study will evaluate the effects of fast-paced assembly-line work on the health of rural women. The fourth study is a comparison of surgical and nonsurgical treatments for CTS.

Prognosis

The prognosis for recovery from repetitive motion disorders depends on the specific disorder, the degree of damage to the nerves and other structures involved, and the patient's compliance with exercise or rehabilitation programs. Most patients experience adequate pain relief from either conservative measures or surgery. Some, however, will not recover full use of the affected body part and must change occupations or give up the activity that produced the disorder.

Resources

BOOKS

National Research Council and Institute of Medicine (IOM). *Musculoskeletal Disorders and the Workplace: Low Back and Upper Extremities.* Washington, DC: National Academy Press, 2001.

"Neurovascular Syndromes: Carpal Tunnel Syndrome." *The Merck Manual of Diagnosis and Therapy*, edited by Mark H. Beers, MD, and Robert Berkow, MD. Whitehouse Station, NJ: Merck Research Laboratories, 2002.

Pelletier, Kenneth R., MD. *The Best Alternative Medicine*, Part II, "CAM Therapies for Specific Conditions: Carpal Tunnel Syndrome." New York: Simon & Schuster, 2002.

"Tendon Problems: Digital Tendinitis and Tenosynovitis." *The Merck Manual of Diagnosis and Therapy*, edited by Mark H. Beers, MD, and Robert Berkow, MD. Whitehouse Station, NJ: Merck Research Laboratories, 2002.

PERIODICALS

Andersen, J. H., J. F. Thomsen, E. Overgaard, et al. "Computer Use and Carpal Tunnel Syndrome: A 1-Year Follow-Up Study." *Journal of the American Medical Association* 289 (June 11, 2003): 2963–2969.

Fuller, David A., MD. "Carpal Tunnel Syndrome." *eMedicine* October 15, 2003 (March 23, 2004). <http://www.emedicine.com/orthoped/topic455.htm>.

Hogan, K. A., and R. H. Gross. "Overuse Injuries in Pediatric Athletes." *Orthopedic Clinics of North America* 34 (July 2003): 405–415.

Kale, Satischandra, MD. "Trigger Finger." *eMedicine* February 25, 2002 (March 23, 2004). <http://www.emedicine.com/orthoped/topic570.htm>.

Kaye, Vladimir, MD, and Murray E. Brandstater, PhD. "Transcutaenous Electrical Nerve Stimulation." *eMedicine* January 29, 2002 (March 23, 2004). <http://www.emedicine.com/pmr/topic206.htm>.

Kern, R. Z. "The Electrodiagnosis of Ulnar Nerve Entrapment at the Elbow." *Canadian Journal of Neurological Sciences/Journal canadien des sciences neurologiques* 30 (November 2003): 314–319.

Kryger, A. I., J. H. Andersen, C. F. Lassen, et al. "Does Computer Use Pose An Occupational Hazard for Forearm Pain; from the NUDATA Study." *Occupational and Environmental Medicine* 60 (November 2003): e14.

Leclerc, A., J. F. Chastang, I. Niedhammer, et al. "Incidence of Shoulder Pain in Repetitive Work." *Occupational and Environmental Medicine* 61 (January 2004): 39–44.

Meals, Roy A., MD. "De Quervain Tenosynovitis." *eMedicine* April 15, 2002 (March 23, 2004). <http://www.emedicine.com/orthoped/topic482.htm>

Nourissat, G., P. Chamagne, and C. Dumontier. "Reasons Why Musicians Consult Hand Surgeons." [in French] *Revue de chirurgie orthopÈdique et rÈparatrice de l'appareil moteur* 89 (October 2003): 524–531.

Stern, Mark, MD, and Scott P. Steinmann, MD. "Ulnar Nerve Entrapment." *eMedicine* 8 January 2004 (March 23, 2004). <http://www.emedicine.com/orthoped/topic574.htm>.

Strober, Jonathan B., MD. "Writer's Cramp." *eMedicine* January 18, 2002 (March 23, 2004). <http://www.emedicine.com/neuro/topic614.htm>.

Strum, Scott, MD. "Overuse Injury." *eMedicine* September 14, 2001 (March 23, 2004). <http://www.emedicine.com/pmr/topic97.htm>.

Tallia, A. F., and D. A. Cardone. "Diagnostic and Therapeutic Injection of the Wrist and Hand Region." *American Family Physician* 67 (February 15, 2003): 745–750.

Valachi, B., and K. Valachi. "Mechanisms Leading to Musculoskeletal Disorders in Dentistry." *Journal of the American Dental Association* 134 (October 2003): 1344–1350.

OTHER

National Institute of Neurological Disorders and Stroke (NINDS). *NINDS Thoracic Outlet Syndrome Information Page*. (March 23, 2004). <http://www.ninds.nih.gov/health_and_medical/disorders/thoracic_doc.htm>.

ORGANIZATIONS

American Academy of Orthopaedic Surgeons (AAOS). 6300 North River Road, Rosemont, IL 60018-4262. (847) 823-7186 or (800) 346-AAOS; Fax: (847) 823-8125. <http://www.aaos.org>.

American Society for Surgery of the Hand (ASSH). 6300 North River Road, Suite 800, Rosemont, IL 60018. (847) 384-8300; Fax: (847) 384-1435. info@hand-surg.org. <http://www.hand-surg.org>.

National Institute for Occupational Safety and Health (NIOSH). Centers for Disease Control and Prevention, 1600 Clifton Road, Atlanta, GA 30333. (404) 639-3534 or (800) 311-3435. <http://www.cdc.gov/niosh/homepage.html>.

National Institute of Arthritis and Musculoskeletal and Skin Diseases (NIAMS) Information Clearinghouse, National

Institutes of Health. 1 AMS Circle, Bethesda, MD 20892-3675. (301) 495-4844 or (877) 22-NIAMS; Fax: (301) 718-6366. NIAMSinfo@mail.nih.gov. <http://www.niams.nih.gov>.

National Institute of Neurological Disorders and Stroke (NINDS). 9000 Rockville Pike, Bethesda, MD 20892. (301) 496-5751 or (800) 352-9424. <http://www.ninds.nih.gov>.

Rebecca J. Frey, PhD

Respite

Definition

Respite literally means a period of rest or relief. Respite care provides a caregiver temporary relief from the responsibilities of caring for individuals with chronic physical or mental disabilities. Respite care is often referred to as a gift of time.

Description

Respite was developed in response to the deinstitutionalization movement of the 1960s and 1970s. Maintaining individuals in their natural homes rather than placing them in long-term care facilities was viewed as beneficial to the individual, the involved family, and society (in terms of lowered health care costs). The primary purpose of respite care is to relieve caregiver stress, thereby enabling them to continue caring for the individual with a disability.

Respite care is typically provided for individuals with disorders related to aging (**dementia**, frail health), terminal illnesses, chronic health issues, or developmental disabilities. More recently, children with behavior disorders have also been eligible for respite care. Respite care is usually recreational and does not include therapy or treatment for the individual with the disability.

Caregivers frequently experience stress in the forms of physical **fatigue**, psychological distress (resentment, frustration, anxiety, guilt, **depression**), and disruption in relations with other family members. The emotional aspects of caring for a family member are often more taxing than the physical demands. Increased caregiver stress may result in health problems such as ulcers, high blood pressure, difficulty sleeping, weight loss or gain, or breathing difficulties.

Types of respite

Length of respite care can be anywhere from a few hours to several weeks. Services may be used frequently or infrequently, such as for emergencies, vacations, one day per week or month, weekends, or everyday.

A variety of facilities provide respite care services. The type of service available is often closely related to the characteristics of the facility, including:

• In-home respite services consist of a worker who comes to the family home while the caregiver is away. These services are usually provided by agencies that recruit, screen, and train workers. This type of respite is usually less disruptive to the individual with the disability, provided there is a good match between the worker and the individual. However, issues of reliability and trustworthiness of the worker can be an additional source of stress for the caregiver.

• Respite centers are residential facilities specifically designed for respite care. Adult day care programs and respite camps also fall into this category. This type of respite offers more peace of mind to the caregiver, and may provide a stimulating environment for the individual with the disability. However, centers usually restrict length of stay and may exclude individuals based on severity of disability.

• Institutional settings sometimes reserve spaces to be used for respite purposes. These include skilled nursing facilities, intermediate care facilities, group homes, senior housing, regular day care or after-school programs for children, and hospitals. Some of these facilities provide higher levels of care, but are less home-like. The individual with the disability may oppose staying in an institutional setting or may fear abandonment.

• Licensed foster care providers can also provide respite services in their homes.

Funding

Costs of respite care present a financial burden to many families. Community mental health centers often fund respite services if the individual meets certain criteria, including eligibility for Medicaid. Wraparound programs (also accessed through community mental health centers) for children with emotional or behavioral disorders also pay for respite services. Veteran's Administration hospitals provide respite care at little or no charge if the individual receiving the care is a veteran (but not if the caregiver is a veteran). Private insurance companies rarely pay for respite, and many respite providers do not accept this form of payment. Some respite facilities have sliding-scale fees. Other facilities operate as a co-op, where caregivers work at the facility in exchange for respite services.

In addition, respite agencies may have difficulty recruiting and retaining qualified employees, because limited funding prevents agencies from offering desirable salaries. The high turnover and unavailability of employees may result in delays in service delivery or family dissatisfaction with services.

Key Terms

Behavior disorders   Disorders characterized by disruptive behaviors such as conduct disorder, oppositional defiant disorder, and attention-deficit/hyperactivity disorder.

Community mental health centers   Organizations that manage and deliver a comprehensive range of mental health services, education, and outreach to residents of a given community.

Deinstitutionalization   The process of moving people out of mental hospitals into treatment programs or halfway houses in local communities. With this movement, the responsibility for care shifted from large (often governmental) agencies to families and community organizations.

Developmental disabilities   Disabilities that are present from birth and delay or prevent normal development, such as mental retardation or autism.

Intermediate care facility   An inpatient facility that provides periodic nursing care.

Medicaid   A program jointly funded by state and federal governments that reimburses hospitals and physicians for the care of individuals who cannot pay for their own medical expenses. These individuals may be in low-income households or may have chronic disabilities.

Skilled nursing facility   An inpatient facility that provides 24-hour nursing services to individuals in need of extended care.

Veteran's Administration hospitals   Medical facilities operated by the federal government explicitly for veterans of the United States military.

Wraparound   A relatively new form of mental health service delivery that strives to accommodate all family members based on self-defined needs, flexibly incorporating both formal and informal community services.

Barriers to using respite services

Recent research suggests that families who use respite tend to have higher levels of perceived stress, lower levels of support from others, and fewer resources. In many of these families, the individuals in need of care have more severe disabilities, problem behaviors such as aggression or self-injury, and communication difficulties; are school-aged; and are more dependent for basic needs such as eating, toileting, and dressing.

It has been well documented that many families eligible for respite care never utilize these services. Research regarding the use, availability, and effectiveness of respite care is still in the preliminary stages. Various reasons for non-utilization of respite include:

• Unfamiliarity: Some families are unaware that such services exist, or may be uncertain about how to access services. This implies a need for improved referral services.

• Funding: Limited funding may prevent some families from receiving services.

• Caregiver qualities: Some caregivers experience guilt or anxiety over allowing someone else to care for their loved one. Being able to maintain one's family independently may be tied to gender roles or cultural customs. Relatives and friends may assist in caregiving, making formal respite unnecessary.

• Care recipient qualities: Occasionally the individual with the disability is opposed to respite care. He or she may not trust strangers or may refuse to leave home. In other instances, the individual may have behaviors, or require physical care, that is too challenging for the respite provider.

• Program qualities: Many researchers believe that respite programs are not adequately meeting the needs of families. In some cases, times that services are offered are inconvenient. Individuals with severe disabilities who pose the most need for services are sometimes excluded.

Many caregivers obtain respite in informal ways not offered by respite services. Some researchers have suggested that respite care should be just one form of service available to caregivers. Other services that may alleviate caregiver stress could include home-delivered meals, transportation assistance, recreational resources, or care skills training.

Resources

BOOKS

Ownby, Lisa L. *Partners Plus: Families and Caregivers in Partnerships: A Family-Centered Guide to Respite Care.* Washington, DC: Child Development Resources, U.S. Department of Education, Office of Educational Research and Improvement, Educational Resources Information Center, 1999.

Tepper, Lynn M. and John A. Toner, eds. *Respite Care: Programs, Problems, and Solutions.*Philadelphia: The Charles Press, 1993.

PERIODICALS

Chan, Jeffrey B., and Jeff Sigafoos. "A Review of Child and Family Characteristics Related to the Use of Respite Care in Developmental Disability Services." *Child and Youth Care Forum* 29, no. 1 (2000): 27-37.

Chappell, Neena L., R. Colin Reid, and Elizabeth Dow. "Respite Reconsidered: A Typology of Meanings Based on the Caregiver's Point of View." *Journal of Aging Studies* 15, no. 2 (2001): 201-216.

ORGANIZATIONS

The Arc National Headquarters, P.O. Box 1047, Arlington, TX 76004. (817) 261-6003; (817) 277-0553 TDD. thearc@metronet.com.<http://www.thearc.org>.

ARCH National Respite Network and Resource Center. Chapel Hill Training-Outreach Project, 800 Eastowne Drive, Suite 105, Chapel Hill, NC 27514. (888) 671-2594; (919) 490-5577. <http://www.chtop.com>.

National Aging Information Center. Administration on Aging, 330 Independence Avenue, SW, Room 4656, Washington, DC 20201. (202) 619-7501. <http://www.aoa.gov/naic>.

National Information Center for Children and Youth with Disabilities. P.O. Box 1492, Washington, DC 20013. (800)-695-0285. <http://www.nichcy.org>.

OTHER

Senior Care Web. <http://www2.seniorcareweb.com>.

Sandra L. Friedrich, MA
Rosalyn Carson-DeWitt, MD

Restless legs syndrome

Definition

Restless legs syndrome (RLS) is a neurological disorder characterized by uncomfortable sensations in the legs and, less commonly, the arms. These sensations are exacerbated (heightened) when the person with RLS is at rest. The sensations are described as crawly, tingly, prickly and occasionally painful. They result in a nearly insuppressible urge to move around. Symptoms are often associated with sleep disturbances.

Description

Restless legs syndrome is a sensory-motor disorder that causes uncomfortable feelings in the legs, especially during periods of inactivity. Some people also report sensations in the arms, but this occurs much more rarely. The sensations occur deep in the legs and are usually described with terms that imply movement such as prickly, creepy-crawly, boring, itching, achy, pulling, tugging and painful.

The symptoms result in an irrepressible urge to move the leg and are relieved when the person suffering from RLS voluntarily moves. Symptoms tend to be worse in the evening or at night.

Restless legs syndrome is associated with another disorder called periodic limb movements in sleep (PLMS). It is estimated that four out of five patients with RLS also suffer from PLMS. PLMS is characterized by jerking leg movements while sleeping that may occur as frequently as every 20 seconds. These jerks disrupt sleep by causing continual arousals throughout the night.

People with both RLS and PLMS are prone to abnormal levels of exhaustion during the day because they are unable to sleep properly at night. They may have trouble concentrating at work, at school or during social activities. They may also have mood swings and difficulty with interpersonal relationships. **Depression** and anxiety may also result from the lack of sleep. RLS affects people who want to travel or attend events that require sitting for long periods of time.

Demographics

As much as 10% of the population of the United States and Europe may suffer from some degree of restless legs syndrome. Fewer cases are indicated in India, Japan and Singapore, suggesting racial or ethnic factors play a role in the disorder. Although the demographics can vary greatly, the majority of people suffering from RLS are female. The age of onset also varies greatly, but the number of people suffering from RLS increases with age. However, many people with RLS report that they had symptoms of the disorder in their childhood. These symptoms were often disregarded as growing pains or hyperactivity.

Causes and symptoms

Restless legs syndrome is categorized in two ways. Primary RLS occurs in the absence of other medical symptoms, while secondary RLS is usually associated with some other medical disorder. Although the cause of primary RLS is currently unknown, a large amount of research into the cause of RLS is taking place. Researchers at Johns Hopkins University published a study in July 2003 suggesting that iron deficiencies may be related to the disorder. They dissected brains from cadavers of people who suffered from RLS and found that the cells in the midbrain were not receiving enough iron. Other researchers suggest that RLS may be related to a chemical imbalance of the neurotransmitter dopamine in the brain. There is also evidence that RLS has a genetic component. RLS occurs three to five times more frequently in an immediate family member of someone who has RLS than in the general population. A site on a chromosome that may

Key Terms

Anemia A condition in which there is an abnormally low number of red blood cells in the bloodstream. It may be due to loss of blood, an increase in red blood cell destruction, or a decrease in red blood cell production. Major symptoms are paleness, shortness of breath, unusually fast or strong heart beats, and tiredness.

Anticonvulsant drugs Drugs used to prevent convulsions or seizures. They often are prescribed in the treatment of epilepsy.

Benzodiazepine drugs One of a class of drugs that have a hypnotic and sedative action, used mainly as tranquilizers to control symptoms of anxiety. Diazepam (Valium), alprazolam (Xanax), and chlordiazepoxide (Librium) are all benzodiazepines.

Dopamine-receptor agonists (DAs) The older class of antipsychotic medications, also called neuroleptics. These drugs primarily block the site on nerve cells that normally receives the brain chemical dopamine.

Opioid Any natural or synthetic substance that produces the same effects as an opiate, such as pain relief, sedation, constipation and respiratory depression. Some opioids are produced by the human body (e.g., endorphins), while others are produced in the laboratory (e.g., methadone).

Periodic Limb Movements in Sleep (PLMS) Random movements of the arms or legs that occur at regular intervals of time during sleep.

contain a gene for RLS has been identified by molecular biologists.

In many people, other medical conditions play a role in RLS and the disorder is therefore termed secondary RLS. People with peripheral neuropathies (injury to nerves in the arms and legs) may experience RLS. Such neuropathies may result from diabetes or alcoholism. Other chronic diseases such as kidney disorders and rheumatoid arthritis may result in RLS. Iron deficiencies and blood anemias are often associated with RLS and symptoms of the disease usually decrease once blood iron levels have been corrected. Attention deficit/hyperactivity disorder has also been implicated in RLS. Pregnant women often suffer from RLS, especially in the third trimester. Some people find that high levels of caffeine intake may result in RLS.

The symptoms of RLS are all associated with unpleasant feelings in the limbs. The words used to describe these feelings are various, but include such adjectives as deep-seated crawling, jittery, tingling, burning, aching, pulling, painful, itchy or prickly. They are usually not described as a muscle cramp or numbness. Most often the sensations occur during periods of inactivity. They are characterized by an urge to get up and move. Such movements include stretching, walking, jogging or simply jiggling the legs. The feelings worsen in the evening.

A variety of symptoms are associated with RLS, but may not be characteristic of every case. Some people with RLS report involuntary arm and leg movements during the night. Others have difficulty falling asleep and are sleepy or fatigued during the day. Many people with RLS

have leg discomfort that is not explained by routine medical exams.

Diagnosis

Restless legs syndrome cannot currently be diagnosed using any laboratory tests or via a routine physical examination. Diagnosis is based on information given to a doctor by the patient regarding his or her symptoms. Usually the doctor takes a complete medical history as well as a family history. The International Restless Legs Syndrome Study group has proposed a set of criteria that can be used while taking a medical history in order to diagnose RLS:

- a compelling urge to move the arms and legs

- restlessness that manifests itself in pacing, tossing and turning and/or rubbing the legs

- symptoms that worsen when the patient is resting and are relieved when the patient is active

- symptoms that worsen at the end of the day

In addition, a physical examination will be made to identify if there are any other medical conditions, such as neurological disorders or blood disorders that may be causing secondary RLS. A doctor who suspects a patient has RLS may suggest that the person spend the night in a sleep clinic to determine whether the patient also suffers from PLMS.

Treatment

Treatment for restless legs syndrome is generally two-pronged, consisting of making lifestyle changes and using medications to relieve some of the symptoms. Lifestyle changes involve making changes to the diet, exercising and performing other self-directed activities, and practicing good sleep hygiene. Although the United States Food and Drug Administration has not yet approved any drugs for treating RLS, four classes of pharmaceuticals have been found effective for treating RLS: dopaminergic agents, **benzodiazepines**, opioids and **anticonvulsants**.

Lifestyle changes

Simple changes to the diet have proven effective for some people suffering from RLS. Vitamin deficiencies are a common problem in RLA patients. In patients with RLS, most physicians will check the levels of blood serum ferritin, which can indicate low iron storage. If these levels are below 50 mcg/L, then supplemental iron should be added to the diet. Other physicians have found that supplements of vitamin E, folic acid and B vitamins, and magnesium provide relief to symptoms or RLS. Reducing or eliminating caffeine and alcohol consumption has been effective in other patients.

Many who suffer from RLS find that **exercise** and massage help reduce symptoms. Walking or stretching before bed, taking a hot bath and using massage or acupressure help improve sleep. Practicing relaxation techniques such as mediation, yoga and biofeedback have also been found to be useful.

Good sleep hygiene includes having a restful, cool sleep environment and sleeping during consistent hours every night. Often people who suffer from RLS find that going to sleep later at night and sleeping later into the morning result in a better sleep.

Pharmaceuticals

Dopaminergic agents are the first type of drug prescribed in the treatment of RLS. Most commonly doctors prescribe dopamine-receptor agonists that are used to treat **Parkinson's disease** such as Mirapex (pramipexole), Permax (pergolide) and Requip (ropinirole). Sinemet (carbidopa/levodopa), which is a drug that adds dopamine to the nervous system, is also commonly prescribed. Sinemet has been used the more frequently than other drugs in treating RLS, but recently a problem known as augmentation has been associated with its use. When augmentation develops, symptoms of RLS will return earlier in the day and increasing the dose will not improve the symptoms.

Benzodiazepines are drugs that sedate and are typically taken before bedtime so that a patient with RLS can sleep more soundly. The most commonly prescribed sedative in RLS is Klonopin (clonazepam).

Opioids are synthetic narcotics that relieve **pain** and cause drowsiness. They are usually taken in the evening. The most commonly used opioids prescribed for RLS include Darvon or Darvocet (propoxyphene), Dolophine (methadone), Percocet (oxycodone), Ultram (Tramadol) and Vicodin (hydrocodone). One danger associated with opioids is that they can be addicting.

Anticonvulsants are drugs that were developed to prevent **seizures** in patients with **epilepsy** and **stroke**. Some RLS patients who report pain in their limbs have reported that these drugs, particularly **Gabapentin** (neurontin), are useful for relieving symptoms.

A few drugs have been found to worsen symptoms of RLS and they should be avoided by patients exhibiting RLS symptoms. These include anti-nausea drugs such as Antivert, Atarax, Compazine and Phenergan. Calcium channel blockers that are often used to treat heart conditions should be avoided. In addition, most anti-depressants tend to exacerbate symptoms of RLS. Finally, antihistamines such as Benadryl have been found to aggravate RLS symptoms in some people.

Clinical trials

A broad spectrum of **clinical trials** are currently underway to study RLS. The Restless Legs Syndrome Foundation maintains a website that lists a variety of studies throughout the United States that are currently recruiting volunteers. The studies test the effects of a variety of treatments including intravenous iron supplements, exercise and sleeping aids on RLS. More information can be found at <http://www.rls.org/frames/home_frame.htm>.

The National Institutes of Health support three clinical trials to gain information about RLS. The first study investigates the effects of the drug Ropinirole, a dopamine-receptor agonist, on spinal cord reflexes and on symptoms of restless legs syndrome. A second study is testing whether or not sensorimotor gating (the brain's ability to filter multiple stimuli) is deficient in patients who suffer from RLS. The goal of the third study is to improve understanding of neurological conditions associated with RLS by taking careful histories and following the treatment provided by primary car physicians. Information on all three trials can be found at <http://clinicaltrials.gov/search/term=Restless%20Legs%20Syndrome> or by calling the Patient Recruitment and Public Liaison Office at 1-800-411-1222 or sending an electronic message to prpl@mail.cc.nih.gov.

Prognosis

RLS is usually compatible with an active, healthy life when symptoms are controlled and nutritional deficits are corrected.

Resources
BOOKS
Cunningham, Chet. *Stopping Restless Legs Syndrome.* United Research Publishers, 2000.

OTHER

"Do You have Restless Legs Syndrome?" *Restless Leg Syndrome Foundation.* (January 23, 2003). <http://www.rls.org/frames/home_frame.htm>.

"Facts about Restless Legs." *National Sleep Foundation.* (June 2003). <http://www.sleepfoundation.org/publications/fact_rls.cfm>.

"Facts About Restless Legs Syndrome (RLS)." *National Heat Blood and Lung Institute.* (October 1996). <http://www.nhlbi.nih.gov/health/public/sleep/rls.htm>.

Mayo Clinic Staff. "Restless Legs Syndrome." (July 23, 2002). <http://www.mayoclinic.com/invoke.cfm?objectid=3E2E9266-6525-4125-923345C17FB0E20F>.

National Institute of Neurological Disorders and Stroke. *NINDS Restless Legs Syndrome Information Page.* (July 1, 2001). <http://www.ninds.nih.gov/health_and_medical/disorders/restless_doc.htm>.

ORGANIZATIONS

RLS Foundation, Inc. 819 Second Street SW, Rochester, MN 55902. (507) 287-6465; Fax: (507) 287-6312. rlsfoundation@rls.org. <http://www.rls.org>.

National Center on Sleep Disorders Research (NCSDR). Two Rockledge Center, Suite 7024, 6701 Rockledge Drive, MSC 7920, Bethesda, MD 20892. (301) 435-0199; Fax: (301) 480-3451.

Juli M. Berwald, PhD

Retrovirus-associated myelopathy *see*
Tropical spastic paraparesis

Rett syndrome

Definition

Rett syndrome (RS) is a neurological disease of children that is also referred to as Rett's disorder or by the compound name of **autism**, **dementia**, **ataxia**, and loss of purposeful hand use. Named for the Austrian pediatrician who first described it, RS is sometimes grouped together with other childhood neurological disorders under the category of pervasive developmental disorders (PDDs) or autistic spectrum disorders. RS is classified by the *Diagnostic and Statistical Manual of Mental Disorders*, Fourth Edition (DSM-IV), as a developmental disorder of childhood. More recently, Rett syndrome has been categorized along with Rubinstein-Taybi syndrome (RSTS), Coffin-Lowry syndrome (CLS), and several other rare disorders as a chromatin disease. Chromatin is the easily stained part of a cell nucleus that contains the cell's DNA, RNA, and several proteins that maintain its structure.

Description

RS was first described by an Austrian pediatrician, Andreas Rett, in 1966. His article attracted little attention, however, because it appeared in a German-language medical journal that was not widely read outside Europe. In 1983, a Swedish researcher named Bengt Hagberg published a follow-up study in the English-language *Annals of Neurology*, which led to worldwide recognition of RS as an identifiable neurological disorder.

RS has a distinctive onset and course. The affected child—almost always a girl—develops normally during the first five months of life. After the fifth month, head growth slows down and the child loses whatever purposeful hand movements she had developed during her first five months. After 30 months, the child frequently develops repetitive hand-washing or hand-wringing gestures; 50–80% of children with the disorder will eventually have **seizures**. RS is also associated with varying degrees of **mental retardation**.

The doctors who first studied RS attributed it to the breakdown or destruction of brain tissue. Later research indicated, however, that it is caused by the failure of the infant's brain to develop normally. This developmental failure is in turn associated with a genetic mutation affecting production of a key protein that organizes the structure of chromatin. Changes in chromatin structure lead to inappropriate activation of the genes that regulate brain development. About 80% of patients who meet the updated 2002 criteria for "classic" RS have this mutation on one of their two X chromosomes.

Demographics

According to the National Institute of Neurological Disorders and Stroke (NINDS), RS affects between one in 10,000 and one in 15,000 female infants. It is thought to occur in all races and ethnic groups with equal frequency. Although Rett syndrome is associated with a genetic mutation, less than 0.5% of reported cases are recurrences within families. Almost all cases represent sporadic (new) mutations of the gene responsible for the syndrome. The risk that the parents of a daughter with RS will have a second child with the disorder is less than 1%.

The reason that almost all patients with RS are female is that the mutation that causes the disorder is located on the X chromosome. While boys have an X and a Y chromosome, girls have two X chromosomes, only one of which is active in any given body cell. The other X chromosome is turned off in a process known as X inactivation, which helps to explain why the symptoms of RS vary from patient to patient. According to mathematical probability, the X chromosome with the mutation will be active in about half the girl's cells, with the healthy X chromosome active in the other half. If by chance a majority of the girl's cells have an active healthy X chromosome, she will have only mild symptoms of RS. On the other hand, if the X chromosome with the mutation is active in a majority of the girl's cells, she will have more severe symptoms. Since boys have only one X chromosome, they have no "backup" healthy X chromosome to compensate for one that contains the mutation. As a result, boys affected by the mutation usually die shortly before or after birth. The few cases of boys surviving with RS involve another genetic disorder known as Klinefelter's syndrome, in which the boy is born with three or more sex chromosomes, two or more Xs and a Y. If one of the X chromosomes contains the RS mutation, the boy may develop RS.

Causes and symptoms

RS is the first neurological disorder in humans to be traced to defects in a protein that controls the expression of other genes. The molecular cause of Rett's disorder is a genetic mutation on the long arm of the X chromosome (Xq28) at a locus known as MECP2. Dr. Huda Zoghbi at Baylor College of Medicine and her collaborator, Dr. Uta Francke at Stanford University, discovered the gene in 1999. The gene contains instructions for the formation of a protein known as methyl cytosine-binding protein 2 or MeCP2, which is crucial to the normal development of the human brain. The mutation associated with RS results in insufficient production of MeCP2. When this key protein is lacking, other genes are "turned on" or remain active at inappropriate points in the brain's development. These activated genes interfere with the normal pattern of brain maturation. The discovery of the MECP2 gene showed that RS should be understood as a genetic interference with normal brain development rather than the result of tissue loss or destruction.

The areas of the brain that are most severely affected by the lack of MeCP2 are the frontal, motor, and temporal portions of the brain cortex; the brain stem; the base of the forebrain; and the basal ganglia. These parts of the brain control such basic functions as movement, breathing, and speech. In addition, the disruption of the normal pattern of brain development in RS affects the child's emotions and ability to learn. RS is now known to be one of the most common causes of mental retardation in girls.

The symptoms of RS are usually described in terms of four stages in the child's development.

STAGE 1, EARLY ONSET (SIX TO 18 MONTHS OF AGE) The early symptoms of RS are not always noticeable in stage 1. The infant may not make eye contact with family members and may not show much interest in toys. She may be considered a "good baby" because she is so calm and quiet. She may also be able to use single words or word combinations before she loses the ability to speak in stage

2. On the other hand, there may also be noticeable hand-wringing and slowing of head growth in this early stage.

STAGE 2, RAPID DETERIORATION (ONE TO FOUR YEARS) The second stage may be either rapid or gradual in onset. The child loses her ability to speak and to make purposeful hand movements—a condition known as **apraxia**. Hand-to-mouth movements may appear, as well as hand-wringing or hand-clapping gestures. These movements may be nearly constant while the child is awake, but disappear during sleep. There may be noticeable episodes of breath holding, air swallowing, and hyperventilating (rapid shallow breathing). The child may have trouble sleeping, and may become irritable or agitated. If she is able to walk, she will start to look unsteady on her feet (ataxia) and may have periods of trembling or shaking. Some girls completely lose the ability to walk in stage 2 and move by crawling or "bottom scooting." Slowed growth of the child's head is usually most noticeable during this stage.

STAGE 3, PLATEAU (TWO TO 10 YEARS) Motor problems and seizures often appear during this stage. The child's behavior, however, often shows some improvement, with less irritability and crying. She may show greater interest in her surroundings, and her attention span and communication skills often improve.

STAGE 4, LATE DETERIORATION OF MOTOR SKILLS (USUALLY AFTER 10 YEARS OF AGE) In stage 4, patients with RS gradually lose their mobility; some stop walking, while others have never learned to walk. There is, however, no loss of cognitive or communication skills, and the repetitive hand movements may decrease. Seizures and breathing problems typically lessen in severity by late adolescence. The spine, however, begins to develop an abnormal sideways curvature (scoliosis), which is usually more severe in girls that have never learned to walk. The patient may also develop muscle rigidity, or **spasticity**. Puberty begins at the same age as in most girls.

Other symptoms associated with RS include a greater risk of bone fractures due to low bone density in spite of adequate calcium in the diet; constipation, which results from poor muscle tone in the digestive tract, scoliosis, and the side effects of anticonvulsant medications; excessive salivation and drooling; gastroesophageal reflux disease (GERD), which results from poor muscle tone in the esophagus; and crying or emotional agitation, which is thought to result from frustration with the inability to communicate.

Diagnosis

The diagnosis of RS is clinical, which means that it is based on external observation of the patient's symptoms rather than on the results of laboratory tests or imaging

Key Terms

Apraxia Inability to carry out ordinary purposeful movements in the absence of paralysis.

Ataxia Loss or failure of muscular coordination, particularly of the arms or legs.

Autism A severe developmental disorder of childhood with onset before three years of age. RS is sometimes categorized as an autistic spectrum disorder because it shares some features with autism, including communication problems, difficulties with social interaction, and abnormal muscle tone.

Basal ganglia Groups of nerve cell bodies located deep within the brain that govern movement as well as emotion and certain aspects of cognition (thinking).

Brain stem The stalk-like portion of the brain that connects the cerebral hemispheres and the spinal cord. The brain stem receives sensory information and controls such vital functions as blood pressure and respiration.

Bruxism Involuntary clenching or grinding of teeth, usually during sleep. Bruxism is considered a supportive criterion of RS.

Cerebral cortex The thin layer of gray matter that covers the surface of the cerebral hemispheres of the brain. It controls movement, perception, behavioral responses, the higher mental functions, and the integration of these activities.

Chromatin The readily stainable portion of a cell nucleus, consisting of DNA, RNA, and various proteins. It coils and folds itself to form chromosomes during the process of cell division. RS is sometimes described as a chromatin disease.

Dementia An overall decline in a person's intellectual function, including difficulties with language, simple calculations, judgment, organizational abilities, and abstract thinking skills as well as loss of memory.

Hyperventilation A pattern of rapid but shallow breathing that is frequently found in patients with Rett syndrome.

Hypotonia Reduced muscle tone. It is one of the earliest symptoms of Rett syndrome.

Klinefelter's syndrome A genetic disorder in males characterized by the presence of two or more X chromosomes instead of the normal XY pattern. The few male patients diagnosed with Rett syndrome who have lived past infancy also have Klinefelter's syndrome.

Kyphosis An abnormal convex (outward) curvature of the upper portion of the spinal column, sometimes called a humpback or hunchback.

Mutation A spontaneous change in the sequence of nucleotides in a chromosome or gene. Mutations may affect the number and structure of chromosomes or cause deletions of part of a chromosome. Rett syndrome is caused by a mutation on the long arm of the X chromosome.

Pervasive developmental disorders (PDDs) A category of childhood disorders that includes Rett syndrome. The PDDs are sometimes referred to collectively as autistic spectrum disorders.

Psychomotor Referring to skills that involve physical movement as well as a mental component.

Scoliosis An abnormal lateral (sidewise) curvature of the spine. Many patients with RS develop scoliosis after puberty.

Spasticity A condition in which the muscles become hypertonic or stiff and the patient's movements awkward or clumsy. Many patients with RS develop spasticity in adult life.

Storage diseases Diseases in which too much of a substance (usually fats, glycogen, or certain enzymes) builds up in specific cells of the body and causes metabolic or tissue disorders.

Vasomotor Referring to the regulation of the diameter of blood vessels.

X inactivation The process in which each cell in a girl's body selects at random and turns off one of its two X chromosomes. X inactivation is one reason why some patients with RS have more severe symptoms than others.

studies. In some cases, however, the child's doctor may order blood or urine tests or an electroencephalogram (EEG) to rule out **epilepsy** or other disorders. The doctor will observe the affected child—usually over a period of several hours or days at various intervals—and interview the parents. In most cases, the diagnosis cannot be made with certainty until the child is three to five years old. A diagnosis of RS can be made by a pediatrician or primary care physician, but should be confirmed by a pediatric **neurologist** (specialist in disorders of the nervous system in children) or developmental pediatrician. In addition to ordering genetic testing, a specialist who is evaluating a child for RS will use several different types of criteria.

Diagnostic criteria

The diagnostic criteria for RS, which were first established in 1985, were revised by an international committee in 2001–2002 in order to improve the consistency of diagnosis as well as take recent genetic discoveries into account. The criteria are divided into three groups: necessary criteria, which must be present for the doctor to make the diagnosis; supportive criteria, which are present in many patients with RS; and exclusion criteria, which rule out a diagnosis of RS.

Necessary criteria include the following:

- child is apparently normal before and around the time of birth
- psychomotor development (development of skills that involve the brain's regulation of motor activity) is either normal for the first six months or is slightly delayed from birth
- circumference of child's head at birth is normal
- head growth slows down after birth
- child loses purposeful hand motions between six and 30 months
- child makes repeated gestures, most commonly hand wringing or squeezing, clapping or tapping, and washing or rubbing motions
- child withdraws socially, loses ability to communicate in words, and loses cognitive skills
- ability to walk is impaired or lost

Supportive criteria include the following:

- disturbed breathing (hyperventilation, air swallowing, breath holding) when awake
- bruxism (grinding the teeth during sleep)
- disturbed sleeping pattern from early infancy
- muscle wasting and loss of muscle tone
- scoliosis or kyphosis
- retarded growth
- hands and feet that are very small compared to the rest of the child's body
- vasomotor disturbances

Exclusion criteria include the following:

- enlargement of the internal organs or other signs of storage diseases
- cataract formation or damage to the retina of the eye
- evidence of brain damage before or shortly after birth
- identification of a metabolic or other progressive neurological disorder
- damage to the nervous system resulting from an infectious disease or head trauma

About 15% of children who are evaluated for RS have RS-like symptoms, or have the MECP2 mutation without fulfilling all the diagnostic criteria. These children are said to have "variant" or "atypical" RS. Children below the age of three years who show some of the signs of RS but do not yet meet the full criteria are said to have "provisional" RS.

Genetic testing

It is important to understand that even though RS is associated with mutations in the MECP2 gene, the syndrome sometimes occurs without the mutation. Conversely, the mutation can occur without producing the symptoms of RS. Genetic testing can identify about 80% of RS cases but is not sufficient to use alone to make the diagnosis. Researchers think that the remaining 20% of cases may be caused either by mutations in other parts of the gene or by genes that have not yet been identified.

Treatment team

Treatment for patients with RS is highly individualized because the severity of specific symptoms varies from patient to patient; for example, some may never have seizures. In almost all cases, however, the treatment team for a child with RS will include a neurologist, an orthopedic surgeon, a physical therapist, an occupational therapist, a dietitian, and a speech-language therapist in addition to a pediatrician and a dentist. In some cases, the treatment team may include a psychiatrist who specializes in childhood and adolescent psychiatry. Most patients will also have a case manager to coordinate treatments.

When the patient reaches puberty, she should be seen by a developmental pediatrician and an orthodontist. **Respite** and in-home caregivers may also be added to the treatment team for adults with RS.

Treatment

There is no cure for RS; treatment is intended to ease the symptoms and to keep the patient mobile as long as possible. It will include most or all of the following:

- Medications. A patient with RS may be given drugs for breathing problems and difficulties with muscle control. One medication that is useful is baclofen (Lioresal), a muscle relaxant. Patients with seizures are given anticonvulsant (anti-seizure) medications.
- Special diets. Many patients with RS have a poor appetite and problems swallowing. The patient may need an assessment by a dietitian to plan meals that are appealing as well as nutritionally sound. Patients with

seizures that cannot be controlled by medications may benefit from a special high-fat, low-carbohydrate diet known as a ketogenic diet.

- Physical therapy. Physical therapy of patients with RS is focused on maintaining or improving the patient's balance and ability to walk; maintaining full range of motion whenever possible; and preventing the muscle contractures that lead to deformities in adult life.

- Splints and braces. Hand or elbow splints may be used to reduce repetitive hand movements and increase the child's purposeful use of her dominant hand. Patients who develop kyphosis (humpback) or scoliosis may be fitted for spinal braces.

- Occupational therapy.

- Speech therapy. Some patients with RS are taught to communicate with body language; others use eye blinking, communication boards, or electronic devices.

- Complementary and alternative therapies. Music therapy has been successfully used in patients with RS, as well as hydrotherapy, equine therapy (horseback riding), and acupuncture.

Clinical trials

As of late summer 2003, there are no open **clinical trials** for RS at the National Institutes of Health (NIH). There are, however, two medical centers funded by the NIH that evaluate patients for RS and conduct research on the disorder; contact information for the Blue Bird Circle Rett Center and the Kennedy Krieger Institute is listed under Resources.

Prognosis

It is difficult to predict the severity or the course of RS in any specific individual. Although the symptoms of RS are disabling, most patients survive into the 40s and 50s. Little is known about patients' long-term prognosis after age 40 because the disorder has been studied intensively only since the mid-1980s.

What is known about the short-term prognosis of middle-aged adults with RS is encouraging, however. Their mental state stabilizes and they are often able to continue to learn as well as improve the use of their hands. They make better eye contact with others. In addition, patients are usually less irritable, sleep better, and have fewer seizures and breathing problems. The chief additional problem for adults with RS is decreased mobility. After the early adult years, the patient's muscles may become rigid or spastic, causing joint deformities and increased difficulty in walking.

Special concerns

Educational and social needs

Most patients with RS can benefit from special educational programs. Education in the public schools is available in most areas until the patient is 21. After that age, the patient may be able to attend sheltered workshops or day centers, depending on where she lives. In the last few years, some young women with milder forms of RS have been able to attend classes at local community colleges or find employment with the help of a job coach.

It is important for patients with RS to participate in community activities and social events precisely because they have a fairly long life expectancy. Personal accounts of adults with RS indicate that they enjoy travel, church or synagogue activities, volunteer work, swimming, camping, music, sports events, and similar outings.

Legal issues

The most pressing long-term concern for patients with RS is working out a life plan for ongoing care, since many are likely to outlive their parents. The parents of a girl diagnosed with RS should consult an estate planner, an attorney, and a certified public accountant (CPA) in order to draft a life plan and letter of intent. A letter of intent is not a legally binding document, but it gives the patient's siblings and other relatives or caregivers necessary information on providing for her in the future. The attorney can help the parents decide about such matters as guardianship as well as guide them through the legal process of appointing a guardian, which varies from state to state.

Resources
BOOKS

American Psychiatric Association. *Diagnostic and Statistical Manual of Mental Disorders*, 4th edition, text revision. Washington, DC: American Psychiatric Association, 2000.

Martin, John H. *Neuroanatomy: Text and Atlas*, 3rd ed. New York: McGraw-Hill, 2003.

Parker, James N., MD, and Philip M. Parker, PhD, eds. *The Official Parent's Sourcebook on Rett Syndrome.* San Diego, CA: ICON Health Publications, 2002.

"Psychiatric Conditions in Childhood and Adolescence." *The Merck Manual of Diagnosis and Therapy*, edited by Mark H. Beers, MD, and Robert Berkow, MD. Whitehouse Station, NJ: Merck Research Laboratories, 1999.

Thoene, Jess G., editor. *Physicians' Guide to Rare Diseases.* Montvale, NJ: Dowden Publishing Company, 1995.

PERIODICALS

Amir, R. E., I. B. Van den Veyver, M. Wan, et al. "Rett Syndrome Is Caused by Mutations in X-Linked MECP2, Encoding Methyl-CpG-Binding Protein 2." *Nature Genetics* 23 (October 1999): 185–188.

Ausio, J., D. B. Levin, G. V. De Amorim, et al. "Syndromes of Disordered Chromatin Remodeling." *Clinical Genetics* 64 (August 2003): 83–95.

Bumin, G., M. Uyanik, I. Yilmaz, et al. "Hydrotherapy for Rett Syndrome." *Journal of Rehabilitation Medicine* 35 (January 2003): 44–45.

Chen, R. Z., S. Akbarian, M. Tudor, and R. Jaenisch. "Deficiency of Methyl-CpG Binding Protein-2 in CNS Neurons Results in a Rett-Like Phenotype in Mice." *Nature Genetics* 27 (March 2001): 327–331.

Hagberg, B., J. Aicardi, K. Dias, and O. Ramos. "A Progressive Syndrome of Autism, Dementia, Ataxia, and Loss of Purposeful Hand Use in Girls: Rett's Syndrome: Report of 35 Cases." *Annals of Neurology* 14 (October 1983): 471–479.

Hagberg, B., F. Hanefeld, A. Percy, and O. Skjeldal. "An Update on Clinically Applicable Diagnostic Criteria in Rett Syndrome. Comments to Rett Syndrome Clinical Criteria Consensus Panel Satellite to European Paediatric Neurology Society Meeting, Baden Baden, Germany, September 11, 2001." *European Journal of Paediatric Neurology* 6 (2002): 293–297.

Hendrich, Brian, and Wendy Bickmore. "Human Diseases with Underlying Defects in Chromatin Structure and Modification." *Human Molecular Genetics* 10, no. 20 (2001): 2233–2242.

Isaacs, J. S., M. Murdock, J. Lane, and A. K. Percy. "Eating Difficulties in Girls with Rett Syndrome Compared with Other Developmental Disabilities." *Journal of the American Dietetic Association* 103 (February 2003): 224–230.

Kadyan, V., A. C. Clairmont, R. J. George, and E. W. Johnson. "Intrathecal Baclofen for Spasticity Management in Rett Syndrome." *American Journal of Physical Medicine and Rehabilitation* 82 (July 2003): 560–562.

Liebhaber, G. M., E. Riemann, and F. A. Baumeister. "Ketogenic Diet in Rett Syndrome." *Journal of Child Neurology* 18 (January 2003): 74–75.

Magalhaes, M. H., J. Y. Kawamura, and L. C. Araujo. "General and Oral Characteristics in Rett Syndrome." *Special Care in Dentistry* 22 (July-August 2002): 147–150.

Moldavsky, M., D. Lev, and T. Lerman-Sagie. "Behavioral Phenotypes of Genetic Syndromes: A Reference Guide for Psychiatrists." *Journal of the American Academy of Child and Adolescent Psychiatry* 40 (July 2001): 749–761.

Rett, A. "Rett Syndrome. History and General Overview." *American Journal of Medical Genetics. Supplement* 1 (1986): 21–25.

Rett, A. "On an Unusual Brain Atrophy Syndrome in Hyperammonemia in Childhood." [in German] *Wiener medizinische Wochenschrift (1946)* 116 (September 10, 1966): 723–726.

Van den Veyver, I. B., and H. Y. Zoghbi. "Genetic Basis of Rett Syndrome." *Mental Retardation and Developmental Disabilities Research Reviews* 8 (2002): 82–86.

Yasuhara, A., and Y. Sugiyama. "Music Therapy for Children with Rett Syndrome." *Brain and Development* 23 (December 2002) (Suppl 1): S82–S84.

ORGANIZATIONS

American Academy of Child and Adolescent Psychiatry. 3615 Wisconsin Avenue, NW, Washington, DC 20016-3007. (202) 966-7300. Fax: (202) 966-2891. (February 25, 2004). <http://www.aacap.org>.

Blue Bird Circle Rett Center, Baylor College of Medicine, Department of Pediatrics, One Baylor Plaza, Room 319C, Houston, TX 77030. (888) 430-7388 or (713) 798-RETT. (February 25, 2004).<http://bluebirdrett.bcm.tmc.edu>.

International Rett Syndrome Association (IRSA). 9121 Piscataway Road, Suite 2-B, Clinton, MD 20735. (301) 856-3334 or 1-800-818-RETT. Fax: (301) 856-3336. (February 25, 2004). <http://www.rettsyndrome.org>

Kennedy Krieger Institute, Department of Neurogenetics, 707 North Broadway, Baltimore, MD 21205. (800) 873-3377 x 29-409 or (443) 923-2778. (February 25, 2004). <http://www.kennedykrieger.org>.

National Institute of Child Health and Human Development (NICHD). National Institutes of Health (NIH), Bldg. 31, Room 2A32, Bethesda, MD 20892-2425. (800) 370-2943 or (301) 496-5133. (February 25, 2004). <http://www.nichd.nih.gov>.

National Organization for Rare Disorders (NORD). 55 Kenosia Avenue, P. O. Box 1968, Danbury, CT 06813-1968. (800) 999-6673 or (203) 744-0100. Fax: (203) 798-2291. (February 25, 2004). <http://www.rarediseases.org>.

Rett Syndrome Research Foundation (RSRF). 4600 Devitt Drive, Cincinnati, OH 45246. (513) 874-3020. Fax: (513) 874-2520. (February 25, 2004). <http://www.rsrf.org>.

OTHER

National Institute of Neurological Disorders and Stroke (NINDS). *Rett Syndrome Fact Sheet.* NIH Publication No. 01-4863. Bethesda, MD: NINDS, 2003.

Rebecca J. Frey, PhD

Reye syndrome

Definition

Reye syndrome is a serious, potentially fatal condition that strikes children and adolescents who have just recovered from a viral infection, especially when that illness has been treated with aspirin or aspirin-containing products. Reye syndrome causes damage to the liver and brain.

Description

Reye syndrome is a relatively rare disease. Since the late 1980s, when concern regarding aspirin use in children became more widely publicized, fewer than 20 cases of

Reye syndrome have been reported annually. This is down from a peak of over 600 cases in 1980. Although researchers have not been able to state this definitively, the decreased incidence of Reye syndrome has been commonly attributed to a greatly decreased use of aspirin-containing products in children.

When Reye syndrome strikes, it can be a devastating illness. The death rate from the disease used to be as high as 50–60%. Better, faster methods of diagnosis have allowed earlier identification of the disorder, allowing the death rate to drop to 30–35%. Younger children seem to have a higher risk of death. Even those children who recover may be faced with lifelong disability, depending on the degree of brain damage suffered. Long-term problems may include behavior problems, attention disorders, **mental retardation**, blindness, **seizures**, varying degrees of paralysis, and learning difficulties.

Demographics

Reye syndrome primarily strikes children and adolescents who have recently recovered from a viral infection, particularly chicken pox or influenza. Because the frequency of most viral infections peaks in the winter months, Reye syndrome is most common in January, February, and March. In the United States, the most common age for Reye syndrome is six to eight years. Reye syndrome is extremely rare in individuals over the age of 18.

Causes and symptoms

Scientists do not feel convinced that the true cause of Reye syndrome has been defined. Although there is a clear-cut association between recent viral infection and the disease, and between use of aspirin-containing products and the disease, the actual mechanism of the condition has not been fully delineated. There may also be an association between the development of Reye syndrome and exposure to pesticides and/or aflatoxin (a toxin produced by a fungus that infests grains, peanuts, soybeans, and corn that have been stored in warm, moist conditions).

The underlying problem in Reye syndrome seems to be dysfunction of the small, energy-producing structures within the body's cells (the mitochondria). The blood becomes more acidic, ammonia levels increase, and sugar levels drop. Large quantities of fat are deposited throughout many organs of the body, most significantly, the liver. The fatty deposits in the liver interfere with normal liver functioning. Swelling and increased pressure in the brain puts pressure on the delicate brain tissues, resulting in damage.

Reye syndrome begins within about a week of recovery from a viral illness. Vomiting and listlessness are

---

Key Terms

Aflatoxin   A toxin produced by a fungus that infests grains, peanuts, soybeans, and corn that have been stored in warm, moist conditions.

Decerebrate posture   Stiff, rigid posture indicative of severe damage to brain stem.

Decorticate posture   A stiff, rigid posture indicative of damage to nerve tracts that run between spinal cord and brain.

Electroencephalogram (EEG)   A test in which electrodes applied to the scalp allow the electrical activity of the brain to be recorded.

Mitochondria   Small, energy-producing structures within the body's cells.

---

some of the earliest symptoms, although they are not necessarily universal in every patient. Children tend to become sleepy, disoriented, confused, and even combative. Reye syndrome can progress very quickly. Within hours, symptoms can become more severe, with loss of consciousness, seizures, stupor, and coma, all signaling critical illness.

Reye syndrome is graded I through V at the time of diagnosis, in order to determine a level of severity. Grades I through III are considered mild to moderate, while grades IV and V are considered critically ill. Criteria for this grading is as follows:

- Grade I: Child is quiet, sleepy, vomiting, and there is some blood evidence of a drop in liver functioning.

- Grade II: Child is confused, delirious, combative, with overly-active reflexes, breathing quickly.

- Grade III: Child is in a light coma, may have seizures, pupils still responsive to light, is in decorticate posture (stiff, rigid posture indicative of damage to nerve tracts that run between spinal cord and brain).

- Grade IV: Child is in a deepening coma, experiencing seizures, pupils nonresponsive to light, has abnormal reflexes, is in decerebrate posture (stiff, rigid posture indicative of severe damage to brain stem).

- Grade V: Child is in a deep coma, pupils are fixed and dilated (abnormally enlarged, do not constrict when exposed to light), no normal reflexes, alternates between decerebrate posture and completely limp, flaccid muscles, cannot breathe independently, EEG reading lacks normal waves.

Diagnosis

There is no specific test to diagnose Reye syndrome. Diagnosis is suggested by a number of different abnormalities, including:

- extremely elevated liver enzymes (20–30 times normal)

- increases in blood ammonia (three times normal)

- low blood sugar

- high blood acidity

- blood clotting abnormalities

- abnormal electroencephalogram (EEG, a test in which electrodes applied to the scalp allow the electrical activity of the brain to be recorded)

- abnormal liver **biopsy**, revealing large quantities of fat deposited within the liver

Treatment team

Children with Reye syndrome are usually cared for in a hospital, with more severely ill children requiring care in an intensive care unit. Health care providers may include pediatric intensivists, neurologists, and gastroenterologists (to closely monitor liver function).

Treatment

There is no cure for Reye syndrome. Treatment is considered supportive, meaning that treatment is given to address the specific complications, in order to try to prevent progression of the liver and brain damage and permanent effects.

Medications such as steroids and/or diuretics may be given to try to relieve brain swelling; at the same time, fluid intake should be restricted to prevent further swelling. Glucose is given to increase blood sugar levels. Vitamin K, platelet transfusions, and frozen plasma may be given to improve a bleeding disorder. Seriously ill patients will probably need to be on a ventilator.

Recovery and rehabilitation

Even children who seem to have made a complete recovery may actually demonstrate significant neuropsychological deficits with specific testing. Depending on the actual deficits, physical therapy, occupational therapy, speech and language therapy, and educational interventions may be necessary.

Prognosis

Prognosis depends on the severity of the brain swelling. The liver functioning is usually fully recovered, but brain damage will leave permanent deficits. When Reye syndrome is diagnosed earlier in its course, aggressive treatment can be started to slow the progress of damaging brain swelling, improving the patient's chance of complete recovery. There is a higher risk of death or of permanent damage when there is a delay in diagnosis and therefore in treatment. When Reye syndrome is not diagnosed and treated quickly, death can occur within only days of the syndrome's onset. Death rates from Reye syndrome are currently about 30–35%.

Special concerns

Reye syndrome can be almost completely prevented by parental awareness of the dangers of administering any aspirin-containing substances to their children. This includes aspirin itself, as well as various cold and flu preparations that may contain salicylates or salicylic acid (the chemical names for aspirin). Many common over-the-counter medications for upset stomach also contain salicylates. Parents should carefully read the list of active ingredients and/or consult a physician or pharmacist before giving their children over-the-counter medicines. Making sure that children are immunized yearly against the flu (influenza vaccine) and considering giving children the chicken pox vaccine may also help decrease the risk of Reye syndrome.

Resources

BOOKS

Gascon, Generoso G., and Pinar T. Ozand. "Aminoacidopathies and Organic Acidopathies, Mitochondrial Enzyme Defects, and Other Metabolic Errors." In *Textbook of Clinical Neurology*, edited by Christopher G. Goetz. Philadelphia: W.B. Saunders Company, 2003.

Rudolph, Jeffrey A., and William F. Balistreri. "Reye Syndrome and the Mitochondrial Hepatopathies." In *Nelson Textbook of Pediatrics*, edited by Richard E. Behrman, et al. Philadelphia: W.B. Saunders Company, 2004.

Wachtel, Tom J. "Reye's Syndrome." In *Ferri's Clinical Advisor: Instant Diagnosis and Treatment*, edited by Fred F. Ferri. St. Louis: Mosby, 2004.

WEBSITES

National Institute of Neurological Disorders and Stroke (NINDS). *Reye Syndrome Fact Sheet.* (April 27, 2004). <http://www.ninds.nih.gov>.

ORGANIZATIONS

National Reye's Syndrome Foundation, Inc. (419) 636-2679 or (800) 233-7393; Fax: (419) 636-9897. nrsf@reyes syndrome.org. <http://www.reyessyndrome.org/default.htm>.

Rosalyn Carson-DeWitt, MD

Rivastigmine *see* **Cholinesterase inhibitors**

S

Sacral nerve root cysts *see* **Perineural cysts**

Sacral radiculopathy *see* **Radiculopathy**

Saint Vitus Dance *see* **Sydenham's chorea**

Salivary gland disease *see* **Cytomegalic inclusion body disease**

▌Sandhoff disease

Definition

Sandhoff disease is a relatively rare, genetically inherited disease that results in the progressive deterioration of the **central nervous system**. In Sandhoff disease, abnormal lipid (fat) accumulation due to a storage defect causes damage to the brain as well as other organs of the body.

Description

Sandhoff disease is an autosomal recessive disorder, meaning that having an affected offspring requires both unaffected parents to be carriers. Parents who carry the disorder will have a 25% risk of having an affected offspring in subsequent pregnancies. This disease is similar to a related disorder known as Tay-Sachs disease, although Sandhoff disease is more severe.

Demographics

As Sandhoff disease is a recessive disorder, males and females are affected with equal frequency. This disorder is more common in people with non-Jewish descent, unlike Tay-Sachs disease, which is prevalent mainly in individuals with Jewish ancestry.

Causes and symptoms

Sandhoff disease is caused by mutations in two different genes that encode subunits that make up a protein called hexosaminidase. Hexosaminidase is an enzyme that breaks down certain fats in the brain. This enzyme is either composed of an alpha and a beta subunit (HexA) or two beta subunits (HexB). Sandhoff disease is caused by a mutation in a gene that is distinct from the gene that causes Tay-Sachs disease. In Tay-Sachs disease, a mutation that affects the alpha subunit of the enzyme causes a deficiency in HexA. Sandhoff disease is caused by mutations that affect the beta subunit, rendering both the HexA and HexB enzymes deficient. A deficiency of this enzyme leads to the accumulation of GM2 ganglioside, a fatty material found in the brain.

The beta subunit is encoded by a gene localized to chromosome 5, while the alpha subunit is encoded by a gene on chromosome 13. There is also another gene on chromosome 5 that encodes an activator that is required for either enzyme to be functional. Similar symptoms are observed in diseases arising from mutations that affect any of these three genes. Only biochemical genetic analysis of enzyme activity can pinpoint the cause and specify the disorder. However, Sandhoff disease can be distinguished from Tay-Sachs disease clinically by virtue of skeletal system or abdominal organ involvement (if present) in the later disease.

At birth, infants tend to be without symptoms and usually do not develop them until approximately six months of age. The symptoms begin with motor deficits (lack of normal movement) and a characteristic startle reaction to various sounds. Babies with Sandhoff disease progressively deteriorate in terms of motor function, and they often have **seizures** and **myoclonus**. Myoclonus is abnormal, exaggerated muscle contractions. Blindness can also be part of the symptoms. The loss of motor function includes the ability to swallow, and the affected infant has an increased risk for inhaling feedings into the lungs, frequently leading to pneumonia.

A typical physical feature of Sandhoff disease is the presence of cherry-red spots in the back of the eyes. Additionally, affected children have an abnormally enlarged head and appear to have a doll-like appearance.

Diagnosis

Because Sandhoff disease and Tay-Sachs disease have similar clinical symptoms, distinguishing them requires biochemical analysis. This involves a test to measure enzyme activity of the two hexosaminidase enzymes. If the enzyme activity results indicate that there is no hexosaminidase activity, it means that the patient has Sandhoff disease. If, however, there is still B subunit activity, then this indicates that the patient might have Tay-Sachs disease.

Treatment

There is no cure for Sandhoff disease, and treatment is based on lessening the symptoms once they begin. Medication is usually given to reduce seizures, for example, and a feeding tube may be inserted to prevent aspiration of feedings into the lungs.

Recovery and rehabilitation

Emphasis is placed on comfort rather than recovery, due to the progressive nature of Sandhoff disease. Because of the nature of the disorder, rehabilitation is not usually applicable to help with improving the motor deficits that develop. Physical therapy may be helpful to maintain muscle tone and skeletal alignment for as long as possible, while positional strategies and devices provided by an occupational therapist may increase comfort as symptoms progress.

Clinical trials

The National Institute of Diabetes and Digestive and Kidney Diseases (NIDDK) is sponsoring, as of February 2004, a study to evaluate children with glycosphingolipid (GSL) storage disorders (such as Sandhoff disease) to investigate changes that occur in the brain that are responsible for nervous system degeneration. In this study, patients will receive medical treatment for their disorder. Contact the National Institute of Diabetes and Digestive and Kidney Diseases (NIDDK), located at 9000 Rockville Pike, Bethesda, Maryland, 20892, Recruiting: Patient Recruitment and Public Liaison Office, (800) 411-1222 or prpl@mail.cc.nih.gov.

Prognosis

The prognosis for Sandhoff disease is poor. Affected babies usually do not survive past the age of three and typically, death occurs due to complications associated with respiratory infections.

Special concerns

Children who are affected with Sandhoff disease will require full time supervision and caretaking responsibilities. Psychological counseling for family members is often helpful. Genetic counseling for reproductive risks is recommended. There are also several support groups operated and comprised of other families nationwide with Sandhoff disease.

Resources
BOOKS

Icon Health Publications. *The Official Parent's Sourcebook on Sandhoff Disease: A Revised and Updated Directory for the Internet Age.* New York: Icon Group International, 2002.

Nussbaum, Robert L., Roderick R. McInnes, and Huntington F. Willard. *Genetics in Medicine.* Philadelphia : Saunders, 2001.

PERIODICALS

Gilbert, F., R. S. Kucherlapati, R. P. Creagan, M. J. Murnane, G. J. Darlington, and F. H. Ruddle. "Tay-Sachs' and Sandhoff's diseases: the assignment of genes for hexosaminidase A and B to individual human chromosomes." *Proc. Nat. Acad. Sci.* 72 (1975): 263–267, 1975.

Neufeld, E. F. "Natural history and inherited disorders of a lysosomal enzyme, beta-hexosaminidase." *J. Biol. Chem.* 264 (1989): 10927–10930.

OTHER

"What every family should know: Sandhoff disease." *The National Tay-Sachs & Allied Diseases Association.* (February 1, 2004). <http://www.ntsad.org/pages/sandhoff.htm>.

"NINDS Sandhoff Disease Information Page." *National Institute of Neurological Disorders and Stroke.* (February 1, 2004). <http://www.ninds.nih.gov/health_and_medical/disorders/sandhoff.htm>.

ORGANIZATIONS

National Tay-Sachs and Allied Diseases Association. 2001 Beacon Street Suite 204, Brighton, MA 02135. (617) 277-4463. (617) 277-0134. (800) 90-NTSAD (906-8723). info@ntsad.org. <http://www.ntsad.org>.

National Organization for Rare Disorders (NORD). P.O. Box 1968 (55 Kenosia Avenue), Danbury, CT 06813-1968. (203) 744-0100. (203) 798-2291. (800) 999-NORD (6673). orphan@rarediseases.org. <http://www.rarediseases.org>.

Bryan Richard Cobb, PhD

Schilder's disease

Definition

Schilder's disease is a form of **multiple sclerosis** that strikes in childhood.

Description

Schilder's disease is a very rare progressive degenerative disease that affects children. It resembles multiple sclerosis both in its symptoms (difficulties with movement and speech) and its pathology (widespread demyelination of the brain). Demyelination refers to the destruction of the myelin that normally encases nerve fibers. Myelin is the fatty white substance that wraps around nerve fibers, providing insulation and allowing nerve signals to move quickly. Without myelin, nervous transmission is significantly slowed. As the disease progresses, larger and larger patches of demyelination occur, interfering with motor movement, speech, personality, hearing and vision. Ultimately, the vital functions (respiration, heart rate, blood pressure) are affected, leading to the individual's death.

Demographics

Schilder's disease is exceedingly rare. Because there are no specific criteria for the diagnosis, there continues to be debate among researchers and clinicians regarding the most appropriate way to definitively diagnose the disease and collect data on its frequency and incidence. Some sources suggest that there have only been nine cases of definitively diagnosed Schilder's disease since it was originally described in the German medical literature in 1912.

Most patients with Schilder's disease are diagnosed between the ages of seven and twelve years of age.

Causes and symptoms

The underlying cause of Schilder's disease is unknown. Symptoms of the disease are caused by widespread patches of demyelination throughout the brain and spinal cord, resulting in slowed, faulty nervous transmission.

Symptoms of Schilder's disease include weakness of one side of the body (hemiparesis), slowness of movement (psychomotor retardation), paralysis of all four extremities (quadraparesis), **seizures**, difficulty with speech (**dysarthria**), visual and hearing impairment, irritability, memory problems, personality changes, and gradual loss of awareness and responsiveness. Over time, patients become unable to maintain their nutritional status and become increasingly thin and malnourished. Bowel and bladder function are often lost as the disease progresses.

Some children have a relentlessly progressive course of the disease, culminating in death. Other children have remissions and exacerbations, with each subsequent exacerbation more severe and each remission less complete, until death supervenes.

Diagnosis

Because researchers and clinicians have not been able to delineate a clear-cut list of criteria for the diagnosis of Schilder's disease, definitive diagnosis is difficult. EEG studies may show some abnormalities. **MRI** studies will certainly reveal demyelination. Other lab studies (blood tests, test on cerebrospinal fluid obtain via lumbar puncture, brain **biopsy**) are usually performed in an effort to rule out some other cause for the patient's symptoms, such as an infectious, malignant, or metabolic condition; in Schilder's disease, these will all come back normal.

Treatment team

The treatment team for a child with Schilder's disease usually consists of neurologists, specialists in multiple sclerosis, and rheumatologists. Support from physical therapists, occupational therapists, and speech and language therapists can help a child maintain as much functioning as possible.

Treatment

There is no cure for Schilder's disease. Treatments are aimed at slowing the inexorable course of the disease, and are similar to treatments used for multiple sclerosis, such as high dose steroids, beta interferon, and immunosuppressants.

Key Terms

Demyelination Destruction of the myelin that should normally wrap around nerve fibers.

Dysarthria Disturbances of speech and communication.

Hemiparesis Weakness of one side of the body.

Myelin The fatty white substance that wraps around nerve fibers, providing insulation and allowing for speedier nervous transmission.

Psychomotor retardation Slowing of movement and speech.

Quadriparesis Weakness of all four limbs.

Prognosis

Schilder's disease is uniformly fatal.

Resources

BOOKS

Ferri, Fred F., ed. *Ferri's Clinical Advisor: Instant Diagnosis and Treatment.* St. Louis: Mosby, 2004.

Goetz, Christopher G., ed. *Textbook of Clinical Neurology.* Philadelphia: W. B. Saunders Company, 2003.

PERIODICALS

Fernández-Jaén, A. "Schilder's diffuse myelinoclastic sclerosis." *Review of Neurology* 33, no. 1 (July 1, 2001): 16–21.

Kotil, K. "Human Prion Diseases." *British Journal of Neurosurgery* 16, no. 5 (October 1, 2002): 516–519.

WEBSITES

National Institute of Neurological Disorders and Stroke (NINDS). *NINDS Schilder's Disease Information Page.* July 24, 2001. <http://www.ninds.nih.gov/health_and_medical/disorders/schilder's.htm>.

ORGANIZATIONS

Multiple Sclerosis Association of America. 706 Haddonfield Road, Cherry Hill, NJ 08002. 856-488-4500 or 800-532-7667; Fax: 856-661-9797. msaa@msaa.com. <http://www.msaa.com>.

Multiple Sclerosis Foundation. 6350 North Andrews Avenue, Ft. Lauderdale, FL 33309-2130. 954-776-6805 or 888-MSFocus (673-6287); Fax: 954-351-0630.

National Multiple Sclerosis Society. 733 Third Avenue, 6th Floor, New York, NY 10017-3288. 212-986-3240 or 800-344-4867 (FIGHTMS); Fax: 212-986-7981. nat@nmss.org. <http://www.nationalmssociety.org>.

Rosalyn Carson-DeWitt, MD

Schizencephaly

Definition

Schizencephaly, or "split brain," is a neurological disease caused by abnormal development of the brain, leading to the characteristic appearance of abnormal clefts in either one or both cerebral hemispheres. The exact etiology is unknown, although it is classified as a type of neuronal migration disorder and thought to be due to a defect in development that occurs during the period of one to seven months of fetal gestation.

Description

Schizencephaly may have different forms. The appearance of the abnormal schizencephalic brain varies depending on the size and extent of the clefts. Clefts may be unilateral or bilateral and usually extend from the surface of the brain to the fluid-filled ventricles. Clefts are usually located next to the Sylvian fissure, but may be located in any part of the hemispheres. Separation of the walls of the cleft is referred to as open-lip schizencephaly, whereas apposed walls are referred to as closed-lip schizencephaly.

Schizencephaly differs from **porencephaly**, another developmental disorder that is due to early injuries to the developing fetal brain. Porencephaly results from injured brain tissue that subsequently dissolves and leaves a fluid-filled area known as a porencephalic cyst. This cyst can resemble the cleft seen in schizencephaly. Whereas schizencephaly is thought to be a primary disorder of development or neuronal migration, porencephaly is thought to be due to secondary brain damage, although the distinction is not entirely clear. Some theories of schizencephaly also propose early brain injury as contributory, but at an earlier stage of development than in porencephaly. Differentiation between the two often requires brain imaging such as **magnetic resonance imaging (MRI)** to identify the nature of the brain tissue lining the cleft. In porencephaly, scar tissue and white matter is often present, whereas in schizencephaly, gray matter lines the cleft.

Demographics

Schizencephaly is a rare disorder and the incidence is unknown. It usually is noticed in infancy or childhood, although it may be diagnosed in adulthood with the onset of **seizures**.

Causes and symptoms

The cause of schizencephaly is unknown, although environmental and genetic factors have been proposed. Various theories exist as to the timing and nature of the defect in development. Early injury to the brain during the second trimester of pregnancy has been proposed to cause the characteristic clefts. These insults may be due to infection, poor blood flow causing **stroke**, or genetic abnormalities. The earlier onset of injury leading to absence of scar tissue around the defect presumably differentiates schizencephaly from porencephaly. A mutation in the EMX2 gene has been associated with schizencephaly in some familial cases, providing evidence for genetic causes. EMX2 is a transcription factor on human chromosome 10 that is important in early brain formation in mice and flies. The clefts in schizencephaly are often lined by normal brain tissue, but may often be surrounded by abnormal brain tissue that has an unusually high density of folding (polymicrogyria). Schizencephaly may also be associated with abnormal nerve clusters called heterotopias in different parts of the brain. Polymicrogyria and heterotopias are thought to be due to defective neuronal migration, and their association with schizencephaly suggests a common underlying mechanism.

Symptoms

Symptoms can vary widely depending on the extent and the size of the cleft. Patients may show developmental delay that can range from mild to severe. Bilateral and open-lip clefts are associated with more severe delay. Affected individuals may have small heads (**microcephaly**) or increased pressure due to fluid accumulation inside the brain, known as **hydrocephalus**. Paralysis of the limbs may be present. The paralysis may be on one or both sides of the body depending on the location of the clefts. Abnormal muscle tone, including decreased tone (**hypotonia**) and increased tone (**spasticity**), can be seen. Some patients may have only seizures. Seizures usually present before three years of age, but patients may present with seizures in later life as their only symptom and then be diagnosed with schizencephaly by brain imaging.

Diagnosis

Diagnosis is made by imaging of the brain. A computed tomography scan (**CT**) or **MRI** demonstrates the abnormal clefts, which may be bilateral or unilateral, open or closed lip. The clefts may appear symmetric or asymmetric. MRI may show evidence of polymicrogyria lining the clefts. There is no genetic testing available at this time for schizencephaly.

Treatment team

Treatment for patients with schizencephaly differs among patients due to the wide variety of clinical manifestations and symptoms. The team responsible for medical care may include a pediatrician and pediatric **neurologist**. A pediatric neurosurgeon may be involved in performing a shunt procedure for hydrocephalus. An orthopedic surgeon may perform surgeries to improve the mobility of spastic limbs. Physical and occupational therapists can help with improving mobility. A case manager may help in coordinating care and treatments.

Treatment

There is no cure for schizencephaly at this time. The treatment of schizencephaly is directed towards the symptoms caused by the abnormally formed brain. Seizures may require anticonvulsant drug therapy. Seizures that cannot be controlled with medications may be treated by surgical removal of the abnormal tissue surrounding the cleft. With complications of hydrocephalus, a surgical shunt procedure may be necessary to relieve fluid accumulation and pressure.

Recovery and rehabilitation

Due to the congenital nature of schizencephaly, symptoms tend to be unchanging and there is little recovery. Physical therapy may be useful in relieving symptoms of spasticity or paralysis and in improving mobility and ambulation. Occupational therapists may help maintain hand function in those with impaired ability.

Clinical trials

A clinical trial funded by the National Institutes of Health is underway to identify the genes responsible for schizencephaly and other developmental brain disorders associated with **epilepsy**. Contact information for the Walsh laboratory is listed under Resources.

Prognosis

The prognosis for individuals with schizencephaly depends on the amount of neurologic deficiency associated with the malformation. Some patients with unilateral clefts may only have seizures and no other cognitive or motor abnormalities. Seizures may respond to medications or require surgery if unmanageable. Patients with severe **mental retardation** and paralysis will often require lifelong dependent care and may have a shortened lifespan as a result of infections such as pneumonias. Bilateral clefts are associated with earlier onset of seizures and seizures that are more difficult to treat.

Special Concerns

Due to developmental disability, individuals with schizencephaly may benefit from special education programs. Various state and federal programs are available to help individuals and their families with meeting these needs.

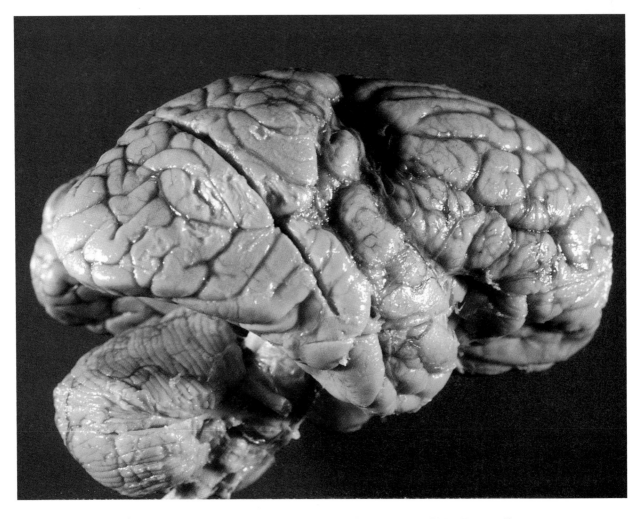

A gray-matter lined cleft in a schizencephalic brain. *(Custom Medical Stock Photo. All Rights Reserved.)*

Key Terms

Neuronal migration   A step of early brain development in which nerve cells travel over large distances to different parts of the brain.

Sylvian fissure   The lateral fold separating the brain hemisphere into the frontal and temporal lobes.

Transcription factor   A protein that acts to regulate the expression of genes.

Ventricle   The spaces in the cerebral hemispheres containing cerebrospinal fluid, a nutrient-rich fluid that bathes the brain.

Resources

BOOKS

Menkes, John H., MD, and Harvey Sarnat, MD, eds. *Childhood Neurology*, 6th edition. Philadelphia: Lippincott Williams & Wilkins, 2000.

"Congenital Anomalies of the Nervous System." *Nelson Textbook of Pediatrics*, 17th edition, edited by Richard E. Behrman, MD, Robert M. Kliegman, MD, and Hal B. Jenson, MD. Philadelphia, PA: Saunders 2004.

PERIODICALS

Guerrini, R., and R. Carrozzo. "Epilepsy and Genetic Malformations of the Cerebral Cortex." *American Journal of Medical Genetics* 106 (2001): 160–173.

Ross, M. E., and C. A. Walsh. "Human Brain Malformations and Their Lessons for Neuronal Migration." *Annual Review of Neuroscience* 24 (2001): 1041–1070.

WEBSITES

National Institutes of Neurological Disorders and Stroke (NINDS). *Schizencephaly Information Page.* (February

26, 2004). <http://www.ninds.nih.gov/ health_and_medical/disorders/schizencephaly.htm>.

National Institutes of Neurological Disorders and Stroke (NINDS). *Cephalic Disorders Information Page.* (February 26, 2004). <http://www.ninds.nih.gov/ health_and_medical/pubs/cephalic_disorders.htm>.

ORGANIZATIONS

March of Dimes Birth Defects Foundation. 1275 Mamaroneck Avenue, White Plains, NY 10605. (914) 428-7100 or (888) MODIMES; Fax: (914) 428-8203. askus@ marchofdimes.com. <http://www.marchofdimes.com>.

National Information Center for Children and Youth with Disabilities. P.O. Box 1492, Washington, DC 20013-1492. (202) 884-8200 or (800) 695-0285; Fax: (202) 884-8441. nichcy@aed.org. <http://www.nichcy.org>.

National Institute of Child Health and Human Development (NICHD). Bldg. 31, Rm. 2A32, Bethesda, MD 20892-2425. (301) 496-5133 or (800) 370-2943. NICHDClearinghouse@mail.nih.gov. <http://www.nichd.nih.gov>.

Walsh Lab Web Site. 4 Blackfan Circle, Boston, MA 02115. (617) 667-0813; Fax: (617) 667-0815. cwalsh@ bidmc.harvard.edu. <http://walshlab.bidmc.harvard.edu/>.

Peter T. Lin, MD

Schizophrenia

Definition

Schizophrenia is a collection of related psychiatric disorders of unknown etiology that follow a specific pattern of behavior. Typical behavior seen in schizophrenia includes psychotic episodes in which there is a severe mental disturbance and perceptions of reality are distorted. Psychotic episodes may also involve hallucinations. Schizophrenics often have delusions about personal identity, immediate surroundings or society, and paranoia. Schizophrenia has a component of heredity, but many factors other than genetics are involved. Schizophrenia is treated with antipsychotic medication.

Description

Schizophrenia involves a specific type of disordered thinking and behavior. It could be described as the splitting of the mind's cognitive functions pertaining to thought, perception, and reasoning from the appropriate emotional responses. Family history of schizophrenia increases an individual's chance of having the disorder, but the exact mode of inheritance is unknown. Only some schizophrenic patients have detectable anatomical brain abnormalities. The cause of schizophrenia has not been determined, yet drugs effective in its treatment have been identified.

Schizophrenia is treated with antipsychotic drugs that primarily act on receptors in the brain for the **neurotransmitters** dopamine and serotonin. These neurotransmitters are chemicals that the brain uses to communicate normal functioning behavior. Receptors for neurotransmitters are sites on the surface of neurons that bind to the neurotransmitters and allow the communication. In schizophrenia, some of the communication mediated by the neurotransmitters dopamine and serotonin and their receptors is abnormal. By inhibiting the activity of these receptors, antipsychotics are effective at decreasing some of the bizarre behavior patterns associated with schizophrenia. Unfortunately, the medication necessary for schizophrenic patients also has severe and pronounced adverse effects, mostly affecting the control of movement. Schizotypal personality disorder is a milder form of the disease.

Demographics

Schizophrenia is estimated to afflict 1% of the world's population, whereas schizotypal personality disorder afflicts 2–3%. Approximately 2.7 million people have schizophrenia in the United States. The incidence of schizophrenia among parents, children, and siblings of patients with the disease is 15%. The rate of adopted children with schizophrenic parents is also 15%. However, the disease is not caused entirely by genetic factors, as identical twins have only a 30–50% tendency to have the same schizophrenic illness. Schizophrenia occurs equally in males and females. The disease may be seen at any age, but the average age for the initiation of treatment is from 28–34 years. Schizophrenia is associated with low economic status, probably due to a lack of proper health care during fetal development.

Causes and symptoms

The cause of schizophrenia is unknown. Some patients display specific physical abnormalities in the brain that are associated with the disease. These include atrophy or degeneration in some brain areas and enlargement of fluid-filled cavities called ventricles. Schizophrenics also have abnormalities in chemical neurotransmitters the brain normally uses to communicate information, specifically the neurotransmitters dopamine and serotonin and their receptors. The imbalance in the activity of these communication components is complex, with overactivity in some parts of the brain and decreased activity in others responsible for different symptoms. The symptoms of schizophrenia are divided into three types: the positive, negative, and disorganized symptoms.

Positive symptoms

Positive symptoms reflect the presence of distinctive behaviors. There are many different positive symptoms of schizophrenia. Schizophrenic patients may experience

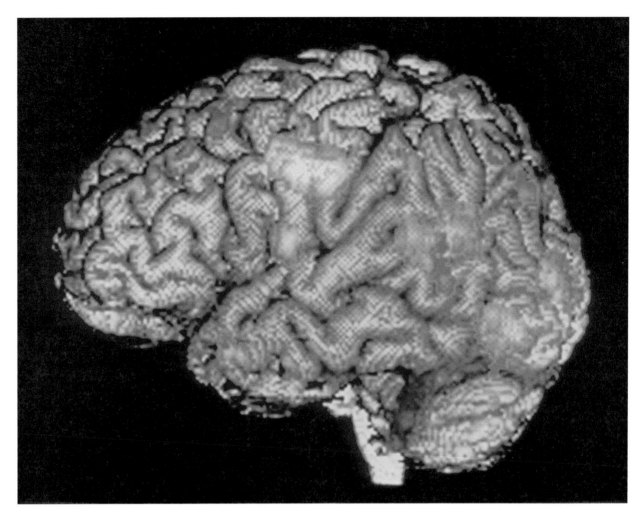

A colored PET scan of the left side of a schizophrenic male patient during a hallucination. The visual and auditory regions of the brain (at the right and the upper center, respectively) are active, confirming that he both saw and heard colored talking heads during the hallucination. *(Wellcome Department of Cognitive Neurology/SPL/Photo Researchers, Inc. Reproduced by permission.)*

strange or paranoid delusions that are out of touch with reality such as the belief that others are persecuting them, or that others are controlling their minds. Schizophrenic patients may have disturbing or frightening hallucinations. The most common hallucinations are auditory, but may also be visual. Other positive symptoms include sensitivity and fearful reaction to ordinary sights, sounds, or smells, along with agitation, tension, and the inability to sleep (insomnia).

Negative symptoms

Negative symptoms reflect the absence of normal social and interpersonal behaviors. Negative symptoms of schizophrenia are varied. Schizophrenic patients often have a reduction in their ability to experience appropriate emotions, or express their emotions. This reduced expressiveness often leads to periods of withdrawal from others. Patients may also experience a lack of motivation, energy,

and ability to experience pleasure. Schizophrenic patients often have poverty of speech, and will not speak readily with others.

Disorganized symptoms

Schizophrenic patients may have confused thinking and speech, which makes it difficult for them to communicate effectively with others. Disorganized behaviors such as unnecessary, repetitive movements are also common.

Diagnosis

Schizophrenics often initially display prodromal signs, which are signs preceding a psychotic episode. Schizophrenic prodromal signs may include social isolation, odd behavior, lack of personal hygiene, and blunted emotions. The prodromal phase is followed by one or more separate psychotic episodes, which are characterized by severe mental disturbances and distorted perceptions of reality. Physicians examining this set of behaviors first attempt to exclude disorders of mood that respond to antidepressants, such as manic **depression**. Sometimes schizophrenia is diagnosed through the patient's response to different therapeutic regimens. Schizophrenic symptoms are not affected by antidepressants, but rather are alleviated by antipsychotics.

Once other disorders have been excluded, the criteria for a diagnosis of schizophrenia is that a patient be continuously ill for at least six months, and that there be one psychotic phase followed by one residual phase of odd behavior. During the psychotic phase, one or more of three groups of psychotic symptoms must be present. The three groups are bizarre delusions, hallucinations, and a disordered or incoherent thought pattern.

Treatment team

Schizophrenic patients are diagnosed and treated by psychiatrists. A licensed therapist performs rehabilitation therapy. Treatment teams from supportive agencies may help with everyday living.

Treatment

Schizophrenia is treated with antipsychotic drugs used in the lowest effective doses. The antipsychotic drugs work mainly to antagonize (inhibit) dopamine and serotonin receptors in specific areas of the brain that are in dysfunction. Classical antipsychotics function primarily on dopamine receptors and have more side effects than modern, atypical antipsychotics that also work on serotonin receptors. The newer, atypical antipsychotics are the treatment of choice because of their comparative lack of side effects, but classical antipsychotics may still be used if a patient is already doing well on the drug. The positive, psychotic symptoms of schizophrenia respond better to antipsychotic treatment than the negative symptoms.

Recovery and rehabilitation

Although antipsychotic drug treatment is necessary for schizophrenic patients, it is not enough for rehabilitation alone. Rehabilitation also requires supportive psychotherapy. Various psychosocial treatments are available for varying stages in the disease, and each patient requires a unique treatment regimen. Doctor and therapist appointments for medication management and psychological healing are necessary in all stages of recovery, even when symptoms are under control. Peer support groups are also very important for rehabilitation. Assertive community treatment (ACT) programs are available for patients who have a severe and unstable course of illness. These programs provide intensive services within a patient's home

---

Key Terms

Etiology   The cause or origin of disease.

Neurotransmitter   Chemicals that act as messengers between cells of the nervous system. Neurotransmitters are released from the axon of one neuron and bind to a specific site such as a receptor in the dendrite of an adjacent neuron, triggering a nerve impulse.

Prodromal   Symptomatic of the approaching onset of an attack or a disease.

---

on a day-to-day basis. ACT teams can follow a patient through all courses of illness and assist them in normal living activities. Patients who are in the later stages of recovery and have few lingering symptoms may get involved with programs designed to help them achieve personal goals pertaining to work, education, and social interactions.

Clinical trials

Most **clinical trials** performed by the National Institute of Mental Health (NIMH) as of January 2004 are centered around three new atypical antipsychotics: olanzapine, risperidone, and aripiprazole. Many clinical trials are being conducted in the United States in different phases. Some studies of schizophrenic patients examine the causes of and potential treatments for negative symptoms as a group, specific symptoms such as cognitive dysfunction, schizophrenia in different age groups such as childhood-onset psychosis, and schizophrenia in different phases of disease course such as first-episode psychosis. Conventional antipsychotics that have excellent initial effects on first episodes also have severe side effects, and hence are associated with eventual patient noncompliance and relapses. The newer antipsychotics may alleviate this problem. Because of this, an NIMH clinical study scheduled to end in June 2004 is examining the role of new atypical antipsychotics in treatment of first psychotic schizophrenic episodes. Clinical trials also examine the ability of specific areas of the brain to function after cognitive stimulation in schizophrenic patients, or analyze DNA samples from families of patients with schizophrenia.

Prognosis

The prognosis for schizophrenia is varied. A diagnosis of schizophrenia does not necessarily mean that the patient will experience a life-long illness. Over a time period of 25–30 years, approximately one-third of schizophrenic patients experience remission or even recovery. Recovery may be in the form of a lack of symptoms or learning to

---

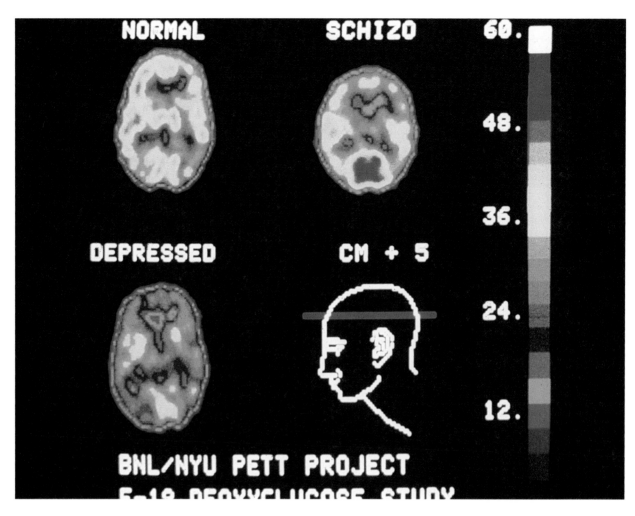

PET scans of normal, schizophrenic, and depressed human brains. *(© NIH/Science Source/Photo Researchers, Inc. Reproduced by permission.)*

live acceptably with some minor symptoms. For this reason, an early negative prognosis should be avoided. However, schizophrenia can be a severe and even dangerous disorder. A wide range of outcomes has been reported, including opposite extremes of full recovery to severe incapacity. A significant proportion of schizophrenic patients have resultant negative outcomes, including an increased mortality rate mostly associated with suicide. Suicide, accidents, and disease are common among patients with schizophrenia, along with an approximate 10-year decrease in lifespan.

Special concerns

A special concern for patients with schizophrenia is the importance of patient compliance even when symptoms have lessened or ceased. It is extremely important for patients to remain in close contact with their treatment team, take all medications consistently, and keep all appointments associated with therapy in order to prevent relapse.

Resources

BOOKS

Neve, Kim A., and Rachael L. Neve, eds. *The Dopamine Receptors.* Totowa, NJ: Humana Press Inc., 1997.

Thomas, Clayton L., ed. *Taber's Cyclopedic Medical Dictionary.* Philadelphia: F. A. Davis Company, 1993.

Zigmond, Michael J., Floyd E. Bloom, Story C. Landis, James L. Roberts, and Larry R. Squire, eds. *Fundamental Neuroscience.* New York: Academic Press, 1999.

OTHER

Weiden, Peter J., Patricia L. Scheifler, Joseph P. McEvoy, Allen Frances, and Ruth Ross, eds. *A Guide For Patients and Families.* Expert Consensus Treatment Guidelines for Schizophrenia, 1999.

WEBSITES

Internet Mental Health. *American Description of Diagnostic Criteria for Schizophrenia.* (April 4, 2004). <http://www.mentalhealth.com>.

National Institute of Mental Health. *Clinical Trials.* (April 4, 2004). <http://clinicaltrials.gov>.

Mental Health: A Report of the Surgeon General Chapter 4. (April 4, 2004). <http://www.schizophrenia.com/research/surg.general.2002.htm>.

ORGANIZATIONS

National Alliance for the Mentally Ill. Colonial Place Three, 2107 Wilson Blvd., Suite 300, Arlington, VA 22201. (703) 524-7600 or (800) 950-6264; Fax: (703) 524-9094. info@nami.org. <http://www.nami.org>.

National Hopeline Network Crisis Center. 201 N. 23rd Street, Suite 100, Purcellville, VA 20132. (540) 338-5756 or (800) 784-2433. Reese@hopeline.com. <http://www.hopeline.com>.

National Institutes of Mental Health. 6001 Executive Blvd., Room 8184, MSC 9663, Bethesda, MD 20892. (301) 443-4513 or (866) 615-6464; (301) 443-4279. nimhinfo@od.nih.gov. <http://www.nimh.nih.gov>.

National Mental Health Association. 2001 N. Beauregard Street, 12th Floor, Alexandria, VA 22311. (703) 684-7722 or (800) 969-6642; (703) 684-5968. <http://nmha.org>.

National Mental Health Consumer Self Help Clearinghouse. 1211 Chestnut Street, Suite 1207, Philadelphia, PA 19107. (215) 751-1810 or (800) 553-4539; Fax: (215) 636-6312. info@mhselfhelp.org. <http://www.mhselfhelp.org>.

Maria Basile, PhD

Sciatica

Definition

Sciatica is **pain** in the lower back that can radiate down the buttocks and leg and occasionally into the foot. The pain is a result of inflammation of the sciatic nerve, usually from a herniated vertebral disk, although other causes are common. Sciatica is one of the frequently reported causes of lower **back pain**.

Description

Sciatica, also known as lumbago or lumbar **radiculopathy**, causes pain as a result of pressure on the sciatic nerve. The sciatic nerve is formed from lumbar roots that emerge from the spinal column. It rises into the pelvis, and travels down the buttocks, the leg, and into the foot. Occurring on both the left and right side of the body, these nerves are the largest in the body, with a diameter as great as a finger; they branch at several points along their path. Sciatica occurs when these nerves become irritated, most often because of a herniated vertebral disk that puts pressure on the sciatic nerve as it emerges from the spinal column.

Sciatica causes pain that may be constant or intermittent and it may include numbness, burning, or tingling. Coughing, sneezing, bending over, or lifting heavy objects

---

Key Terms

Herniated disk   A condition in which part or all of the soft, central portion of an intervertebral disk is forced through a weakened part of the disk, resulting in back pain and leg pain caused by nerve root irritation.

Sciatic nerve   The nerve controlling the muscles of the back of the knee and lower leg, and providing sensation to the back of the thigh, part of the lower leg, and the sole of the foot.

---

may increase the pain. In some cases, there is weakening of muscles in the buttocks, legs, and/or feet.

Demographics

Sciatica is one of the most common forms of back pain. It occurs in about 5% of people who visit their doctor for back pain and in 1–3% of the general adult population. It is most common in people who are between 30 and 50 years of age, as those are the ages most prone to herniating vertebral disks. After age 30, the tough exterior of the vertebral disks undergoes a natural thinning, making it easier for the gel-like inner core to rupture it. After the age of 50, the interior of the vertebral disk becomes slightly hardened, making it less likely to protrude out.

Causes and symptoms

Pressure on the sciatic nerve can result from poor posture, muscle strain, pregnancy, wearing high heels, or being overweight. A herniated disk in the lumbar spine is the most common cause of sciatica. Herniated disks occur when the gel-like inner core of a vertebral disk (*nucleus puposus*) ruptures through the tougher outer section (*annulus*) of the disk. This extrusion puts pressure on the nerve root, causing it to function improperly. Another common cause of sciatica is lumbar spinal stenosis, or narrowing of the spinal canal, which puts pressure on the roots making up the sciatic nerve. Degenerative disk disease causes sciatica when the disk weakens enough to allow excessive movement of the vertebrae near the sciatic nerve. In addition, the degenerated disk may leak irritating proteins in the vicinity of the nerve. Although isthmic spondylolisthesis is relatively common in adults, it only occasionally causes sciatica. This occurs when a vertebra develops a stress fracture and slips, slightly impinging on the sciatic nerve as it exits the spine. **Piriformis syndrome** causes sciatica when the sciatic muscle is irritated as it runs under the piriformis muscle in the buttocks. Finally, sacroiliac joint dysfunction can put pressure on the sciatic nerve, leading to sciatica.

Diagnosis

A physician will perform a physical exam on a patient complaining of sciatica in order to try to identify the part of the nerve that is irritated. This exam may include squatting, walking, standing on toes, and leg raising tests. Most commonly, lifting the leg to a 45° angle while holding it straight helps localize the pain. Other tests that may be performed include x ray to look for stress fractures in bones and **magnetic resonance imaging (MRI)** or computerized tomography (**CT**) to look at softer tissues and ligaments. A nerve conduction velocity test and **electromyography** may also aid in diagnosis.

Treatment

In most cases, conservative treatments are effective for sciatica. A short period of rest, coupled with the application of cold packs and heat packs to the affected area, reduces inflammation of the nerve. Non-steroidal anti-inflammatory medicines can also be taken to decrease inflammation. Injection of corticosteriods may also be recommended to decrease swelling of the nerve. Physical therapy and short walks are also recommended.

If after three or more months, sciatica continues and become progressively worse, surgical techniques can be used to relieve the pressure on the sciatic nerve. Surgery is often very effective in relieving pain, although results can vary depending upon the cause of the sciatica. Overall, about 90% of patients undergoing surgery for sciatica pain receive some relief.

Recovery and rehabilitation

Usually, sciatica improves within a few weeks. In cases of severe injury to the nerve, such as laceration or other trauma, recovery may be not possible or may be limited. The extent of disability may vary from partial to complete loss of movement or sensation in the affected leg. Nerve pain may also persist.

Clinical trials

A recent drug trial found that the drug Remicade (infliximab), which is used to treat arthritis, is often effective for treating sciatica. The drug reduces the level of a chemical called tumor necrosis factor alpha, which plays an important role in the inflammatory response of the body. It is thought that this factor is also critical to sciatica.

The National Institutes of Health (NIH) are conducting three ongoing studies on the treatment of sciatica. One study investigates the effects of the antidepressants desipramine and benztropine on sciatica. A second looks at the effects of magnets on sciatica. A third investigates the role of two drugs, nortriptyline and MS Contin (a type of morphine), as treatment for sciatica. Contact information for these studies is the National Institute for Dental and Craniofacial Research (NIDCR), 9000 Rockville Pike, Bethesda, MD 20892; the toll-free number is (800) 411-1222.

Resources

BOOKS

Credit, Larry P., Sharon G. Hartunian, and Margaret J. Nowak. *Relieving Sciatica.* Vonore, TN: Avery Publishing Group, 2000.

Fishman, Loren, and Carol Ardman. *Back Pain: How to Relieve Low Back Pain and Sciatica.* New York: W.W. Norton and Company, 1997.

OTHER

Hochschuler, Stephen H. "What You Need to Know about Sciatica." *SpineHealth.com.* February 12, 2004 (April 4, 2004). <http://www.spine-health.com/topics/cd/d_sciatica/sc01.html>.

"Sciatica." *American Association of Orthopaedic Surgeons.* February 12, 2004 (April 4, 2004). <http://orthoinfo.aaos.org/fact/thr_report.cfm?Thread_ID=167&topcategory=Spine>.

"Sciatica." *Harvard Medical Schools Consumer Health Information.* February 12, 2004 (April 4, 2004). <http://www.intelihealth.com/IH/ihtIH/WSIHW000/9339/25686.html>.

ORGANIZATIONS

American Academy of Orthopaedic Surgeons. 6300 North River Road, Rosemont, IL 60018-4262. (847) 823-7186 or (800) 346-AAOS; Fax: (847) 823-8125. <http://www.aaos.org>.

National Institute of Arthritis and Musculoskeletal and Skin Diseases. Office of Communications and Public Liaison, National Institute of Health, Bldg. 31, Room 4C02 31 Center Dr. MSC 2350. Bethesda, MD 20892-2350. (301) 496-8190; Fax: (301) 480-2814. <http://www.niams.nih.gov/>.

Juli M. Berwald, PhD

Sciatic neuropathy

Definition

Sciatica is a term given to any painful condition of the leg that originates in the lower back and descends down the leg. Because it tends to involve a single nerve tract it is designated as mononeuropathy (localized nerve disorder).

The cause of this **pain** is the neuropathy defined by the inflammation and swelling of the large sciatic nerve that originates from the exit of an intervertebral nerve plexus between one of the large lumbar vertebral discs. A portion of the sciatic nerve also originates from the sacrum. The name for the region from which this nerve emanates is the sacral plexus. It encompasses the lumbar vertebra L 4– 5 through the sacral vertebra S 1–3. The intervertebral nerves join to form one of the larger nerve tracts in the body, the sciatic nerve. This nerve tract winds over the pelvic bones and down the proximal posterior side of the femurs (either right or left). From there it branches into the tibial and common peroneal nerve. Further branching produces the deep peroneal nerve.

An inflammation or irritation of this nerve can produce pain that ranges anywhere from mild discomfort to extreme distress. Many sufferers describe a constant pain that does not ease with change in body position or conventional medications. The pain can originate from a small area of the lower back to running along the hip, and down the leg past the ankle to the foot.

Additional symptoms of sciatic neuropathy that distinguish it from **peripheral neuropathy** include sensation changes. These occur on the soles of the foot and up the leg. They may include numbness and tingling and even a burning sensation. Difficulty in walking is common and, in serious conditions, there may be an inability to move the foot or knee.

Description

The most common source of inflammation of the sciatic nerve and its branches is injury to an intervertebral disc. This neuritis (nerve inflammation) may occur when pressure on the disc forces it to rupture, squeezing some of the softer more gelatinous interior against the nerve. In turn, this constant pressure begins to irritate the sciatic nerve until eventual swelling from inflammation occurs. The irritation is transmitted to the brain and the patient experiences constant or intermittent pain of varying degrees.

Depending on the degree of herniation to the disc, the pain may eventually go away or the patient may consider lower back surgery. Surgery is the most extreme form of treatment for this condition, as most cases will be relieved with **exercise** and anti-inflammatory medications. Healing may be slow and take up to six weeks.

A common source of sciatic neuropathy is wounding of the sciatic nerve. This condition presents itself when a person has been forced to lie down for extended lengths of time. The resulting pressure on the nerve and lack of movement produces neuropathy. This condition is often confused with tibial nerve dysfunction or common nerve dysfunction.

Wounds to the sciatic nerve may result from fractures of the pelvis, gunshots, or blunt objects such as a bat or stick. Car injuries may often produce damage to the sciatic nerve. Physiological damage can also result from diabetes or an abscess.

Another possible cause of pressure on the sciatic nerve is that imposed by a tumor. Again, surgery may be considered to treat this form of sciatica. The physician may offer alternative therapies to treat the tumor, but therapies are case dependent and vary widely. In cases where tumors are present, the primary cause of the sciatica usually requires treatment that is are not aimed specifically at resolving the sciatica.

Direct trauma to the sciatic nerve may also produce inflammation. A fall or a puncture from an injection could produce insult to the nerve tissues and result in sciatica. In these cases, the treatment is simple and effective. Movement and anti-inflammatory medications usually improve the situation until it eventually resolves.

Demographics

While there varying demographics regarding sciatica, there are conditions that may alert a physician to look for underlying cause of the condition. People under 20 or over 55 are often examined for additional symptoms of other disorders. Associated pain in the back of the chest is a concern along with recent major injury as the type sustained from a traffic injury.

Included in the groups of patients who receive additional examination when they complain of sciatica are those who have lost weight recently, have had cancer, are on steroids, have worsening pain, and those who have developed other nervous system disorders in the past.

Causes and symptoms

As previously noted, the most common cause of sciatica is a "slipped" or herniated disk, also called a prolapsed intervertebral disk (PID) or a herniated nucleus pulposus. Any trauma or injury to the nerve will result in swelling and inflammation. While this healing condition persists, the nerve will respond with pain, which in turn, will often reduce normal movement.

Rarely, sciatic neuropathy has been reported after surgical procedures that required the patient to be immobilized in the operating room for long periods of time or in positions that may have irritated the sciatic nerve.

Diagnosis

Sciatica is in itself a symptom of some other condition which must be diagnosed by a physician. The root causes of the disorder may vary. Only a professional who is trained in recognizing the information provided by the patient and laboratory results can determine if or whether the condition is an isolated symptom or a symptom of a more general or serious disorder of the patient.

Although the diagnosis is based primarily upon symptoms of pain, the physician will usually test for muscle strength, reflexes and flexibility while considering a diagnosis of sciatic neuropathy. Areas of spinal problems that may cause sciatic nerve irritation or compression are usually visible on **MRI** or **CT** images. Occasionally, further nerve function tests may be necessary.

Treatment team

Physicians are the first contact to be made in a treatment team. It is the physician who must first make the diagnosis. A radiologist or laboratory technician may take x rays of the area to look for bone spurs of disk protrusions. Once the diagnosis is made the pharmacist may be called to provide appropriate medication for treatment. In more severe cases, a physical therapist may be used to keep the patient active and performing physical tasks that help reduce the pain. With intractable pain, a neurosurgeon may be consulted for surgery.

Treatment

The immediate treatment of most cases of sciatica is to recommend medications specific to the inflammation. Staying active is also highly recommended, while avoiding activities that put pressure on the back. Studies have found that a simple combination of anti-inflammatory medication such as ibuprofen and mild exercise, such as walking, are effective treatment for most cases of common sciatica. Sometimes an epidural injection (an injection to the epidural space of the spine) may provide pain relief. Surgery for a herniated disk is an aggressive alternative, and includes more risk.

Recovery and rehabilitation

The majority of patients suffering with sciatica recover in a few weeks to six or seven weeks. While the pain may be intense for some sufferers, it is usually temporary. With treatment, person has an excellent chance for reduction or resolution of the neuropathy pain of sciatica.

Clinical trials

A large clinical trial testing the effectiveness of new drug therapies is being conducted by the National Institute of Dental and Craniofacial Research (NIDCR). This may seem like an unlikely group to sponsor such a trial, but any study that examines the effectiveness of medication on nerves may be of great aid to patients suffering from sciatica. Information on additional **clinical trials** can be found at the United States government website for clinical trials: <http://www.clinicaltrials.gov>.

Prognosis

The prognosis for the pain relief of most cases of sciatica is excellent. With a combined use of anti-inflammatory drugs and mild exercise, such as walking, sciatica can be reduced and even eliminated. If the underlying cause is more serious, the prognosis varies with the degree of severity and type of condition.

Special concerns

One of the myths associated with sciatica is the need to rest in bed. In fact, mild exercise is one of the best treatments for the pain. Prolonged sitting is a primary cause of many cases of sciatica. If a job requires extended periods of sitting, it is wise to take short walks or perform mild stretches to keep compression of the lower lumbar vertebrae from occurring.

Resources

BOOKS

Burn, Lois. *Back and Neck Pain: The Facts.* New York: Oxford University Press, 2000.

Fishman, Lauren, and Carol Ardman. *Back Pain: How to Relieve Low Back Pain and Sciatica.* New York: W. W. Norton & Company, 1999.

OTHER

National Library of Medicine. "Sciatica." *MEDLINE plus.* (February 11, 2004). <http://www.nlm.nih.gov/medlineplus/sciatica.html>.

ORGANIZATIONS

American Chronic Pain Association (ACPA). P.O. Box 850, Rocklin, CA 95677. (916) 632-0922 or (800) 533-3231; Fax: (916) 632-3208. ACPA@pacbell.net. <http://www.theacpa.org/>.

National Institute of Arthritis and Musculoskeletal and Skin Dieseases (NIAMS). National Institutes of Health, Bldg. 31, Rm. 4C05, Bethesda, MD 20892. (301) 496-8188; Fax: (540) 862-9485. ncpoa@cfw.com. <http://www.niams.nih.gov/index.htm>.

Brook Ellen Hall, PhD

Seizure disorder *see* **Epilepsy**

Seizures

Definition

A seizure is a sudden change in behavior characterized by changes in sensory perception (sense of feeling) or motor activity (movement) due to an abnormal firing of nerve cells in the brain. **Epilepsy** is a condition characterized by recurrent seizures that may include repetitive muscle jerking called convulsions.

Description

Seizure disorders and their classification date back to the earliest medical literature accounts in history. In 1964, the Commission on Classification and Terminology of the International League Against Epilepsy (ILAE) devised the first official classification of seizures, which was revised again in 1981. This classification is accepted worldwide and is based on electroencephalographic (EEG) studies. Based on this system, seizures can be classified as either focal or generalized. Each of these categories can also be further subdivided.

Focal seizures

A focal (partial) seizure develops when a limited, confined population of nerve cells fire their impulses abnormally on one hemisphere of the brain. (The brain has two portions or cerebral hemispheres—the right and left hemispheres.) Focal seizures are divided into simple or complex based on the level of consciousness (wakefulness) during an attack. Simple partial seizures occur in patients who are conscious, whereas complex partial seizures demonstrate impaired levels of consciousness.

Generalized seizures

A generalized seizure results from initial abnormal firing of brain nerve cells throughout both left and right hemispheres. Generalized seizures can be classified as follows:

- Tonic-clonic seizures: This is the most common type among all age groups and is categorized into several phases beginning with vague symptoms hours or days before an attack. These seizures are sometimes called grand mal seizures.

- Tonic seizures: These are typically characterized by a sustained nonvibratory contraction of muscles in the legs and arms. Consciousness is also impaired during these episodes.

- Atonic seizures (also called "drop attacks"): These are characterized by sudden, limp posture and a brief period of unconsciousness and last for one to two seconds.

- Clonic seizures: These are characterized by a rapid loss of consciousness with loss of muscle tone, tonic spasm, and jerks. The muscles become rigid for about 30 seconds during the tonic phase of the seizure and alternately contract and relax during the clonic phase, which lasts 30–60 seconds.

- Absence seizures: These are subdivided into typical and atypical forms based on duration of attack and level of consciousness. Absence (petit mal) seizures generally begin at about the age of four and stop by the time the child becomes an adolescent. They usually begin with a brief loss of consciousness and last between one and 10 seconds. People having a petit mal seizure become very quiet and may blink, stare blankly, roll their eyes, or move their lips. A petit mal seizure lasts 15–20 seconds. When it ends, the individual resumes whatever he or she was doing before the seizure began, will not remember the seizure, and may not realize that anything unusual happened. Untreated, petit mal seizures can recur as many as 100 times a day and may progress to grand mal seizures.

- Myoclonic seizures: These are characterized by rapid muscular contractions accompanied with jerks in facial and pelvic muscles.

Subcategories are commonly diagnosed based on EEG results. Terminology for classification in infants and newborns is still controversial.

Causes and symptoms

Simple partial seizures can be caused by congenital abnormalities (abnormalities present at birth), tumor growths, head trauma, **stroke**, and infections in the brain or nearby structures. Generalized tonic-clonic seizures are associated with drug and alcohol abuse, and low levels of blood glucose (blood sugar) and sodium. Certain psychiatric medications, antihistamines, and even antibiotics can precipitate tonic-clonic seizures. Absence seizures are implicated with an abnormal imbalance of certain chemicals in the brain that modulate nerve cell activity (one of these **neurotransmitters** is called GABA, which functions as an inhibitor). Myoclonic seizures are commonly diagnosed in newborns and children.

Symptoms for the different types of seizures are specific.

Partial seizures

SIMPLE PARTIAL SEIZURES Multiple signs and symptoms may be present during a single simple partial seizure. These symptoms include specific muscles tensing and then alternately contracting and relaxing, speech arrest, vocalizations, and involuntary turning of the eyes or head. There could be changes in vision, hearing, balance, taste, and smell. Additionally, patients with simple partial seizures may have a sensation in the abdomen, sweating,

Key Terms

Electroencephalograph (EEG)   An instrument that measures the electrical activity of the brain. The EEG traces the electrical activity in the form of wave patterns onto recording paper. Wave patterns that have sudden spikes or sharp waves strongly suggest seizures. An EEG with a seizure-type wave pattern is called an epileptiform EEG.

Hallucination   False sensory perceptions. A person experiencing a hallucination may "hear" sounds or "see" people or objects that are not really present. Hallucinations can also affect the senses of smell, touch, and taste.

Illusion   A misperception or misinterpretation in the presence of a real external stimulus.

paleness, flushing, hair follicles standing up (piloerection), and dilated pupils (the dark center in the eye enlarges). Seizures with psychological symptoms include thinking disturbances and **hallucinations**, or illusions of memory, sound, sight, time, and self-image.

COMPLEX PARTIAL SEIZURES Complex partial seizures often begin with a motionless stare or arrest of activity; this is followed by a series of involuntary movements, speech disturbances, and eye movements.

Generalized seizures

Generalized seizures have a more complex set of signs and symptoms.

TONIC-CLONIC SEIZURES Tonic-clonic seizures usually have vague prodromal (pre-attack) symptoms that can start hours or days before a seizure. These symptoms include anxiety, mood changes, irritability, weakness, **dizziness**, lightheadedness, and changes in appetite. The tonic phases may be preceded with brief (lasting only a few seconds in duration) muscle contractions on both sides of affected muscle groups. The tonic phase typically begins with a brief flexing of trunk muscles, upward movement of the eyes, and pupil dilation. Patients usually emit a characteristic vocalization. This sound is caused by contraction of trunk muscles that forces air from the lungs across spasmodic (abnormally tensed) throat muscles. This is followed by a very short period (10–15 seconds) of general muscle relaxation. The clonic phase consists of muscular contractions with alternating periods of no movements (muscle atonia) of gradually increasing duration until abnormal muscular contractions stop. Tonic-clonic seizures end in a final generalized spasm. The affected person can lose consciousness during tonic and clonic phases of seizure.

Tonic-clonic seizures can also produce chemical changes in the body. Patients commonly experience lowered carbon dioxide (hypocarbia) due to breathing alterations, increased blood glucose (blood sugar), and elevated level of a hormone called prolactin. Once the affected person regains consciousness, he or she is usually weak, and has a **headache** and muscle **pain**. Tonic-clonic seizures can cause serious medical problems such as trauma to the head and mouth, fractures in the spinal column, pulmonary edema (water in the lungs), aspiration pneumonia (a pneumonia caused by a foreign body being lodged in the lungs), and sudden death. Attacks are generally one minute in duration.

TONIC SEIZURES Tonic and atonic seizures have distinct differences but are often present in the same patient. Tonic seizures are characterized by nonvibratory muscle contractions, usually involving flexing of arms and relaxing or flexing of legs. The seizure usually lasts less than 10 seconds but may be as long as one minute. Tonic seizures are usually abrupt and patients lose consciousness. Tonic seizures commonly occur during non-rapid eye movement (non-REM) sleep and drowsiness. Tonic seizures that occur during wakeful states commonly produce physical injuries due to abrupt, unexpected falls.

ATONIC SEIZURES Atonic seizures, also called "drop attacks," are abrupt, with loss of muscle tone lasting one to two seconds, but with rapid recovery. Consciousness is usually impaired. The rapid loss of muscular tone could be limited to head and neck muscles, resulting in head drop, or it may be more extensive, involving muscles for balance and causing unexpected falls with physical injury.

CLONIC SEIZURES Generalized clonic seizures are rare and seen typically in children with elevated fever. These seizures are characterized by a rapid loss of consciousness, decreased muscle tone, and generalized spasm that is followed by jerky movements.

ABSENCE SEIZURES Absence seizures are classified as either typical or atypical. The typical absence seizure is characterized by unresponsiveness and behavioral arrest, abnormal muscular movements of the face and eyelids, and lasts less than 10 seconds. In atypical absence seizures, the affected person is generally more conscious, the seizures begin and end more gradually, and do not exceed 10 seconds in duration.

MYOCLONIC SEIZURES Myoclonic seizures commonly exhibit rapid muscular contractions. Myoclonic seizures are seen in newborns and children who have either symptomatic or idiopathic (cause is unknown) epilepsy.

Demographics

Approximately 1.5 million persons in the United States suffer from a type of seizure disorder. The annual incidence (number of new cases) for all types of seizures is 1.2 per 1,000 and, for recurrent seizures, is 0.54 per 1,000. Isolated seizures may occur in up to 10% of the general population. Approximately 10–20% of all patients have intractable epilepsy (epilepsy that is difficult to manage or treat). It is estimated that 45 million people in the world are affected by seizures. Seizures affect males and females equally and can occur among all age groups. There seems to be a strong genetic correlation, since seizures are three times more prevalent among close relatives than they are in the general population.

Children delivered in the breech position have increased prevalence (3.8%) of seizures when compared to infants delivered in the normal delivery position (2.2%). Seizures caused by fever have a recurrence rate of 51% if the attack occurred in the first year of life, whereas recurrence rate is decreased to 25% if the seizure took place during the second year. Approximately 88% of children who experience seizures caused by fever in the first two years experience recurrence.

Approximately 45 million people worldwide are affected by epilepsy. The incidence is highest among young children and the elderly. High-risk groups include persons with a previous history of brain injury or lesions.

Diagnosis

Patients seeking help for seizures should first undergo an EEG that records brain-wave patterns emitted between nerve cells. Electrodes are placed on the head, sometimes for 24 hours, to monitor brain-wave activity and detect both normal and abnormal impulses. Imaging studies such as **magnetic resonance imaging** (**MRI**) and computed axial tomography (**CT**)—that take still "pictures"—are useful in detecting abnormalities in the temporal lobes (parts of the brain associated with hearing) or for helping diagnose tonic-clonic seizures. A complete blood count (CBC) can be helpful in determining whether a seizure is caused by a neurological infection, which is typically accompanied by high fever. If drugs or toxins in the blood are suspected to be the cause of the seizure(s), blood and urine screening tests for these compounds may be necessary.

Antiseizure medication can be altered by many commonly used medications such as sulfa drugs, erythromycin, warfarin, and cimetidine. Pregnancy may also decrease serum concentration of antiseizure medications; therefore, frequent monitoring and dose adjustments are vital to maintain appropriate blood concentrations of the antiseizure medication—known as the therapeutic blood concentration. Diagnosis requires a detailed and accurate history, and a physical examination is important since this may help identify neurological or systemic causes. In cases in which a **central nervous system** (CNS) infection (i.e., meningitis or encephalitis) is suspected, a lumbar puncture (or spinal tap) can help detect an increase in immune cells (white blood cells) that develop to fight the specific infection.

Treatments

Treatment is targeted primarily to:

- assist the patient in adjusting psychologically to the diagnosis and in maintaining as normal a lifestyle as possible

- reduce or eliminate seizure occurrence

- avoid side effects of long-term drug treatment

Simple and complex partial seizures respond to drugs such as **carbamazepine**, **valproic acid** (valproate), phenytoin, **gabapentin**, **tiagabine**, **lamotrigine**, and **topiramate**. Tonic-clonic seizures tend to respond to valproate, carbamazepine, phenytoin, and lamotrigine. Absence seizures seem to be sensitive to ethosuximide, valproate, and lamotrigine. Myoclonic seizures can be treated with valproate and clonazepam. Tonic seizures seem to respond favorably to valproate, **felbamate**, and clonazepam.

People treated with a class of medications called barbiturates (Mysoline, Mebral, **phenobarbital**) have adverse cognitive (thinking) effects. These cognitive effects can include decreased general intelligence, attention, memory, problem solving, motor speed, and visual motor functions. The drug phenytoin (Dilantin) can adversely affect speed of response, memory, and attention. Other medications used for treatment of seizures do not have substantial cognitive impairment.

Surgical treatment may be considered when medications fail. Advances in medical sciences and techniques have improved methods of identifying the parts of the brain that generate abnormal discharge of nerve impulses. Surgical treatment now accounts for about 5,000 procedures annually. The most common type of surgery is the focal cortical resection. In this procedure, a small part of the brain responsible for causing the seizures is removed. Surgical **intervention** may be considered a feasible treatment option if:

- the site of seizures is identifiable and localized

- surgery can remove the seizure-generating (epileptogenic) area

- surgical procedure will not cause damage to nearby areas

Prognosis

About 30% of patients with severe seizures (starting in early childhood), continue to have attacks and usually never achieve a remission state. In the United States, the prevalence of treatment-resistant seizures is about one to two per 1,000 persons. About 60–70% of persons achieve a five-year remission within 10 years of initial diagnosis. Approximately half of these patients become seizure-free. Usually the prognosis is better if seizures can be controlled by one medication, the frequency of seizures decreases, and there is a normal EEG and neurological examination prior to medication cessation.

People affected by seizure have increased death rates compared with the general population. Patients who have seizures of unknown cause have an increased chance of dying due to accidents (primarily drowning). Other causes of seizure-associated death include abnormal heart rhythms, water in the lungs, or heart attack.

Prevention

There are no gold standard recommendations for prevention, since seizures can be caused by genetic factors, blood abnormalities, many medications, illicit drugs, infection, neurologic conditions, and other systemic diseases. If a person has had a previous attack or has a genetic propensity, care is advised when receiving medical treatment or if diagnosed with an illness correlated with possible seizure development.

Resources

BOOKS

Goetz, Christopher G . *Textbook of Clinical Neurology.* 1st edition. Philadelphia: W. B. Saunders Company, 1999.

Goldman, Lee, and others. *Cecil Textbook of Medicine.* 21st edition. Philadelphia: W. B. Saunders Company, 2000.

Goroll, Allan H. *Primary Care Medicine.* 4th edition. Philadelphia: Lippincott Williams and Wilkins, 2000.

PERIODICALS

Dodrill, C. R., C. G. Matthew. "The role of Neuropsychology in the Assessment and Treatment of Persons with Epilepsy." *American Psychologist* (September 1992).

ORGANIZATIONS

Epilepsy Foundation. 4351 Garden City Drive, Landover, MD 20785-7223. (800) 332-1000. <http://www.efa.org>.

Laith Farid Gulli, MD
Alfredo Mori, MD, FACEM

Septo-optic dysplasia

Definition

Septo-optic dysplasia (SOD) is a rare, congenital disorder. Findings include optic nerve hypoplasia with a thin or absent septum pellucidum and/or corpus callosum and pituitary dysfunction. Optic nerve hypoplasia is mandatory for the diagnosis of SOD.

Description

SOD also known as DeMorsier's syndrome is a combination of optic nerve underdevelopment (hypoplasia) with abnormalities of a part of the brain called the septum pellucidum and/or corpus callosum. Endocrine disorders such as dwarfism, decreased thyroid gland function (hypothyroidism), dehydration, delayed or precocious puberty and reduced blood sugar may occur from dysfunction of the pituitary gland of the brain. SOD has also been associated with congenital architectural brain anomalies.

Causes and symptoms

The cause of SOD is thought to be related to intrauterine viral infections or diabetes during pregnancy. Antiseizure medications, alcohol and illicit drugs have also been linked to SOD. In addition vascular abnormalities and uncommonly genetics are thought to play a role.

Patients afflicted with SOD can present at any age depending on the severity of the symptoms. Signs and symptoms such as failure to thrive, prolonged jaundice, body temperature dysregulation, decreased blood sugar, small genitalia or muscular flaccidity can herald the diagnosis of SOD in newborns.

Older children may complain of visual difficulties and be found to have strabismus (crossed eyes), nystagmus (involuntary, jerky eye movements) or inability to fixate on an object. In addition pupillary and color vision abnormalities may be noted. The optic nerves will appear small and grey or pale in color and can be surrounded by a yellowed halo signifying hypoplasia or atrophy.

A large percentage of SOD patients will have endocrine disorders. By far growth hormone deficiencies are the most common in patients with optic nerve hypoplasia. Growth hormone deficiency can lead to reduced blood sugar, while abnormal levels of reproductive hormones can result unusual pubertal development. Reduced levels of thyroid-stimulating hormone will cause suboptimal thyroid gland functioning (hypothyroidism). Other endocrine problems include increased urination, dehydration and death.

In some instances patients will have behavioral and cognitive problems resulting from brain maldevelopment or endocrinologic disorders.

Diagnosis

Suspicion for the diagnosis of SOD is based on clinical findings described above. In addition **magnetic resonance imaging (MRI)** of the brain focusing on the visual

Key Terms

Corpus callosum The largest commissure connecting the right and left hemispheres of the brain.

Septum pellucidum Two-layered thin wall separating the right and the left anterior horn of lateral ventricle.

pathways, hypothalamus-pituitary region and other midline structures and septum pellucidum is invaluable for solidifying the diagnosis.

Treatment team

Pediatricians, endocrinologists, optometrists, ophthalmologists, neuro-ophthalmologists and neurologists can all contribute to patient care.

Treatment

SOD is treated symptomatically. Hormone deficiencies are managed with hormone replacement therapy while the best possible visual acuity is achieved with corrective spectacle lenses.

Recovery and rehabilitation

Patients with extremely poor vision may benefit from a low vision specialist. He or she may be able to prescribe a visual apparatus to maximally improve visual function.

Special concerns

Patients with severe visual **depression** may have difficulty obtaining a driver's license or gainful employment.

Resources
BOOKS

Liu, Grant T., Nicholas J. Volpe, and Steven L. Galetta. *Neuro-Ophthalmology Diagnosis and Management,* 1st ed. Philadelphia, PA: W. B. Saunders Company, 2001.

PERIODICALS

Campbell, Carrie. "Septo-optic dysplasia: a literature review." *Optometry* 72, no. 7 (July 2003): 417-426.

ORGANIZATIONS

National Organization for Rare Disorders. PO Box 1968, Danbury, CT 06813-1968. 202-744-1000 or 800-999-NORD; Fax: 203-798-2291. orphan@rarediseases.org. <http://www.rarediseases.org>.

National Eye Institute. National Institute of Health, Bldg. 31, Rm. 6A32, Bethesda, MD 20892-2510. 301-496-5248. 2020@b31.nei.nih.gov. <http://www.nei.nih.gov>.

Adam J. Cohen, MD

Shaken baby syndrome

Definition

Shaken baby syndrome is a severe form of head injury caused by the forcible shaking of a child. The force is sufficient to cause the brain to bounce against the baby's skull, causing injury or damage to the brain.

Description

Shaking an infant forcibly transfers a great deal of energy to the infant. When the shaking occurs as the infant is being held, much of the force is transferred to the neck and the head. The force can be so great that the brain can move within the skull, rebounding back and forth from one side of the skull to the other. The bashing can be very destructive to the brain, causing bruising, swelling, or bleeding. Bleeding of the brain is also called intracerebral hemorrhage. The force of shaking can also damage the neck.

As its name implies, shaken baby syndrome can often be a result of deliberate abuse. The brain damage can also be the result of an accident. The force and length of the force necessary to cause shaken baby syndrome is debatable. What is clear is that not much time is needed, since most shaking events likely tend to last only 20 seconds or less. It is the explosive violence of the shaking that exacts the damage.

Demographics

Reliable statistics on the prevalence of shaken baby syndrome do not exist. Estimates in the United States approach 50,000 cases each year. Nearly 25% of infants with shaken baby syndrome die from the brain injuries sustained. The victims of this syndrome range in age from just a few days to five years, with an average age of six to eight months. Statistics point to men as the usual perpetrators, typically young men (i.e., early 20s). Females who shake babies tend to be caregivers. As reliable statistics emerge, it would not be unexpected to find the actual number of cases greatly exceeds these crude estimates. Abuse of children is a hidden event, so many cases of abuse, including shaken baby syndrome, are not reported or are presented in some other form (such as a fall or an accident).

Causes and symptoms

The cause of the brain, neck, and spine damage that can result from shaken baby syndrome is brute force. The violent shaking of a baby by a much stronger adult conveys a tremendous amount of energy to the infant. Part of the reason for the damage is because an infant's head is much larger than the rest of the body, in relation to an older child or an adult. This, combined with neck muscles that are still developing and are incapable of adequately supporting the head, can make shaking an explosively destructive event. The amount of brain damage depends on how hard the shaking is and how long an infant is shaken. If accidental, the force and length of the head trauma similarly determines the extent of injury.

The normal tossing and light "horse play" that can occur between an adult and an infant is not sufficient to cause shaken baby syndrome.

The damage to the brain can have dire consequences that include permanent and severe brain damage or death. Other symptoms that can develop include behavioral changes, lack of energy or motivation, irritable behavior, loss of consciousness, paling of the skin color or development of a bluish tinge to the skin, vomiting, and convulsions. These symptoms are the result of the destruction of brain cells that occurs directly due to the trauma of the blow against the skull, and secondarily as a result of oxygen deprivation and swelling of the brain. The banging of the brain against the sides of the skull causes the inflammation and swelling as well as internal bleeding. Increased intracranial pressure can be damaging to the structure and function of the brain.

Additionally, because the neck and head can absorb a tremendous amount of energy due to the shaking force of the adult, bones in the neck and spine can be broken and muscles can be torn or pulled. The eyes can also be damaged by the explosive energy of shaking. Retinal damage occur in 50–80% of cases. The damage can be so severe as to permanently blind an infant.

Shaken baby syndrome is also known as abusive head trauma, shaken brain trauma, pediatric **traumatic brain injury**, **whiplash** shaken infant syndrome, and shaken impact syndrome.

Diagnosis

Diagnosis depends on the detection of a blood clot below the inner layer of the dura (a membrane that surrounds the brain), but external to the brain. The clot is also known as a **subdural hematoma**. Two other critical features of shaken baby syndrome that are used in diagnosis are brain swelling and hemorrhaging in the eyes.

An infant may also have external bruising on parts of the body that were used to grip him or her during shaking. Bone or rib fractures can also be apparent. However, these external features may not always be present. Diagnosis can also involve the nondestructive imaging of the brain using the techniques of computed tomography (**CT**), skull x ray, or **magnetic resonance imaging (MRI)**. Typically, these procedures are done after an infant has been stabilized and survival is assured.

Treatment team

Treatment in an emergency setting typically involves nurses and emergency room physicians. A neurosurgeon is usually consulted when shaken baby syndrome is suspected. Depending on the extent of injury, neurosurgeons can become involved if surgery for brain repair is needed.

Police officers and **social workers** also become involved in cases of shaken baby syndrome, who work to ensure that the child is placed in a safe environment.

Treatment

Initially, treatment is provided on an emergency basis. Life-saving measures can include stopping internal bleeding in the brain and relieving pressure that can build up in the brain because of bleeding and swelling of the brain.

Recovery and rehabilitation

If the infant survives the initial injury from shaken baby syndrome, rehabilitation focuses on recovering as much function as possible. Physical and occupational therapies can offer exercises for caregivers to provide the child, as well as any supportive or positional devices required. The full effects of the brain injury sustained in infants who survive shaken baby syndrome may not become apparent until delays in developmental milestones such as sitting alone, walking, or acquiring speech are noticed.

Clinical trials

As of May 2004, there are no **clinical trials** on shaken baby syndrome underway or recruiting participants in the United States. However, agencies such as the National Institute of Neurological Disorders and Stroke fund studies that seek to better understand the basis of the damage. Other agencies attempt to lessen the occurrence of the syndrome through counseling, anger management, and interventions in abusive situations.

Prognosis

The prognosis for children with shaken baby syndrome is usually poor. Twenty percent of cases result in death within the first few days. If an infant survives, he or she will most often be left with intellectual and developmental disabilities such as **mental retardation** or **cerebral palsy**. Damage to the eyes can cause partial or total loss of vision. A survivor will likely require specialized care for the remainder of his or her life.

Resources

BOOKS

Lazoritz, Stephen, and Vincent J. Palusci, eds. *Shaken Baby Syndrome: A Multidisciplinary Approach.* Binghamton, NY: Haworth Press, 2002.

PERIODICALS

Geddes, J. F., and J. Plunkett. "The Evidence Base for Shaken Baby Syndrome." *British Medical Journal* (March 2004): 719–720.

Harding, B., R. A. Risdon, and H. F. Krous. "Shaken Baby Syndrome." *British Medical Journal* (March 2004): 720–721.

OTHER

"NINDS Shaken Baby Syndrome Information Page." *National Institute of Neurological Disorders and Stroke.* May 13, 2004 (May 27, 2004). http://www.ninds.nih.gov/health_and_medical/disorders/shakenbaby.htm>.

ORGANIZATIONS

National Institute for Neurological Diseases and Stroke. P.O. Box 5801, Bethesda, MD 20824. (301) 496-5751 or (800) 352-9424. <http://www.ninds.nih.gov>.

The National Center on Shaken Baby Syndrome. 2955 Harrison Blvd., #102, Ogden, UT 84403. (801) 627-3399 or (888) 273-0071; Fax: (801) 627-3321. dontshake@mindspring.com. <http://www.dontshake.com>.

National Institute of Child Health and Human Development. 31 Center Drive, Rm. 2A32 MSC 2425, Bethesda, MD 20892-2425. (301) 496-5133; Fax: (301) 496-7101. <http://www.nichd.nih.gov>.

The Arc of the United States. 1010 Wayne Avenue, Suite 650, Silver Spring, MD 20910. (301) 565-3842; Fax: (301) 565-3843. info@thearc.org. <http://www.thearc.org>.

Think First Foundation [National Injury Prevention Program]. 5550 Meadowbrook Drive, Suite 110, Rolling Meadows, IL 60008. (847) 290-8600 or (800) 844-6556; Fax: (847) 290-9005. thinkfirst@thinkfirst.org. <http://www.thinkfirst.org>.

Brian Douglas Hoyle, PhD

Shingles

Definition

Shingles is infection by the varicella-zoster virus of the dorsal root ganglia of the spine. Equivalent terms for shingles are herpes zoster, zoster, zona, or acute posterior ganglionitis.

Description

Shingles is an infection of the **central nervous system**, in particular, the dorsal root ganglia of the spine, which migrates through sensory nerves to the skin. There it manifests (usually on the upper trunk) as painful, bumpy, fluid-filled eruptions or vesicles. Shingles may also cause nerve **pain** (neuralgia). The affected areas of skin are those supplied by sensory nerves radiating from the infected dorsal root ganglia. Sensory nerves from these ganglia serve non-overlapping, sharply bounded strips or areas of the skin called dermatomes. Because the left and right sides of the body are divided into separate sets of dermatomes, shingles lesions do not cross the midline of the body.

Demographics

The virus that causes shingles is usually contracted in childhood. It is the same virus that causes chicken pox, which is primarily a disease of childhood because it is highly contagious; that is, few individuals live to adulthood without contracting chicken pox. (This statement applies to the temperate zones of the world. For unknown reasons, chicken pox and shingles are less prevalent in tropical regions.) The virus that causes both chicken pox and shingles can, however, be contracted by an individual for the first time in adulthood. First infection, at whatever age it occurs, is called primary infection. Primary infection does not cause shingles; shingles arises from reactivation of virus introduced to the body by an earlier, primary infection.

Shingles arises in individuals who have already had chicken pox, and especially in people with weakened immune systems, such as the elderly or people receiving chemotherapy or bone marrow transplantation. Persons with **AIDS** are also vulnerable to shingles. Shingles incidence increases steadily with age. Among 10–19 year olds, the rate per 1,000 persons per year is only 1.38. In the 30–49 age range, it rises to 2.29 cases of shingles per 1,000 persons per year. By age 60–79, almost seven cases occur per 1,000 people per year, and this increases to 10 in the 80–89 age group.

Causes and symptoms

Shingles is caused by the varicella-zoster virus (VZV), also known as HHV-3. VZV is genetically similar to the herpes simplex viruses, the type of viruses that

Key Terms

Ganglion A mass of nerve cells usually found outside the central nervous system, from which axons arrive from the periphery and proceed to the spinal cord or brain; plural form: ganglia .

Herpes simplex An infection caused by the herpes simples virus, affecting the skin and nervous system and producing small, temporary, often-painful blisters on the skin and mucous membranes.

Hemiparesis Muscle weakness of one side of the body.

Neuralgia Pain along a nerve pathway.

Vesicle A small, raised lesion filled with clear fluid.

causes cold sores and genital herpes. Herpes simplex virus also takes up permanent residence in sensory nerve ganglia, but not in the dorsal root ganglia of the spine, as does VZV. In chicken pox, the virus is inhaled and begins replicating in the upper respiratory tract before spreading to the liver and other body systems.

Following primary infection, VZV remains as a symptomless infection in the dorsal root ganglia of the spinal cord. It may or may not become active again, that is, begin reproducing, later in life. Reactivation occurs more often in older people, probably as a result of decreased immune response with age. Reactivation may be symptomless, but usually causes shingles. Repeat episodes of shingles are rare (occurring in less than 4% of patients) because the immune system's response to VZV is boosted by a first shingles episode.

Chills, fever, malaise, gastrointestinal problems, and pain in the affected skin areas may precede appearance of skin eruptions by several days. Viral particles travel away from the spinal cord along the sensory nerves toward the skin, causing inflammation of those nerves, which may be painful. On the fourth or fifth day, skin vesicles begin to appear. The affected area is usually hypersensitive, and disabling pain (described as sharp, stabbing, or burning) may occur in the affected area. About the fifth day after appearing, the vesicles begin to crust or scab and the disease resolves within the next two weeks. There may be no visible aftereffects, although slight scarring from the vesicles may occur.

Especially in elderly patients, pain may persist for months or years after shingles has otherwise resolved. This pain, postherpetic neuralgia, is caused by damage to the dorsal root ganglia that renders them either spontaneously active (perceived as chronic pain) or hypersensitive to slight stimuli such as light touch.

VZV can become active in the cranial nerves as well as in the spinal ganglia. Involvement of branches of the trigeminal nerve (fifth cranial nerve) is most common. When the ophthalmic branch of the trigeminal nerve is involved, this condition is called herpes zoster ophthalmicus. It can cause swelling of the eyelid, pain, and other complications involving the eye. Herpes zoster ophthalmicus can also lead to weakness or partial paralysis (hemiparesis) on the opposite side of the body from the nerve affected, possibly by inducing irritation of the blood vessels in the brain. Infection of cranial nerves by reactivated VZV can also affect the hearing. When this occurs, it is usually associated with facial palsy and is known as Ramsay-Hunt syndrome.

Large amounts of free virus (i.e., virus not held inside cells) is present in the fluid-filled vesicles or bumps that erupt on the skin during shingles. Thus, people who are not resistant to VZV are easily infected by contact with persons having an outbreak of shingles. A particular strain of VZV can remain latent for decades and then reappear as a new epidemic.

Diagnosis

Diagnosis is based on history and symptoms. The person must have initially had chicken pox in order to have shingles. Definite diagnosis is difficult before eruption of the characteristic vesicles or bumps on the skin. Often persons with early shingles mistake the reddened, painful area as an accidental burn. Once vesicles appear, however, they are hard to mistake because of their dermatome-bounded distribution on the body. In children, shingles (VZV reactivation) must be differentiated from chicken pox (primary VZV infection). This is normally not difficult, as chicken pox vesicles occur widespread on the body and shingles lesions are usually limited to one area on the person's midsection. Herpes simplex virus can also produce vesicle eruptions similar to those of shingles. If there is doubt about which virus is present, virus from the patient can be cultured.

Treatment team

Unless there are complications such as in a person with AIDS, or a child with leukemia, a primary physician can usually treat shingles.

Treatment

Treatment for shingles is primarily with **antiviral drugs**, traditionally acyclovir but, more recently, famcyclovir and valacyclovir. Additionally, a live attenuated-virus vaccine for chicken pox has been licensed since

1995. The vaccine was developed to immunize children undergoing cancer treatment because chicken pox can cause severe complications in such children.

The pain associated with shingles, and with the postherpetic neuralgia that may linger (especially in older patients, after the condition has otherwise resolved), is best treated using combination therapy based on antivirals, antidepressants, corticosteroids, opioids (morphine), and topical agents (applied directly to the skin). The inexpensive amino acid lysine has also been reported to ease the symptoms of both herpes simplex infections and shingles.

Recovery and rehabilitation

Recovery from shingles for the otherwise healthy patient is straightforward and generally requires no special rehabilitation aid or therapy.

Clinical trials

As of mid 2004, several **clinical trials** related to shingles are recruiting patients. One is sponsored by the National Center for Research Resources, University of Texas, and titled "Randomized Study of Two Doses of Oral Valacyclovir in Immunocompromised Patients with Uncomplicated Herpes Zoster." The study seeks to investigate the efficacy of higher-than-standard doses of valacyclovir by assessing quality of life, pain level, and utilization of medical resources of patients treated with a higher-than-standard dose of valacylovir as compared to a control group treated with the standard dose. Contact information is University of Texas Medical Branch, Galveston, Texas, 77555-0209; Stephen K. Tyring is the recruiter, telephone: (281) 333-2288.

Another trial recruiting patients as of 2004 is sponsored by the Baylor College of Medicine, Texas Children's Hospital, and titled "Valacyclovir in Immunocompromised Children." The study seeks to learn how the body handles valacyclovir, its efficacy in treating immunocompromised children with shingles, and the side effects of such treatment. The recruiting inquiries in Pennsylvania is Children's Hospital of Philadelphia, Pennsylvania, 19104; Donna Sylvester, RN, phone: (215) 590-3284. The recruiting inquiries in Texas is Texas Children's Hospital, Houston, Texas, 77030; Susan Blaney, MD, phone: (832) 822-4215, e-mail: sblaney@bcm.tmc.edu , or Lisa R Bomgaars, MD, phone: (832) 824-4688, e-mail: lbomgaars@bcm.tmc.edu.

A third study ongoing in 2004 is sponsored by the drug maker NeurogesX and titled "Controlled Study of NGX-4010 for the Treatment of Postherpetic Neuralgia." NGX-4010 consists of a capsaicin dermal (skin) patch. Capsaicin is the active substance in chili peppers, and is used, paradoxically, both as an irritant and for pain relief. The purpose of this clinical trial is to evaluate the efficacy of a capsaicin patch for relief of postherpetic neuralgia. Contact information varies by state but can viewed at the National Institutes of Health Web site at <http://www.clinicaltrials.gov/ct/show/NCT00068081?order=3>.

Prognosis

Generally, the prognosis for persons with shingles is good. Shingles is almost never a life-threatening disease in otherwise healthy patients, and usually resolves without treatment in a few weeks. However, postherpetic neuralgia, which occurs more often in elderly patients, can be disabling and difficult to treat.

Persons who have an impaired immune system , such as those deficient in cytotoxic T lymphocytes, persons undergoing immune suppression (e.g., for organ transplant), and persons who have AIDS or leukemia may suffer more serious effects from shingles, as the reactivated virus sometimes disseminates from the dorsal root ganglia to other parts of the body. In these cases, complications can resemble those for primary infection of adults with VZV, namely, viral pneumonia, male sterility, acute liver failure, and (in pregnant women) birth defects.

Resources

BOOKS

Glaser, Ronald, and James F. Jones, (eds). *Herpes Virus Infections.* New York: Marcel Dekker, Inc., 1994.

Strauss, James H., and Ellen G. Strauss. *Viruses and Human Disease.* New York: Academic Press, Elsevier Science, 2002.

PERIODICALS

Ho, Charles C., "Use of Combination Therapy for Pin Relief in Acute and Chronic Herpes Zoster." *Geriatrics* (Dec. 1, 2001).

Johns Hopkins Medical Institutions. "Opioid Medications a Good Bet for Shingles-Related Pain." *Ascribe Higher Education News Service* (Oct. 7, 2002).

Madison, Linda K. "Shingles Update: Common Questions in Caring for a Patient with Shingles." *Orthopaedic Nursing* (Jan. 1, 2000).

"New Therapies Reduce Morbidity from Herpes Zoster." *Ophthalmology Times* (Jan. 1, 1999).

Sheff, Barbara, "Microbe of the Month: Varicella-Zoster Virus." *Nursing* (Nov. 1, 2000).

Smith, Angela D. "Lysine for Herpes Simplex Infections." *Medical Update* (Nov. 1, 2001).

OTHER

"NINDS Shingles Information Page." *National Institute of Neurological Disorders and Stroke.* April 28, 2004 (May 27, 2004). <http://www.ninds.nih.gov/health_and_medical/disorders/shingles_doc.htm>.

Larry Gilman, PhD

Shy-Drager syndrome *see* **Multiple system atrophy**

Single Proton Emission Computed Tomography

Definition

Single proton (or photon) emission computed tomography (SPECT) allows a physician to see three-dimensional images of a person's particular organ or body system. SPECT detects the course of a radioactive substance that is injected, ingested, or inhaled. In neurology, a SPECT scan is often used to visualize the brain's cerebral blood flow and thereby, indicate metabolic activity patterns in the brain.

Purpose

SPECT can locate the site of origin of a seizure, can confirm the type of seizure that has occurred, and can provide information that is useful in the determination of therapy. Other uses for SPECT include locating tumors, monitoring the metabolism of oxygen and glucose, and determining the concentration of neurologically relevant compounds such as dopamine.

Currently, a clinical trial is underway in the United States to evaluate the potential of SPECT to study brain receptors for the neurotransmitter acetylcholine. The study will help to determine the usefulness of the technique in charting the progress of the brain deterioration associated with **Parkinson's disease**.

Precautions

The exposure to **radiation**, particularly to the thyroid gland, is minimized as described below in the sections on preparation and aftercare.

Description

Since its development in the 1970s, single proton emission computed tomography has become a critical and routine facet of a clinician's diagnostic routine. A SPECT scan is now a typical part of the diagnosis of coronary artery disease, cancer, **stroke**, liver disease, bone and spinal abnormalities, and lung maladies.

SPECT produces two-dimensional and three-dimensional images of a target region in the body by detecting the presence and location of a radioactive compound given prior to the test. The photon emissions of the radioactive compound can be detected in a manner that is similar to the detection of x rays in computed tomography (**CT**). The

Key Terms

Half-life The time required for half of the atoms in a radioactive substance to decay.

Radioisotope One of two or more atoms with the same number of protons but a different number of neutrons with a nuclear composition. In nuclear scanning, radioactive isotopes are used as a diagnostic agent.

Seizure A sudden attack, spasm, or convulsion.

image produced is a compilation of data collected over time following introduction of the tracer.

The radioactive compound that is introduced typically loses its radioactive potency rapidly (this is expressed as the half-life of a compound). For example, gamma-emitting compounds can have a half-life of just a few hours. This is beneficial for the patients, as it limits the contact time with the potentially damaging radioisotope.

The emitted radiation is collected by a gamma-camera through thousands of round or hexagonal channels that are arranged in parallel in a part of the machine called the collimator. Only gamma rays can pass through the channels. At the other end of the channel, the radiation contacts a crystal of sodium iodide. The interaction produces a photon of light (hence, the name of the technique). The light is subsequently detected and the time and body location of the light-producing radiation is stored computationally. At the end of the SPECT scan, the stored information can be integrated to produce a composite image.

Typically, a patient is stationary. The SPECT scanner can move completely around the patient. Usually the patient will lie on a bed with their head restrained in a holder. Scans are taken for periods up to six hours following the injection of the tracer.

Monitoring of the heartbeat (electrocardiogram), respiration, and blood pressure are accomplished just prior to the start of the scan, five minutes after the introduction of the tracer, and 30–60 minutes after injection. Blood and urine samples are often collected towards the end of the scan.

Preparation

On the night before a scan, the patient takes an oral dose of potassium iodide. This protects the thyroid gland from the radioactive tracer. If a patient is allergic to potassium iodide, potassium perchlorate can be taken instead. Just prior to a scan, small radioisotope markers that contain the element 99Tc are attached with adhesive to the patient's head. Two intravenous catheters are usually placed in veins, through which the radioactive tracer is injected, and so that blood samples can be withdrawn during the scan.

Aftercare

Oral doses of potassium iodide or potassium perchlorate are taken daily for four days following a scan. Patients are asked to urinate every two hours for the first 12 hours following the scan to eliminate the tracer from their body as quickly as possible.

Risks

The use of radiation poses a risk of cellular or tissue damage. However, the injection of the radioactive tracer results in the swift movement of the tracer through the body, and its rapid elimination.

Normal results

The image of the target region of the body is compared to an image of the healthy target region. Analysis of the images by a qualified physician determines the result.

Resources

BOOKS

Brant, Thomas. *Neurological Disorders: Course and Treatment,* 2nd. ed. Philadelphia: Academic Press, 2002.

OTHER

"Psychopharmacology—The Fourth Generation of Progress." *Positron and Single Photon Emission Tomography. Principles and Applications in Psychopharmacology.* American College of Neuropsychopharmacology. (January 27 2004). <http://www.acnp.org/g4/GN401000088/CH087.html>

Brian Douglas Hoyle, PhD

Sixth nerve palsy

Definition

Cranial nerve six supplies the lateral rectus muscle allowing for outward (abduction) eye movement. A sixth nerve palsy, also known as abducens nerve palsy, is a neurological defect resulting from an impaired sixth nerve or the nucleus that controls it. This may result in horizontal double vision (diplopia) with in turning of the eye and decreased lateral movement.

Description

Isolated sixth nerve palsies usually manifest as a horizontal diplopia worse when looking towards the affected eye, with a decreased ability to abduct. Since the sixth nerve only innervates the lateral rectus muscle, isolated palsies will only manifest in this fashion.

Demographics

Sixth nerve palsies have no predilection for males or females and can occur at any age.

Causes and symptoms

For all intensive purposes causes of abducens nerve palsy can be classified as congenital or acquired. Isolated congenital sixth nerve palsy is quite uncommon. If congenital the usual presentation is accompanied by other cranial nerve deficits as seen with Duane's retraction or **Moebius syndromes**. Strabismus, commonly known as "lazy eye," may mimic the appearance of abducens nerve palsy and may go undetected until adulthood because of compensatory mechanisms allowing for alignment of the eyes when focusing. Abduction deficits may also result from **myasthenia gravis**, thyroid eye disease, inflammation and orbital fractures which imitate sixth nerve palsies.

A myriad of causes resulting in abducens nerve palsies have been reported. In order to better differentiate these one must take into account the patient's age and underlying illnesses. In children trauma and tumors were reported as the most common causes. Therefore if no trauma has occurred one must consider a tumor of the **central nervous system** in the pediatric population. Other causes include idiopathic intracranial hypertension, inflammation following viral illness or immunization, **multiple sclerosis**, fulminant ear infections, Arnold-Chiari malformations and meningitis.

New onset palsies in adults can stem from myasthenia gravis, diabetes, meningitis, microvascular disease (atherosclerotic vascular disease) or giant cell arteritis (arterial inflammation). Other causes include **Lyme disease**, syphilis, cancers, autoimmune disorders, central nervous system tumors, and vitamin deficiencies.

Children may be found to have head tilt or in-turning of the affected eye, with reduction of outward gaze. They will very rarely complain of double vision, while adults may describe two images, side by side (horizontal diplopia), which are furthest apart when looking towards the affected eye. Covering of one eye, no matter which one is covered, and gazing away from the affected eye will resolve their diplopia. Patients may also note muscle weakness, possibly heralding myasthenia gravis, or **headache** and jaw **pain**, raising the possibility of giant cell arteritis.

Optic nerve swelling or jumpy eye movements (nystagmus) may occur at any age and warrants immediate work-up for a central nervous system tumor.

Key Terms

Multiple sclerosis   A slowly progressive CNS disease characterized by disseminated patches of demyelination in the brain and spinal cord, resulting in multiple and varied neurologic symptoms and signs, usually with remissions and exacerbations.

Myasthenia gravis   A disease characterized by episodic muscle weakness caused by loss or dysfunction of acetylcholine receptors.

Strabismus   Deviation of one eye from parallelism with the other.

Diagnosis

Diagnosis of sixth nerve palsy is based on history and clinical findings. Once the diagnosis has been established the work-up should be tailored based on the patient's age and medical history.

Pediatric patients with no apparent trauma should undergo **magnetic resonance imaging** of the brain with contrast enhancement to rule out a central nervous system structural lesion (tumor or aneurysm). If the imaging is without abnormal findings a lumbar puncture (spinal tap) should be done to exclude increased intracranial pressure or infection. If this is normal, consideration of a post-viral or post-immunization palsy may be safely entertained.

Isolated abducens palsies in the adult population should be approached in a more conservative manner. If a patient is known to have diabetes, high blood pressure, or atherosclerotic vascular disease, a small **stroke** is likely. If diplopia worsens or no improvement occurs at eight weeks time, a more extensive work-up including magnetic resonance imaging of the brain with contrast and blood work to exclude infections, autoimmune disorders, vitamin deficiencies, or inflammation is warranted. A potentially devastating, blinding disorder known as cranial arteritis may occur in patients usually over 50 years of age. Headache, jaw pain worsened with chewing, night sweats, fevers, weight loss, or muscle aches necessitate blood work to rule out this inflammatory disorder.

Treatment team

Ophthalmologists, neuro-ophthalmologists, optometrists, neurologists, and pediatricians are medical specialists who can evaluate and diagnose a patient with a sixth nerve palsy. Usually an optometrist or ophthalmologist will initially see a patient complaining of diplopia or displaying findings of sixth nerve palsy. A referral will then likely be made to a **neurologist** or neuro-ophthalmologist for evaluation and work-up.

Treatment

Treatment of sixth nerve palsies is dictated by the underlying causes. Older patients who are thought to have had a mini-stroke are observed for several months, because of likely spontaneous resolution. Causes related to masses of the central nervous system or systemic disease should be managed and treated promptly by the appropriate specialist.

Children who are at risk for amblyopia can be treated with patching to reduce the risk of permanent visual loss. Older patients may elect to use a prism incorporated into a spectacle to reduce or eliminate their double vision. Prisms or fogging of one eye are excellent options for the older patient being observed for spontaneous resolution of their palsy.

If diplopia persists for greater than six months and prisms cannot realign the images surgical intervention is an option. Depending on the amount of lateral rectus muscle function one or two surgical options are used. If muscle function remains, weakening of the medial rectus muscle and tightening of the affected lateral rectus muscle may resolve the patient's complaint. If no function exists then a muscle transposition surgery can help restore some abduction ability.

Botulinum toxin may also be used to weaken the medial rectus muscle of the affected eye. This weakening effect is short-lived and repeat injections are necessary.

Clinical trials

As of November, 2003, no **clinical trials** regarding abducens nerve palsies were underway.

Prognosis

Isolated abducens nerve palsies in the older population are usually related to a small stroke and resolve within several months. Palsies related to trauma or brain masses have a guarded prognosis and recovery, if any, may take up to one year. Treatment of systemic disorders, such as myasthenia gravis, have an excellent prognosis, while inflammation related to multiple sclerosis is likely to improve as well. Unfortunately there are no hard and fast rules regarding recovery of any sixth nerve palsy.

Special concerns

Patients afflicted with a sixth nerve palsy should refrain from driving unless an eye patch is used. In addition certain types of employment may warrant a medical leave or temporary change of duties.

Resources

BOOKS

Beers, Mark H., and Robert Berkow, eds. *The Merck Manual of Diagnosis and Therapy.* Whitehouse Station, NJ: Merck Research Laboratories, 1999.

Burde, Ronald M., Peter J. Savino, and Jonathan D. Trobe. *Clinical Decisions in Neuro-Ophthalmology,* 3rd ed. St. Louis: Mosby, 2002.

Liu, Grant T., Nicholas J. Volpe, and Steven L. Galetta. *Neuro-Ophthalmology Diagnosis and Management,* 1st ed. Philadelphia: W. B. Saunders Company, 2001.

Adam J. Cohen, MD

Sjogren-Larsson syndrome

Definition

Sjogren-Larsson syndrome is an inherited condition resulting in thickened, dry, rough skin (ichthyosis), **mental retardation**, and stiff, rigid muscles (**spasticity**). Although not all the manifestations of the disease may be immediately evident at birth, the disease is not considered to be progressive.

Description

Originally identified in Swedish patients, Sjogren-Larsson is a rare genetic disorder. The condition is more common in places where intermarriage within families is traditional, such as among the Haliwa Native Americans of Halifax and Warren counties in North Carolina, and in Vasterbotten and Norrbotten Counties in Sweden.

Demographics

The frequency of Sjogren-Larsson syndrome in the United States is unknown. In Sweden, 0.4 of every 100,000 babies is born with the condition. There is no increased association with a particular race or sex.

Causes and symptoms

Sjogren-Larsson syndrome is inherited in an autosomal recessive fashion, meaning that an affected child has received a faulty gene from both the mother and the father. The disorder has been traced to a variety of defects on chromosome 17, resulting in a defective or deficient enzyme called fatty aldehyde dehydrogenase and an inability to appropriately metabolize compounds called fatty alcohols. Fatty alcohols and fatty aldehydes accumulate and cause water loss from the skin, leading to the severely dry, thickened skin characteristic of the disease.

Key Terms

Ichthyosis Dry, thickened, rough, coarse skin, sometimes with evident scaling.

Myelin The coating on nerves that helps speed the electrical transmission along them.

Spasticity Stiff, rigid, dysfunctional muscles.

Most babies with Sjogren-Larsson syndrome are born prematurely. They often have noticeably reddened skin at birth (erythema), with fine scales evident. Over the course of the first year, the skin becomes increasingly dry, rough, scaly, and thickened. The skin is often itchy. Neurological signs become obvious when the child is late or completely misses reaching various developmental milestones (sitting, crawling, pulling to a stand, vocalizing). The muscles are stiff and rigid, prohibiting normal motor development. Some children are able to walk with braces, but others must rely on a wheelchair throughout life. Mild to moderate mental retardation also becomes evident over time. Language is usually quite delayed. About 40% of children with Sjogren-Larsson syndrome suffer from **seizures**. Other characteristics of people with Sjogren-Larsson syndrome include short stature, poor eyesight, sensitivity to light resulting in squinting, defective tooth enamel, coarse and brittle hair, curved spine (hunchback), and unusually widely-spaced eyes.

Diagnosis

Sjogren-Larsson syndrome can be diagnosed by demonstrating greatly decreased activity of the deficient enzyme, or by identifying one of the genetic defects known to cause Sjogren-Larsson syndrome. **MRI** of the brain will reveal problems with myelin, the whitish material that normally forms a sheath around nerves, allowing for quick conduction of nerve messages. Skin biopsies will reveal a variety of abnormalities characteristic of Sjogren-Larsson syndrome. An EEG (electroencephalogram) will reveal disordered electrical patterns throughout the brain.

Treatment team

A child with Sjogren-Larsson syndrome will usually require diagnostic and treatment help from a team of professionals, including a **neurologist**, orthopedic surgeon, dermatologist, and ophthalmologist. Most children with Sjogren-Larsson syndrome need to be placed in a special educational setting.

Treatment

There are no treatments that can cure Sjogren-Larsson syndrome. A number of lotion or cream preparations (including mineral oil, urea, and vitamin D-3) may help improve itching and flaking, decrease the speed of skin turnover, and soften the skin. Sauna treatments and frequent showering and bathing may improve moisture levels in the skin.

Spasticity is sometimes improved through various surgical procedures. Braces may help increase mobility.

Recovery and rehabilitation

Most children with Sjogren-Larsson syndrome will benefit from services by a physical therapist (to help improve mobility), occupational therapist (to help improve ability to attend to activities of daily living), and speech and language therapist (to help develop both receptive and expressive language).

Prognosis

People with Sjogren-Larsson syndrome will not be able to live independently. They will require care throughout their lives. They may live to an adult age. The disease is not progressive, so the level of disability identified will remain constant.

Special concerns

In families who have an increased risk of Sjogren-Larsson disease, prenatal diagnosis can be accomplished through amniocentesis, chorionic villi sampling, or fetal skin **biopsy**.

Resources

BOOKS

"Disorders of Keratinization." In *Nelson Textbook of Pediatrics*, edited by Richard E. Behrman, et al. Philadelphia: W. B. Saunders Company, 2004.

PERIODICALS

Haddad, F. S., M. Lacour, J. I. Harper, and J. A. Fixsen. "The orthopaedic presentation and management of Sjogren-Larsson syndrome." *J Pediatr Orthop* 19, no. 5 (September-October 1999): 617-19.

Lacour, M. "Update on Sjogren-Larsson syndrome." *Dermatology* 193, no. 2 (1996): 77-82

ORGANIZATIONS

Foundation for Ichthyosis & Related Skin Types, Inc. (F.I.R.S.T.). 650 N. Cannon Avenue, Suite 17, Lansdale, PA 19446. 215-631-1411; Fax: 215-631-1413. info@scalyskin.org. <http://www.scalyskin.org/>.

Rosalyn Carson-DeWitt, MD

Sleeping sickness *see* **Encephalitis lethargica**

Sleep apnea

Definition

Sleep apnea, or sleep-disordered breathing, is a condition in which breathing is briefly interrupted or even stops episodically during sleep. Because repeated arousal or even full awakening when breathing stops disturbs sleep, individuals suffering from sleep apnea are often drowsy during the day. Complications from an insufficient amount of oxygen reaching the brain are serious and even potentially life threatening. Sleep apnea appears to be far more common than was initially realized when it was first described in 1965.

Description

The syndrome of sleep apnea is subdivided into two types: central and obstructive. Central sleep apnea, in which the brain does not properly signal respiratory muscles to begin breathing, is much less common than obstructive sleep apnea. In the latter condition, there are repeated episodes of upper airway obstruction during sleep, typically reducing blood oxygen saturation.

A distinctive form of obstructive sleep apnea is known as the Pickwickian syndrome, named after the protagonist in Charles Dickens' *Pickwick Papers*. Like that character, individuals with the Pickwickian syndrome are overweight, with large necks, fat buildup around the soft tissues of the neck, and loss of muscle tone with aging. When the neck muscles relax during sleep, these characteristics allow the windpipe to collapse during breathing, which usually causes loud snoring.

When the individual with obstructive sleep apnea attempts to inhale, this causes suction that collapses the windpipe and blocks air flow for 10–60 seconds. The resulting fall in blood oxygen level signals the brain to awaken the person enough to tighten the upper airway muscles and reopen the windpipe, resulting in a snort or gasp before snoring resumes. The entire cycle may occur repeatedly, as often as hundreds of times each night.

Demographics

Approximately 6–7% of the population of the United States, or 18 million Americans, are thought to have sleep apnea, but only 10 million have symptoms, and only 0.6 million have yet been diagnosed. In Americans aged 30–60 years, obstructive sleep apnea affects nearly one in four men and one in 10 women; men are twice as likely as

Key Terms

Central sleep apnea A less-common form of sleep apnea in which the brain does not properly signal respiratory muscles to begin breathing.

Continuous positive airway pressure (CPAP) A device that keeps the airway open during sleep by delivering pressurized air through a mask over the nose or over both the nose and mouth.

Obstructive sleep apnea The most common form of sleep apnea characterized by repeated episodes of upper airway obstruction during sleep.

Pickwickian syndrome A distinctive form of obstructive sleep apnea associated with being overweight, having a large neck, fat buildup around the soft tissues of the neck, and loss of muscle tone with aging.

Polysomnography (PSG) A test done at a specialized sleep center in which breathing, brain waves, heartbeat, muscle tension, and eye movement are monitored during sleep through wires attached to the skin; additional testing may include oxygen levels and audio and/or video recordings.

Sleep apnea (sleep-disordered breathing) A condition in which breathing is briefly interrupted or even stops episodically during sleep.

Tracheostomy A surgical procedure that makes an opening in the windpipe to bypass the obstructed airway.

Uvulopalatopharyngoplasty (UPPP) A surgical procedure to remove excess tissue at the back of the throat and relieve airway obstruction.

women to have sleep apnea. As sleep apnea seldom occurs in premenopausal females, it is suggested that hormones may play some role in the disorder.

Other predisposing factors include age, as nearly 20–60% percent of the elderly may be affected; overweight status or obesity; or use of alcohol or sedatives. Based on a 1995 study, elderly African Americans are more than twice as likely as elderly whites to suffer from sleep apnea. Some families appear to have increased incidence of sleep apnea.

Causes and symptoms

Causes of central sleep apnea include various severe and life-threatening lesions of the lower brainstem, which controls breathing. Examples include bulbar **poliomyelitis**, a form of polio affecting the brainstem; degenerative diseases; **radiation** treatment to the neck, damaging the lower brainstem; and severe arthritis of the cervical spine and/or base of the skull, putting pressure on the lower brainstem.

Symptoms of central sleep apnea include cessation of breathing during sleep, often causing frequent awakenings and complaints of insomnia. In central sleep apnea, breathing patterns may also be disrupted during wakefulness. Other symptoms may relate to the underlying neurological condition affecting the brainstem, and may include difficulty swallowing, change in voice, or limb weakness and numbness.

Normally, muscles in the upper throat keep this part of the airway open, allowing air to enter the lungs. Although these muscles relax somewhat during sleep, they retain enough tone to keep the passage open. If the passage is narrow, relaxation of throat muscles during sleep can obstruct, or block, the passage and hinder or prevent air from flowing into the lungs.

Individuals with obstructive sleep apnea may have airway obstruction because of excessive relaxation of throat muscles or because of an already narrowed passage.

Because many patients with obstructive sleep apnea have no major structural defects in the airway and are not obese, other factors such as disordered control of ventilation and changes in lung volume during sleep may play a role in causing the condition.

Soon after falling asleep, the patient with obstructive sleep apnea typically begins snoring heavily. The snoring continues for some time and may become louder before the apnea, during which breathing stops for 10–60 seconds. A loud snort or gasp ends the apnea, followed by more snoring in a recurrent pattern. Decreased oxygen level in the blood during the apneas may cause decreased alertness and other symptoms, while disturbance of the sleep pattern at night may cause daytime drowsiness.

Those with the Pickwickian syndrome have a large neck or collar size, nasal obstruction, a large tongue, a narrow airway, or certain shapes of the palate and jaw.

While patients with sleep apnea may not be aware of the problem, their spouse may seek medical assistance because they are frequently awakened by their partner's snoring, which may be described as loud, squeaky, or raspy. In other cases, the patient may seek help for **fatigue**, difficulty staying awake during the day, or falling asleep at inappropriate times.

Because of restless sleep and decreased oxygen supply to the brain, patients with sleep apnea may complain of impaired mental function, slowed reaction times, problems concentrating, memory loss, poor judgment, personality changes such as irritability or **depression**, morning headaches, and decreased interest in sex.

Additional symptoms may include excessive sweating during sleep, bedwetting, nightmares, dry mouth when awakening caused by sleeping with the mouth open, development of high blood pressure, and frequent upper respiratory infections. Young children with sleep apnea may have visible inward movement of the chest during sleep, learning problems, growth or developmental problems, and hyperactive behavior.

Drinking alcohol before bedtime or taking sleeping pills may increase the risk of apneic episodes, as may breathing through the mouth rather than the nose during sleep.

Severe obstructive sleep apnea may cause pulmonary hypertension, or increased pressure in lung arteries, eventually leading to heart failure. Other complications may include increased risk of cardiovascular disease, **stroke**, heart arrhythmias or irregular heartbeats, and disorders of immune function.

Diagnosis

Although sleep apnea has been more widely diagnosed in the past decade, experts estimate that at least 90–95% of cases remain undiagnosed. Reasons for this include vague, slowly developing symptoms that largely occur when the patient is sleeping; limited knowledge of the disease by physicians; and expensive, specialized testing needed for definitive diagnosis.

Talking to the patient and the spouse or parent is an important first step, but it may not be sufficient. Similarly, the physical examination often fails to reveal distinctive abnormalities. Helpful diagnostic aids may include a questionnaire asking about typical symptoms and sleep habits, and a detailed inspection of the mouth, neck, and throat. Arterial blood gases may reveal low oxygen or high carbon dioxide levels in the blood.

More recently, it has been recognized that obstructive sleep apnea can occur even in individuals of normal weight who lack the other distinctive features of the Pickwickian syndrome. Up to 40% of people with obstructive sleep apnea are not obese.

When sleep apnea is suspected from characteristic symptoms and physical appearance, in many other cases, an overnight polysomnography (PSG) testing at a specialized sleep center may be suggested. During this test, breathing, brain waves, heartbeat, muscle tension, and eye movement are monitored through wires attached to the skin while the patient sleeps. Oxygen levels can be monitored through a device applied to a fingertip, and audio and/or video recordings may provide additional diagnostic information.

After the test, a physician trained in PSG testing analyzes the recordings to determine if sleep apnea or other conditions are present. In some cases, PSG can also be done at home after a sleep technologist attaches the wires and instructs the parent or other responsible adult on how to record sleep activity. Although portable PSG tests are less expensive and more convenient, they are subject to lost or inadequate recording, technical problems, and slightly lower diagnostic accuracy. Patients with inconclusive results on home studies and those with negative studies but persistent symptoms should have standard PSG testing in a sleep center.

Treatment team

The internist or family practitioner is often the first physician consulted because the earliest symptoms of sleep apnea are typically vague. If sleep apnea is suspected, the patient is usually referred to a **neurologist** or specialist in sleep disorders. Ear, nose, and throat specialists can help determine if there are characteristic abnormalities of the jaw or palate contributing to the problem, and in some cases they may perform corrective surgery if indicated. Lung specialists should manage severe cases of sleep apnea that result in pulmonary hypertension. Technicians involved in the diagnosis and treatment of sleep apnea may include PSG technicians and respiratory therapists.

Treatment

For mild cases of sleep apnea, simple measures may suffice, such as losing weight through a diet and **exercise** program, or preventing the person from sleeping on their back. More severe cases may need assisted breathing devices to wear at night or surgery to correct airway obstruction. Individuals with sleep apnea should avoid sedatives, sleeping pills, narcotics, and alcohol, especially at bedtime, as these **central nervous system** depressants can prevent them from awakening enough to keep breathing.

General suggestions to promote better sleep include good sleep habits, going to bed at a regular time each night, and arising at the same time each morning rather than sleeping late on weekends. Keeping the bedroom at a comfortable temperature is conducive to better sleep. Exercising 20–30 minutes each day, at least five to six hours before bedtime, may be helpful both for sleeping better and for weight loss.

Caffeine and related stimulants found in coffee, tea, chocolate, and some diet drugs and **pain** relievers should be avoided. Smoking disrupts sleep by causing early morning awakening in response to nicotine withdrawal. Alcohol reduces the amount of time spent in deep sleep and rapid eye movement (REM) sleep and proportionately increases time spent in the lighter stages of sleep, which are less refreshing.

To relax before bedtime, taking a warm bath, reading, or other restful bedtime ritual may be helpful. Sleeping until the sun rises helps the body's internal biological clock reset itself, as does daily exposure to an hour of morning sunlight. When unable to sleep despite these measures, it is better to read, watch television, or listen to soothing music rather than lying in bed awake, which can cause anxiety and worsen insomnia.

To keep the airway open during sleep, some individuals with obstructive sleep apnea need a device called nasal CPAP, or continuous positive airway pressure, which delivers air through a mask over the nose or over both the nose and mouth. This is considered to be the most effective and widely used therapy.

Complications of CPAP may include nasal congestion or dryness, discomfort related to wearing the mask, and feelings of claustrophobia. To relieve these problems, heated humidifiers to moisturize and warm the air, better fitting and more comfortable masks, or applying steroids within the nasal passages may be helpful. In patients who find it difficult to exhale against the increased pressure of CPAP, bilevel positive-pressure therapy may be equally effective.

Some investigators are studying mechanical devices inserted into the mouth during sleep to open the airway by moving the jaw forward. Although these oral appliances appear to prevent daytime sleepiness and sleep disordered breathing, they do not seem to be as effective as nasal CPAP. However, they may be a reasonable option for patients who are unwilling or unable to use nasal CPAP.

Obstructive sleep apnea in children may be caused by enlarged tonsils and adenoids and can be corrected by tonsillectomy. In adults, surgery to remove airway obstruction may be needed, depending on the anatomical structure. Excess tissue at the back of the throat may be removed in a procedure called an uvulopalatopharyngoplasty, or UPPP. Some cases may require repairing a deviated nasal septum, or other surgery to remove blockage of the nose or upper throat. Surgery to correct obstructive sleep apnea seems to be most effective when it is tailored to the individual's specific anatomical obstruction.

As a last resort, a tracheostomy can be performed, making an opening in the windpipe to bypass the obstructed airway during sleep. During the day, a valve over the opening is closed so the person can speak, and at night, the valve is opened to bypass the obstruction.

If brainstem injury or disease impairs respiratory drive, causing central sleep apnea, mechanical ventilation on a respirator may be needed to ensure continued breathing.

Medications being tested in sleep apnea include Provigil, a nonaddictive drug that improves daytime alertness. Side effects may include nausea and headaches. Decongestants may reduce airway obstruction related to nasal congestion. Results of a controlled trial published in November 2003 suggest that the cholinesterase inhibitor physostigmine may reduce apnea episodes.

Clinical trials

The National Institutes of Neurological Disorder and Stroke, the National Heart, Lung, and Blood Institute (NHLBI), and the National Institute on Aging all support sleep apnea research.

The National Institute of Child Health and Human Development (NICHD) is recruiting children and adolescents with obstructive sleep apnea or other obesity-related diseases for a trial of orlistat (Xenical, Hoffmann LaRoche). By preventing the action of digestive enzymes, this drug interferes with the absorption of approximately one-third of dietary fat. Study subjects may receive active medication or placebo, but all will be enrolled in a weight loss program, including nutrition education, behavioral self-monitoring strategies, and promotion of physical activity.

The APPLES study (apnea positive pressure long-term efficacy study), sponsored by the NHLBI, is recruiting patients with obstructive sleep apnea to determine the effectiveness of nasal CPAP therapy as compared with a similar-appearing control device that does not administer air delivered under positive pressure. Outcomes studied in this trial include mental function, mood, daytime sleepiness, and quality of life. Contact information is the office of study chair William C. Dement, MD, PhD, (650) 723-8131, or <http://apples.stanford.edu>.

The NHLBI is also planning a study of the outcomes of sleep disorders in men aged 65 years and older. It will look at whether sleep disorders such as obstructive sleep apnea are associated with increased risk of cardiovascular disease, falls, decreased physical function, impaired mental function, decreased bone density, fractures, and death.

Prognosis

Treating sleep apnea by eliminating the obstruction usually prevents and reverses complications such as pulmonary hypertension, high blood pressure, and heart disease. Individuals with obstructive sleep apnea who are unable or unwilling to tolerate CPAP may suffer from abnormal heart rhythms, reduced alertness, and sleep deprivation.

Left untreated, sleep apnea can profoundly reduce daytime functioning, work performance, social relationships, and quality of life. If patients fall asleep while driving or engaging in another potentially hazardous activity during the day, sleep apnea may be fatal. Severe, untreated sleep apnea doubles or even triples the risk of automobile accidents compared with the general population. These individuals are also at risk of sudden death from respiratory arrest during sleep.

Children with unrecognized obstructive sleep apnea may experience problems with learning, development, and behavior, as well as failure to grow, heart problems, and high blood pressure. Daytime sleepiness may cause personality changes, poor school performance, and difficulties with interpersonal relationships. Lagging development may lead to frustration and even depression.

Until additional research is carried out, it remains unclear if there is a "safe" number of apnea episodes, or how sleep apnea interacts with other causes of lung or heart failure. It appears that most patients with sleep apnea and heart or lung failure also have underlying diseases such as obstructive lung disease caused by smoking or asthma, severe obesity, or coronary artery disease.

Central sleep apnea usually has a poor prognosis related to the underlying injury or disease affecting the brainstem. Most patients with central sleep apnea require prolonged mechanical ventilation, which can also lead to many serious complications.

Special concerns

Sleep apnea is difficult to diagnose without expensive testing, can aggravate or cause heart and lung problems, often reduces function and quality of life, and may require invasive surgical procedures or long-term use of nasal CPAP. For all these reasons, prevention of obstructive sleep apnea is a worthwhile goal.

Weight reduction in overweight individuals and decreasing intake of alcohol and sedatives have independent health benefits as well as reducing risk of developing obstructive sleep apnea. In children with enlargement of the tonsils and adenoids, corrective surgery may reduce upper respiratory infections while preventing sleep apnea.

In experiments in rats, intermittent decreases in blood oxygen levels during sleep, similar to those seen with obstructive sleep apnea, cause degenerative changes in the hippocampus, a brain region involved in memory and learning. These degenerative changes in the brain are associated with deficits in maze learning. If similar changes occur in obstructive sleep apnea, this might explain decreased mental function observed with this disorder. Brain degeneration related to episodic decreases in oxygen levels would be another important reason to ensure that obstructive sleep apnea is diagnosed and effectively treated.

Although it is well recognized that sleep apnea is more common in men than in women, a study in October 2003 also suggested that men are far more likely than women to seek treatment at a specialized sleep clinic. Research is ongoing to determine the cause of gender differences in sleep apnea and to increase referrals of women to sleep centers where they may obtain appropriate care.

Resources

PERIODICALS

Boyer, S., and V. Kapur. "Role of Portable Sleep Studies for Diagnosis of Obstructive Sleep Apnea." *Current Opinion in Pulmonary Medicine* 2003 Nov 9(6): 465–70.

Durand, E., F. Lofaso, S. Dauger, G. Vardon, C. Gaultier, and J. Gallego. "Intermittent Hypoxia Induces Transient Arousal Delay in Newborn Mice." *Journal of Applied Physiology* 96 (March 2004): 1216–1222.

Fitzpatrick, M. F., H. McLean, A. M. Urton, A. Tan, D. O'Donnell, and H. S. Driver. "Effect of Nasal or Oral Breathing Route on Upper Airway Resistance during Sleep." *European Respiratory Journal* 22, no. 5 (November 2003): 827–32.

Gozal, D., B. W. Row, et al. "Temporal Aspects of Spatial Task Performance during Intermittent Hypoxia in the Rat: Evidence for Neurogenesis." *European Journal of Neuroscience* 2003 Oct 18(8): 2335–42.

Hedner, J., H. Kraiczi, Y. Peker, and P. Murphy. "Reduction of Sleep-Disordered Breathing after Physostigmine." *American Journal of Respiratory and Critical Care Medicine* (2003) 168: 1246–1251.

Jordan, A. S., and R. D. McEvoy. "Gender Differences in Sleep Apnea: Epidemiology, Clinical Presentation and Pathogenic Mechanisms." *Sleep Medicine Review* 2003 Oct 7(5): 377–89.

Jordan, A. S., D. P. White, and R. B. Fogel. "Recent Advances in Understanding the Pathogenesis of Obstructive Sleep Apnea." *Current Opinion in Pulmonary Medicine* 2003 Nov 9(6): 459–64.

Kao, Y. H., Y. Shnayder, and K. C. Lee. "The Efficacy of Anatomically Based Multilevel Surgery for Obstructive Sleep Apnea." *Otolaryngology Head Neck Surgery* 2003 Oct 129(4): 327–35.

Lim, J., T. Lasserson, J. Fleetham, and J. Wright. "Oral Appliances for Obstructive Sleep Apnea." *Cochrane Database Systems Review* 2003 (4): CD004435.

Moyer, C. A., S. S. Sonnad, S. L. Garetz, J. I. Helman, and R. D. Chervin. "Quality of Life in Obstructive Sleep Apnea: A Systematic Review of the Literature." *Sleep Medicine* 2001 Nov 2(6): 477–91.

Qureshi, A., and R. D. Ballard. "Obstructive Sleep Apnea." *Journal of Allergy and Clinical Immunology* 2003 Oct 112(4): 643–51.

Wolk, R., A. S. Shamsuzzaman, and V. K. Somers. "Obesity, Sleep Apnea, and Hypertension." *Hypertension* 2003 Nov 10.

WEBSITES

Clinical Trials (March 2, 2004). <http://www.clinicaltrials.gov/ct/action/GetStudy>.

HealthFinder PO Box 1133, Washington, DC 20013-1133. (March 1, 2004). <http://www.healthfinder.gov/search/default.asp?ct=HFDocs&so=Rank%5Bd%5D%2CDocTitle&doclang=1&page=1&q1=sleep&apnea>.

National Institute of Neurological Disorders and Stroke NIH Neurological Institute. PO Box 5801, Bethesda, MD 20824. (800) 352-9424. (March 2, 2004). <http://www.ninds.nih.gov/search.htm?Text2=%27Sleep+apnea%27&Text1=Sleep+apnea>.

National Sleep Foundation. *When You Can't Sleep: The ABCs of ZZZs.* 2002. February 22, 2004 (March 2, 2004). <http://www.sleepfoundation.org/publications/ZZZs.cfm>

Stanford University Medical Center 300 Pasteur Drive, Stanford, CA 94305. (650) 723-4000. (March 2, 2004). <http://www.stanford.edu/~dement/childapnea.html>.

U.S. National Library of Medicine 8600 Rockville Pike, Bethesda, MD 20894. (March 2, 2004). <http://www.nlm.nih.gov/medlineplus/ency/article/003997.htm>.

OTHER

Apneos Corporation 2033 Ralston Avenue #41, Belmont, CA 94002. (650) 591-2895. (March 2, 2004). <http://www.apneos.com>.

ORGANIZATIONS

The American Lung Association. 61 Broadway, 6th Floor, New York, NY 10006. (212) 315-8700. (March 2, 2004). <http://lungusa.org/diseases/sleepapnea.html>.

The Sleep Apnea Society of Alberta. c/o 911-78 Avenue SW, Calgary, AB T2V0T7. (800) 817-5337. (March 2, 2004). <http://www.sleep-apnea.ab.ca/prognosis.htm>.

Laurie Barclay

▌ Social workers

Definition

A social worker is a helping professional who is distinguished from other human service professionals by a focus on both the individual and his or her environment. Generally, social workers have at least a bachelor's degree from an accredited education program and in most states they must be licensed, certified, or registered. A Master's in Social Work is required for those who provide psychotherapy or work in specific settings such as hospitals or nursing homes.

Description

Social workers comprise a profession that had its beginnings in 1889 when Jane Addams founded Hull House and the American settlement house movement in Chicago's West Side. The ethics and values that informed her work became the basis for the social work profession. They include respect for the dignity of human beings, especially those who are vulnerable, an understanding that people are influenced by their environment, and a desire to work for social change that rectifies gross or unjust differences.

The social work profession is broader than most disciplines with regard to the range and types of problems addressed, the settings in which the work takes place, the levels of practice, interventions used, and populations served. It has been observed that social work is defined in its own place in the larger social environment, continuously evolving to respond to and address a changing world. Although several definitions of social work have been provided throughout its history, common to all definitions is the focus on both the individual and the environment, distinguishing it from other helping professions.

Social workers may be engaged in a variety of occupations ranging from hospitals, schools, clinics, police departments, public agencies, and court systems to private practices or businesses. They provide the majority of mental health care to persons of all ages in this country, and in rural areas they are often the sole providers of services. In general, they assist people to obtain tangible services, help communities or groups provide or improve social and health services, provide counseling and psychotherapy with individuals, families, and groups, and participate in policy change through legislative processes. The practice of social work requires knowledge of human development and behavior, of social, economic and cultural institutions, and of the interaction of all these factors.

Resources
PERIODICALS

Gibelman, Margaret. "The Search for Identity: Defining Social Work—Past, Present, Future." *Social Work* 44, no. 4. (1999).

ORGANIZATIONS

National Association of Social Workers. 750 First St. NE, Washington, D.C. 20002-4241. <http://www.naswdc.org>.

OTHER

National Association of Social Workers. *Choices: Careers in Social Work.* (2002). <http://www.naswdc.org/pubs/choices/choices.htm>.

National Association of Social Workers. *Professional Social Work Centennial: 1898–1998, Addams' Work Laid the Foundation.* 1998 (2002). <http://www.naswdc.org/nasw/centennial/addams.htm>.

Judy Leaver, MA
Rosalyn Carson-DeWitt, MD

Sodium oxybate

Definition

Sodium oxybate is primarily used to treat cataplexy attacks (episodes of weak or paralyzed muscles) in patients with **narcolepsy**, a condition that causes excessive sleepiness.

Purpose

There is no known cure for narcolepsy. Sodium oxybate is specifically indicated only for the treatment of cataplexy; it does not promote wakefulness or relieve excessive sleepiness, the main symptom of narcolepsy.

Description

Sodium oxybate is also sold in the United States under the name Xyrem. It is a Schedule III, federally controlled substance. Sodium oxybate has a high potential for abuse and is commonly known by its non-medical name, GHB. Patients who are prescribed sodium oxybate should use care when storing and disposing of the medication and its containers.

Recommended dosage

Sodium oxybate is taken as an oral solution, mixed with water. Physicians prescribe it in varying dosages. Sodium oxybate is usually taken in two divided doses, the first administered at bedtime and the second 2.5–4 hours later. As the medication induces sleep quickly, an alarm clock is sometimes needed to wake the person for the second dose. Typical adult daily dosages range from .17–.31 oz (5–9 g). If the first half of a daily divided dose is missed, it should be taken as soon as possible. If the second half of a daily divided dose is missed, that dose should be skipped and no more sodium oxybate should be taken until the following day. Two doses of sodium oxybate should never be taken at the same time.

Sodium oxybate works quickly, relaxing muscles and inducing sleep. As food will decrease the amount of sodium oxybate absorbed into the body, patients should not take the medication with meals.

Precautions

Sodium oxybate may be habit forming and has a high potential for non-medical abuse. When taking the medication, it is important to follow physician instructions precisely.

Sodium oxybate is sleep inducing and takes effect quickly. It should, therefore, be taken only at bedtime and while in bed. It may also cause clumsiness and impair clarity of thinking. It can exacerbate the side effects of alcohol and other medications. A physician should be consulted before taking sodium oxybate with certain non-prescription medications. Patients should avoid alcohol and **central nervous system** (CNS) depressants (medications that can make one drowsy or less alert, such as antihistimines, sleep medications, and some **pain** medications) while taking sodium oxybate because they can exacerbate the side effects.

Sodium oxybate may not be suitable for persons with a history of hypopnea (abnormally slow breathing), **sleep apnea**, liver or kidney disease, **depression**, metabolic disorders, high blood pressure, angina (chest pain), or irregular heartbeats and other heart problems.

Before beginning treatment with sodium oxybate, patients should notify their physician if they have a history of consuming a large amount of alcohol or a history of drug use. In these cases, dependence on sodium oxybate may be more likely to develop.

Patients who become pregnant while taking sodium oxybate should contact their physician immediately. Taking sodium oxybate while pregnant may cause fetal harm.

Side effects

Research indicates that sodium oxybate, when used under a physician's direction, is generally well tolerated. However, sodium oxybate may case a variety of usually mild side effects. These side effects usually do not require medical attention, and may diminish with continued use of the medication. They include:

- flu-like feeling
- abdominal pain
- difficulty sleeping
- nightmares
- nervousness or anxiety
- depression
- diarrhea
- dry mouth
- runny nose
- neck pain or stiffness

Key Terms

Cataplexy A sudden and dramatic loss of muscular strength without loss of consciousness; one symptom of narcolepsy.

Narcolepsy A serious sleep disorder characterized by excessive daytime sleepiness, sudden uncontrollable attacks of REM sleep, and attacks of cataplexy.

• **back pain**

• nausea or vomiting

• **headache**

Other, uncommon side effects of sodium oxybate can be potentially serious. A patient taking soduim oxybate who experiences any of the following symptoms should immediately contact their physician:

• sleepwalking

• change in vision

• ringing or pounding in the ears

• problems with memory

• numbness or tingling feelings on the skin

• disorientation, **fainting**, or loss of consciousness

• irregular heartbeat

• shortness of breath

• hives, rashes, or bluish patches on the lips and skin

• chest pain

• severe headache

Interactions

Sodium oxybate may have negative interactions with some anticoagulants (blood thinners), antidepressants, antifungals, antibiotics, asthma medications, barbiturates, and monoamine oxidase inhibitors (MAOIs). Seizure prevention medications **diazepam** (Valium), **phenobarbital** (Luminal, Solfoton), phenytoin (Dilantin), propranolol (Inderal), and rifampin (Rifadin, Rimactane) may also adversely react with sodium oxybate.

Resources

BOOKS

Parker, James N., and Philip N. Parker. *The Official Patient's Sourcebook on Narcolepsy.* San Diego: ICON Health, 2002.

OTHER

"Sodium Oxybate (Systemic)." *Medline Plus.* National Library of Medicine. May 13, 2004 (May 27, 2004).

<http://www.nlm.nih.gov/medlineplus/druginfo/uspdi/500407.html>.

"Xyrem (Sodium Oxybate) Oral Solution Medication Guide." *U.S. Food and Drug Administration Center for Drug Evaluation and Research.* May 13, 2004 (May 27, 2004). <http://www.fda.gov/cder/drug/infopage/xyrem/medicationguide.htm>.

ORGANIZATIONS

Center for Narcolepsy. 701B Welch Road; Room 146, Palo Alto, CA 94304-5742. (650) 725-6517; Fax: (650) 725-4913. <http://www-med.stanford.edu/school/Psychiatry/narcolepsy/>.

Adrienne Wilmoth Lerner

Sotos syndrome

Definition

Sotos syndrome is a genetic condition causing excessive growth and a distinctive head and facial appearance. It has in the past been known as cerebral gigantism. It is often accompanied by delayed development, low muscle tone, and impaired speech.

Description

Sotos syndrome was first described in 1964 and is primarily classified as an overgrowth syndrome, which means that the individual affected with it experiences rapid growth. A number of different symptoms occur in Sotos syndrome; however, it primarily results in rapid growth beginning in the prenatal period and continuing through the infancy and toddler years and into the elementary school years. It is also strongly associated with the bones developing and maturing more quickly (advanced bone age), a distinctive appearing face, and developmental delay.

The excessive prenatal growth often results in the newborn being large with respect to length and head circumference; weight is usually average. The rapid growth continues through infancy and into the youth years with the child's length/height and head circumference often being above the 97th percentile, meaning that out of 100 children of the same age, the child is longer/taller and has a larger head than 97 others. The rate of growth appears to decrease in later childhood and adolescence and final heights tend to be within the normal ranges.

The facial features of individuals with Sotos syndrome change over time. In infants and toddlers, the face is round with the forehead being prominent and the chin small. As the child grows older and becomes an adolescent, the face becomes long with the chin being more prominent, usually with a pointed or square shape. In

Key Terms

Advanced bone age   The bones, on x ray, appear to be those of an older individual.

Congenital   Refers to a disorder which is present at birth.

Failure to thrive   Significantly reduced or delayed physical growth.

Jaundice   Yellowing of the skin or eyes due to excess of bilirubin in the blood.

Karyotype   A standard arrangement of photographic or computer-generated images of chromosome pairs from a cell in ascending numerical order, from largest to smallest.

Tumor   An abnormal growth of cells. Tumors may be benign (noncancerous) or malignant (cancerous).

adults, faces are usually long and thin. The head remains large from birth through adulthood.

Hypotonia is present at birth in nearly every child with Sotos syndrome. Hypotonia means that there is significantly less tone in the muscles. Bodies with hypotonia are sometimes referred to as "floppy." Muscle tone improves as the child grows older, but even in adults, it is still present to some degree. Hypotonia affects many aspects of the baby's development. It can cause difficulty in sucking and swallowing, and many babies are diagnosed with failure to thrive in the newborn period. This, however, usually lasts for about three to four months and then goes away. Hypotonia makes attaining fine motor skills (grasping, playing with toys, babbling) and gross motor skills (rolling, crawling, walking) difficult and these developmental milestones are usually delayed. Speech is also affected by hypotonia but as the child grows older and the hypotonia resolves or goes away, speech improves. Although the child may have delayed development, intellect typically is borderline to normal. Special attention may be needed in certain subjects, such as reading comprehension and arithmetic. Severe **mental retardation** is rarely seen.

There are a number of other features that have been associated with Sotos syndrome, including jaundice in the newborn period, coordination problems, and a tendency for clumsiness. Behavioral problems and emotional immaturity are commonly reported. About half of the children with Sotos syndrome will experience a seizure associated with fever. Dental problems such as early eruption of teeth, excessive wear, discoloration, and gingivitis are common. Teeth may also be aligned incorrectly due to changes in the facial structure.

Infections tend to develop in the ear, upper respiratory tract, and urinary tract. In some children, hearing may be disrupted due to recurrent ear infections and in these situations, a referral to an otolaryngologist (a doctor specializing in the ear, nose, and throat) may be necessary for assessment of hearing. Urinary tract infections occur in about one out of five children with Sotos syndrome. These have been associated with structural problems of the bladder and ureters; consequently, if urinary tract infections occur, the child should undergo further evaluations.

Congenital heart problems and development of tumors have been reported in individuals with Sotos syndrome. However, the information regarding the actual risks of these problems is not definitive and medical screening for these conditions is not routinely recommended.

Genetic profile

Sotos syndrome is for the most part a sporadic condition, meaning that a child affected by it did not inherit it from a parent. In a very few families, autosomal dominant inheritance has been documented, which means that both a parent and his/her child is affected by Sotos syndrome. The cause of Sotos syndrome is not known and the gene(s) that are involved in it have not been identified.

Demographics

Sotos syndrome is described by different groups as being both "fairly common" and "rare." A 1998 article in the *American Journal of Medical Genetics* states that over 300 cases of Sotos syndrome have been published and probably many more are unpublished. As of 2001, incidence numbers had not been determined. Sotos syndrome occurs in both males and females and has been reported in several races and countries.

Signs and symptoms

A variety of clinical features are associated with Sotos syndrome.

- Newborns are large with respect to length and head circumference; weight is usually average. The rapid growth continues through infancy and into childhood with the child's length/height and head circumference often being above the 97th percentile. The rate of growth appears to decrease in later childhood and adolescence.

- Respiratory and feeding problems (due to hyoptonia) may develop in the neonatal period.

- Infants have a round face with prominent forehead and small chin. As the child grows into adolescence and then adulthood the face becomes long and thin, and the chin becomes more prominent.

- Hypotonia is present at birth. This affects the development of fine and gross motor skills, and developmental milestones are usually delayed. Speech is also affected by hypotonia but as the child grows older and the hypotonia resolves or goes away, speech improves.

- Intellect typically is borderline to normal.

- Behavioral problems and emotional immaturity are commonly reported.

- Dental problems such as early eruption of teeth, excessive wear, discoloration, and gingivitis are common.

Diagnosis

Diagnosis of Sotos syndrome is based upon clinical examination, medical history, and x ray data. There are no laboratory tests that can provide a diagnosis. The clinical criteria that are considered to be diagnostic for Sotos syndrome are excessive growth during the prenatal and postnatal period, advanced bone age, developmental delay, and a characteristic facial appearance. It should be noted that although features suggestive of Sotos syndrome may be present at birth or within 6-12 months after birth, making a diagnosis in infancy is not clear cut and may take multiple evaluations over several years.

There are many conditions and genetic syndromes that cause excessive growth; consequently, a baby and/or child who has accelerated growth needs to be thoroughly examined by a physician knowledgeable in overgrowth and genetic syndromes. The evaluation includes asking about health problems in the family as well as asking about the growth patterns of the parents and their final height. In some families, growth patterns are different and thus may account for the child's excessive growth. The child will also undergo a complete physical examination. Additional examination of facial appearance, with special attention paid to the shape of the head, width of the face at the level of the eyes, and the appearance of the chin and forehead is necessary as well. Measurement of the head circumference, arm length, leg length, and wing span should be taken. Laboratory testing such as chromosome analysis (karyotype) may be done along with testing for another genetic syndrome called fragile-X. A bone age will also be ordered. Bone age is determined by x rays of the hand. If the child begins to lose developmental milestones or appears to stop developing, metabolic testing may be done to evaluate for a metabolic condition.

Treatment and management

There is no cure or method for preventing Sotos syndrome. However, the symptoms can be treated and managed. In the majority of cases, the symptoms developed by individuals with Sotos syndrome are treated and managed the same as in individuals in the general population. For example, physical and occupational therapy may help with muscle tone, speech therapy may improve speech, and behavioral assessments may assist with behavioral problems.

Managing the health of a child with Sotos syndrome includes regular measurements of the growth parameters, i.e., height, head circumference, and weight, although excessive growth is not treated. Regular eye and dental examinations are also recommended. Medical screening for congenital heart defects and tumors is not routinely recommended, although it has been noted that symptoms should be evaluated sooner rather than later.

Prognosis

With appropriate treatment, management, and encouragement, children with Sotos syndrome can do well. Adults with Sotos syndrome are likely to be within the normal range for height and intellect. Sotos syndrome is not associated with a shortened life span.

Resources

BOOKS

Anderson, Rebecca Rae, and Bruce A. Buehler. *Sotos Syndrome: A Handbook for Families.* Omaha, NB: Meyer Rehabilitation Institute, 1992.

Cole, Trevor R.P. "Sotos Syndrome." In *Management of Genetic Syndromes,* edited by Suzanne B. Cassidy and Judith E. Allanson. New York: Wiley-Liss, 2001, pp. 389–404.

PERIODICALS

Sotos Syndrome Support Association Quarterly Newsletter.

ORGANIZATIONS

Sotos Syndrome Support Group. Three Danda Square East #235, Wheaton, IL 60187. (888) 246-SSSA or (708) 682-8815. <http://www.well.com/user/sssa/>.

WEBSITES

Genetic and Rare Conditions Site. <http://www.kumc.edu/gec/support/>.

The Family Village. <http://www.familyvillage.wisc.edu/index.htmlx>.

Cindy L. Hunter, CGC

Spasticity

Definition

Spasticity is a form of muscle overactivity. A spastic muscle is one in which a muscle resists being stretched out, and the resistance to stretch is greater the faster the muscle is moved. Spasticity is often used as an umbrella term for other forms of muscle overactivity that often occur at the same time in the same patient.

Description

Spasticity occurs following damage to the neurons, or nerve cells, that send signals from the brain to the muscles to cause movement. These neurons, which run from the brain through the spinal cord, are called upper motor neurons, and damage to them produces an upper motor neuron syndrome. The upper motor neuron syndrome may be caused by **stroke**, **traumatic brain injury**, **spinal cord injury**, **multiple sclerosis**, or numerous other less common causes of damage to the motor neurons. Damage to the brain occurring prior to or shortly after birth is called **cerebral palsy** (CP), which is the most common cause of an upper motor neuron syndrome in children.

The other forms of muscle overactivity common in the upper motor neuron syndrome are:

- Clonus, a relatively slow rhythmic contraction and relaxation of a muscle, typically occurring after a stimulus such as movement or while attempting to hold the muscle still. Clonus can be mild or severe in intensity.

- Spasms, strong and sustained contractions of muscles, which are often painful.

- Increased reflexes, in which the normal reflexes (such as knee extension in response to tapping) are greatly exaggerated.

Together, all these forms of muscle overactivity can cause significant disability in a patient, interfering with dressing, bathing, feeding, mobility, and other activities of daily living. The upper motor neuron syndrome also involves weakness and loss of dexterity, which may be even more disabling to the patient, and may be much less amenable to treatment.

Clinical patterns and problems

Spasticity may affect any muscle or group of muscles, but common patterns are often seen. Each causes its own set of impairments. For instance, the forearm may be drawn up and in toward the chest, making it difficult to put on or take off a shirt. The thighs may be pulled close together, not only making dressing difficult, but narrowing the base of support for standing and walking. The fingers may be clenched tight, driving the nails into the palm and preventing access for cleaning, resulting in infections and skin breakdown. One of the most common patterns is termed equinus, in which the calf muscles tighten, preventing the ankle from flexing completely and leading to walking on the toes.

When the muscle that is overactive is also very strong, it can lead to more severe complications, including partial

Key Terms

Equinus Excess contraction of the calf, causing toe walking.

dislocation. Hip dislocation is a common complication of spasticity in cerebral palsy. A constant imbalance in the forces across a joint due to spasticity can cause the bone to form new tissue in response, leading to bony deformities.

Inactivity brought on by disability can lead to a host of other problems, including pressure sores, osteoporosis, respiratory infections, and social isolation.

Contracture

The resistance to stretch that characterizes spasticity may be mild and infrequent, or it may be severe and quite frequent. In the latter case, the patient can rarely attain a fully stretched position for the muscle, and the muscle spends more time than normal in a partially shortened position. When this occurs, a muscle can develop contracture. A contracture is the loss of full range of motion of a joint due to changes in the soft tissues (muscles and tendons) surrounding that joint. In contracture, the muscle fibers remodel themselves to accommodate this shorter length, thus shortening the muscle overall. In addition, the muscle may develop more fibrous tissue that cannot stretch as much, further increasing its resistance to stretch.

A muscle that develops contracture becomes almost impossible to stretch out to its full length, further worsening the clinical problems of the person with spasticity.

Treatments

Spasticity or other forms of muscle overactivity should be treated if they interfere with function, comfort, or care, or have the potential to lead to deformity that will later require treatment. Treatments available include physical therapy, oral medications, chemical denervation, intrathecal baclofen, neurosurgery, and orthopedic surgery.

Physical therapy

Physical therapy includes daily stretching exercises to maintain the full range of motion for the affected muscles. In mild spasticity, this may be the only treatment needed, while in severe spasticity, it is a part of the full therapy plan. Physical therapy also includes instructions in how to perform activities that are energy-efficient and do not worsen spasticity, including ways to transfer in and out of bed, sitting positions, and hygiene activities.

Bracing may be used to support a weak muscle, or to prevent excess contraction of a spastic muscle. A knee-ankle-foot brace is common to help correct equinus, for instance. Serial casting may be used to stretch out a contractured muscle, with a series of casts at increasing joint angles applied over time. The physical therapist also provides advice on assistive equipment such as wheelchairs and walkers.

Oral medications

Four main medications are used to treat spasticity and other forms of muscle overactivity. Each causes sedation, and thus their uses are limited in patients for whom excess sedation is a significant problem. Oral medications are typically most useful in patients with mild, widespread spasticity, or those for whom sedation is not a problem. They may also be useful at night, to improve comfort during sleep.

Benzodiazepines include **diazepam** and clonazepam. They are most commonly used in spinal cord injury and multiple sclerosis, and may be especially effective against painful spasms. They also reduce anxiety, which may be useful in some patients. Typical side effects include weakness, sedation, and confusion.

Oral baclofen is primarily used for patients with spinal cord injury or multiple sclerosis (MS). A special caution with baclofen is that sudden withdrawal may cause **seizures** and hallucinations. Tizanidine is also used widely in those with spinal cord injury or MS, and is also used in other patients. It is less likely to cause weakness than some other oral medications.

Dantrolene sodium is used for patients with stroke, cerebral palsy, MS, and spinal cord injury. It is somewhat less likely to cause confusion and sedation than other medications, and may be more effective against clonus than some of the other medications. Diarrhea is a side effect in some patients, and monitoring for liver damage is required.

Chemodenervation

Chemodenervation refers to use of a chemical to prevent a nerve from stimulating its target muscle. This reduces spasticity. Chemodenervation is performed with phenol, ethyl alcohol, or **botulinum toxin**. Chemodenervation is most appropriate in patients with localized spasticity in one or two large muscles or several small muscles.

Phenol and ethyl alcohol are injected directly onto the nerve, causing the nerve fiber to degenerate so that it cannot send messages to the muscle. Benefits may last from a month to six months or more, when the nerve regrows. Advantages of the procedure are that the chemicals are inexpensive and can be used repeatedly. Disadvantages are that the injection requires a high degree of skill, may cause

pain due to damage to nerves carrying sensory information, and has a somewhat unpredictable duration of action.

Botulinum toxin is injected into the overactive muscle. It prevents the nerve endings from releasing the chemical they use to stimulate the muscle. The effect lasts approximately three months. Benefits include a simpler and easier injection procedure, with more predictable and reproducible results, with no risk of pain. Disadvantages include high cost and the potential to develop antibodies against the toxin after repeat injections, rendering it ineffective.

Intrathecal baclofen

Intrathecal baclofen (ITB) delivers baclofen directly to the spinal cord, via a tube from an implanted pump. It is most commonly used in patients with widespread spasticity, especially children with cerebral palsy. The pump is implanted in the wall of the abdomen, and the tube is inserted between the vertebrae in the lower or mid-back, releasing the drug into the space surrounding the spinal cord. This allows a much smaller amount of baclofen to be used than if delivered orally, reducing side effects. The baclofen is contained in a reservoir within the pump, and is refilled approximately every three months. The dose can be adjusted to match activities, for instance, increasing at night to aid sleep and decreasing in the morning to increase stiffness slightly to aid getting out of bed. Risks include pump failure and sudden withdrawal from baclofen, which can be dangerous or even fatal, as well as surgery and anesthesia risks. Benefits include reduced spasticity without excess sedation.

Neurosurgery

Selective dorsal rhizotomy (SDR) is used to treat spasticity in cerebral palsy. During SDR, certain overactive nerves entering the spinal cord are cut, reducing the activity that leads to spasticity. Children receiving SDR tend to be able to walk more normally, assuming they have good underlying strength before the operation. SDR is a major surgery requiring general anesthesia. Long-term results indicate children receiving SDR require slightly fewer orthopedic surgeries later in life.

Orthopedic surgery

This type of surgery is performed on muscle or bone, in order to correct deformity, including contracture. The most common surgery is tendon lengthening to treat equinus. In this procedure, the Achilles tendon is cut and the leg is placed in a cast in a more normal position. The tendon regrows to a longer length, reducing the equinus. Other tendon lengthening procedures are performed at the hips and knees. An osteotomy may also be performed to remove abnormal bone growth.

Resources

BOOKS

Glenn, J. Whyte. *The Practical Management of Spasticity.* Philadelphia: Lea & Febiger, 1990.

Mayer, N. H., and D. M. Simpson. *Spasticity: Etiology, Evaluation, Management, and the Role of Botulinum Toxin.* New York: WE MOVE, 2002.

ORGANIZATIONS

WE MOVE. 204 West 84th Street, New York, NY 10024. (212) 875-8389 or (800) 437-MOV2. wemove@wemove.org. <http://www.wemove.org>.

Richard Robinson

SPECT scan *see* **Single proton emission computed tomography**

Speech synthesizer

Definition

A speech synthesizer is a computerized device that accepts input, interprets data, and produces audible language.

It is capable of translating any text, predefined input, or controlled nonverbal body movement into audible speech. Such inputs may include text from a computer document, coordinated action such as keystrokes on a computer keyboard, simple action such as directional interpretation of a joystick, or basic functions such as eye, head, or foot movement.

Purpose

According to a study by the American Speech and Hearing Association, approximately 1.5 million people in the United States are unable to communicate through vocal language; this number does not include hearing impaired. A speech synthesizer can provide an electronic means of verbal communication for individuals who are unable to speak or have visual impairments. Since spoken language is the primary means of communication in most societies, it is often essential for people who are unable to speak on their own to capture that ability.

Individuals with motor neuron disease (MND) often lose their ability to speak due to weakened vocal cords. MND is a classification for disorders that cause muscle weakness and wasting such as **amyotrophic lateral sclerosis** (ALS), progressive bulbar palsy (PBP), **primary lateral sclerosis** (PLS), and progressive muscular atrophy (PMA). In patients with **cerebral palsy**, the area of the brain controlling vocal muscles is damaged resulting in speech loss.

Speech synthesizers can also be useful for people who are visually impaired. Although they may be able to produce oral speech, they are unable to read or produce written text in a non-Braille format. In the example of a student who is visually impaired, the ability to take notes during a lecture and to then review those notes later is not possible. However, with a speech synthesizer, the student can type lecture notes into a laptop and have a text-to-speech software program read them back for review and revision. Without this technology, the more time-consuming method of transcribing audio-recorded lectures into Braille is used.

Precautions

There are many considerations involved in selecting a method for speech synthesis. Key factors are the type of technology used, costs, and equipment. Technology can be overpriced or can quickly become obsolete. When considering the purchase of a speech synthesizer, it is important to determine the reliability of the manufacturer as well as policies regarding maintenance and upgrades of equipment or software. The most cost-effective tools are a laptop computer equipped with appropriate software and hardware. Unfortunately, many insurance companies will not cover the purchase of speech synthesizers or related assistive communication devices.

Description

There are many technologies involved in the production of speech with speech synthesizers. The two most definitive segments are how the user inputs information to be spoken and how the sounds for the words are actually interpreted and produced.

The first step to produce the speech is the composition of text to be spoken. In some cases, it is as simple as loading a computer text file into a software program. In other cases, a more complicated input system is required.

There are many different input devices, but the most prevalent is a keyboard or other similar typing board (such as a touchscreen). Patients with severe mobility restrictions may instead use a joystick device. Special input devices are created that act as switches. These switches are programmed to accept and decipher the motions of the user, even blinking of the eyes. Essentially any muscular movement can be interpreted as a switch and programmed to produce language.

The second step is deciphering the input and producing the desired audio speech. Data is gathered or assembled through the input device until the user indicates that the information is complete. The computer then interprets and speaks the words, phrases, or sentences. Complicated logic is involved when translating written text into spoken language. For example, there are many words that are spelled the same, but pronounced differently in different contexts. The software must make that determination.

Depending on the device, multiple shortcuts may be available to the user. Examples include:

- storing phrases or sentences to reuse at a later time

- translation of abbreviations such as ASAP, which can also be programmed to speak the full phrase, i.e., "as soon as possible"

- software programs that "guess" what the user wants to say and predicts the output as input is gathered; if correct, the user can acknowledge the completion, thereby speeding up the entry of data

Preparation

Even with the advanced technology available for speech synthesizers, a bottleneck of information often occurs with the input. A typical spoken conversation takes place at a rate of 150–200 words per minute. While some individuals can become proficient at touch-typing, allowing for greater success with interactive conversations, many individuals are challenged to produce even 15 words per minute with communication devices.

The typical setup for individuals who use a computer or touchscreen includes a computer, keyboard, monitor, and speakers. In many cases, this equipment can be attached to a wheelchair or bed frame, allowing the user access to "speech" at any time. Other users may simply carry a laptop, batteries, and the necessary connection cables.

For those users unable to manipulate a computer or keyboard-style input device, there is a period of learning and acclimation required to become accustomed to the switch-style inputs. The user must learn how to complete the step-by-step process of composing thoughts into text for output.

A major challenge for individuals who are visually impaired is the presence of graphics in text. Because graphics typically lack a textual equivalent, they are not recognized and spoken by the synthesizer. This may cause the user to miss some information on the screen.

Aftercare

Once an individual has selected a speech synthesis device, there is little follow-up necessary. Hardware and software updates frequently evolve and so there is potential to upgrade devices periodically. Depending on the underlying cause of speech loss, some patients may need to change devices as they lose or regain the ability to speak or move.

Normal results

Through a speech synthesizer, non-vocal users can communicate with spoken words and people who are visually impaired can hear written text. The challenge of becoming proficient with these devices may be greater for some individuals based on physical restrictions.

Resources

BOOKS

Holmes, John, and Wendy Holmes. *Speech Synthesis and Recognition*, 2nd Edition. New York: Taylor & Francis, 2002.

PERIODICALS

Pausch, Randy, and Ronald D. Williams. "Giving CANDY to Children: User-Tailored Gesture Input Driving an Articulator-Based Speech Synthesizer." *Communications of the ACM* 35 n5 (May 1992): 58–67.

Sasso, Len. "Voices from the Machine." *Electronic Musician* February 1, 2004.

WEBSITES

Maxey, H. David. "Smithsonian Speech Synthesis History Project." *National Museum of Natural History, Smithsonian Institute.* July 1, 2002 (cited March 23, 2003 [June 3, 2004]). <http://www.mindspring.com/~ssshp/ssshp_cd/dk_779.htm#V>.

Olshan, Michael. "Voice Lessons: Speaking with ALS." *American Speech-Language-Hearing Association.* 2004 (cited March 23,2004 [June 3, 2004]). <http://www.asha.org/public/speech/disorders/als-voice-lessons-speaking-with-als.htm>.

"Speech Synthesis." *Wikipedia.* March 23, 2004 (cited March 26, 2004 [June 3, 2004]). <http://en.wikipedia.org/wiki/Speech_synthesis>.

"What is MND?" *Motor Neuron Diesease Association.* March 26, 2004 (cited March 26, 2004 [June 3, 2004]). <http://www.mndassociation.org/full-site/what/index.htm>.

ORGANIZATIONS

American Speech-Language-Hearing Association. 10801 Rockville Pike, Bethesda, MD 20852. (800) 638-8255. actioncenter@asha.org. <http://www.asha.org>.

Motor Neuron Disease Association. P.O. Box 246, Northampton NN1 2PR, United Kingdom. 01604 250505; Fax: 01604

638289/624726. enquiries@mndassociation.org.
<http://www.mndassociation.org>.

Stacey L. Chamberlin

Spinal cord tumors *see* **Brain and spinal tumors**

Spinal surgery *see* **Laminectomy**

Spinal cord infarction

Definition

Spinal cord infarction (sometimes called spinal **stroke**) refers to injury to the spinal cord due to oxygen deprivation.

Description

Spinal cord infarction occurs when one of the three major arteries that supply blood (and therefore oxygen) to the spinal cord is blocked. As a result of such an occlusion, the spinal cord is deprived of oxygen, resulting in injury and destruction of the very vulnerable nerve fibers. The resulting disability will depend on what level of the spinal cord suffers the injury; everything below the area of the occlusion will be affected.

Demographics

Spinal cord infarction is a relatively rare condition, affecting about 12 in 100,000 people in the population.

Causes and symptoms

A variety of conditions can result in occlusion of the spinal arteries and spinal cord infarction, including:

- atherosclerosis of the aorta

- a dissecting aortic aneurysm (as well as surgical accidents that occur when clipping aortic aneurysms)

- a tumor or abscess impinging on an artery

- blockages in smaller blood vessels due to diabetes, polyarteritis nodosa, systemic **lupus** erythematosus, neurosyphilis, tuberculous meningitis, pneumococcal meningitis

- severe low blood pressure

- blood clots

- vasculitis

Rare cases of spinal cord infarction have resulted from conditions that exert pressure on the spine (pregnancy, back injury, **exercise**), resulting in the core of a spinal disc (nucleus pulposus) extruding out of the disc and entering into a spinal artery, resulting in a blockage of blood flow.

Depending on the mechanism underlying the spinal cord infarction, the symptoms may begin abruptly and acutely or slowly and gradually. Specific symptoms depend on where in the spinal cord the infarction occurs. Symptoms can include **pain**; paraplegia; quadriplegia; initially limp, floppy muscles that become tightly contracted (spastic) over the next several days; initial loss of reflexes, which become overactive (hyperreflexia) over the next several days; loss of the sense of pain and temperature; and loss of bladder and bowel control.

Diagnosis

Diagnosis is often made by excluding other conditions that might account for the patient's symptoms. Although many tests will not actually reveal spinal cord infarction as the reason for a patient's loss of function, it is important that a variety of tests are performed in order to search for potentially reversible causes of disability. **MRI** scanning may be helpful in this effort; it may not actually reveal images indicative of spinal cord infarction, however.

Treatment team

Individuals with spinal cord infarction are usually cared for by neurologists, physiatrists, physical therapists, and occupational therapists. Complications of spinal cord infarction may require consultation with urologists and pulmonologists.

Treatment

Once an individual has suffered a spinal cord infarction, there are no treatments that will reverse the damage. Some degree of functioning may return as the acute inflammation decreases. Underlying conditions that may have predisposed the individual to spinal cord infarction should certainly be addressed and treated.

Recovery and rehabilitation

Rehabilitation will involve teaching the individual new ways of being as independent as possible, based on the new limitations rendered by the disabilities of spinal cord infarction. The efforts of physical and occupational therapists will be crucial in this endeavor.

Prognosis

The prognosis of spinal cord infarction tends to be very poor. There is a high risk of death, either during the acute phase of infarction or over the long term, particularly due to blood clots in the lungs (pulmonary emboli) or infection of bladder, lungs, or skin ulcerations secondary to inactivity and debilitation. Disability is significant, with a risk of paraplegia or quadriplegia.

Special concerns

The sudden loss of normal functioning and independence that can occur due to spinal cord infarction can prompt severe **depression**. Supportive psychotherapy can be an important adjunctive aid to optimal recovery.

Resources
BOOKS

Hauser, Stephen L. "Diseases of the Spinal Cord." *Harrison's Principles of Internal Medicine*, edited by Eugene Braunwald, et al. NY: McGraw-Hill Professional, 2001.

Perron, Andrew D., and J. Stephen Huff. "Spinal Cord Disorders." *Rosen's Emergency Medicine: Concepts and Clinical Practice*, 5th ed., edited by Lee Goldman, et al. St. Louis: Mosby, Inc., 2002.

Pryse-Phillips, William, and T. Jock Murray. "Infectious diseases of the nervous system." *Noble: Textbook of Primary Care Medicine*, edited by John Noble, et al. St. Louis: W. B. Saunders Company, 2001.

WEBSITES

National Institute of Neurological Disorders and Stroke (NINDS). *NINDS Spinal Cord Infarction Information Page.* January 28, 2003. (June 3, 2004). <http://www.ninds.nih.gov/health_and_medical/disorders/spinal_infarction.htm>.

ORGANIZATIONS

Christopher Reeve Paralysis Foundation / Paralysis Resource Center. 500 Morris Avenue, Springfield, NJ 07081. 973-379-2690 or 800-225-0292; Fax: 973-912-9433. info@crpf.org; research@crpf.org. <http://www.christopherreeve.org>.

National Spinal Cord Injury Association. 6701 Democracy Blvd. #300-9, Bethesda, MD 20817. 301-214-4006 or 800-962-9629; Fax: 301-881-9817. info@spinalcord.org. <http://www.spinalcord.org>.

Rosalyn Carson-DeWitt, MD

Spinal cord injury

Definition

Spinal cord injury is damage to the spinal cord that causes loss of sensation and motor control.

Description

Approximately 10,000 new spinal cord injuries (SCIs) occur each year in the United States. About 250,000 people are currently affected. Spinal cord injuries can happen to anyone at any time of life. The typical patient, however, is a man between the ages of 19 and 26, injured in a motor vehicle accident (about 50% of all SCIs), a fall (20%), an act of violence (15%), or a sporting accident (14%). Most SCI patients are white, but the nonwhite fraction of SCI patients is larger than the nonwhite fraction of the general population. Alcohol or other drug abuse plays an important role in a large percentage of all spinal cord injuries. Six percent of people who receive injuries to the lower spine die within a year, and 40% of people who receive the more frequent higher injuries die within a year.

Short-term costs for hospitalization, equipment, and home modifications are approximately $140,000 for an SCI patient capable of independent living. Lifetime costs may exceed one million dollars. Costs may be three to four times higher for the SCI patient who needs long-term institutional care. Overall costs to the American economy in direct payments and lost productivity are more than $10 billion per year.

Causes and symptoms

The spinal cord is about as big around as the index finger. It descends from the brain down the back through hollow channels of the backbone. The spinal cord is made of nerve cells (neurons). The nerve cells carry sensory data from the areas outside the spinal cord (periphery) to the brain, and they carry motor commands from brain to periphery. Peripheral neurons are bundled together to make up the 31 pairs of peripheral nerve roots. The peripheral nerve roots enter and exit the spinal cord by passing through the spaces between the stacked vertebrae. Each pair of nerves is named for the vertebra from which it exits. These are known as:

- C1-8. These nerves enter from the eight cervical or neck vertebrae.

- T1-12. These nerves enter from the thoracic or chest vertebrae.

- L1-5. These nerves enter from the lumbar vertebrae of the lower back.

- S1-5. These nerves enter through the sacral or pelvic vertebrae.

- Coccygeal. These nerves enter through the **coccyx** or tailbone.

Peripheral nerves carry motor commands to the muscles and internal organs, and they carry sensations from these areas and from the body's surface. (Sensory data from the head, including sight, sound, smell, and taste, do not pass through the spinal cord and are not affected by most SCIs.) Damage to the spinal cord interrupts these signals. The interruption damages motor functions that allow the muscles to move, sensory functions such as feeling heat and cold, and autonomic functions such as urination, sexual function, sweating, and blood pressure.

Spinal cord injuries most often occur where the spine is most flexible, in the regions of C5-C7 of the neck, and T10-L2 at the base of the rib cage. Several physically distinct types of damage are recognized. Sudden and violent jolts to nearby tissues can jar the cord. This jarring causes a temporary spinal concussion. Concussion symptoms usually disappear completely within several hours. A spinal contusion or bruise is bleeding within the spinal column. The pressure from the excess fluid may kill spinal cord neurons. Spinal compression is caused by some object, such as a tumor, pressing on the cord. Lacerations or tears cause direct damage to cord neurons. Lacerations can be caused by bone fragments or missiles such as bullets. Spinal transection describes the complete severing of the cord. Most spinal cord injuries involve two or more of these types of damage.

PARALYSIS AND LOSS OF SENSATION The extent to which movement and sensation are damaged depends on the level of the spinal cord injury. Nerves leaving the spinal cord at different levels control sensation and movement in different parts of the body. The distribution is roughly as follows:

- C1-C4: head and neck

- C3-C5: diaphragm (chest and breathing)

- C5-T1: shoulders, arms and hands

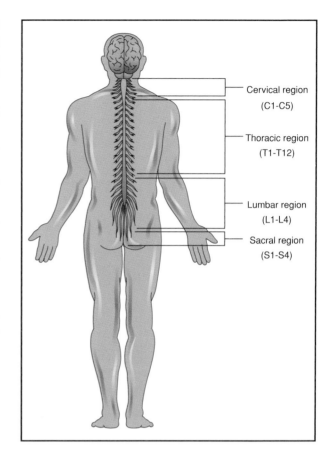

The extent of sensory and motor loss resulting from a spinal cord injury depends on the level of the injury because nerves at different levels control sensation and movement in different parts of the body. The distribution is as follows: C1-C4: head and neck; C3-C5: diaphragm; C5-T1: shoulders, arms, and hands; T2-T12: chest and abdomen (excluding internal organs); L1-L4: abdomen (excluding internal organs), buttocks, genitals, upper legs; L4-S3: legs; S2-S4: genitals, muscles of the perineum. *(Illustration by Electronic Illustrators Group.)*

- T2-T12: chest and abdomen (excluding internal organs)

- L1-L4: abdomen (excluding internal organs), buttocks, genitals, and upper legs

- L4-S1: legs

- S2-S4: genitals and muscles of the perineum

Damage below T1, which lies at the base of the rib cage, causes **paralysis** and loss of sensation in the legs and trunk below the injury. Injury at this level usually does no damage to the arms and hands. Paralysis of the legs is called paraplegia. Damage above T1 involves the arms as well as the legs. Paralysis of all four limbs is called quadriplegia or tetraplegia. Cervical or neck injuries not only cause quadriplegia but also may cause difficulty in breathing. Damage in the lower part of the neck may leave enough diaphragm control to allow unassisted breathing.

Patients with damage at C3 or above, just below the base of the skull, require mechanical assistance to breathe.

Symptoms also depend on the extent of spinal cord injury. A completely severed cord causes paralysis and loss of sensation below the wound. If the cord is only partially severed, some function will remain below the injury. Damage limited to the front portion of the cord causes paralysis and loss of sensations of **pain** and temperature. Other sensation may be preserved. Damage to the center of the cord may spare the legs but paralyze the arms. Damage to the right or left half causes loss of position sense, paralysis on the side of the injury, and loss of **pain** and temperature sensation on the opposite side.

DEEP VENOUS THROMBOSIS Blood does not flow normally to a paralyzed limb that is inactive for long periods. The blood pools in the deep veins and forms clots, a condition known as **deep vein thrombosis**. A clot or thrombus can break free and lodge in smaller arteries in the brain, causing a **stroke**, or in the lungs, causing **pulmonary embolism**.

PRESSURE ULCERS Inability to move also leads to pressure ulcers or bed sores. Pressure ulcers form where skin remains in contact with a bed or chair for a long time. The most common sites of pressure ulcers are the buttocks, hips, and heels.

SPASTICITY AND CONTRACTURE A paralyzed limb is incapable of active movement, but the muscle still has tone, a constant low level of contraction. Normal muscle tone requires communication between the muscle and the brain. Spinal cord injury prevents the brain from telling the muscle to relax. The result is prolonged muscle contraction or **spasticity**. Because the muscles that extend and those that bend a joint are not usually equal in strength, the involved joint is bent, often severely. This constant pressure causes deformity. As the muscle remains in the shortened position over several weeks or months, the tendons remodel and cause permanent muscle shortening or contracture. When muscles have permanently shortened, the inner surfaces of joints, such as armpits or palms, cannot be cleaned and the skin breaks down in that area.

HETEROTOPIC OSSIFICATION Heterotopic ossification is an abnormal deposit of bone in muscles and tendons that may occur after injury. It is most common in the hips and knees. Initially heterotopic ossification causes localized swelling, warmth, redness, and stiffness of the muscle. It usually begins one to four months after the injury and is rare after one year.

AUTONOMIC DYSREFLEXIA Body organs that regulate themselves, such as the heart, gastrointestinal tract, and glands, are controlled by groups of nerves called autonomic nerves. Autonomic nerves emerge from three different places: above the spinal column, in the lower back

from vertebrae T1-L4, and from the lowest regions of the sacrum at the base of the spine. In general, these three groups of autonomic nerves operate in balance. Spinal cord injury can disrupt this balance, a condition called autonomic dysreflexia or autonomic hyperreflexia. Patients with injuries at T6 or above are at greatest risk.

In autonomic dysreflexia, irritation of the skin, bowel, or bladder causes a highly exaggerated response from autonomic nerves. This response is caused by the uncontrolled release of norepinephrine, a hormone similar to adrenaline. Uncontrolled release of norepinephrine causes a rapid rise in blood pressure and a slowing of the heart rate. These symptoms are accompanied by throbbing **headache**, nausea, **anxiety**, sweating, and goose bumps below the level of the injury. The elevated blood pressure can rapidly cause loss of consciousness, **seizures**, cerebral hemorrhage, and **death**. Autonomic dysreflexia is most often caused by an over-full bladder or bladder infection, impaction or hard impassable fecal mass in the bowel, or skin irritation from tight clothing, **sunburn**, or other irritant. Inability to sense these irritants before the autonomic reaction begins is a major cause of dysreflexia.

LOSS OF BLADDER AND BOWEL CONTROL Bladder and bowel control require both motor nerves and the autonomic nervous system. Both of these systems may be damaged by SCI. When the autonomic nervous system triggers an urge to urinate or defecate, continence is maintained by contracting the anal or urethral sphincters. A sphincter is a ring of muscle that contracts to close off a passage or opening in the body. When the neural connections to these muscles are severed, conscious control is lost. In addition, loss of feeling may prevent sensations of fullness from reaching the brain. To compensate, the patient may help empty the bowel or bladder by using physical maneuvers that stimulate autonomic contractions before they would otherwise begin. However, the patient may not be able to relax the sphincters. If the sphincters cannot be relaxed, the patient will retain urine or feces.

Retention of urine may cause muscular changes in the bladder and urethral sphincter that make the problem worse. Urinary tract infection is common. Retention of feces can cause impaction. Symptoms of impaction include loss of appetite and nausea. Untreated impaction may cause perforation of the large intestine and rapid overwhelming infection.

SEXUAL DYSFUNCTION Men who have sustained SCI may be unable to achieve an erection or ejaculate. Sperm formation may be abnormal too, reducing fertility. Fertility and the ability to achieve orgasm are less impaired for women. Women may still be able to become pregnant and deliver vaginally with proper medical care.

Key Terms

Autonomic nervous system The part of the nervous system that controls involuntary functions such as sweating and blood pressure.

Botulinum toxin Any of a group of potent bacterial toxins or poisons produced by different strains of the bacterium *Clostridium botulinum.*

Computed tomography (CT) An imaging technique in which cross-sectional x rays of the body are compiled to create a three-dimensional image of the body's internal structures.

Magnetic resonance imaging (MRI) An imaging technique that uses a large circular magnet and radio waves to generate signals from atoms in the body. These signals are used to construct images of internal structures.

Motor Of or pertaining to motion, the body apparatus involved in movement, or the brain functions that direct purposeful activity.

Motor nerve Motor or efferent nerve cells carry impulses from the brain to muscle or organ tissue.

Peripheral nervous system The part of the nervous system that is outside the brain and spinal cord. Sensory, motor, and autonomic nerves are included.

Postural drainage The use of positioning to drain secretions from the bronchial tubes and lungs into the trachea or windpipe.

Range of motion (ROM) The range of motion of a joint from full extension to full flexion (bending) measured in degrees like a circle.

Sensory nerves Sensory or afferent nerves carry impulses of sensation from the periphery or outward parts of the body to the brain. Sensations include feelings, impressions, and awareness of the state of the body.

Voluntary An action or thought undertaken or controlled by a person's free will or choice.

Diagnosis

The location and extent of spinal cord injury is determined with **computed tomography scans** (CT scans), **magnetic resonance imaging** (MRI) scans, and x rays. X rays may be enhanced with an injected contrast dye.

Treatment

A person who may have a spinal cord injury should not be moved. Treatment of SCI begins with **immobilization**. This strategy prevents partial injuries of the cord from severing it completely. Use of splints to completely immobilize suspected SCI at the scene of the injury has helped reduce the severity of spinal cord injuries in the last two decades. Intravenous methylprednisone, a steroidal anti-inflammatory drug, is given during the first 24 hours to reduce inflammation and tissue destruction.

Rehabilitation after spinal cord injury seeks to prevent complications, promote recovery, and make the most of remaining function. Rehabilitation is a complex and long-term process. It requires a team of professionals, including a **neurologist**, physiatrist or rehabilitation specialist, physical therapist, and occupational therapist. Other specialists who may be needed include a respiratory therapist, vocational rehabilitation counselor, social worker, speech-language pathologist, nutritionist, special education teacher, recreation therapist, and clinical psychologist. Support groups provide a critical source of information, advice, and support for SCI patients.

Paralysis and loss of sensation

Some limited mobility and sensation may be recovered, but the extent and speed of this recovery cannot be predicted. Experimental electrical stimulation has been shown to allow some control of muscle contraction in paraplegia. This experimental technique offers the possibility of unaided walking. Further development of current control systems will be needed before useful movement is possible outside the laboratory.

The physical therapist focuses on mobility, to maintain range of motion of affected limbs and reduce contracture and deformity. Physical therapy helps compensate for lost skills by using those muscles that are still functional. It also helps to increase any residual strength and control in affected muscles. A physical therapist suggests adaptive equipment such as braces, canes, or wheelchairs.

An occupational therapist works to restore ability to perform the activities of daily living, such as eating and grooming, with tools and new techniques. The occupational therapist also designs modifications of the home and workplace to match the individual impairment.

A pulmonologist or respiratory therapist promotes airway hygiene through instruction in assisted coughing techniques and postural drainage. The respiratory professional also prescribes and provides instruction in the use of ventilators, facial or nasal masks, and tracheostomy equipment where necessary.

Pressure ulcers

Pressure ulcers are prevented by turning in bed at least every two hours. The patient should be turned more frequently when redness begins to develop in sensitive areas. Special mattresses and chair cushions can distribute weight more evenly to reduce pressure. Electrical stimulation is sometimes used to promote muscle movement to prevent pressure ulcers.

Spasticity and contracture

Range of motion (ROM) exercises help to prevent contracture. Chemicals can be used to prevent **contractures** from becoming fixed when ROM **exercise** is inadequate. Phenol or alcohol can be injected onto the nerve or **botulinum toxin** directly into the muscle. Botulinum toxin is associated with fewer complications, but it is more expensive than phenol and alcohol. Contractures can be released by cutting the shortened tendon or transferring it surgically to a different site on the bone where its pull will not cause as much deformity. Such tendon transfers may also be used to increase strength in partially functional extremities.

Heterotopic ossification

Etidronate disodium (Didronel), a drug that regulates the body's use of calcium, is used to prevent heterotopic ossification. Treatment begins three weeks after the injury and continues for 12 weeks. Surgical removal of ossified tissue is possible.

Autonomic dysreflexia

Autonomic dysreflexia is prevented by bowel and bladder care and attention to potential irritants. It is treated by prompt removal of the irritant. Drugs to lower blood pressure are used when necessary. People with SCI should educate friends and family members about the symptoms and treatment of dysreflexia, because immediate attention is necessary.

Loss of bladder and bowel control

Normal bowel function is promoted through adequate fluid intake and a diet rich in fiber. Evacuation is stimulated by deliberately increasing the abdominal pressure, either voluntarily or by using an abdominal binder.

Bladder care involves continual or intermittent catheterization. The full bladder may be detected by feeling its bulge against the abdominal wall. Urinary tract infection is a significant complication of catheterization and requires frequent monitoring.

Sexual dysfunction

Counseling can help in adjusting to changes in sexual function after spinal cord injury. Erection may be enhanced through the same means used to treat erectile dysfunction in the general population.

Prognosis

The prognosis of SCI depends on the location and extent of injury. Injuries of the neck above C4 with significant involvement of the diaphragm hold the gravest prognosis. Respiratory infection is one of the leading causes of death in long-term SCI. Overall, 85% of SCI patients who survive the first 24 hours are alive 10 years after their injuries. Recovery of function is impossible to predict. Partial recovery is more likely after an incomplete wound than after the spinal cord has been completely severed.

Prevention

Risk of spinal cord injury can be reduced through prevention of the accidents that lead to it. Chances of injury from automobile accidents, the major cause of SCIs, can be significantly reduced by driving at safe speeds, avoiding alcohol while driving, and using seat belts.

Resources

BOOKS

Bradley, Walter G., et al., eds. *Neurology in Clinical Practice.* 2nd ed. Boston: Butterworth-Heinemann, 1996.

Martini, F. *Fundamentals of Anatomy and Physiology.* Englewood Cliffs, NJ: Prentice Hall, 1989.

Yarkony, Gary M., ed. *Spinal Cord Injury: Medical Management and Rehabilitation.* Gaithersburg, MD: Aspen Publishers, Inc., 1994.

ORGANIZATIONS

The National Spinal Cord Injury Association. 8300 Colesville Road, Silver Spring, Maryland 20910. (301) 588-6959. <http://www.erols.com/nscia>.

Richard Robinson

Spinal muscular atrophy

Definition

Spinal muscular atrophies (SMAs) are a wide group of genetic disorders characterized by primary degeneration of anterior horn cells of the spinal cord, resulting in progressive muscle weakness. The most common form of spinal muscular atrophy is childhood proximal SMA. Other forms of SMAs include X-linked recessively inherited bulbospinal SMA, distal SMAs, scapuloperoneal SMAs, and others such as facioscapulohumeral, scapulohumeral, oculopharyngeal, and Ryukyuan SMAs.

Description

SMAs present with diverse symptoms and differ in age of onset, mode of inheritance, distribution of muscle weakness, and progression of symptoms.

Childhood proximal SMA is subdivided into three clinical groups: type I, type II, and type III SMA. SMA type IV designates adult form of proximal SMA. Although it is now apparent that the phenotype of SMA associated with mutations of the survival motor neuron (SMN1) gene spans a continuum without a clear delineation of subtypes, the classification is useful for prognosis and management.

SMA I (acute infantile SMA, Werdnig-Hoffman disease) manifests by decreased fetal movements in the last trimester of pregnancy in about one third of cases. About 65% of affected infants are floppy at birth, while delayed motor milestones are characteristic in all affected children by the age of six months. In addition to muscle weakness, clinical features include head lag, poor sucking and swallowing, weak cry, proximal limb weakness, and lack of reflexes. Affected children never raise their head, roll over, or walk. Sometimes weakness of the face and jaw muscles, finger tremor, and respiratory difficulty occur. Orthopedic abnormalities such as congenital dislocation of the hip, chest wall asymmetries, and flexion contractures are present in 25% of affected newborns.

SMA II (intermediate SMA) usually manifests itself between six and 12 months of age. Although poor muscle tone may be evident at birth or within the first few months of life, patients with SMA II may gain motor milestones slowly. Eighty percent are able to sit independently, although they are not able stand or walk alone. Limb girdle weakness, twitching, lack of reflexes, and weakness of tongue, face, and neck muscles are seen. **Tremors** affecting the upper extremities, musculoskeletal deformities, and respiratory failure occur.

SMA III (chronic SMA, Kugelberg-Welander disease) presents with the onset of symptoms after the age of 18 months. Patients walk independently, but may fall frequently or have trouble walking up and down stairs between age two to three years. Muscular weakness is present on both sides of the body, and the legs are more severely affected than the arms. Difficulty swallowing and difficulty speaking may occur in later stages of the disorder.

SMA IV manifests as muscle weakness usually in the second or third decade of life. The findings are similar to those described for SMA III.

Bulbospinal muscular atrophy (Kennedy disease) manifests as muscle weakness between the ages of 20 and 40 years. Weakness and atrophy in the lower extremities are usually followed by problems with the pectoral girdle, facial muscles, distal limb, and bulbar muscles. Muscle cramps on exertion often precede the weakness by several years. Fine tremors of the face are present in over 90% of patients. Type 2 diabetes mellitus, hand tremor, and infertility can also occur. Bulbar involvement predisposes the person with spinal muscular atrophy to recurrent aspiration pneumonia, due to weakening of the muscles necessary for efficient swallowing.

Other less common forms of SMAs include distal SMAs (10% of all SMA cases) and scapuloperoneal SMA (7% of all SMA cases). Distal SMAs are a group of disorders that manifest most commonly soon after birth, with muscle wasting in the hands and feet. Later in life, abnormal gait and foot deformities are seen. Similar clinical signs occur in adult-onset forms. Scapuloperoneal SMA has a characteristic pattern of muscle weakness, usually involving the heart and sensory neuropathy (Davidenkow's syndrome).

Demographics

SMAs are one of the most common groups of neuromuscular diseases in children, with an incidence of four to 10 per 100,000 live births. Other SMAs have a lower incidence, as a rule less than one per 100,000 live births.

Causes and symptoms

Spinal muscular atrophies are genetic diseases. Types I, II, and III SMAs have been mapped to chromosome 5q11.2-13.3. In 1994, the survival motor neuron (SMN1) gene was identified as responsible for SMA when mutations occur. The SMN1 gene has a duplicate copy called the SMN2 gene, but it is not able to compensate for the defects in the SMN1 gene. There is evidence that type I SMA is caused by deletion of the SMN1 gene, whereas type III is associated with a conversion event of SMN1 into SMN2, leading to an increased number of SMN2 genes. In addition to bulbospinal muscular atrophy, which has been shown to be caused by a defect in the androgen receptor gene, six other SMAs have already been mapped to corresponding chromosomal locations.

Inheritance pattern for most forms of SMA is autosomal recessive, meaning that both parents are carriers of the disorder, and the chance of having a child affected with the disorder is 25% with each pregnancy. Familial forms of the disorder that occur later in life are usually due to an autosomal recessive or autosomal dominant inheritance pattern.

Diagnosis

Diagnosis is based on the clinical presentation, family history, and genetic testing. The genetic test is based on the fact that approximately 95–98% of individuals with a clinical diagnosis of childhood SMA lack exon 7 in both copies of the SMN1 gene. Likewise, all patients with bulbospinal muscular atrophy have a defect in the androgen receptor gene.

Key Terms

Atrophy Wasting or degeneration of tissues.

Contractures Abnormal, usually permanent, stiffness or contractions of a muscle due to wasting of muscle fibers, extensive scar tissue over a joint, or other factors.

Distal muscles Muscles farthest away from the center of the body, such as muscles in the fingers and toes.

Proximal muscles Muscles closest to the center of the body, such as muscles used in breathing and sitting upright.

An electromyelogram may reveal damaged nerve impulses secondary to muscle fiber degeneration. Sensory nerve conduction studies are normal in all forms of SMA, the exceptions being bulbospinal muscular atrophy and Davidenkow's syndrome. Muscle **biopsy** is critical in the diagnosis of childhood SMA. If performed, it reveals atrophy of muscle fibers with a characteristic form of muscle fiber type grouping.

Treatment team

A multidisciplinary approach is essential for providing care and treatment of a person with spinal muscular atrophy, including specialists in the fields of neurology, physical therapy, occupational therapy, respiratory therapy, surgery, and genetic counseling.

Treatment

As no specific treatment is available for spinal muscular atrophies, the resulting complications of muscle deterioration are managed as best as possible. Treatment in severe childhood SMA includes prescription of antibiotics for respiratory infections and tube feeding in children with profound difficulty in sucking and swallowing. In children with SMA II, the goals of conservative therapy include maintaining the sitting posture, preserving or improving function, and reducing progression of deformity. This is achieved by regular active **exercise** monitored by physical therapists, gentle traction to prevent contractures (stiff muscles near the joints), splinting, bracing, and the use of spinal positioning devices and upright mobility systems. Orthopedic surgical interventions such as tendon transfer or spinal surgery can prevent disability in patients with expected prolonged survival.

Recovery and rehabilitation

As there is no recovery from spinal muscular atrophies, the emphasis is placed upon maintaining muscle function and mobility for as long as possible. Physical therapy is an integral part of maintaining movement in persons with spinal muscular atrophies. In children, range of motion exercises keep muscles and joints moving, while reaching games provide stimulation and aid in coordination. Water therapy also provides an enjoyable medium for working the muscles and joints.

As muscle weakness progresses and affects posture, occupational therapy can provide assistive devices and strategies to maintain positioning and movement, such as specialized wheelchairs and reaching devices. Respiratory therapy is also important to teach parents the chest therapy exercises and maneuvers that are necessary to remove accumulated secretions and mucous from the lungs.

Normal education should be encouraged for children with spinal muscular atrophies, especially in the more slowly progressive forms, as intelligence is preserved and even superior in many children with SMA.

Clinical trials

Riluzole, **gabapentin**, albuterol, phenylbutyrate, and thyrotropin-releasing hormone have so far been tested and have shown potential effects on improvement of muscle strength in children with SMA. Many different controlled trials are needed to confirm these preliminary findings.

Prognosis

Progressive muscle weakness usually leads to death by age four for persons with SMA I. Muscle weakness progresses at varying rates in SMA II, and many persons survive into adulthood. The life expectancy of patients with SMA III is close to that of the healthy population. Progression of the adult-onset SMAs is usually slow, and patients are ambulatory until late in the disease. Lifespan is only slightly reduced.

Special concerns

Genetic counseling is important in SMA, since prenatal and preimplantation genetic diagnoses offer the parents the possibility to prevent the disease.

Resources

BOOKS

"Disorders of Upper and Lower Motor Neurons," chapter 80 in *Neurology in Clinical Practice*, edited by Walter G. Bradley, Robert B. Daroff, Gerald Fenichel, and Joseph Jankovic. Burlington, MA: Butterworth Heinemann, 2003.

PERIODICALS

Zerres, K., S. Rudnik-Schoneborn, E. Forrest, et al. "A Collaborative Study on the Natural History of Childhood and Juvenile Onset Proximal Spinal Muscular Atrophy (Type II and III SMA): 569 Patients." *J Neurol Sci.* 146 (February 1997): 67–72.

OTHER

"NINDS Spinal Muscular Atrophy Information Page." National Institute of Neurological Disorders and Stroke. May 5, 2004 (May 27, 2004). <http://www.ninds.nih.gov/health_and_medical/disorders/sma.htm>.

"Understanding Spinal Muscular Atrophy: A Comprehensive Guide." *Families of Spinal Muscular Atrophy.* May 5, 2004 (May 27, 2004). <http://www.fsma.org/booklet.shtml#taking>.

ORGANIZATIONS

Families of SMA. PO Box 196, Libertyville, IL 60048-0196. (847) 367-7623 or (800) 886-1762. sma@fsma.org. <http://www.fsma.org>.

Borut Peterlin, MD, PhD

Spina bifida

Definition

Spina bifida belongs to a group of disorders known as neural tube defects (NTDs). These all involve problems in the development and closure of the neural tube, a structure in the human fetus that begins forming very early in a pregnancy. The neural tube eventually becomes the spinal column. When the neural tube does not close properly, it can lead to spina bifida, a disruption in the spinal column. Spina bifida occurs to varying degrees of severity, and in various forms.

Description

Spina bifida is also known by the name spinal dysraphism. It generally occurs in two major types. One types is spina bifida cystica or spina bifida aperta, which involves a sac filled with spinal contents along the spine. The other type is spina bifida occulta, in which the spinal cord stays inside the spinal canal and there is no sac.

Spina bifida ranges from having no or mild effects, to having severe effects and a significant impact upon a person's life. Physical symptoms can include weakness of limbs, paralysis, lack of bowel or bladder control, learning problems, **hydrocephalus**, **seizures**, central apnea, clubfeet, impaired vision, and latex sensitivity.

Depending upon the involvement of the spinal problem, spina bifida can also have psychological and emotional impacts upon the affected person and his or her family.

Demographics

Spina bifida is fairly common; it is thought to occur in about one in 2,000 live births in the United States. NTDs in general occur in about one in 1,000 live births in the United States. Many areas have an even higher prevalence, for somewhat unknown reasons. A population with a higher prevalence for NTDs is the United Kingdom, with an estimated rate of 2.8 per 1,000 live births in the 1970s. A similar study in Ireland at that time estimated the rate to be about 7.1 per 1,000 live births. Through the advent of prenatal screening, prenatal diagnosis, pregnancy management options, and unknown factors the prevalence in the British Isles has fallen somewhat in recent years.

Higher rates of NTDs have been reported in the northwest British Isles, with lower rates in the southeast. In Canada, higher prevalence rates for NTDs have been reported in the eastern region of the country, as compared to the western region. A higher prevalence of NTDs has been seen in China in the provinces north of the Yangtze River, and these may be as much as six times higher than in the southern provinces. Pockets of higher prevalence have also been seen in India, but these do not fit any clear geographic areas or regions.

In the United States, people of Hispanic ancestry have a higher chance for NTDs than other ethnic groups. Conversely, African Americans and some Asians have a lower risk than other ethnic groups. When those with high NTD risks immigrate to other countries, they do not keep their high risk for NTDs. When those with low NTD risks migrate, they tend to maintain their low risk status, as a group.

Spina bifida has been reported in males and females roughly equally.

Causes and symptoms

Spina bifida occurs because the neural tube, around the area of the spine, fails to close during fetal development. A multifactorial cause for this has been assumed, because multiple factors seem to be involved. It may best be described as an interaction between multiple genes and the environment. Many aspects of this interaction are still not well understood. As well, an exact neurological cause for spina bifida has not been identified.

Spina bifida can run in families. Multiple genes may be involved because identical twins, those with the exact same genetics, have been studied at length. Spina bifida also occurs as part of genetic syndromes and chromosome disorders.

Numerous families with NTDs have been studied to help identify recurrence risks. Generally, the risk is 3–5% for a couple to have another child with an NTD if they already have one. If a parent has an NTD, they have a 3–5% chance to have a child with one. If two or more children

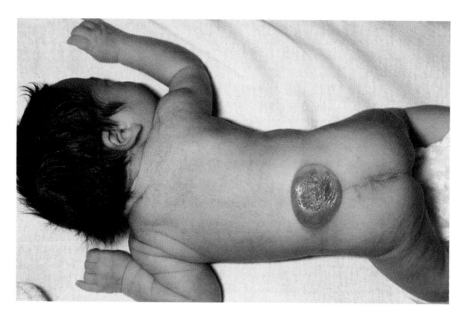

An infant with spina bifida. *(© Custom Medical Stock Photo. Reproduced by permission.)*

already have NTDs, the risk is 6–9% for another one. If an NTD is in other more distant family members, the risk is somewhat higher than the average population, but probably not higher than 0.5%.

Environmental factors are also important in spina bifida. For example, taking the B vitamin folic acid before pregnancy conception has been shown to significantly reduce a woman's risk of having a child with the condition. Additionally, some medications can increase a woman's risk for spina bifida; these include some anti-seizures medications. As it turns out, many of these medications naturally reduce the levels of folic acid in one's body.

Neurological symptoms of spina bifida are varied. Many of them relate back to the early embryo's development, and how spina bifida occurs at this time. Three cell layers develop in the very early embryo; these are the ectoderm, mesoderm, and endoderm. The mesoderm normally sends signals to a region of the ectoderm to make it develop into neural tissue. Eventually, the neural ectoderm folds to form a tube, which runs for most of the length of the embryo. The top of the neural tube eventually forms the brain and top of the spinal column. The bottom of the neural tube eventually forms the lower back and bottom of the spinal column. This happens through very careful and controlled cell movements. The neural tube is usually completed forming by about 18 to 26 days after ovulation.

Failure of the neural tube to close causes spina bifida, and this disrupts the spinal column's structure and functioning. This disruption can be mild, as in spina bifida occulta. It may also be more severe with a large sac or cyst present, as in spina bifida cystica.

In about 80–90% of spina bifida cases, there is a cyst with parts of the spinal cord and spinal wall present. This is called a myelomeningocele (or meningomyelocele). This type of spina bifida can happen in a relatively high or low position on one's back. It often causes problems with bladder and bowel functioning, and sometimes paralysis or limb weaknesses. A neuropathic bladder can sometimes affect kidney functioning as well.

When a developing baby cannot move their limbs well *in utero*, this sometimes leads to feet and legs that turn inward, or clubfoot. As a result, some children with spina bifida are born with clubfoot.

Myelomeningoceles often cause spinal fluid to not flow properly through the system, and hydrocephalus may be a result. Head ultrasound scans may show hydrocephalus in about 90% of newborns with spina bifida. It is often associated with an **Arnold-Chiari malformation**, Type II. This occurs when the medulla pushes downward below the foramen magnum, and overlaps the spinal cord. This malformation is present in about 70% of people who have a meningomyelocele; it can cause distortion of the medulla and midbrain, as well as central apnea.

Hydrocephalus can eventually cause increased pressure to develop in the brain. This may ultimately lead to one's brain not being able to grow properly, and cause learning problems. Seizures may also be present. Learning problems are not a certainty with spina bifida, but when present they vary greatly. Their severity is impossible to predict. However, hydrocephalus and seizures put one at a higher risk for learning problems. Surveys on intellectual development have shown that children with hydrocephalus have lower IQs than their siblings without the condition.

In about 5% of spina bifida cases, there is no spinal tissue in the cyst wall; these are called meningoceles. Hydrocephalus is not usually present in this type of spina bifida, and a neurological examination may even be perfectly normal.

Optic atrophy and squinting may occur in people who have spina bifida, and a result of these may be poorer vision.

There is an association between spina bifida and latex sensitivity. Many have attributed this to the fact that people with the condition have a higher exposure to latex, since they may be in hospitals more often. Interestingly, a study in 2000 showed that 22% of children with spina bifida still had latex sensitivity, despite efforts to maintain latex-free environments for them.

Spina bifida occulta may cause mild symptoms, or none at all. Sometimes the only signs of it may in the lower spine area as a dimple, a small tuft of hair, or a small growth. If one has an imaging scan and a tethered spinal cord is noted, this can sometimes be a sign of spina bifida occulta as well.

Diagnosis

A early time to find spina bifida is during a detailed prenatal ultrasound scan, especially between 16 and 20 weeks gestation (from the last menstrual period). Ultrasounds cannot identify every structural problem in a developing baby, so some cases of spina bifida (especially mild forms) may be missed. However, it is a risk-free method to use that gives immediate results.

Prenatal blood screening is often offered to women between 15 and 21 weeks in a pregnancy. This screening measures the levels of various chemicals naturally found in a mother's blood, including alpha-fetoprotein (AFP). For this reason, the screening is often called AFP screening. AFP is a protein normally made by a developing fetus, so it is naturally present in maternal serum and called MS-AFP. When a fetus has spina bifida, the levels of MS-AFP may be higher than usual because it leaks out of the hole in the spine. If a woman's AFP screen comes back abnormal with a high MS-AFP value, she often is at a higher risk for having a baby with spina bifida. This may prompt her physician to offer her a detailed ultrasound, as well as other medical options that might give her more information about the baby.

One option to find spina bifida is a procedure called amniocentesis. Amniocentesis involves removing a small amount of fluid from around the baby, using a fine needle. This fluid naturally contains AFP, which may also be elevated if the baby has spina bifida. There is a small risk of miscarriage, about one in 200, with this procedure. As such, every women usually receives proper counseling through their doctor or a genetic counselor before having the test done.

Sometimes, spina bifida can only be seen at birth. A physical examination usually identifies spina bifida cystica fairly easily, especially if the sac is large. Spina bifida occulta can be more difficult to find, but clues can be a dimple in the lower back, a tuft of hair, or a small growth.

Once spina bifida is seen outwardly, imaging scans like x rays, ultrasound, **magnetic resonance imaging (MRI)**, or computed tomography (**CT**) can be helpful to see the extent of it. It is also a good way to identify whether someone has associated neurological complications like hydrocephalus.

Since spina bifida may occur as part of some genetic conditions, a medical geneticist should be involved to thoroughly examine a child with spina bifida. Identifying a particular syndrome in a child can help them receive more personalized medical care, and can help families identify a cause for why the spina bifida happened. It can also help to give families specific information about the chance of it happening again, for them or for other family members.

Some genetic testing, like chromosome studies, may identify a diagnosis or cause for the spina bifida. Abnormal genetic test results cannot be changed or reversed, but may provide answers about why the spina bifida occurred.

Treatment team

Treatment for people with spina bifida is highly dependent upon their symptoms. A multi-disciplinary team and approach is extremely helpful. Some hospitals offer day-long clinics devoted to people with spina bifida, which makes things much easier for families in terms of coordinating multiple appointments.

A treatment team for someone with spina bifida may include a **neurologist**, neurosurgeon, surgeon, **neuropsychologist**, medical geneticist, genetic counselor, orthopedic surgeon, physiatrist, physical therapist, occupational therapist, speech therapist, registered dietitian, social worker, nephrologist, ophthalmologist, audiologist, and a primary care provider. A neonatologist and pediatric specialists in those fields may be available to aid in the care for children. Those specializing in early childhood and development are particularly helpful, especially for issues related to attending school. Above all, good communication between the various specialists to coordinate care is essential.

Treatment

There is no known cure for spina bifida. Treatment primarily focuses on dealing with symptoms as they arise, since they vary so greatly from person to person.

Key Terms

Arnold-Chiari malformation, Type II Change in the brain when the medulla pushes downward below the foramen magnum, and overlaps the spinal cord.

Central apnea Abnormal breathing as a result of the medulla being pushed down, such as from an Arnold-Chiari malformation, Type II.

Chromosome Located in most cell nuclei, the genetic structure that contains all genes and DNA that make up an organism.

Clubfoot Abnormal positioning of the feet and legs, when they are turned inward towards each other.

Computed tomography (CT) scan Three-dimensional internal image of the body, created by combining x-ray images from different planes using a computer program.

Cyst Sac of tissue filled with fluid, gas or semi-solid material.

Foramen magnum Large opening in the back of the skull, where the spinal cord connects with the brain.

Hydrocephalus A state when fluid builds up in the brain, which may cause increased internal pressure and enlarged head size.

Magnetic resonance imaging (MRI) scan Three-dimensional internal image of the body, created using magnetic waves.

Medulla (spinalis) Elongated, cylindrical portion of the nervous system, which is contained in the spinal canal.

Neuropathic bladder Improper or lack of bladder function, due to a nerve problem.

Syndrome A well-recognized pattern of health problems or birth defects.

Ultrasound Two-dimensional internal image of the body, created using sound waves.

Ventriculoatrial (VA) shunt Tube that is placed from the brain to the chest cavity, in order to drain fluid.

Ventriculoperitoneal (VP) shunt Tube that is placed from the brain to the abdomen, in order to drain fluid.

X ray Two-dimensional internal image of the body, using radioactive waves.

Surgery to correct the spinal problem in spina bifida cystica is often done. This involves carefully tucking the spinal contents back into the spinal column, and closing the covering back up. This often happens shortly following birth to reduce the risk of developing an infection, and requires some time to heal afterward. Surgery has not been known to allow someone to regain functions they would not have had otherwise like movement, bowel, or bladder control.

A child with spina bifida is often carefully watched for signs of hydrocephalus. This may be done by measuring head circumference (which may enlarge) or with periodic head ultrasound or CT scans. If hydrocephalus is found, a procedure to put in a ventriculoperitoneal (VP) or ventriculoatrial (VA) shunt may be done. If a shunt is placed, it must be continually monitored and may need to be adjusted. Some people have their shunts removed later if the hydrocephalus never returns, and some people have a shunt for their entire lives.

Medications are widely available to treat those who develop seizures, and these may need periodic adjustments. Those who have problems with bowel or bladder

control may require surgery, medications, or may never fully have these functions.

Babies and children with clubfoot often need to see an orthopedic surgeon and physiatrist, both of whom can recommend ways to correct them. Wearing braces on the legs can turn the feet back to their usual position, and this may be the only thing required. Sometimes surgery is necessary.

Surgery to correct the spinal problem during a pregnancy is experimental and not widely available. Since 1997, about 200 fetuses have had closure of myelomeningoceles during pregnancy. Since the surgery is so new, exact success rates, safety and long-term effects of the procedure are still not known as of early 2004.

Recovery and rehabilitation

Therapies and rehabilitation may be quite involved or relatively brief for people with spina bifida, depending on the severity of symptoms. Physical therapy is extremely important and can be ongoing. Speech and occupational therapies may be helpful if learning problems or delayed development are noted.

For those with wheelchairs, ramps and other assistive devices are helpful in their homes and places they frequent.

Clinical trials

As of early 2004, two **clinical trials** are under way in the United States to study spina bifida. National Institute of Child Health and Human Development (NICHD) sponsors both of these studies. One study is devoted to the genetics of spina bifida, recruiting many family members of an affected person to analyze and compare selected genes. The other study is attempting to identify the effectiveness and safety of spina bifida surgery during pregnancies. More information can be found at <http://www.clinicaltrials.gov>.

Prognosis

Prognosis in spina bifida is extremely varied and unpredictable. Years ago with far less intervention and fewer treatments available, someone with severe spina bifida had a high chance to die from complications. Mortality may still be high in complex cases even today. Conversely, those with a mild form of spina bifida may never even know they have it unless they have an internal imaging scan for an unrelated reason. As such, they may never have complications related to spina bifida and would have an average life span.

Today, there are far more options for helping those with spina bifida. Information can be learned during a pregnancy, allowing parents to make decisions and potentially prepare before birth. These treatments and therapies help maintain a better quality of life for those with spina bifida, and continue to offer hope.

Special concerns

Many couples who find their child has spina bifida during a pregnancy experience an array of emotional and psychological issues. They may be wondering how and why this happened, and may want some immediate answers. They also may be feeling guilt or wondering whether they could have caused it to happen. Issues related to these pregnancies, such as continuation or interrupting a pregnancy, can be complex and should be treated with sensitivity and care.

An important aspect of good prenatal care is regular folic acid supplementation, because this is known to reduce the risk for NTDs significantly. This can be gained through a prenatal vitamin, a separate supplement, or a healthy diet. Many breakfast cereals, breads, and other foods are now being supplemented with folic acid.

The current recommendation is for all women in their reproductive years to take 0.4 milligrams of folic acid daily, especially from about three to four months before conception. A woman with an affected child should take 4 milligrams of folic acid daily, beginning at least three to four months prior to conception. The reason for taking folic acid before conception is because the fetal spine forms very early, sometimes before a woman even knows she is pregnant.

Another tricky issue is managing the pregnancy of a woman with **epilepsy** or a seizure disorder. Many anti-seizure medications, like Depakote, cause an increased risk for NTDs and spina bifida. However, the risk of a woman having a seizure during pregnancy is also significant. The art is to find a balance between these two risks, in a way that makes everyone feel the most comfortable.

Resources

BOOKS

Lutkenhoff, Marlene. *Spinabilities: A Young Person's Guide to Spina Bifida.* Woodbine House, 1997.

Lutkenhoff, Marlene. *Children with Spina Bifida: A Parent's Guide*, 1st ed. Woodbine House, 2003.

Sandler, Adrian. *Living with Spina Bifida: A Guide for Families and Professionals.* University of North Carolina Press, 2004.

PERIODICALS

Frey, Lauren, and W. Allen Hauser. "Epidemiology of Neural Tube Defects." *Epilepsia* 44, Suppl. 3 (2003): 4–13.

Zipitis, Christos S., and Constantinos Paschalides. "Caring for a child with spina bifida: understanding the child and carer." *Journal of Child Health Care* 7, no. 2 (2003): 101–112.

WEBSITES

Children with Spina Bifida: A Resource Page for Parents. <www.waisman.wisc.edu/~rowley/sb-kids/index.htmlx>.

March of Dimes. <www.modimes.org>.

National Institute of Neurological Disorders and Stroke. <www.ninds.nih.gov/index.htm>.

ORGANIZATIONS

Association for Spina Bifida & Hydrocephalus (U.K.). ASBAH House, 42 Park Road, Peterborough, United Kingdom PE1 2UQ. (01733) 555988. (01733) 555985. info@asbah.org. <http://www.asbah.org>.

Spina Bifida and Hydrocephalus Association of Canada. 977-167 Lombard Avenue, Winnipeg, Manitoba, Canada R3B 0V3. 204-925-3650 or 800-565-9488; Fax: 204-925-3654. spinab@mts.net. <http://www.sbhac.ca/index.php?page=main>.

Spina Bifida Association of America. 4590 MacArthur Boulevard N.W., Suite 250, Washington, DC 20007-4226.

202-944-3285 or 800-621-3141; Fax: 202-944-3295. sbaa@sbaa.org. <http://www.sbaa.org>.

Deepti Babu, MS, CGC

Spinocerebellar ataxia

Definition

Spinocerebellar **ataxia** is a genetically inherited disorder characterized by abnormal brain function that represents a varied group of disorders. It is most commonly inherited as a dominant trait, which means that any individual who is a carrier of one of the many different gene mutations is affected. It also means that a carrier will have a 50% percent chance of having an affected offspring, regardless of the genetic background of the reproductive mate. In this group of disorders, the brain and spinal cord degenerate.

Description

Individuals affected with spinocerebellar ataxia develop a degenerative condition that affects a region in the base of the brain called the **cerebellum** located behind the brainstem. The primary function of the cerebellum is to coordinate the body's ability to move. Loss of this quintessential function leads to a progressive atrophy, or wasting away of muscles. The spine also atrophies and this can lead to **spasticity**.

Spinocerebellar ataxia can be physically devastating and the progressive loss of the ability to coordinate movements in emotional complications and significant lifestyle changes. The adverse effects involve the legs, hands, and the speech. Currently, there are 11 types of spinocerebellar ataxia. As there are many different genes mutations that cause this disease, there are different names for each type. The different types have numerical assignments as nomenclature. For example, Spinocerebellar ataxia type 1 is also known as SCA1. The numbers span from 1-25 (there is no SCA9) and are designated based on the time at which they were identified and characterized. Spinocerebellar ataxia is the same disease as spinal cerebellar ataxia.

Demographics

There are several gene mutations on different chromosomes that cause Spinocerebellar ataxia and the frequency of these gene within different populations varies considerably. In fact, due to the number of different types it is often difficult to estimate the incidence of a specific type in a specific population. In general, the incidence is thought to be approximately one to five per 100,000 people. There is no known predilection for sex. As with virtually all autosomal dominant disorders, males and females are equally likely to inherit a defective gene.

Causes and symptoms

Spinocerebellar ataxia is caused by a genetic defect that involves an expansion in the DNA sequence called a trinucleotide repeat expansion for SCA types 1-3, 6-10, 12, and 17. In general, the type of DNA expansion involves three DNA letters (nucleotides). In these cases, the sequence CAG (C=cytosine, A=adenine, G=guanine) is repeated above the normal repeat length. The normal repeat number differs for different types, as does the expanded repeat sizes. By repeating this sequence of DNA too many times, function of the protein it encodes can be disrupted. Other types of repeat expansions that cause SCA have been discovered. For example, SCA10 involves an ATTCT repeat expansion of the SCA10 gene and SCA8 involves an expansion in the SCA8 gene with the nucleotides CTG repeated. Finally, SCA14 involves a mutation in a gene that does not involve a trinucleotide repeat expansion.

The most common types are SCA1 (6%), SCA2 (14%), SCA3 (21%), SCA6 (15%), SCA7 (5%), and SCA8 (2–5%). Age of onset for all of these types is on average from 20–30 years of age except for SCA6, which usually occurs between the ages of 40 and 50. People with SCA8 usually develop symptoms between in their late 30s. SCA2 patients usually develop **dementia** and slow eye movements. SCA8, which has a normal lifespan, and SCA1 patients are both characterized as having active reflexes. SCA7 patients develop visual loss. SCA3 is also known as **Machado-Joseph disease**.

In SCA types 1–3 and 7, there can be an earlier age of onset with increased severity (called anticipation) as the defect is passed from one generation to the next. This means that children can be more severely affect at an earlier age than their affected parent. The size of the repeat of nucleotides in the affected genes is thought to correlate with the severity and age of onset in offspring. As the repeat size expands, the severity worsens and age of onset becomes earlier compared with the affected parent. However, repeat size does not predict the exact age of onset or the specific symptoms that will develop.

Penetrance refers to the likelihood that individuals with a genetic defect will develop the disease. In spinocerebellar ataxia, the penetrance is quite high; however, there are rare cases in which people do not develop symptoms. The reason for the lack of complete penetrance is currently unknown.

Key Terms

Ataxia   A condition marked by impaired muscular coordination, most frequently resulting from disorders in the brain or spinal cord.

Atrophy   The progressive wasting and loss of function of any part of the body.

Autosomal dominant   A pattern of inheritance in which only one of the two copies of an autosomal gene must be abnormal for a genetic condition or disease to occur. An autosomal gene is a gene that is located on one of the autosomes or non-sex chromosomes. A person with an autosomal dominant disorder has a 50% chance of passing it to each of their offspring.

Penetrance   The degree to which individuals possessing a particular genetic mutation express the trait that this mutation causes. One hundred percent penetrance is expected to be observed in truly dominant traits.

Trinucleotide repeat expansion   A sequence of three nucleotides that is repeated too many times in a section of a gene.

Affected individuals initially develop poor coordination of movement, which is the definition of ataxia. Developing poor movement coordination in patients is manifested clinically by difficulty in walking, abnormalities in hand or eye movements, and speech difficulties. Generally, the age of onset is usually after 18 years old, making it typically an adult-onset disorder. The severity of progressive degeneration depends primarily on the underlying defect.

Diagnosis

The diagnosis of spinocerebellar ataxia is initially suspected by the adult-onset of symptoms. An **MRI** scan can detect atrophy (wasting) of the cerebellum, a typical finding in patients with spinocerebellar ataxia. A clinical evaluation involves an extensive neurological examination. Genetic testing is a critical component of the diagnosis, as symptoms among the various types of spinocerebellar ataxia are similar. A molecular genetic test to determine the gene that has the trinucleotide repeat expansion can be helpful in quickly identifying other carriers in the family. Once the genetic defect is characterized, family members can also be tested. Unfortunately, genetic testing is not always 100% informative. There are rare cases of spinocerebellar ataxia diagnosed clinically that cannot be explained by any of the known genetic defects. It is estimated that in approximately 50–60% of Caucasian persons with a dominant familial form of cerebellar ataxia, DNA testing can provide a definitive diagnosis.

Treatment team

For people who begin to show symptoms and are later diagnosed with spinocerebellar ataxia, a careful evaluation by a **neurologist** is usually required. Treatment is based on lessening the symptoms as they develop. A fulltime caretaker and nursing support will eventually be required in the later stages of the disease. Psychological counseling is often needed depending on the family, the patient, and their needs.

Treatment

There is no cure for spinocerebellar ataxia. There is also no treatment to slow the progression of the disease. Treatment, therefore, remains supportive. Drugs that help control **tremors** are not effective for treating cerebellar tremors. Although dietary factors are not proven to be helpful, vitamin supplementation is recommended.

Recovery and rehabilitation

Researchers assume that physical therapy does not slow the progression of loss of coordination or muscle wasting. However, people with spinocerebellar ataxias are encouraged to remain as active as possible. Occupational therapy can be helpful in developing ways to accommodate the patient in performing daily activities. Walkers and other devices can assist in allow the patient to have mobility. Other modifications such as ramps for a wheelchair, heavy eating utensils, and raised toilet seats can make patients more independent. Speech therapy and computer-based communication aids often help as the person loses his or her ability to speak.

Clinical trials

As of early 2004, there are no approved **clinical trials** for the treatment or cure of spinocerebellar ataxia. There is, however, a clinical trial to determine the maximum tolerated dose of a drug called idebenone in children, adolescents, and adults with Friedreich's Ataxia, a disorder related to spinocerebellar ataxia (contacts: Patient Recruitment and Public Liaison Office, Building 61, 10 Cloister Court, Bethesda, Maryland 20892-4754; toll free: 1-800-411-1222). Additionally, there is also an ongoing study to determine the efficacy of high-dose intravenous immunoglobulin therapy in patients with cerebellar degeneration that are already enrolled.

Prognosis

There are many factors that determine the prognosis of an affected individual. These factors depend on the type of genetic mutation, the size of the repeat expansion, anticipation, and the age at which symptoms develop. Although these factors can help determine the prognosis, the exact age of onset and the specific symptoms are difficult to determine, especially for carriers with no symptoms. Ultimately, as with all progressive degenerative disorders, the disease is fatal. In the case of spinocerebellar ataxia, persons usually die one to two decades after symptoms develop. The prognosis for SCA11 and SCA6 is typically less severe, with a very slow worsening of symptoms, and persons with SCA8 and SCA11 have a normal lifespan.

Special concerns

Genetic testing of at-risk family members can be performed when an affected individual has a known genetic mutation. Testing of high-risk family members without symptoms raises many issues. For example, individuals who test negative usually feel guilty that they did not inherit the genetic defect, and parents who are affected feel guilty that they passed on the gene defect. These experiences can have a significant impact on the family dynamics, particularly in adult-onset disorders. Additionally, it is often unclear when (or if) family members who test positive for the mutation will develop symptoms and how severe the symptoms will be. It is generally considered not useful to test children with no symptoms. These issues and others are usually carefully evaluated by family members with the help of a genetic counselor.

Resources

BOOKS

Pulst, Stefan, M. *Neurogenetics.* New York: Oxford University Press, 1999.

OTHER

"NINDS Ataxias and Cerebellar/Spinocerebellar Degeneration Information Page." *National Institute of Neurological Disorders and Stroke.* (February 11, 2004). <http://www.ninds.nih.gov/health_and_medical/disorders/ataxia.htm>.

"Spinocerebellar ataxia." *National Center for Biotechnology Information.* (February 14, 2004). <http://www.ncbi.nlm.nih.gov/books/bv.fcgi?call=bv.View..ShowSection&rid=gnd.section.218>.

ORGANIZATIONS

National Ataxia Foundation (NAF). 2600 Fernbrook Lane, Suite 119, Minneapolis, MN 55447. (612) 553-0020; Fax: (612) 553-0167. naf@mr.net. <http://www.ataxia.org>.

National Society of Genetic Counselors (NSGC). 233 Canterbury Drive, Wallingford, PA 19086-6617. (610) 872-7608; Fax: (610) 872-1192. nsgc@aol.com. <http://www.nsgc.org>.

WE MOVE (Worldwide Education and Awareness for Movement Disorders). 204 West 84th Street, New York, NY 10024. (212) 875-8389 or (800) 437-MOV2 (6683). wemove@wemove.org. <http://www.wemove.org>.

Bryan Richard Cobb, PhD

Status epilepticus

Definition

Status epilepticus is a term describing a state of continuous seizure activity. In the past, 30 minutes of continuing seizure or frequent attacks that prevent recovery was required for the definition of status to be met. However, since most **seizures** last less than four to five minutes, it is now understood that any seizure that continues five minutes or longer should be potentially considered as status epilepticus, and managed accordingly.

Description

Nearly all types of seizures have the potential of occurring in a continuous or repeated fashion. There are two general categories: generalized status and focal status, depending on the clinical features of the situation. Generalized status can preferentially manifest with tonic, clonic, absence, and/or myoclonic seizures. Hence, status can be merely a prolongation of commonly observed individual seizure types. Non-convulsive status epilepticus can manifest with sustained or repeating complex partial seizures with a change in mental status, or simply as a focal seizure with limited physical signs but without alteration of consciousness. Status can occur in individuals who have **epilepsy** already. However, in some cases, the first seizure that a person experiences can be status epilepticus.

Demographics

The epidemiology of status epilepticus varies depending on the study. However, in the United States the incidence is approximately up to 40 per 100,000 individuals. Therefore more than 100,000 cases of status occur annually. Up to 10% of all first-time seizures are situations of status epilepticus. The mortality of status epilepticus is roughly 20%. Those most at risk are the very young or the elderly. The causes of death vary depending on the age of the patient, presence of medical complications, duration of

Key Terms

Absence A type of seizure that causes brief (shorter than 30 seconds) episodes of staring.

Clonic A type of seizure characterized by rhythmic jerking of the arms and legs.

Myoclonic A type of seizure that causes brief muscle jerks of the whole body or a limb.

Tonic A type of seizure characterized by episodes of stiffening in all the limbs for up to one or two minutes.

the uncontrollable seizures, and the underlying cause of the status epilepticus.

Causes and symptoms

The exact pathophysiology of why a seizure evolves into status is complex and not fully understood. However, status epilepticus has many causes, some of which are the same as causes of seizures in general. In infants, status can occur in the setting of perinatal **hypoxia** or anoxia (low oxygen or lack of oxygen) that injures the brain. Also, illness such as meningitis that can cause seizures can also be severe enough to cause status epilepticus. Metabolic disorders of infancy and childhood that can be causes of epilepsy can also produce status epilepticus. In adults, infections of the brain, strokes, brain tumors, and severe head trauma can cause seizures and hence status epilepticus.

Clinically, status epilepticus is basically a prolonged seizure situation. Individual seizures occurring frequently enough to impair full recovery to baseline function can be a manifestation of status epilepticus as well. A limited seizure such as an arm jerking without alteration of consciousness is called a simple or focal seizure. If it occurs continuously, the term epilepsy partialis continua is used. This is the least serious of the different types of status epilepticus. The more dangerous type is, of course, generalized tonic/clonic status. This is because cardiac arrhythmias or blood pressure changes can be life threatening. Also, breathing and oxygenation can be compromised, and patients may require ventilator assistance. Complex partial seizures and absence seizures are manifested with an alteration of consciousness. When these particular seizures become status, patients may simply appear confused or agitated. Since they are not having convulsions, they may be misdiagnosed as having a psychiatric symptom. Nevertheless, prompt and accurate diagnosis is important for proper management.

Diagnosis

When convulsions are occurring, status is typically easily recognized. However, subtle status, as in complex partial or absence status, may necessitate an electroencephalogram (EEG) for diagnosis. The EEG is not only used for initial diagnosis, but is often left running for longer periods to monitor response to treatment. The recognition of seizure activity is only one of the urgent tasks in the care of the patient. The other major issue is to rapidly identify the cause of seizures and the status epilepticus. This involves testing blood for at least glucose, electrolytes, liver function, and illicit substances. Very low blood glucose or extreme changes in sodium, for example, can cause seizures. Infections such as meningitis can cause status. Rapidly assessed levels of older, commonly used seizure medications such as phenytoin, **Phenobarbital**, **carbamazepine**, and valproic acid are sometimes sought in cases where there is no available history from the patient. Indeed, one of the most frequent causes of status is low anticonvulsant levels in a patient with a history of epilepsy.

Treatment team

Patients in status epilepticus will often necessitate a **neurologist** to guide the management from the emergency department through the rest of the hospital stay. **Social workers** are important for discharge plans because many patients who survive status epilepticus may need skilled nursing or rehabilitation to fully recover prior to being discharged home.

Treatment

The treatment of status depends on identifying quickly the underlying cause, if any. In cases of hypoglycemia, thiamine must be administered just prior to glucose supplementation. This is because some individuals, alcoholics for example, may be deficient in thiamine and a correction of glucose levels without thiamine supplementation can cause a condition known as Wernicke's **encephalopathy**. Sodium must be corrected slowly or a condition called central pontine myelinolysis can occur. A computed tomography (**CT**) scan of the brain is often ordered to evaluate for any brain trauma. A lumbar puncture may be performed to determine if there is meningitis so appropriate antibiotics can be used. Overall, in cases that an identifiable cause of status can be found, the key to successful treatment is the management of the underlying cause itself. There are published guidelines for the treatment of seizures themselves. Initially, a sedative such as lorazepam or **diazepam** is given, which can stop many seizures at least temporarily while a longer-acting anticonvulsant such as phenytoin takes effect. If seizures persist, then the addition of Phenobarbital is typically added. Since this particular medication, when fully loaded, causes respiratory **depression**, an anesthesiologist is consulted to manage ventilator assistance. Status epilepticus is managed and treated in an intensive care unit with EEG monitoring to continually assess the response to seizure medications. When Phenobarbital fails to stop the ongoing seizures, a number of other medications are considered, such as a midazolam drip or propofol. Anesthetic dosages of these particular medications are usually effective in suppressing seizure activity. Approximately every 24 hours, the dosage is reduced to determine if seizures recur or not. The severity of status can vary widely. Sometimes, it is effectively treated within one to two hours and other times the status is severe and extremely resistant to treatment and lasts for weeks. In such cases, the mortality rate is significant because of risk of medical complications such as pneumonia and blood clots.

Recovery and rehabilitation

The recovery from status epilepticus will depend on its duration. If status can be effectively stopped in a relatively short period of time, complete neurological recovery is possible. The longer the seizures persist, the greater the chance of cerebral injury. Also, the longer the status epilepticus, the more difficult it is to stop. A complication of status epilepticus can actually be the development of epilepsy in a percentage of cases.

Prognosis

The prognosis with status epilepticus will depend on the duration of status and co-existing medical problems. The prognosis is good for recovery if status can be stopped in a relatively short period of time (hours) and there are no complications such as infection, active cardiac problems, or other active medical issues. However, prognosis for complete recovery is less favorable as status persists for long periods of time. Co-existing medical problems will complicate management and chance for a negative outcome.

Special concerns

It is important to be on the lookout for subtle status situations that may go unrecognized. An EEG is a relatively easy way to rule in or rule out presence of active seizures. It is crucial to respond urgently to status epilepticus because the longer the seizures continue the more difficult they are to stop.

Resources
BOOKS

Browne, T. R., and G. L. Holmes. *Handbook of Epilepsy*, 2nd edition. Philadelphia: Lippinocott Williams & Wilkins, 2000.

Engel, Jr., J., and T. A. Pedley. *Epilepsy: A Comprehensive Textbook*. Philadelphia: Lippincott-Raven, 1998.

Hauser, W. A., and D. Hesdorffer. *Epilepsy: Frequency, Causes, and Consequences*. New York: Demos Publications, 1990.

Wyllie, E. *The Treatment of Epilepsy: Principles and Practice*, 3rd edition. Philadelphia: Lippincott Williams & Wilkins.2001.

PERIODICALS

Epilepsy Foundation of America's Working Group on Status Epilepticus. "Treatment of Convulsive Status Epilepticus: Recommendations of the JAMA." *Journal of the American Medical Association* 270 (1993): 854–859.

Hesdorffer, D. C., G. Logroscino, G. Cascino, J. F. Annegers, and W. A. Hauser. "Risk of Unprovoked Seizure after Acute Symptomatic Seizure: Effect of Status Epilepticus." *Annals of Neurology* 44 (1998): 908–912.

ORGANIZATIONS

American Epilepsy Society. 342 North Main Street, West Hartford, CT 06117-2507. (860) 586-7505. <http://www.aesnet.org>.

Epilepsy Foundation of America. 4351 Garden City Drive, Landover, MD 20785-7223. (800) 332-1000. <http://www.epilepsyfoundation.org>.

Internation League Against Epilepsy. Avenue Marcel Thiry 204, B-1200, Brussels, Belgium. + 32 (0) 2 774 9547; Fax: + 32 (0) 2 774 9690. <http://www.epilepsy.org>.

Roy Sucholeiki, MD

Steele-Richardson-Olszewski syndrome *see*
Progressive supranuclear palsy

Stiff person syndrome

Definition

Stiff person syndrome (SPS) is an extremely rare progressive neurological disorder characterized by persistent rigidity and spasms of certain voluntary muscles, especially those of legs and feet. In some cases, muscles of the neck, trunk, and shoulders may also be involved. SPS may begin as recurring (intermittent) episodes of stiffness and spasms, often precipitated by surprise or minor physical contact.

Description

SPS is a rare progressive neurological disorder characterized by constant painful contractions and spasms of voluntary muscles, particularly the muscles of the back and upper legs. In 1956, scientists at the Mayo Clinic also coined the term stiff man syndrome, and clearly described the stiff person syndrome as a neurological disorder. The rigidity, which is characterized by tightness and stiffness, begins slowly over several months at the axial muscles, especially the thoracic and lumbar spine, and spreads to the legs. The stiffness may worsen when the affected individual is anxious or exposed to sudden motion or noise. Affected muscles may become twisted and contracted, resulting in bone fractures in the most severe cases.

Another abnormality in SPS is called co-contraction: when the person attempts to contract a muscle to move in one direction, muscles that pull in the opposite direction are involuntarily activated. Individuals with SPS may have difficulty making sudden movements and may have a stiff-legged unsteady gait (manner of walking). The muscle contractions are usually reduced with extra rest.

Eventually, persons with stiff person syndrome may develop a hunched posture (kyphosis) or a swayback (lordosis).

Demographics

The frequency of SPS worldwide or in the United States is unknown, but the syndrome is rare. Unlike many autoimmune diseases, which have a higher incidence in women, SPS is found more frequently in men, occurring in men in approximately 70% of all cases. The syndrome also occurs in children younger than three years, most commonly in infants. Onset in adults is most frequent in the third to fifth decades of life.

Causes and symptoms

The cause of stiff person syndrome is unknown, however, researchers theorize that SPS may be an autoimmune disorder. An autoimmune disorder involves a malfunction of the immune system, where the body produces antibodies against its own tissues. Antibodies are proteins produced by the body as part of its defense against foreign bacteria, viruses, or other harmful substances. Other autoimmune disorders such as diabetes, pernicious anemia (a chronic, progressive blood disorder), and thyroiditis (inflammation of the thyroid gland) may occur more frequently in patients with SPS.

Often SPS, antibodies are produced against glutamic acid decarboxylase (GAD), an enzyme largely found in the **central nervous system**. However, GAD antibodies alone appear to be insufficient to cause SPS, as some persons with stiff person disease do not have the GAD antibodies, and GAD antibodies are associated with a number of diseases.

Symptoms may occur gradually, spreading from the back and legs to involve the arms and neck. Initially, the patient has an exaggerated upright posture and may experience back discomfort, stiffness or **pain** in the entire back,

Key Terms

Antibody Proteins produced by the immune system in response to the introduction of foreign molecules called antigens. Antibodies neutralize these molecules to prevent infection or disease.

Autoimmune disorder A large group of diseases characterized by abnormal functioning of the immune system that produces antibodies against its own tissues.

Kyphosis Posterior curvature of the spine, creating a humpback appearance.

Lordosis Anterior curvature of the spine, creating a swayback appearance.

which worsens with tension or stress. Some persons with SPS, in the early stages, show brief episodes of rather dramatic severe worsening that resolve spontaneously within hours or days. Later in the disease, upper limb muscles also begin to be involved, particularly when the person is stimulated, surprised, angered, upset, or frightened. This sort of stimulation may evoke painful severe spasms in the upper arm and leg muscles that resolve slowly. The person with SPS begins to move very slowly because rapid movement induces severe spasms. Even the lower extremities may become involved when moved rapidly. In the end stages of the disease, few muscles in the body are spared. However, facial and pharyngeal muscles may be especially affected.

Babies and young children are less rigid between attacks. Involvement of lower arm and leg muscles is often more evident, particularly during muscle spasms.

Diagnosis

During physical examination, the physician who suspects SPS looks for stiffness, rigidity or increased tone, spasm, or pain. The areas of involvement may include the face, neck, abdomen, or arms, but more typically the legs or lumbar spine are involved. Evaluation may include tests to rule out other causes of stiffness such as **multiple sclerosis**. When overwhelming anxiety and fear overshadow the stiffness, it may be difficult to distinguish SPS from an emotional disorder.

Laboratory procedures assess the presence of specific autoantibodies called anti-GAD, which are found at high levels in the blood of a person with SPS. These examinations include immunocytochemistry, Western blotting, ELISA (enzyme-linked immunosorbent assay), and radioimmunoassay (RIA). The last two procedures have the advantage of quantitatively assessing the amount of anti-GAD antibody a patient produces.

Electromyography (EMG) is an important diagnostic tool to determine an abnormal firing pattern in the muscles sometimes seen in persons with SPS. The EMG findings of SPS may be subtle in patients who are fully treated for symptoms of SPS. Except for global muscle stiffness, results of a neurological examination are usually normal. Results of conventional computed tomography and **magnetic resonance imaging** of the brain are also normal.

Treatment team

The treatment team for a person with SPS is often composed of physical and occupational therapists, nutritionists, neurosurgeons, and neurologists.

Treatment

SPS is clinically elusive, but potentially treatable. Traditional treatment for SPS starts with medications such as baclofen or a **benzodiazepine**. Commonly used benzodiazepines are **diazepam** (Valium) or lorazepam (Ativan). Both benzodiazepine and baclofen act increasing the activity of the central inhibitory systems. Although no studies have been performed, tizanidine (Zanaflex) may be a less sedating alternative, and prednisone is also a commonly prescribed drug for treatment of SPS.

In some patients, plasmapheresis, a process of filtering the blood to remove excess antibodies, has been demonstrated to be useful in removing anti-GAD antibodies from the bloodstream. In the hospital setting, intravenous immunoglobulin (IVIG) has also been used in the treatment of SPS.

Recovery and rehabilitation

Physical therapy and occupational therapy are critical to the recovery of patients under treatment. Medical treatment can make the patient feel weak, a feeling that may be alleviated by therapy. The person with SPS may also have problems with voluntary movements and fine motor skills. Occupational and physical therapists devise strategies to compensate for these weaknesses during the common daily activities of living.

Clinical trials

In 2004 there were two open **clinical trials** recruiting patients entitled "Cause, Development, and Progression of Stiff-Person Syndrome" and "Diagnostic Evaluation of Patients with Neuromuscular Disease," sponsored by National Institute of Neurological Disorders and Stroke (NINDS). For further and updated information, visit the website <www.clinicaltrials.gov>, sponsored by the National Institutes of Health.

Prognosis

There is no cure for SPS and the long-term prognosis is variable. Many patients have a slow course of the disorder that is mostly without symptoms, punctuated by occasional episodes of stiffness. Other patients may have a much more aggressive course, rapidly progressing to the late stages of disease. Other forms of the disease have been described that are accompanied by brain disorders and other central nervous system abnormalities, but whether they are separate diseases or different manifestations of the same disease is unclear. Management of the disorder with drug therapy usually provides significant improvement and relief of symptoms.

Special concerns

Many of the medications prescribed for SPS are not indicated during pregnancy. Elderly persons with SPS may have increased chances of falling and injury because of concurrent disability from other causes. As with all autoimmune disorders, dietary changes are sometimes helpful. For best results, dietary changes should be made under the supervision of a physician experienced in nutritional medicine.

Resources

BOOKS

Icon Health Publications. *The Official Patient's Sourcebook on Stiff-Person Syndrome: A Revised and Updated Directory for the Internet Age.* San Diego: Icon Group International, 2002.

Larsen, Povl K., J. Egeberg, and A. Schousboe. *Glutamate and GABA Receptors and Transporters.* Taylor & Francis, 2001.

PERIODICALS

Gerschlager, W. et al. "Quality of life in stiff person syndrome." *Movement Disorders* 17 (2002): 1064–1067.

OTHER

"NINDS Stiff-Person Syndrome Information Page." *National Institute of Neurological Disorders and Stroke.* (March 11, 2004). <http://www.ninds.nih.gov/health_and_medical/disorders/stiffperson_doc.htm>.

ORGANIZATIONS

National Rehabilitation Information Center (NARIC). 4200 Forbes Boulevard; Suite 202, Lanham, Maryland 20706-4829. (301) 562-2400 or (800) 346-2742; (301) 562-2401. naricinfo@heitechservices.com. <http://www.naric.com>.

National Organization for Rare Disorders (NORD). 55 Kenosia Avenue, Danbury, Connecticut 06813-1968. (203) 744-0100; Fax: (203) 798-2291. orphan@rarediseases.org. <http://www.rarediseases.org>.

National Institute of Arthritis and Musculoskeletal and Skin Diseases (NIAMS). Bldg. 31, Rm. 4C05, Bethesda,

Maryland 20892-2350. (301) 496-8188.
NIAMSInfo@mail.nih.gov. <http://www.nih.gov/niams>.

Bruno Verbeno Azevedo
Iuri Drumond Louro, MD, PhD

Striatonigral degeneration

Definition

Striatonigral degeneration is a neurodegenerative disease caused by disruption of two areas, the striatum and substantia nigra, which work together to enable movement and balance.

Description

Striatonigral degeneration was described in 1961 and 1964. However, since the disorder has common manifestations seen in multiple diseases (e.g., the Shy-Drager syndrome, where autonomic nervous system failure predominates, and sporadic olivopontocerebellar degeneration, where **cerebellum** deficits predominate), it was necessary to clarify the nomenclature. In 1999, the name striatonigral degeneration was replaced with the accepted new names: multiple system atrophy-Parkinson (MSA-P), if **Parkinson's disease** symptoms predominate, or MSA-cerebellum (MSA-C), if cerebellar **ataxia** is the main feature. Patients who have MSA have characteristic pathological changes in common, but in variable degrees. Affected neurons in the brain have inclusion bodies that cause neuronal loss, by a mechanism of programmed cell death called apoptosis. The presence of inclusion bodies in neurons causes a reaction to self-destruct following a programmed sequence of chemical reactions that promotes cell death.

Demographics

The prevalence of MSA-P is difficult to establish with accuracy since the disorder is frequently misdiagnosed in the United States and internationally. It is estimated to account for 5–22% of cases in patients with Parkinson's or Parkinson-like disorders. Approximately 80% of patients present with MSA-P symptoms and 20% exhibit symptoms of cerebellar ataxia (MSA-C subtype). It is estimated that the prevalence of this disorder is 1.9–4.9 cases per 100,000. The age range of diagnosis is between 33 and 76 years of age. MSA-P has never been identified in a person younger than 30 years. The mean survival time after the onset of symptoms is 7–9 years. There is no racial predilection, and males and females are affected equally.

The mean age of diagnosis is 53 years. For the majority of MSA-P affected persons, the full clinical picture evolves within five years after onset of symptoms.

Causes and symptoms

The cause of MSA has not been identified. MSA occurs in the general population in a sporadic manner. The disorder is degenerative and progressively worsens. The natural history of the disorder is chronic, symptoms progressively worsen, and the disorder often results in death, after multiple treatment efforts.

Common symptoms of MSA-P (which may be asymmetric) include bradykinesia (slowness of movement) characterized by an irregular jerky postural tremor. It is uncommon for the tremor to occur at rest. Additionally, patients often exhibit rigidity, postural instability, and a characteristic quivering high-pitched **dysarthria**. Many patients with MSA-P also develop orofacial and craniocervical **dystonia**. Patients with the MSA-C subtype also develop gait and limb ataxia, eye abnormalities, and scanning dysarthria. Other symptoms can include **depression**, emotional lability (fluctuations of emotional state), hyperreflexia, extensor plantar (sole) response, **myoclonus**, or laryngeal stridor. Failure of the autonomic nervous system (ANS) is a characteristic of both subtypes (MSA-P and MSA-C), which primarily consists of urogenital problems and **orthostatic hypotension**. ANS failure causes early male erectile dysfunction and urinary dysfunction, causing problems with frequency, urgency, retention, and incontinence. Additionally, patients frequently develop postprandial (after food) postural hypotension and episodes of syncope (loss of consciousness), due to lack of oxygen to the brain (cerebral hypoperfusion).

Diagnosis

No specific lab tests are indicated. High-resolution neuroimaging studies may demonstrate neuronal abnormalities and/or atrophy in the brain. The diagnosis is based on history, physical examination, and family history (to detect genetic correlations). A definite diagnosis can be obtained by pathological examination of brain neurons. A probable diagnosis is made by the presence of ANS failure, poor response to medications, or cerebellar dysfunction (cerebellar ataxia). Neuroimaging studies using **magnetic resonance imaging (MRI)** indicate that that there is volume loss (neuronal loss) in associated areas in the brain (the striatum and substantia nigra). Functional neuroimaging techniques (which take images of neuron function) indicate that neuron receptor binding is defective and there is low metabolism (low level of vital chemical reactions).

Key Terms

Ataxia Muscular incoordination and irregularity of muscular action.

Autonomic nervous system (ANS) Consists of neurons that are not under one's conscious control. The ANS is comprised of two subdivisions called the parasympathetic nervous system, which slows heart rate, increases intestinal and gland activity, and relaxes the sphincter muscles; and the sympathetic nervous system, which accelerates heart rate, raises blood pressure, and constricts blood vessels.

Cerebellar ataxia Disorders of the cerebellum that cause a loss of muscular coordination.

Dysarthria Nerve damage that causes disturbances in muscular control, resulting in impaired speech articulation.

Dyskinesias A group of disorders characterized by involuntary movements of muscles.

Dystonia Abnormal tone in a group of muscles.

Hyperreflexia An increased reaction to reflexes.

Incontinence Inability to control excretory functions such as defecation and urination.

Laryngeal stridor Constriction of the voice box, causing vocal hoarseness.

Myoclonus Spasm or twitching of a muscle or a group of muscles.

Orthostatic hypotension A reduction of blood pressure (systolic blood pressure that occurs when the heart contracts or diastolic pressure that occurs when the heart muscle relaxes).

Paresis A slight paralysis.

Parkinson's disease A neurodegenerative disorder characterized by slowness of voluntary movements, mask-like facial expression, and a rhythmic tremor of the limbs and stooped posture.

Receptor A structure located on the outside of a cell's membrane that causes the cell to attach to specific molecules; the molecules are then internalized, taken inside the cell.

Striatum Area located deep within the brain.

Substantia nigra An area located in the middle portion of the brain that can become depleted of a specific neurotransmitter called dopamine, causing symptoms of Parkinson's disease.

Syncope Loss of consciousness.

Tremor An involuntary movement characterized by quivering and trembling.

Treatment team

The treatment team can typically include a **neurologist** and respiratory care providers, when management of breathing difficulties requires professional intervention. A physical therapist can help with postural and movement difficulties. An audiologist is utilized for speech and eating difficulties.

Treatment

No surgical treatment exists for striatonigral degeneration, and pharmacological treatment is not effective in the long term. Approximately 30% of patients demonstrate initial improvement with a medication called levodopa-carbidopa. However, symptomatic improvement is temporary; approximately 90% patients are unresponsive to levodopa in the long term. Dystonia can be treated with **botulinum toxin**, which tends to control involuntary muscular movements. Affected persons who develop failure of the autonomic nervous system may develop orthostatic hypotension. Patients who develop low blood pressure symptoms should avoid activities such as overeating, straining at stool passage, and exposure to extreme heat. Elevating the

head of the bed, use of pressure stockings, and increased sodium intake (which causes water retention, which in turn stabilizes blood pressure) are treatments for hypotension. Additionally, medication to correct hypotension can be prescribed, including fludrocortisone, ephedrine, and midodrine. Medication to treat postprandial hypotension (octreotide) or bladder symptoms (oxybutynin) can be given when needed. Overall, however, the result of medical treatment for MSA is poor.

Recovery and rehabilitation

Rehabilitation can include patient, family, and caretaker education concerning the possibilities of respiratory failure, aspiration pneumonia, trauma, and syncope. Patients can develop paresis of the larynx or pharynx, central chronic respiratory failure (a chronic respiratory failure due to destruction of neurons in the brain), or sudden death. Patients require physical therapy to help maintain mobility and prevent permanent muscular contractures. Speech therapy can improve speech impairments and difficulty with swallowing (dysphagia) mechanisms. Dysphagia may necessitate tube placement and feedings.

Patients eventually require occupational therapy to limit handicap from disability. A wheelchair is indicated depending on liability to falls due to gait (walking) ataxia and postural instability. Psychological support is necessary for the patient and family member caretakers.

Clinical trials

Clinical trials are being done to find methods to prevent and treat MSA-P. The Mayo Clinic in Rochester, Minnesota, currently has projects and investigations concerning new techniques for diagnosis using **PET** scan technology. This technology is likely to be available in the near future.

Prognosis

The disorder is degenerative and the mean survival time in confirmed cases is seven years. The range of survival for persons with MSA-P is 2–15 years. Approximately 50% of affected patients who receive levodopa develop side effects that can include **dyskinesia** of orofacial and neck muscles.

Special concerns

Episodes of syncope can cause severe trauma, usually from falls. Patients are advised to lie or sit down when symptoms appear. Family members and caretakers should be aware of the syncope and the dangers associated with falls and trauma.

Resources

PERIODICALS

Wenning, Gregor, and Werner Poewe. "Multiple System Atrophy." *The Lancet Neurology* 3:2 (February 2004).

WEBSITES

National Organization for Rare Disorders (NORD). (May 23, 2004). <http://www.rarediseases.org>.

The Mayo Clinic. *Clinical Information.* (May 23, 2004). <http://www.mayoresearch.mayo.edu>.

ORGANIZATIONS

Worldwide Education & Awareness for Movement Disorders (WE MOVE). 204 West 84th Street, New York, NY 10024. (212) 875-8312 or (800) 437-6682; Fax: (212) 875-8389. wemove@wemove.org. <http://www.wemove.org>.

Laith Farid Gulli, MD
Nicole Mallory, MS, PA-C

▌Stroke

Definition

A stroke is the sudden death of brain cells in a localized area due to inadequate blood flow.

Description

A stroke occurs when blood flow is interrupted to part of the brain. Without blood to supply oxygen and nutrients and to remove waste products, brain cells quickly begin to die. Depending on the region of the brain affected, a stroke may cause paralysis, speech impairment, a loss of memory and reasoning ability, coma, or death. A stroke is also sometimes called a brain attack or a cerebrovascular accident (CVA).

Some important stroke statistics include:

- More than half a million people in the United States experience a new or recurrent stroke each year.

- Stroke is the third leading cause of death in the United States and the leading cause of disability.

- Stroke kills about 150,000 Americans each year, or almost one out of three stroke victims.

- Three million Americans are currently permanently disabled from stroke.

- In the United States, stroke costs about $30 billion per year in direct costs and loss of productivity.

- Two-thirds of strokes occur in people over age 65.

- Strokes affect men more often than women, although women are more likely to die from a stroke.

- Strokes affect blacks more often than whites, and are more likely to be fatal among blacks.

Stroke is a medical emergency requiring immediate treatment. Prompt treatment improves the chances of survival and increases the degree of recovery that may be expected. A person who may have suffered a stroke should be seen in a hospital emergency room without delay. Treatment to break up a blood clot, the major cause of stroke, must begin within three hours of the stroke to be effective. Improved medical treatment of all types of stroke has resulted in a dramatic decline in death rates in recent decades. In 1950, nine in 10 people died from stroke, compared to slightly less than one in three today.

Causes and symptoms

Causes

There are four main types of stroke. Cerebral thrombosis and cerebral embolism are caused by blood clots that block an artery supplying the brain, either in the brain itself or in the neck. These account for 70–80% of all strokes. Subarachnoid hemorrhage and intracerebral hemorrhage occur when a blood vessel bursts around or in the brain.

Cerebral thrombosis occurs when a blood clot, or thrombus, forms within the brain itself, blocking the flow of blood through the affected vessel. Clots most often form due to "hardening" (atherosclerosis) of brain arteries. Cerebral thrombosis occurs most often at night or early in the morning. Cerebral thrombosis is often preceded by a **transient ischemic attack** (TIA), sometimes called a "mini-stroke." In a TIA, blood flow is temporarily interrupted, causing short-lived stroke-like symptoms. Recognizing the occurrence of a TIA and seeking immediate treatment are important steps in stroke prevention.

Cerebral embolism occurs when a blood clot from elsewhere in the circulatory system breaks free. If it becomes lodged in an artery supplying the brain, either in the brain or in the neck, it can cause a stroke. The most common cause of cerebral embolism is atrial fibrillation, a disorder of the heartbeat. In atrial fibrillation, the upper chambers (atria) of the heart beat weakly and rapidly, instead of slowly and steadily. Blood within the atria is not completely emptied. This stagnant blood may form clots within the atria, which can then break off and enter the circulation. Atrial fibrillation is a factor in about 15% of all strokes. The risk of a stroke from atrial fibrillation can be dramatically reduced with daily use of anticoagulant medication.

Hemorrhage, or bleeding, occurs when a blood vessel breaks, either from trauma or excess internal pressure. The vessels most likely to break are those with preexisting defects such as an aneurysm. An aneurysm is a "pouching out" of a blood vessel caused by a weak arterial wall. Brain **aneurysms** are surprisingly common. According to autopsy studies, about 6% of all Americans have them. Aneurysms rarely cause symptoms until they burst. Aneurysms are most likely to burst when blood pressure is highest, and controlling blood pressure is an important preventive strategy.

Intracerebral hemorrhage affects vessels within the brain itself, while subarachnoid hemorrhage affects arteries at the brain's surface, just below the protective arachnoid membrane. Intracerebral hemorrhages represent about 10% of all strokes, while subarachnoid hemorrhages account for about 7%.

In addition to depriving affected tissues of blood supply, the accumulation of fluid within the inflexible skull creates excess pressure on brain tissue, which can quickly lead to death. Nonetheless, recovery may be more complete for a person who survives hemorrhage than for one who survives a clot, because the blood deprivation effects are usually not as severe.

Death of brain cells triggers a chain reaction in which toxic chemicals created by cell death affect other nearby cells. This is one reason why prompt treatment can have such a dramatic effect on final recovery.

Risk factors

Risk factors for stroke involve age, sex, heredity, predisposing diseases or other medical conditions, and lifestyle choices, including:

- Age and sex. The risk of stroke increases with increasing age, doubling for each decade after age 55. Men are more likely to have a stroke than women.

- Heredity. Blacks, Asians, and Hispanics all have higher rates of stroke than do whites, related partly to higher blood pressure. People with a family history of stroke are at greater risk.

- Diseases. Stroke risk is increased for people with diabetes, heart disease (especially atrial fibrillation), high blood pressure, prior stroke, or TIA. Risk of stroke increases tenfold for someone with one or more TIAs.

- Other medical conditions. Stroke risk increases with obesity, high blood cholesterol level, or high red blood cell count.

- Lifestyle choices. Stroke risk increases with cigarette smoking (especially if combined with the use of oral contraceptives), low level of physical activity, alcohol consumption above two drinks per day, or use of cocaine or intravenous drugs.

Symptoms

Symptoms of an embolic stroke usually come on quite suddenly and are at their most intense right from the start, while symptoms of a thrombotic stroke come on more gradually. Symptoms may include:

- blurring or decreased vision in one or both eyes

- severe headache

- weakness, numbness, or paralysis of the face, arm, or leg, usually confined to one side of the body

- dizziness, loss of balance or coordination, especially when combined with other symptoms

Diagnosis

The diagnosis of stroke is begun with a careful medical history, especially concerning the onset and distribution of symptoms, presence of risk factors, and the exclusion of other possible causes. A brief neurological exam is performed to identify the degree and location of any deficits such as weakness, incoordination, or visual losses.

Once stroke is suspected, a computed tomography **(CT) scan** or **magnetic resonance imaging (MRI)** scan is performed to distinguish a stroke caused by blood clot from one caused by hemorrhage, a critical distinction that guides therapy. Blood and urine tests are done routinely to look for possible abnormalities.

Other investigations that may be performed to guide treatment include an electrocardiogram, **angiography**, ultrasound, and electroencephalogram.

Treatment team

Stroke treatment involves a multidisciplinary team. Physicians are responsible for caring for the stroke survivor's general health and providing guidance aimed at preventing a second stroke. Neurologists usually lead acute-care stroke teams and direct patient care during hospitalization. The team may include a physiatrist (a specialist in rehabilitation), a rehabilitation nurse, a physical therapist, an occupational therapist, a speech-language pathologist, a social worker, a psychologist, and a vocational counselor.

Treatment

Emergency treatment

Emergency treatment of stroke from a blood clot is aimed at dissolving the clot. This "thrombolytic therapy" is currently performed most often with tissue plasminogen activator, or t-PA. This t-PA must be administered within three hours of the stroke event. Therefore, patients who awaken with stroke symptoms are ineligible for t-PA therapy, as the time of onset cannot be accurately determined. The t-PA therapy has been shown to improve recovery and decrease long-term disability in selected patients. The t-PA therapy carries a 6.4% risk of inducing a cerebral hemorrhage, and is not appropriate for patients with bleeding disorders, very high blood pressure, known aneurysms, any evidence of intracranial hemorrhage, or incidence of stroke, head trauma, or intracranial surgery within the past three months. Patients with clot-related (thrombotic or embolic) stroke who are ineligible for t-PA treatment may be treated with heparin or other blood thinners, or with aspirin or other anti-clotting agents in some cases.

Emergency treatment of hemorrhagic stroke is aimed at controlling intracranial pressure. Intravenous urea or mannitol plus hyperventilation are the most common treatments. Corticosteroids may also be used. Patients with reversible bleeding disorders such as those due to anticoagulant treatment should have these bleeding disorders reversed, if possible.

Surgery for hemorrhage due to aneurysm may be performed if the aneurysm is close enough to the cranial surface to allow access. Ruptured vessels are closed off to prevent rebleeding. For aneurysms that are difficult to reach surgically, endovascular treatment may be used. In this procedure, a catheter is guided from a larger artery up into the brain to reach the aneurysm. Small coils of wire are discharged into the aneurysm, which plug it up and block off blood flow from the main artery.

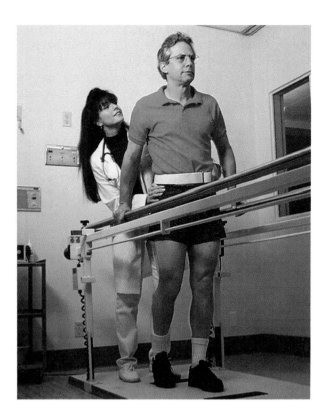

A man who suffered a stroke is helped with his rehabilitation by a physical therapist. *(© 1993 ATC Productions. Custom Medical Stock Photo. Reproduced by permission.)*

Recovery and rehabilitation

Rehabilitation refers to a comprehensive program designed to help the patient regain function as much as possible and compensate for permanent losses. Approximately 10% of stroke survivors are without any significant disability and able to function independently. Another 10% are so severely affected that they must remain institutionalized for severe disability. The remaining 80% can return home with appropriate therapy, training, support, and care services.

Rehabilitation is coordinated by a team that may include the services of a **neurologist**, a physiatrist, a physical therapist, an occupational therapist, a speech-language pathologist, a nutritionist, a mental health professional, and a social worker. Rehabilitation services may be provided in an acute care hospital, rehabilitation hospital, long-term care facility, outpatient clinic, or at home.

The rehabilitation program is based on the patient's individual deficits and strengths. Strokes on the left side of the brain primarily affect the right half of the body, and vice versa. In addition, in left-brain-dominant people, who constitute a significant majority of the population, left-brain strokes usually lead to speech and language deficits, while right-brain strokes may affect spatial perception. Patients

Key Terms

Aneurysm A pouch-like bulging of a blood vessel.

Atrial fibrillation A disorder of the heartbeat associated with a higher risk of stroke. In this disorder, the upper chambers (atria) of the heart do not completely empty when the heart beats, which can allow blood clots to form.

Cerebral embolism A blockage of blood flow through a vessel in the brain by a blood clot that formed elsewhere in the body and traveled to the brain.

Cerebral thrombosis A blockage of blood flow through a vessel in the brain by a blood clot that formed in the brain itself.

Intracerebral hemorrhage A cause of some strokes in which vessels within the brain begin bleeding.

Subarachnoid hemorrhage A cause of some strokes in which arteries on the surface of the brain begin bleeding.

Tissue plasminogen activator (tPA) A substance that is sometimes given to patients within three hours of a stroke to dissolve blood clots within the brain.

with right-brain strokes may also deny their illness, neglect the affected side of their body, and behave impulsively.

Rehabilitation may be complicated by cognitive losses, including diminished ability to understand and follow directions. Poor results are more likely in patients with significant or prolonged cognitive changes, sensory losses, language deficits, or incontinence.

Preventing complications

Rehabilitation begins with prevention of stroke recurrence and other medical complications. The risk of stroke recurrence may be reduced with many of the same measures used to prevent stroke, including quitting smoking and controlling blood pressure.

One of the most common medical complications following stroke is deep venous thrombosis, in which a clot forms within a limb immobilized by paralysis. Clots that break free can often become lodged in an artery feeding the lungs. This type of pulmonary embolism is a common cause of death in the weeks following a stroke. Resuming activity within a day or two after the stroke is an important preventive measure, along with use of elastic stockings on the lower limbs. Drugs that prevent clotting may be given, including intravenous heparin and oral warfarin.

Weakness and loss of coordination of the swallowing muscles may impair swallowing (dysphagia), and allow food to enter the lower airway. This may lead to aspiration pneumonia, another common cause of death shortly after a stroke. Dysphagia may be treated with retraining exercises and temporary use of pureed foods.

Depression occurs in 30–60% of stroke patients. Antidepressants and psychotherapy may be used in combination.

Other medical complications include urinary tract infections, pressure ulcers, falls, and **seizures**.

Types of rehabilitative therapy

Brain tissue that dies in a stroke cannot regenerate. In some cases, other brain regions may perform the functions of that tissue after a training period. In other cases, compensatory actions may be developed to replace lost abilities.

Physical therapy is used to maintain and restore range of motion and strength in affected limbs, and to maximize mobility in walking, wheelchair use, and transferring (from wheelchair to toilet or from standing to sitting, for instance). The physical therapist advises on mobility aids such as wheelchairs, braces, and canes. In the recovery period, a stroke patient may develop muscle **spasticity** and contractures, or abnormal contractions. Contractures may be treated with a combination of stretching and splinting.

Occupational therapy improves self-care skills such as feeding, bathing, and dressing, and helps develop effective compensatory strategies and devices for activities of daily living. A speech-language pathologist focuses on communication and swallowing skills. When dysphagia is a problem, a nutritionist can advise alternative meals that provide adequate nutrition.

Mental health professionals may be involved in the treatment of depression or loss of thinking (cognitive) skills. A **social worker** may help coordinate services and ease the transition out of the hospital back into the home. Both social workers and mental health professionals may help counsel the patient and family during the difficult rehabilitation period. Caring for a person affected with stroke requires learning a new set of skills and adapting to new demands and limitations. Home caregivers may develop stress, anxiety, and depression. Caring for the caregiver is an important part of the overall stroke treatment program.

Support groups can provide an important source of information, advice, and comfort for stroke patients and for caregivers. Joining a support group can be one of the most important steps in the rehabilitation process.

Clinical trials

As of mid-2004, there were numerous open **clinical trials** for stroke, including:

• "Adjunctive Drug Treatment for Ischemic Stroke Patients," "E-Selectin Nasal Spray to Prevent Stroke Recurrence," "Improving Motor Learning in Stroke Patients," "Aspirin or Warfarin to Prevent Stroke," "Hand **Exercise** and Upper Arm Anesthesia to Improvements Hand Function in Chronic Stroke Patients," "Preliminary Study of Transcranial Magnetic Stimulation for Stroke Rehabilitation," and "Using fMRI to Understand the Roles of Brain Areas for Fine Hand Movements" are all sponsored by the National Institute of Neurological Disorders and Stroke.

• "Preventing Post-Stroke Depression" is sponsored by the National Institute of Mental Health (NIMH).

• "Walking Therapy in Hemiparetic Stroke Patients Using Robotic-Assisted Treadmill Training" is sponsored by the United States Department of Education.

• "Brain Processing of Language Meanings" is sponsored by Warren G. Magnuson Clinical Center.

Updated information on these and other ongoing trials for the study and treatment of stroke can be found at the National Institutes of Health Web site for clinical trials at <http://www.clinicaltrials.org>.

Prognosis

Stroke is fatal for about 27% of white males, 52% of black males, 23% of white females, and 40% of black females. Stroke survivors may be left with significant deficits. Emergency treatment and comprehensive rehabilitation can significantly improve both survival and recovery.

Prevention

Damage from stroke may be significantly reduced through emergency treatment. Knowing the symptoms of stroke is as important as knowing those of a heart attack. Patients with stroke symptoms should seek emergency treatment without delay, which may mean dialing 911 rather than their family physician.

The risk of stroke can be reduced through lifestyle changes, including:

• stopping smoking

• controlling blood pressure

• getting regular exercise

• keeping weight down

• avoiding excessive alcohol consumption

• getting regular checkups and following the doctor's advice regarding diet and medicines

Treatment of atrial fibrillation may significantly reduce the risk of stroke. Preventive anticoagulant therapy may benefit those with untreated atrial fibrillation. Warfarin (Coumadin) has proven to be more effective than aspirin for those with higher risk.

Screening for aneurysms may be an effective preventive measure in those with a family history of aneurysms or autosomal polycystic kidney disease, which tends to be associated with aneurysms.

Resources

BOOKS

Caplan, L. R., M. L. Dyken, and J. D. Easton. *American Heart Association Family Guide to Stroke Treatment, Recovery, and Prevention.* New York: Times Books, 1996.

Warlow, C. P., et al. *Stroke: A Practical Guide to Management.* Boston: Blackwell Science, 1996.

Weiner F., M. H. M. Lee, and H. Bell. *Recovering at Home After a Stroke: A Practical Guide for You and Your Family.* Los Angeles: The Body Press/Perigee Books, 1994.

PERIODICALS

Selman, W. R., R. Tarr, and D. M. D. Landis. "Brain Attack: Emergency Treatment of Ischemic Stroke." *American Family Physician* 55 (June 1997): 2655–2662.

Wolf, P. A., and D. E. Singer. "Preventing Stroke in Atrial Fibrillation." *American Family Physician* (December 1997).

ORGANIZATIONS

National Stroke Association. 9707 E. Easter Lane, Englewood, Co. 80112. (800) 787-6537. (June 3, 2004). <http://www.stroke.org>.

American Heart Association. 7320 Greenville Ave. Dallas, TX 75231. (214) 373-6300. (June 3, 2004). <http://www.americanheart.org>.

Richard Robinson

Sturge-Weber syndrome

Definition

Sturge-Weber syndrome (SWS) is a condition involving specific brain changes that often cause **seizures** and mental delays. It also includes port-wine colored birthmarks (or "port-wine stains"), usually found on the face.

Description

The brain finding in SWS is leptomeningeal angioma, which is a swelling of the tissue surrounding the brain and spinal cord. These angiomas cause seizures in approximately 90% of people with SWS. A large number of affected individuals are also mentally delayed.

Port-wine stains are present at birth. They can be quite large and are typically found on the face near the eyes or on the eyelids. Vision problems are common, especially if a port-wine stain covers the eyes. These vision problems can include glaucoma and vision loss.

Facial features, such as port-wine stains, can be very challenging for individuals with SWS. These birthmarks can increase in size with time, and this may be particularly emotionally distressing for the individuals, as well as their parents. A state of unhappiness about this is more common during middle childhood and later than it is at younger ages.

Genetic profile

The genetics behind Sturge-Weber syndrome are still unknown. Interestingly, in other genetic conditions involving changes in the skin and brain (such as **neurofibromatosis** and **tuberous sclerosis**) the genetic causes are well described. It is known that most people with SRS are the only ones in their family with the condition; there is usually not a strong family history of the disease. However, a gene known to cause SWS has not been identified. For now, SWS is thought to be caused by a random, sporadic event.

Demographics

Sturge-Weber syndrome is a sporadic disease that is found throughout the world, affecting males and females equally. The total number of people with Sturge-Weber syndrome is not known, but estimates range between one in 400,000 to one in 40,000.

Causes and symptoms

People with SWS may have a larger head circumference (measurement around the head) than usual. Leptomeningeal angiomas can progress with time. They usually only occur on one side of the brain, but can exist on both sides in up to 30% of people with SWS. The angiomas can also cause great changes within the brain's white matter. Generalized wasting, or regression, of portions of the brain can result from large angiomas. Calcification of the portions of the brain underlying the angiomas can also occur. The larger and more involved the angiomas are, the greater the expected amount of mental delays in the individual. Seizures are common in SWS, and they can often begin in very early childhood. Occasionally, slight paralysis affecting one side of the body may occur.

Port-wine stains are actually capillaries (blood vessels) that reach the skin's surface and grow larger than usual. As mentioned earlier, the birthmarks mostly occur near the eyes; they often occur only on one side of the

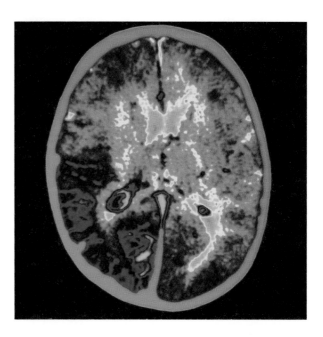

This magnetic resonance image of the brain shows a patient affected with Sturge-Weber syndrome. The front of the brain is at the top. Green colored areas indicate fluid-filled ventricles. The blue area is where the brain has become calcified. *Photo Researchers, Inc.*

face. Though they can increase in size over time, port-wine stains cause no direct health problems for the person with SWS.

Vision loss and other complications are common in SWS. The choroid of the eye can swell, and this may lead to increased pressure within the eye in 33–50% of people with SWS. Glaucoma is another common vision problem seen in SWS, and is more often seen when a person has a port-wine stain that is near or touches the eye.

In a 2000 study about the psychological functioning of children with SWS, it was noted that parents and teachers report a higher incidence of social problems, emotional distress, and problems with compliance in these individuals. Taking the mental delays into account, behaviors associated with **attention-deficit hyperactivity disorder** (ADHD) were noted; as it turns out, about 22% of people with SWS are eventually diagnosed with ADHD.

Diagnosis

Because no genetic testing is available for Sturge-Weber syndrome, all diagnoses are made through a careful physical examination and study of a person's medical history.

Port-wine stains are present at birth, and seizures may occur in early childhood. If an individual has both of these features, SWS should be suspected. A brain **MRI** or **CT scan** can often reveal a leptomeningeal angioma or brain

Key Terms

Calcification A process in which tissue becomes hardened due to calcium deposits.

Choroid A vascular membrane that covers the back of the eye between the retina and the sclera and serves to nourish the retina and absorb scattered light.

Computed tomography (CT) scan An imaging procedure that produces a three-dimensional picture of organs or structures inside the body, such as the brain.

Glaucoma An increase in the fluid eye pressure, eventually leading to damage of the optic nerve and ongoing visual loss.

Leptomeningeal angioma A swelling of the tissue or membrane surrounding the brain and spinal cord, which can enlarge with time.

Magnetic resonance imaging (MRI) A technique that employs magnetic fields and radio waves to create detailed images of internal body structures and organs, including the brain.

Port-wine stain Dark-red birthmarks seen on the skin, named after the color of the dessert wine.

Sclera The tough white membrane that forms the outer layer of the eyeball.

calcifications, as well as any other associated white matter changes.

Treatment

Treatment of seizures in SWS by anti-epileptic medications is often an effective way to control them. In the rare occasion that an aggressive seizure medication therapy is not effective, surgery may be necessary. The general goal of the surgery is to remove the portion of brain that is causing the seizures, while keeping the normal brain tissue intact. Though most patients with SWS only have brain surgery as a final attempt to treat seizures, some physicians favor earlier surgery because this may prevent some irreversible damage to the brain (caused by the angiomas).

Standard glaucoma treatment, including medications and surgery, is used to treat people with this complication. This can often reduce the amount of vision loss.

There is no specific treatment for port-wine stains. Because they contain blood vessels, it could disrupt blood flow to remove or alter the birthmarks.

Prognosis

The prognosis for people with SWS is directly related to the amount of brain involvement for the leptomeningeal angiomas. For those individuals with smaller angiomas, prognosis is relatively good, especially if they do not have severe seizures or vision problems.

Resources

BOOKS

Charkins, Hope. *Children with Facial Difference: A Parent's Guide.* Bethesda, MD: Woodbine House, 1996.

ORGANIZATIONS

The Sturge-Weber Foundation. PO Box 418, Mount Freedom, NJ 07970. (800) 627-5482 or (973) 895-4445. Fax: (973) 895-4846. swfoffice@aol.com. <http://www.sturge weber.com/>.

WEBSITES

"Sturge-Weber Syndrome." *Family Village.* <http://www. familyvillage.wisc.edu/lib_stur.htm>.

Sturge-Weber Syndrome Support Group of New Zealand. <http://www.geocities.com/HotSprings/Spa/1563/>.

Deepti Babu, MS

▌ Stuttering

Definition

Stuttering has no absolute definition that encompasses all the aspects of the disorder. In general, it is a condition in which a person trying to speak has difficulty in expressing words normally. Morphemes (actual individual sounds such as "mm" or the explosive "p") are not easily articulated. Two common symptoms of stuttering are the drawing out of the morpheme as in "mmmmmore" or the repetitious "l-l-l-look" of seemingly simple words.

Stuttering is not to be confused with another speech disorder called cluttering. Cluttering has a much more definitive cause and clearer symptoms. Its neurogenic link has been more thoroughly established, while the roots of stuttering have not. Cluttering involves a rapid speech pattern, while stuttering can take on a variety of levels of complexity.

Description

In the past, researchers and speech therapists assumed that stuttering was a developmental disorder. Increasing evidence points to a genetic cause in many patients, especially males. The results are far from clear and studies are conflicting in their data and conclusions. Many studies are focused on the fact that monozygotic (one egg) twins both seem to stutter when the disorder is present.

Key Terms

Clutter A fluency disorder where speech delivery is either abnormally fast, irregular, or both.

Stutter A speech disorder involving hesitations and involuntary repetitions of certain sounds.

Stuttering is usually identified in children. Unless the situation is extremely stressful, such as speaking in front of a large group of people, or an equally distressing condition is present, very few adults begin to stutter later in life. Stress and anxiety about the inability to easily express thoughts and words is very distressing for the child who stutters and can prolong recovery or even prevent it.

The social anxiety accompanying stuttering is one of the reasons researchers have historically cited the lack of emotional well-being or the production of high anxiety as the root cause of the disorder. While at an early age, when peer pressure and social acceptance is extraordinarily important, the lack of understanding by other children can be very difficult to overcome. At this point, stuttering does become an emotional as well as physical challenge.

Demographics

More than 1% of the population stutters. However, if every person who has, at some time, found themselves stuttering when anxious were included, the condition would be considered a great deal more common. Males are four times more likely than females to stutter. Stuttering is also more common in children than adults.

The Stuttering Foundation of America has provided facts on who is likely to stutter. They describe four of the most common factors that lead to stuttering. The first is genetics. Clinical results indicate that around 60% of those who stutter have a family member who also stutters. A second possible cause for stuttering involves developmental delays. Researchers claim that children with other speech and language problems are more likely to stutter than those who do not.

The third proposed reason for stuttering involves the physiology of the brain. With **magnetic resonance imaging (MRI)** and other such examinations, it appears that some people process speech and language in different regions of the brain than those who do not stutter. Early language acquisition occurs in the Broca's area of the brain, but this ability lasts only for a short time during childhood. After initial speech is acquired, language is learned in other regions of the brain. This may have an influence on those who stutter.

Finally, family dynamics are implicated as reasons for stuttering. Parents with high expectations and little patience may push a child to speak before he or she is ready. Without proper education, some parents may push their children to achieve certain goals by a particular age. If the goal is not, met a child may experience anxiety and it is possible this could result in stuttering.

Causes and symptoms

The actual physiological cause of stuttering is not conclusive.

Neurogenic stutterers are those people who have developed the disorder as a result of some sort of head injury or trauma. Their speech may be repetitious, prolonged, and they may even experience a mental block on certain words or phrases. However, they seem to lack the fears and anxieties of those who are designated as developmental stutterers. The severity of neurogenic stuttering is directly correlated with the degree of brain injury and degree of healing.

Diagnosis

A health professional or speech therapist trained in identifying varying speech disorders makes the diagnosis of stuttering. Stuttering must be isolated from anxious stammering, brain-related cluttering, and a variety of additional speech disorders.

Treatment team

The treatment team for a stutterer is multidisciplinary. Initially, a child's parent or teacher may identify a problem in communication and reading aloud. The pediatrician usually identifies and makes the diagnosis of stuttering as opposed to other vocal disturbances. A neurological consultation may be sought. Occurrences such as head trauma or lesions of the brain must be ruled out as a contributing factor.

Many speech and language pathologists have been trained and licensed to work with stutterers. They can provide exercises, vocal awareness, and support that the stutterer needs to begin a path to recovery. Many schools offer these types of support and are free to the students.

One of the best teams for the treatment of stuttering is the family and friends of the person who stutters. It is likely the stutterer feels embarrassment or guilt over the condition. Family and friends who take the time to understand the condition and show their patience and acceptance can help the person who stutters. Reading books about the condition and aiding in home therapies is a proven method of making the stutterer feel less shame and embarrassment. In turn, the benefits of therapy can be reached more quickly.

Treatment

Most clinicians recommend a holistic approach in which patients are allowed to find their own most useful therapy. A good rapport should exist between the speech therapist and patient.

Significantly, often when the person who stutters focuses on a related task such as singing, the individual fails to show any symptoms. When a prescribed set of words and additional distraction are employed, it appears the stutterer has fewer problems speaking clearly. Singing and rhyming are strategies used by speech therapists as confidence boosters to illustrate that the person has the ability to express language in a natural, easily flowing manner.

Recently, some electrical devices for the treatment of stuttering have come onto the market, but their success is still not well documented. The Delayed Auditory Feedback (DAF) and Frequency-Shifting Auditory Feedback (FAF) are electronic devices that pick up a voice from a microphone, delay the sound for a fraction of a second, and feed the voice back through earphones. Some clinicians claim the feedback machines can significantly reduce or eliminate stuttering.

Recovery and rehabilitation

Recovery from stuttering is unpredictable for several reasons. Many people must come to the aid of the stutterer. Family and friends, the therapist, schoolmates, and a variety of additional environmental conditions must be in place for the stutterer to gain control over the disorder. If all is in place, the chance of significant improvement is excellent.

Clinical trials

As of early 2004, the National Institute on Deafness and Other Communication Disorders and the National Institute of Neurological Diseases and Stroke were sponsoring several **clinical trials** on the nature and treatment of stuttering. Information about the studies can be found at the National Institutes of Health clinical trials website: <http://www.clinicaltrials.gov/ct/search?term=stuttering&submit=Search>.

Prognosis

The prognosis for people who stutter can be very good. The American Society of Stuttering lists some famous people who stutter and have proceeded to make careers in which their voice is an asset. The list includes James Earl Jones, Mel Tillis, Winston Churchill, Marilyn Monroe, Carly Simon, and many more celebrities who make their living by announcing, acting, or singing.

Special concerns

Many childhood stutterers are not receiving adequate treatment because of poverty or financially stretched school resources. The American Institute for Stuttering offers information on seeking financial resources for the treatment of stuttering, training of professionals to treat those who stutter, and additional information about stuttering.

Resources

BOOKS

Guitar, Barry, and Theodore Peters. *Stuttering: An Integrated Approach to Its Nature and Treatment*, 2nd ed. Philadelphia: Lippincott, Williams & Wilkins, 1998.

Kehoe, Thomas. *Multifactoral Stuttering Therapy: A Guide for Persons Who Stutter, Parents, and Speech-Language Pathologists*. Boulder, CO: Casa Futura Technologies, 2002.

Logan, Robert. *The Three Dimensions of Stuttering: Neurology, Behavior, and Emotion*. London: Whurr Publishers, 1998.

OTHER

"How to React When Speaking with Someone Who Stutters." *Stuttering Foundation of America*. April 4, 2004 (June 3, 2004). <http://206.104.238.56/brochures/br_htr.htm>.

"Stuttering." *University of Maryland Medicine*. April 4, 2004 (June 3, 2004). <http://www.umm.edu/ent/stutter.htm>.

ORGANIZATIONS

American Speech-Language-Hearing Association. 10801 Rockville Pike, Rockville, MD 20852. (301) 897-5700 or (800) 638-8255; (301) 571-0457. actioncenter@asha.org. <http://www.nsastutter.org>.

National Stuttering Association. 471 East La Palma Avenue, Suite A, Anaheim Hills, CA 92807. (714) 693-7480 or (800) 364-1677; (714) 630-7707. nsastutter@asha.org. <http://www.nsastutter.org>.

Brook Ellen Hall, PhD

Subacute sclerosing panencephalitis

Definition

Subacute sclerosing panencephalitis (SSPE) is a long-lasting (chronic) infection of the **central nervous system** that causes inflammation of the brain. The infection is caused by an altered form of the measles virus. The symptoms appear years after the initial infection, following reactivation of the latent virus.

Description

SSPE is one of three types of encephalitis that can occur following infection with the measles virus. The other forms are an acute (sudden appearance of symptoms) form that is typically associated with the rash that forms during the measles infection. The other form of SSPE affects the myelin sheath surrounding nerve cells, and is likely part of an autoimmune reaction.

SSPE develops when the measles virus, which is still present but is in an inactive (or latent) form, is reactivated. The appearance of symptoms typically leads to a disease that last from one to three years.

The disease is also known as subacute sclerosing leukencephalitis and Dawson's encephalitis.

Demographics

Children and young adults are primarily affected with SSPE. Males are also more affected than females, with a male-to-female ratio of 4:1. As well, there is a geographical component to the infection, with those in rural areas being much more susceptible (approximately 85% of cases arise in rural environments). Since the measles vaccine has been introduced, the disease has become rare in many areas of the globe, particularly the western world (about one in 1,000,000 people). Fewer than 10 cases per year occur in the United States. However, in the Middle East and India the incidence of the disease remains high (over 20 cases per 1,000,000 people).

Causes and symptoms

The disease is caused by the reactivated form of a mutated measles virus. The inactive form of the virus can be present in the body for up to 10 years following the initial bout of measles before the symptoms of SSPE develop. While normally the measles virus does not infect the brain, the mutated virus is capable of invading the brain.

When symptoms do develop, motor skills and mental faculties become progressively worse. Initial symptoms include a change in behavior, irritability, memory loss, and difficulty in forming thoughts and solving problems. Subsequently, a person can experience involuntary movements and **seizures** (also known as myoclonic spasms), loss of the ability to walk, difficulty speaking, and swallowing difficulty (dysphagia). Blindness can occur. In the final stages of the disease, a patient with SSPE may become mute and can lapse into a coma.

Monitoring the electrical activity of the brain has shown that SSPE causes disruptions that are consistent with the deterioration of the central nervous system. These changes tend to occur in stages, and so can be diagnostic of the progression of the disease. A different pattern of

Key Terms

Antibody A special protein made by the body's immune system as a defense against foreign material (bacteria, viruses, etc.) that enters the body. It is uniquely designed to attack and neutralize the specific antigen that triggered the immune response.

Encephalitis Inflammation of the brain, usually caused by a virus. The inflammation may interfere with normal brain function and may cause seizures, sleepiness, confusion, personality changes, weakness in one or more parts of the body, and even coma.

Seizure A sudden attack, spasm, or convulsion.

brain deterioration has been detected using the techniques of computed tomography and **magnetic resonance imaging**. However, this latter pattern is not yet refined enough for diagnostic use. Examination of brain tissue has shown that the disease is associated with the deterioration of the cortex and loss of white matter.

Diagnosis

SSPE is diagnosed based on the early symptoms, detection of antibodies to the measles virus, detection of protein in the spinal fluid, and the information gained from monitoring of the brain.

Treatment team

Initially, the family physician and local clinicians provide care. With the progression of the disease, specialists such as neurologists can become involved. Nurses are critical for those patients with advanced disease. Family and friends are an important source of care throughout the disease.

Treatment

There is no cure for SSPE. In the past, the primary means of treatment included therapy to curb seizures and the use of supportive measures such as feeding tubes when swallowing becomes difficult. During the 1990s, evidence accumulated in the medical literature to support the contention that SSPE can be stabilized and the progressive deterioration can be slowed by drug therapy. The drugs used lessen the damage inflicted by the immune system (immunomodulators such as the **interferons**), or attack the virus. The drugs used are an orally administered form of the antiviral drug inosine pranobex (oral isoprinosine), oral isoprinosine combined with interferon alpha or beta, and interferon alpha combined with intravenous ribavirin (another antiviral). In particular, the isoprinosine-interferon alpha combination has been reported to produce up to a 50% rate of remission or improvement in symptoms. As promising as these results are, no controlled studies have yet been performed. Therefore, the treatments are not typically used.

Recovery and rehabilitation

As SSPE is almost always fatal, emphasis is placed upon maintaining comfort, rather than rehabilitation.

Clinical trials

There were no **clinical trials** in progress or planned in the United States as of January 2004. However, organizations such as the National Institute for Neurological Diseases and Stroke undertake and fund research aimed at furthering the understanding of the causes, prevention, and treatment of subacute sclerosing panencephalitis and related diseases.

Prognosis

Without treatment, death usually occurs within one to three years following the first appearance of symptoms. Treatment with immunomodulators and **antiviral drugs** has achieved remission of the disease in some cases. As well, remission can occur spontaneously in approximately 5% of cases.

Resources

BOOKS

Icon Health Publications. *The Official Parent's Sourcebook on Subacute Sclerosing Panencephalitis: A Revised and Updated Directory for the Internet Age.* San Diego: Icon Grp. Int., 2002.

PERIODICALS

Forcic, D., M. Baricevic, R. Zgorelec, et al. "Detection and characterization of measles virus strains in cases of subacute sclerosing panencephalitis in Croatia." *Virus Research* (January 1999): 51–56.

Hayashi, M., N. Arai, J. Satoh, et al. "Neurodegenerative mechanisms in subacute sclerosing panencephalitis." *Journal of Child Neurology* (October 2002): 725–730.

OTHER

National Library of Medicine. "Subacute Sclerosing Panencephalitis." *MEDLINE plus.* <http://www.nlm.nih.gov/medlineplus/ency/article/001419.htm> (January 25, 2004).

"Subacute Sclerosing Panencephalitis Information Page." *National Institute of Neurological Disorders and Stroke.* <http://www.ninds.nih.gov/health_and_medical/disorders/subacute_panencephalitis_.htm> (January 26, 2004).

ORGANIZATIONS

National Institute for Neurological Diseases and Stroke (NINDS). 6001 Executive Boulevard, Bethesda, MD 20892. (301) 496-5751 or (800) 352-9424. <http://www.ninds.nih.gov>.

National Organization for Rare Disorders. 55 Kenosia Avenue, Danbury, CT 06813-1968. (203) 744-0100 or (800) 999-6673; Fax: (203) 798-2291. orphan@rarediseases.org. <http://www.rarediseases.org>.

Brian Douglas Hoyle, PhD

Subarachnoid hemorrhage *see* **Aneurysm**

Subcortical arteriosclerotic encephalitis *see* **Binswanger disease**

Subdural hematoma

Definition

A subdural hematoma is a pooling of blood between the dura, which is a leathery membrane just under the skull, and the brain itself. Subdural hematomas usually occur following a head trauma that breaks the blood vessels that surround the brain. The pressure of the accumulated blood on the brain can cause a variety of symptoms including problems with speech, vision, or even a loss of consciousness.

Description

The bony skull encases the brain, protecting it from external damage. Between the skull and the brain itself is a tough leathery tissue, called the dura. This dura serves two purposes, forming a second layer of protection around the brain and providing vasculation that nourishes the brain with blood and spinal fluid. During a severe blunt head trauma, the bridging blood vessels that connect the dura to the skull may tear because of shear forces to the head. The broken vessels bleed into the space between the skull and the dura. This pooling of blood puts pressure on the brain, and it swells in response. Because the skull creates a defined volume, there is no extra room for the brain to swell and therefore, parts of the brain become compressed. This usually has neurological consequences including visual problems, speech dysfunction, and loss of consciousness.

The term subdural hematoma has a variety of synonyms including SDH, subdural hemorrhage, and blood clot on the brain. Physicians may use the adjectives acute, subacute, and chronic to describe the time course and volume of blood in subdural hematomas. Acute describes subdural hematomas that gather a large amount of blood

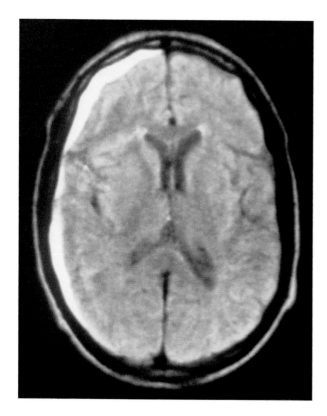

Nuclear magnetic resonance image of the head of a person suffering from a subdural hematoma. The two elongated white areas on the left side of the brain represent the blood that has been lost into the space between the brain and the skull. *(Hammersmith Hospital Medical School / Photo Researchers, Inc.)*

quickly. Subacute refers to subdural hematomas that occur between three and seven days following an injury to the head. In these patients, the blood clots will liquefy and in some cases the various cellular components of the blood clots will form layers that can be visualized using computerized tomography (**CT**). Chronic usually refers to subdural hematomas that produce symptoms two to three weeks following an injury. In these hematomas, the blood clot has become mostly blood serum. Additionally, subdural hematomas are classified as simple or complicated. About half of all cases are simple, which implies that there is no laceration or contusion in the brain. In complicated SDH, the brain has suffered some sort of traumatic injury.

Demographics

SDH can happen to anyone who experiences a head trauma. In the United States, between 15% and 30% of patients suffering from head injuries have SDH. About half of the cases of SDH are simple SDH. The other half of the cases involves other complications such as laceration of the brain, and the mortality rate is much greater in these individuals. SDH is more common in people older than 60

because their blood vessels are more fragile than those in younger people. SDH is also associated with child abuse. People with blood disorders, such as hemophiliacs, people on anticoagulants, and alcoholics, are at higher risk for developing subdural hematomas.

Causes and symptoms

Subdural hematomas are most often caused by head trauma. Rarely, they can occur spontaneously, especially in elderly persons. Often the person will lose consciousness following the trauma, but SDH can occur when the person has remained conscious. Signs indicating the presence of SDH include headaches, **dizziness**, nausea, pupil dilation, slurred speech, and weakness in the limbs. More severe symptoms include loss of consciousness, disorientation, amnesia, trouble with breathing, or even coma.

Diagnosis

Diagnosis of an acute or chronic subdural hematoma is most often accomplished by using a computerized tomography (CT) scan, which is a specialized x ray. The SDH appears as a white crescent shape that lies along the skull. In subacute SDH, the shape of the pooled blood looks more lens-like and **magnetic resonance imaging (MRI)** is recommended to distinguish it from an **epidural hematoma**.

Treatment

In many cases, small subdural hematomas may be treated with observation and a series of CT scans to ensure that the blood is reabsorbing and not becoming calcified. In more severe cases, surgical intervention is necessary. The surgeon will open the skull in a procedure known as a **craniotomy** and remove the blood clot to release the pressure on the brain. The clot is removed with suction and irrigation.

Recovery and rehabilitation

Following surgical removal of a subdural hematoma, a patient will most likely need to remain in the intensive care unit for a period of time. Diuretics to decrease swelling of the brain and **anticonvulsants** to prevent **seizures** will be administered. Some of the complications associated with surgery are swelling of the brain, infection, seizures, memory loss, **headache**, difficulty concentrating, and chronic SDH. In about 50% of the cases, a hematoma may recur following surgery.

Prognosis

The prognosis for someone who has suffered a subdural hematoma depends on the size and severity of the blood clot. Acute SDH may have very high rates of death

Succinamides

Key Terms

Craniotomy A surgical procedure in which part of the skull is removed (then replaced) to allow access to the brain.

Dura matter The strongest and outermost of three membranes that protect the brain, spinal cord, and nerves of the cauda equina.

Skull All of the bones of the head.

and long term disability. Subacute and chronic SDH usually have a better prognosis, with most symptoms abating following surgery. Mortality rates associated with simple SDH approach 20% as compared with 50% for complicated SDH. In all cases, persons who have experienced a subdural hematoma have a high risk of seizures, although this can usually be controlled with medication.

Resources

BOOKS

Greenberg, David A., et. al. *Clinical Neurology,* 5th. ed. New York: McGraw-Hill/Appleton & Lange, 2002.

OTHER

Kiriakopoulos, Elaine T. "Subdural Hematoma." *MEDLINE plus.* National Library of Medicine. <http://www.nlm.nih.gov/medlineplus/ency/article/000713.htm> (November 16, 2002).
"Subdural Hematoma." *University of Missouri Health Care.* <http://www.muhealth.org/~neuromedicine/subdural.shtml> (February 15, 2001).

ORGANIZATIONS

National Institute for Neurological Diseases and Stroke (NINDS). 6001 Executive Boulevard, Bethesda, MD 20892. (301) 496–5751 or (800) 352-9424. <http://www.ninds.nih.gov>.

Juli M. Berwald, PhD

Succinamides

Definition

Succinamides are a sub-class of **anticonvulsants**, indicated for the treatment of **seizures** associated with **epilepsy**.

Purpose

Although there is no known cure for epilepsy, succinamides are used to control and prevent absence (petit mal) seizures associated with the disorder. Succinamides

are most often used in conjunction with other anticonvulsant medications to control other types of seizures (such as other generalized tonic-clonic or grand mal seizures) as part of a comprehensive course of treatment for epilepsy and other disorders.

Description

Succinamides are sold under several names, including ethosuximide (Zarontin) and celontin. Zarontin is the only succinamide that is regularly used in the United States today, as celontin has a higher rate of side effects. Zarontin effectively controls partial seizures, but in some individuals may actually increase the likelihood of generalized seizures. It is often, therefore, prescribed in combination with other anticonvulsants to minimize the chances of generalized seizures.

Recommended dosage

Succinamides are taken orally and are available in tablet or suspension form. For the treatment of epilepsy, succinamides may be taken by both adults and children. Succinamides are prescribed by physicians in varying dosages, but typical total daily dosages range from 250mg to 1.5g.

When beginning a course of treatment that includes succinamides, most physicians recommend a gradual dose-increasing regimen. Patients typically take a reduced dose at the beginning of treatment. The prescribing physician will determine the proper initial dosage, and then will periodically raise the patient's daily dosage until seizure control is achieved.

A double dose of any succinamide should not be taken together. If a daily dose is missed, take it as soon as possible. However, if it is within four hours of the next dose, then skip the missed dose. Physicians typically direct patients to gradually taper their daily dosages when ending treatment that includes succinamides. Stopping the medicine suddenly may cause seizures to return, occur more frequently, or become more severe.

Precautions

A physician should be consulted before taking succinamides with certain non-prescription medications. Persons should avoid alcohol and CNS depressants (medicines that can make one drowsy or less alert, such as antihistimines, sleep medications, and some **pain** medications) while taking succinimides or any other anticonvulsants. They can exacerbate the side effects of alcohol and other medications. Succinamides are not habit-forming.

A course of treatment including succinamides may not be appropriate for persons with gastrointestinal disorders, **stroke**, anemia, mental illness, diabetes, high blood

Key Terms

Absence seizure A type of generalized seizure where the person may temporarily appear to be staring into space and/or have jerking or twitching muscles. Previously called a petit mal seizure.

Epilepsy A disorder associated with disturbed electrical discharges in the central nervous system that cause seizures.

Seizure A convulsion, or uncontrolled discharge of nerve cells that may spread to other cells throughout the brain, resulting in abnormal body movements or behaviors.

Tonic-clonic seizure A type of seizure involving loss of consciousness, generalized involuntary muscular contractions, and rigidity.

presure, angina (chest pain), irregular heartbeats, or other heart problems.

Succinamides may not be suitable for persons with a history of liver or kidney disease. In rare cases, succinamides may cause abnormalities in the blood and abnormal liver or kidney function. Periodic blood, kidney, and liver function tests are advised for all patients using the medicine. To check for rare blood disorders and symptoms of infection, periodic blood tests may be necessary while taking succinamides.

Before beginning treatment with succinamides, patients should notify their physician if they consume a large amount of alcohol, have a history of drug use, are pregnant, nursing, or plan on becoming pregnant. Although succinamides have not been associated with problems during pregnancy, other anticonvulsant medications may cause birth defects. Patients are often advised to use effective birth control while taking succinamides in combination with other anticonvulsants. Women who become pregnant while taking succinamides should contact their physician immediately.

Side effects

Patients should discuss with their physicians the risks and benefits of treatment including succinamides before taking the medication. Succinamides are usually well tolerated, but may case a variety of usually mild side effects. Diziness, nausea, and drowsiness are the most frequently reported side effects. Most side effects do not require medical attention, and usually diminish with continued use of the medication. Possible side effects include:

- unusual tiredness or weakness
- clumsiness
- hiccups
- loss of appetite
- nausea, vomiting, stomach cramps

If any symptoms persist or become too uncomfortable, the prescribing physician should be consulted.

Other, uncommon side effects of succinamides can be serious or could indicate an allergic reaction. Patients who experience any of the following symptoms should immediately contact a physician:

- nightmares and sleeplessness
- rash or bluish patches on skin
- persistent nosebleed
- ulcers or white spots on lips
- extreme mood or mental changes
- shakiness or unsteady walking
- severe unsteadiness or clumsiness
- speech or language problems
- difficulty breathing
- chest pain
- irregular heartbeat
- faintness or loss of consciousness
- severe cramping
- persistant, severe headaches
- persistant sore throat, fever, or pain

Interactions

Succinamides may have negative interactions with some antihistimines, antidepressants, antibiotics, and monoamine oxidase inhibitors (MAOIs). Other medications such as **Diazepam** (Valium), **phenobarbital** (Luminal, Solfoton), nefazodone, metronidazole, and certain anesthetics may react with succinamides.

Resources

BOOKS

Weaver, Donald F. *Epilepsy and Seizures: Everything You Need to Know.* Toronto: Firefly Books, 2001.

OTHER

"Ethosuximide Oral." *Medline Plus.* <http://www.nlm.nih.gov/medlineplus/druginfo/medmaster/a682327.html> (May 1, 2004).

"Zarontin." *RxMed.* <http://www.rxmed.com/b.main/b2.pharmaceutical/b2.1.monographs/CPS-%20Monographs/CPS-%20(General%20Monographs-%20Z)/ZARONTIN.html> (May 1, 2004).

American Epilepsy Society. 342 North Main Street, West Hartford, CT 06117-2507. <http://www.aesnet.org>.

Epilepsy Foundation. 4351 Garden City Drive, Landover, MD 20785-7223. (800) 332-1000. <http://www.epilepsy foundation.org>.

Adrienne Wilmoth Lerner

Sunsetting of eyes *see* **Visual disturbances**

Swallowing disorders

Definition

Swallowing disorders (also called dysphagia) are any conditions that cause impairment of the movement of solids or fluids from the mouth, down the throat, and into the stomach.

Description

Swallowing disorders are a significant source of disability. They can have a severe effect on overall calorie intake and nutritional status, and they can adversely affect an individual's enjoyment of eating and drinking and the ability to participate in related social interactions. Swallowing disorders may affect the ability to swallow liquids, solids, or both. In addition to complicating or preventing intake of liquids and solids, some swallowing disorders may make an individual susceptible to pneumonia, if any portion of the substances being swallowed are directed into the lungs.

Many conditions are associated with swallowing disorders. Any condition that interferes with one or more of the three normal phases associated with swallowing will impair an individual's swallowing ability. The three normal phases include the oral phase, the pharyngeal phase, and the esophageal phase. Oral refers to the mouth; pharyngeal refers to the pharynx (the area of the airway at the back of the mouth, and leading to the esophagus and the lungs); esophageal refers to the esophagus (the tube passageway between the mouth and the stomach).

The oral phase refers to the aspects of swallowing that rely on intact mouth functioning. The oral phase is itself divided into two phases, the oral preparatory phase and the oral transit phase. In the oral preparatory phase, solids are broken into smaller, softer bits through chewing and mixing with saliva. The resulting mass to be swallowed is referred to as the "bolus." The oral transit phase refers to the movement of the bolus to the back of the mouth, through the actions of the tongue.

The pharyngeal phase refers to the transit of the bolus into the pharynx, also called the swallowing reflex. During this phase, it is crucial that breathing cease and that the entry from the pharynx into the larynx (voice box) closes tightly, thus preventing food or fluid from entering into the lungs.

The esophageal phase refers to the transit of the bolus down the esophagus and into the stomach. The esophageal phase is guided primarily by a series of involuntary waves of muscular action, called peristalsis, that move the bolus down the esophagus towards the stomach. At the end of the esophagus is an area called the esophageal sphincter, which must relax sufficiently to allow the bolus to enter the stomach. The esophageal sphincter, however, must also quickly resume appropriate muscle tone to avoid allowing stomach contents to exit the stomach and go back up the esophagus (called reflux).

Of the three phases of swallowing, only the oral phase requires conscious input; both the pharyngeal and the esophageal phases occur outside of voluntary control. The amount of time required for the oral phase varies depending on the individual; some people eat or drink very slowly, chewing many times, while others seem to "inhale" their food. Under normal conditions, the pharyngeal phase is over in about one second, and the esophageal phase takes about three seconds. Various disorders may increase the duration (and relative success) of any of these phases.

Swallowing disorders can be caused by the following:

- mechanical obstruction at any point along the swallowing path
- problems with the nerves and muscles necessary for chewing and moving the food around the mouth
- decreased sensation, leading to inability to feel the food and organize its movement appropriately
- inability of the larynx to close tightly
- problems with coordinating breathing and its cessation
- problems with the involuntary muscle movements necessary for moving the bolus down the esophagus

These problems may occur at the actual level of functioning (for example, muscle defects) or at the level of the brain's organization of these functions.

Complications of swallowing disorders include dehydration, weight loss, malnutrition, social isolation, and aspiration pneumonia.

Causes and symptoms

A huge variety of disorders may cause problems with swallowing, including:

- progressive neurological conditions (such as **Parkinson's disease**, **multiple sclerosis**, **amyotrophic lateral sclerosis**, Huntington's **chorea**, **post-polio syndrome**, **myasthenia gravis**, muscular dystrophy)

Key Terms

Bolus   A mass of a substance to be swallowed.

Esophagus   The tube leading from the back of the mouth, down the throat, and into the stomach.

Larynx   The "voice box," located between the pharynx (upper area of the throat) and the trachea (windpipe).

Peristalsis   Waves of involuntary muscle contraction and relaxation.

Pharynx   The part of the airway that is located at the back of the throat.

- mechanical blockage of the swallowing apparatus (by tumors; abnormal tissue growth called esophageal webs or rings; abnormal outpouchings of areas of the esopahagus called Zenker's diverticula; scar tissue or strictures due to **radiation** therapy, medications, toxic or chemical exposure, ulcers, or smoke inhalation)

- damage to the brain or spinal cord (due to **cerebral palsy** or after **stroke**, **spinal cord injury**, traumatic head injury, or direct injury to any of the structures necessary for swallowing)

- certain medications (nitrates, anticholinergic agents, aspirin, calcium tablets, calcium channel blockers, iron tablets, vitamin C, tetracycline)

- congenital defects (such as cleft palate)

Symptoms of swallowing difficulties include weight loss; dehydration; sensation of having a lump in the throat after having attempted to swallow; drooling; unintentional retention of food within the mouth, despite attempts to swallow; coughing; choking; change in voice; regurgitation of liquids or solids through the nose; difficulty chewing; difficulty breathing or talking while eating, drinking, and swallowing; recurrent bouts of pneumonia.

Diagnosis

A variety of tests can diagnose dysphagia. A thorough neurological examination may reveal deficits involving the cranial nerves responsible for the strength and coordination of the muscles of swallowing. Fiberoptic endoscopy uses a narrow lighted scope to examine the mouth, pharynx, and esophagus. Videofluroscopic swallowing studies require the patient to swallow a solution containing barium; a moving x-ray machine takes images to evaluate the swallowing mechanism. Ultrasound studies can examine the tongue and larynx during swallowing. Scintigraphy involves swallowing a radioactive substance, and then examining images to see if the patient is

aspirating. Manometry is a test that measures the changes in pressure throughout the esophagus during swallowing, in order to evaluate peristalsis.

Treatment team

Neurologists, gastroenterologists, and otorhinolaryngologists may all work with patients suffering from dysphagia. Speech and language therapists are trained to evaluate and help individuals who have swallowing problems.

Treatment

Treatment ranges from simple changes in posture while eating to medications to surgical interventions.

When swallowing problems are mild, learning new eating techniques (smaller bites, more chewing) may be sufficient. Therapists can help individuals learn the most effective head and neck posture for successful swallowing. Exercises to strengthen muscles necessary for swallowing and improve coordination may be helpful. In order to improve their ease of swallowing, some people learn to avoid foods with certain textures, to thin or thicken liquids, or to avoid foods or beverages that are too hot or too cold. Medications may help improve swallowing. **Botulinum toxin** can relax spastic muscle that interfere with swallowing.

When no therapies or medications are helpful, and an individual's nutritional status is seriously compromised, alternative methods of providing nutrition (such as through a feeding or gastrostomy tube directly into the stomach) may be necessary.

Prognosis

Dysphagia can be a very serious condition. Its prognosis depends on how severe the swallowing problems are and how severely they interfere with proper nutrition, as well as on details of the underlying condition responsible for the dysphagia.

Resources

BOOKS

Cohen, Disney, and Henry P. Parkman. "Diseases of the Esophagus." In *Cecil Textbook of Internal Medicine*, edited by Lee Goldman, et al. Philadelphia: W. B. Saunders Company, 2000.

Logemann, Jeri. "Mechanisms of Normal and Abnormal Swallowing." In *Otolaryngology: Head and Neck Surgery*, edited by Charles Cummings, et al. St. Louis: Mosby-Year Book, Inc., 1998.

PERIODICALS

Lind, C. D. "Dysphagia: Evaluation and Treatment." *Gastroenterolgical Clinics of North America* 32, no. 2 (June 2003): 553–575

WEBSITES

American Academy of Otolaryngology—Head and Neck Surgery. *Doctor, I Have Trouble Swallowing.* 2002. <http://www.entnet.org/healthinfo/throat/swallowing.cfm> (June 3, 2004).

National Institute of Neurological Disorders and Stroke (NINDS). *NINDS Swallowing Disorders Information Page.* November 6, 2002. <http://www.ninds.nih.gov/health_and_medical/disorders/swallowing_disorders.htm> (June 3, 2004).

ORGANIZATIONS

American Academy of Otolaryngology—Head and Neck Surgery. One Prince St., Alexandria, VA 22314-3357. 703-836-4444. <http://www.entnet.org/healthinfo/throat/swallowing.cfm>.

Rosalyn Carson-DeWitt, MD

Sydenham's chorea

Definition

Sydenham's **chorea** is an acute but self-limited movement disorder that occurs most commonly in children between the ages of five and 15, and occasionally in pregnant women. It is closely associated with rheumatic fever following a throat infection. The disorder is named for Thomas Sydenham (1624–1689), an English doctor who first described it in 1686. Other names for Sydenham's chorea include simple chorea, chorea minor, acute chorea, rheumatic chorea, juvenile chorea, and St. Vitus' dance. The English word chorea itself comes from the Greek word *choreia*, which means "dance." The disorder takes its name from the rapid involuntary jerking or twitching movements of the patient's face, limbs, and upper body.

Description

Sydenham's chorea is best described as a neurologic complication of rheumatic fever triggered by a throat infection (pharyngitis) caused by particular strains of bacteria known as group A beta-hemolytic streptococci or as GAS bacteria. In general, streptococci are spherical-shaped anaerobic bacteria that occur in pairs or chains. GAS bacteria belong to a subcategory known as pyogenic streptococci, which means that the infections they cause produce pus.

The initial throat infection that leads to Sydenham's chorea is typically followed by a symptom-free period of one to five weeks. The patient then develops an acute case of rheumatic fever (ARF), an inflammatory disease that affects multiple organ systems and tissues of the body. In most patients, ARF is characterized by fever, arthritis in one or more joints, and carditis, or inflammation of the heart. In about 20% of patients, however, Sydenham's chorea is the only indication of ARF. Sydenham's is considered a delayed complication of rheumatic fever; it may begin as late as 12 months after the initial sore throat, and it may start only after the patient's temperature and other physical signs have returned to normal. The average time interval between the pharyngitis and the first symptoms of Sydenham's, however, is eight or nine weeks.

It is difficult to describe a typical case of Sydenham's chorea because the symptoms vary in speed of onset as well as severity. Most patients have an acute onset of the disorder, but in others, the onset is insidious, which means that the symptoms develop slowly and gradually. In some cases, the child's physical symptoms are present for four to five weeks before they become severe enough for the parents to consult a doctor. In other cases, emotional or psychiatric symptoms precede the clumsiness and involuntary muscular movements that characterize the disorder. The psychiatric symptoms that may develop in patients with Sydenham's chorea are one reason why it is sometimes categorized as a PANDAS (pediatric autoimmune neuropsychiatric disorders associated with streptococcal infections) disorder.

Demographics

Both ARF and Sydenham's chorea are relatively uncommon disorders in the United States. According to the Centers for Disease Control and Prevention (CDC), only 1–3% of people with streptococcal throat infections develop ARF; thus, the incidence of ARF in the United States is thought to be about 0.5 per 100,000 patients between five and 17 years of age.

In general, the incidence of Sydenham's chorea is lower in the developed countries than in others, largely because of the widespread use of antibiotics in these countries to treat childhood streptococcal infections in the 1960s and 1970s. In addition, the disorder appears to have been overdiagnosed in the past; whereas at one time doctors thought that as many as half of all patients with ARF developed Sydenham's, present reports estimate that about 26% of ARF patients develop chorea. On the other hand, however, there are signs that the incidence of rheumatic fever is rising again in the United States and Canada; since the late 1980s, outbreaks have been reported at military installations in California and Missouri as well as in various cities in Pennsylvania, Utah, and Ohio. It is thought that this increase is due to more virulent strains of group A streptococci.

With regard to age, the incidence of Sydenham's chorea is higher in childhood and adolescence than in

Key Terms

Anaerobic Able to grow or live in the absence of oxygen.

Antibody An immunoglobulin molecule that interacts with the specific antigen that stimulated the body to produce it.

Anticonvulsant A type of drug given to prevent seizures.

Antigen Any substance that induces the body to produce antibodies and reacts with them.

Basal ganglia (singular, ganglion) Groups of nerve cell bodies located deep within the brain that govern movement as well as emotion and certain aspects of cognition (thinking).

Carditis Inflammation of the heart tissue.

Chorea A term that is used to refer to rapid, jerky, involuntary movements of the limbs or face that characterize several different disorders of the nervous system, including chorea of pregnancy and Huntington's chorea as well as Sydenham's chorea.

Compulsion A repetitive or stereotyped act or ritual.

Hemichorea Chorea that affects only one side of the body.

Insidious Developing in a stealthy or gradual manner.

Obsession A persistent or recurrent thought, image, or impulse that is unwanted and distressing.

Pediatric Autoimmune Neuropsychiatric Disorders Associated with Streptococcal Infections (PANDAS) A group of childhood disorders associated with such streptococcal infections as scarlet fever and strep throat. Sydenham's chorea is considered a PANDAS disorder.

Pharyngitis Inflammation of the throat, accompanied by dryness and pain. Pharyngitis caused by a streptococcal infection is the usual trigger of Sydenham's chorea.

St. Vitus' dance Another name for Sydenham's chorea. St. Vitus was a fourth-century martyr who became the patron saint of dancers and actors during the Middle Ages.

Streptococcus (plural, streptococci) A genus of spherical-shaped anaerobic bacteria occurring in pairs or chains. Sydenham's chorea is considered a complication of a streptococcal throat infection.

adult life. It occurs more frequently in females than in males; the gender ratio is thought to be about two females to one male. Since the peak incidence of rheumatic fever in North America occurs in late winter and spring, Sydenham's chorea is more likely to occur in the summer and early fall. There is no evidence that the disorder selectively affects specific racial or ethnic groups.

About 20% of patients diagnosed with Sydenham's chorea experience a recurrence of the disorder, usually within two years of the first episode. Most women who develop Sydenham's during pregnancy have a history of ARF in childhood or of using birth control pills containing estrogen.

Causes and symptoms

The basic cause of Sydenham's chorea is infection with GAS bacteria, which are usually transmitted from person to person through large droplets produced by coughing or sneezing, or by direct contact. GAS bacteria can also be transmitted through contaminated food, most commonly eggs, milk, or milk products. The bacteria then invade the patient's upper respiratory tract, producing the sore throat that precedes the movement disorder.

The next stage in the development of Sydenham's chorea is an abnormal response of the patient's immune system to the streptococcal infection. Streptococcal antigens resemble nerve tissue antigens. In some people, the immune system produces antibodies against the streptococcal antigens that then cross-react against the tissues in certain regions of the brain—specifically, areas of the brain known as the basal ganglia. The basal ganglia are paired clusters of nerve cells that lie deep within the brain; they serve to regulate a person's movements, although they also play a role in governing emotions and certain aspects of thinking. **Magnetic resonance imaging (MRI)** studies of patients with Sydenham's chorea indicate that the basal ganglia are abnormally large, suggesting that they have been affected by the inflammation caused by the infection.

Some people are at greater risk of developing Sydenham's chorea. The risk factors for the disorder include:

• Living in crowded living conditions, inadequate sanitation, and malnutrition. Streptococcal infections are most common among the poor or homeless.

• Genetic factors. Some families appear to be more susceptible to ARF, although no specific genes have been identified.

• Female gender. Some researchers think there is a link between female sex hormones and susceptibility to Sydenham's, given that girls are more likely than boys to develop the disorder, particularly during puberty. In addition, women who are pregnant or have taken birth control pills containing estrogen are more likely to have recurrences of Sydenham's. The disorder is virtually unknown in sexually mature males.

PHYSICAL SYMPTOMS Although the speed of onset varies, patients with Sydenham's chorea develop rapid and purposeless involuntary motions or gestures that may involve all the muscles of the body, except those around the eyes. Most patients are affected on both sides of the body; however, about 20% have symptoms on only side of the body, a condition called hemichorea. The movements disappear during sleep, but usually become more severe when the child is tired or under stress. The patient's intentional movements such as picking up objects or writing by hand may become clumsy or uncoordinated; in addition, the muscles may become generally weak or lose their tone. In milder cases of Sydenham's, the patient may have only facial grimacing and some difficulty putting on clothes or doing other tasks that require fine coordination. In more severe cases, however, the patient's life may be disrupted by movements that affect large groups of muscles, preventing the patient from walking, going to school, or doing most daily activities.

PSYCHIATRIC SYMPTOMS As has been mentioned earlier, some children develop psychiatric symptoms associated with Sydenham's chorea before the physical symptoms appear. They may start acting unusually restless, aggressive, or hyperemotional. Behavioral or emotional disturbances that have been observed with the disorder include:

• frequent mood changes

• episodes of uncontrollable crying

• behavioral regression, that is, acting like much younger children

• mental confusion

• general irritability

• difficulty concentrating

• impulsive behavior

The most common psychiatric syndrome observed in children with Sydenham's chorea, however, is obsessive-compulsive disorder (OCD). OCD is characterized by obsessions, which are unwanted recurrent thoughts, images, or impulses, and by compulsions, which are repetitive rituals, mental acts, or behaviors. Obsessions in children often take the form of fears of intruders or harm coming to a family member. Compulsions may include such acts as counting silently, washing the hands over and over, insisting on keeping items in a specific order, checking repeatedly to make sure a door is locked, and similar behaviors.

Diagnosis

The diagnosis of Sydenham's chorea is usually based on a combination of a recent history of a streptococcal infection and the doctor's observation of the patient's involuntary movements. Unlike tics, the movements associated with chorea are not repetitive, and unlike the behavior of hyperactive children, the movements are not intentional. The recent onset of the movements rules out a diagnosis of **cerebral palsy**. If Sydenham's is suspected, the physician may ask the patient to stick out the tongue and keep it in that position, or to squeeze the doctor's hand. Many patients with Sydenham's cannot hold their mouth open and keep the tongue out for more than a second or two. Another characteristic of Sydenham's is an inability to grip with a steady pressure; when the patient squeezes the doctor's hand, the strength of the grip will increase and decrease in an erratic fashion. This characteristic is sometimes called the "milking sign."

Although imaging studies are used by researchers to study Sydenham's chorea, they are not ordinarily used by themselves to diagnose the disorder. Blood tests may show elevated levels of antibodies against streptococcal bacteria, or the patient's throat culture may be positive, but more often these tests give negative results by the time the movement disorder develops.

Once the diagnosis has been made, the doctor will evaluate the patient's heart for any indications of damage caused by rheumatic fever. This evaluation includes listening for abnormal heart sounds through a stethoscope and taking x rays to determine whether the heart is enlarged. In some cases, the doctor may order an electrocardiogram (EKG) to assess any irregularities in the patient's heartbeat.

Treatment team

In most cases, a child with Sydenham's chorea will be examined and diagnosed by a pediatrician. A child or adolescent psychiatrist may be consulted if the patient has developed symptoms of OCD. Children with heart murmurs or other signs of carditis may be referred to a pediatric cardiologist for further evaluation.

Treatment

Adequate treatment of a streptococcal throat infection with antibiotics may help to prevent an attack of ARF or Sydenham's chorea.

If the chorea has already developed, most doctors do not advise treating the involuntary movements by themselves unless they are so severe that the child is disabled or at risk of self-injury. The reason for this precaution is that some of the recommended drugs, which are known as dopamine antagonists or neuroleptics, have potentially severe side effects. Dopamine antagonists include such medications as haloperidol (Haldol), risperidone (Risperdal), and pimozide (Orap). Some doctors may prescribe an anticonvulsant (antiseizure) drug, most commonly sodium valproate (Depakene), to lower the risk of injury. If the patient does not respond to the anticonvulsant, the child may be prescribed the lowest effective dose of a neuroleptic. Some doctors may prescribe a benzodiazepine tranquilizer like **diazepam** (Valium) or lorazepam (Ativan) to control the movements. Another type of drug that appears to help some patients with Sydenham's is corticosteroids, which are given to lower the inflammation associated with ARF.

Most doctors recommend ongoing treatment with penicillin to prevent a recurrence of ARF or Sydenham's chorea, although there is some disagreement as to whether this treatment should continue for five years after an acute attack or for the rest of the patient's life. The penicillin may be given orally or by injection. Patients who cannot take penicillin may be given erythromycin or sulfadiazine.

Obsessive-compulsive disorder is treated with a combination of psychotherapy (usually cognitive behavioral therapy, or CBT) and medications (usually selective serotonin reuptake inhibitors or SSRIs).

Recovery and rehabilitation

Most patients with Sydenham's chorea recover after a period of bed rest and temporary limitation of normal activities. In most cases, the symptoms disappear gradually rather than stopping abruptly.

Clinical trials

As of early 2004, the National Institute of Mental Health (NIMH) is recruiting subjects for a study of **magnetic resonance imaging** (**MRI**) in assessing brain structure and function in patients with childhood-onset psychiatric disorders. Sydenham's chorea, as well as other PANDAS disorders, is one of the conditions included in the study.

Prognosis

Sydenham's chorea is a self-limiting disorder that usually runs its course within one to six months, although it occasionally lasts as long as one to two years. In most cases, the patient recovers completely, although the disorder may recur. In a very few cases—about 1.5% of patients diagnosed with Sydenham's—there may be increasing muscle stiffness and loss of muscle tone resulting in disability. This condition is occasionally referred to as paralytic chorea.

Special concerns

Many doctors recommend that children with Sydenham's chorea should not be kept out of school longer than is necessary. Some of the psychological side effects that were once thought to be caused by the chorea itself are now regarded as the result of missing school combined with worry about other people's reactions to the involuntary movements.

Resources

BOOKS

American Psychiatric Association. *Diagnostic and Statistical Manual of Mental Disorders*, 4th edition, text revision. Washington, DC: American Psychiatric Association, 2000.

Martin, John H. *Neuroanatomy: Text and Atlas*, 3rd ed. New York: McGraw-Hill, 2003.

"Sydenham's Chorea (Chorea Minor; Rheumatic Fever; St. Vitus' Dance)." Section 19, Chapter 271 in *The Merck Manual of Diagnosis and Therapy*, edited by Mark H. Beers, MD, and Robert Berkow, MD. Whitehouse Station, NJ: Merck Research Laboratories, 2002.

PERIODICALS

Arnold, P. D., and M. A. Richter. "Is Obsessive-Compulsive Disorder an Autoimmune Disease?" *Canadian Medical Association Journal/Journal de l'association médicale canadienne* 165 (November 13, 2001): 1353–1358.

Bonthius, D. J., and B. Karacay. "Sydenham's Chorea: Not Gone and Not Forgotten." *Seminars in Pediatric Neurology* 10 (March 2003): 11–19.

Cardoso, F., D. Maia, M. C. Cunningham, and G. Valenca. "Treatment of Sydenham Chorea with Corticosteroids." *Movement Disorders* 18 (November 2003): 1374–1377.

Caviness, John M., MD. "Primary Care Guide to Myoclonus and Chorea." *Postgraduate Medicine* 108 (October 2000): 163–172.

Church, A. J., F. Cardoso, R. C. Dale, et al. "Anti-Basal Ganglia Antibodies in Acute and Persistent Sydenham's Chorea." *Neurology* 59 (July 23, 2002): 227–231.

Herrera, Maria Alejandra, MD, and Nestor Galvez-Jiminez, MD. "Chorea in Adults." *eMedicine* 1 February 2002 (April 27, 2004). <http://www.emedicine.com/neuro/topic62.htm>.

Snider, L. A., and S. E. Swedo. "Post-Streptococcal Autoimmune Disorders of the Central Nervous System." *Current Opinion in Neurology* 16 (June 2003): 359–365.

OTHER

American Academy of Child and Adolescent Psychiatry (AACAP). AACAP Facts for Families, No. 60. *Obsessive-Compulsive Disorder in Children and Adolescents*. (April 27, 2004). <http://www.aacap.org/publications/factsfam/ocd.htm>.

National Institute of Neurological Disorders and Stroke (NINDS). *NINDS Sydenham Chorea Information Page*. (April 27, 2004). <http://www.ninds.nih.gov/health_and_medical/disorders/sydenham.htm>.

American Academy of Child and Adolescent Psychiatry (AACAP). 3615 Wisconsin Avenue NW, Washington, DC 20016-3007. (202) 966-7300; Fax: (202) 966-2891. <http://www.aacap.org>.

National Institute of Neurological Disorders and Stroke (NINDS). 9000 Rockville Pike, Bethesda, MD 20892. (301) 496-5751 or (800) 352-9424. <http://www.ninds.nih.gov>.

National Organization for Rare Disorders (NORD). P. O. Box 1968, Danbury, CT 06813-1968. (203) 744-0100 or (800) 999-NORD; Fax: (203) 798-2291. orphan@rarediseases.org. <http://www.rarediseases.org>.

WE MOVE—Worldwide Education and Awareness for Movement Disorders. 204 West 84th Street, New York, NY 10024. (212) 875-8389 or (800) 437-MOV2. wemove@wemove.org. <http://www.wemove.org>.

Rebecca J. Frey, PhD

Syncope *see* **Fainting**

Syphilitic spinal sclerosis *see* **Tabes dorsalis**

Syringomyelia

Definition

The term syringomyelia refers to a collection of differing conditions characterized by damage to the spinal cord that is caused by a formation of abnormal fluid-filled cavities (syrinx) within the cord. In 1827, French physician Charles-Prosper Ollivier d'Angers (1796–1845) suggested the term syringomyelia after the Greek *syrinx*, meaning pipe or tube, and *myelos*, meaning marrow. Later, the term **hydromyelia** was used to indicate a dilatation of the central canal, and syringomyelia referred to cystic cavities separate from the central spinal canal.

Description

The cavities may be a result of **spinal cord injury**, tumors of the spinal cord, or congenital defects. An idiopathic form of syringomyelia (a form of the disorder without known cause) is also described in medical literature. The fluid-filled cavity, or syrinx, expands slowly and elongates over time, causing progressive damage to the nerve centers of the spinal cord due to the pressure exerted by the fluid. This damage results in **pain**, weakness, and stiffness in the back, shoulders, arms, or legs. People with syringomyelia experience different combinations of symptoms. In many cases, the disorder is related to abnormal lesions of the foramen magnum, the opening in the occipital

bone that houses the lower portion of the medulla oblongata, the structure that links the brain and spinal cord. An additional cause of syringomyelia involves a Chiari malformation, a condition in which excess cerebral matter extends downward towards the medulla oblongata, crowding the outlet to the spinal canal. Some familial cases of syringomyelia have been observed, although this is rare. Types of syringomyelia include:

• syringomyelia with fourth ventricle communication

• syringomyelia due to blockage of cerebrospinal fluid (CSF) circulation (without fourth ventricular communication)

• syringomyelia due to spinal cord injury

• syringomyelia and spinal dysraphism (incomplete closure of the neural tube)

• syringomyelia due to intramedullary tumors

• idiopathic syringomyelia

Demographics

Syringomyelia occurs in approximately eight of every 100,000 individuals. The onset is most commonly observed between ages 25 to 40. Rarely, syringomyelia may develop in childhood or late adulthood. Males are affected with the condition more often than females. No geographic difference in the prevalence of syringomyelia is known, and the occurrence of syringomyelia in different races is also unknown. Familial cases have been described.

Causes and symptoms

Most people with syringomyelia experience **headaches**, along with intermittent pain in the arms or legs, usually more severe on one side of the body. The pain may begin as dull or achy and slowly increases, or may occur suddenly, often as a result of coughing or straining. Pain in the extremities frequently becomes chronic. Additionally, numbness and tingling in the arm, chest, or back is often reported. The inability to feel the ground under the foot, or tingling in the legs and feet is also frequently experienced. Weakness of an extremity, leading to clumsiness in grasping objects or difficulty walking may also occur in individuals with syringomyelia. Eventually, functional use of the limb may be lost.

The cause of syringomyelia remains unknown. Not a single clear theory at the present can properly explain the basic mechanisms of cyst formation and enlargement. One theory proposes that syringomyelia results from pulsating CSF pressure between the fourth ventricle of the brain and the central canal of the spinal cord. Another theory suggests that syrinx development, particularly in people with Chiari

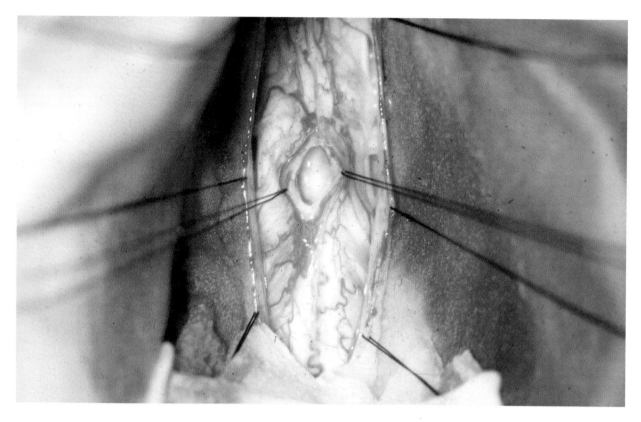

A spinal cord cyst associated with syringomyelia. *(Custom Medical Stock Photo. All Rights Reserved.)*

malformation, occurs after a difference in intracranial pressure and spinal pressure. A third theory contends that syrinx formation is caused by the cerebellar tonsils acting as a piston to produce large pressure waves in the spinal subarachnoid space, and this action forces fluid through the surface of the spinal cord into the central canal. Syringomyelia usually progresses slowly; the course may extend over many years. Infrequently, the condition may have a more acute course, especially when the brainstem is affected.

Diagnosis

Examination by a **neurologist** may reveal loss of sensation or movement caused by compression of the spinal cord. Diagnosis is usually reached by **magnetic resonance imaging (MRI)** of the spine, which can confirm syringomyelia and determine the exact location and extent of damage to the spinal cord. The most common place for a syrinx to develop is in the cervical spine (neck), with the second most common in the thoracic spine (chest and rib areas). The least likely place for a syrinx is in the lumbar spine (lower back). MRI of the head can be useful to determine the presence of any additional lesions present, as well as the presence of **hydrocephalus** (excess CSF in the ventricles of the brain). As the syrinx grows in size, it may

cause scoliosis (abnormal curvature of the spine), which is best determined by x ray of the spine.

Treatment team

Diagnosis and treatment of syringomyelia require specialized physicians, including neurologists, radiologists, neurosurgeons, and orthopedists, along with specialized nurses. Physical therapy is often useful to maximize muscular function and assist with gait (walking).

Treatment

Treatment, usually surgery, is aimed at stopping the progression of spinal cord damage and maximizing functioning. Surgical procedures are often performed if there is an identifiable mass compressing the spinal cord. Additional surgical options to minimize the syrinx include correction of spinal deformities and various CSF-shunting procedures. Fetal spinal cord tissue implantation has recently been used in an attempt to obliterate syrinx. Surgery results in stabilization or modest improvement in symptoms for most patients. Many physicians advocate surgical treatment only for patients with progressive neurological deterioration or pain. Delay in treatment when the condition is progressive may

Key Terms

Cerebrospinal fluid (CSF) The clear fluid that circulates through the brain and spinal cord.

Medulla oblongata The lower part of the brain stem that borders the spinal cord and regulates breathing, heartbeat, and blood flow.

Syrinx Abnormal fluid-filled cavities within the spinal cord.

result in irreversible spinal cord injury, and post-traumatic syringomyelia remains difficult to manage.

Medications (vasoconstrictors) are often prescribed to help reduce fluid formation around the spinal cord. Avoiding vigorous activity that increases venous pressure is often recommended. Certain exercises such as bending the trunk so the chest rests on the thighs may reduce the risk of syrinx expansion. People with progressive symptoms of syringomyelia, whether or not surgically treated, usually are monitored by their physician and have MRI scans completed every six to 12 months.

Recovery and rehabilitation

Despite reports of neurological recovery following surgery, most people achieve stabilization or only mild improvement in symptoms. Syringomyelia in children has a much lower incidence of sensory disturbance and pain than occurs with adolescents and adults, and is associated with a high incidence of scoliosis that is more favorable to surgical treatment. Additionally, all cases of syringomyelia do not progress at the same rate. Some people, usually with milder symptoms, experience stabilization in their symptoms for a period of years. A frequent complication of symptom progression is the person's ongoing need to adjust to evolving functional losses that accompany syringomyelia. These adjustments may result in loss of independence and loss of personal privacy. Rehabilitation may focus on maintaining functionality for as long as practically possible with the use of exercises and adaptive equipment, or, especially in the case of children, may focus on recovery from scoliosis caused by the syringomyelia.

Clinical trials

As of February 2004, the National Institute of Neurological Disorders and Stroke (NINDS) was sponsoring three trials for the study of syringomyelia, including the physiology of syringomyelia, study and surgical reatment of syringomyelia, and genetic analysis of the Chiari I malformation.

Prognosis

The prognosis for persons with syringomyelia depends on the underlying cause of the syrinx and on the type of treatment. Untreated syringomyelia is compatible with long-term survival without progression in 35–50% of cases. In patients treated by shunting for syringomyelia due to spinal cord injury, long-lasting pain relief and improved strength are usually observed. Recent studies have revealed an unsatisfactory long-term prognosis due to high rates of syrinx recurrence in other forms of syringomyelia. Surgery (posterior fossa decompression) in syringomyelia associated with a Chiari malformation is described as a surgically safe procedure with a considerable chance of clinical improvement. In pediatric syringomyelia, surgery is effective in improving or stabilizing scoliosis.

Resources

BOOKS

Anson, John A., Edward C. Benzel, and Issam A. Awad. *Syringomyelia & the Chiari Malformation.* Rolling Hills, IL: American Association of Neurological Surgeons, 1997.

Icon Health Publications Staff. *The Official Patient's Sourcebook on Syringomyelia: A Revised and Updated Directory for the Internet Age.* San Diego: Icon Group International, 2002.

Klekamp, Joerg. *Syringomyelia: Diagnosis & Treatment* New York: Springer-Verlag, 2001.

PERIODICALS

Brodbelt, A. R., and M. A. Stoodley. "Post-traumatic Syringomyelia: A Review." *J Clin Neurosci.* 10, no. 4 (July 2003): 401–408.

Todor, D. R., T. M. Harrison, and T. H. Milhorat. "Pain and Syringomyelia: A Review." *Neurosurg Focus* 8, no. 3 (2000): 1–6.

OTHER

"Syringomyelia Fact Sheet." *National Institute of Neurological Disorders and Stroke.* February 10, 2004 (April 4, 2004). <http://www.ninds.nih.gov/health_and_medical/pubs/syringomyelia.htm>.

ORGANIZATIONS

American Syringomyelia Alliance Project (ASAP). P.O. Box 1586, Longview, TX 75606-1586. (903) 236-7079 or (800) ASAP-282 (272-7282); Fax: (903) 757-7456. info@asap.org. <http://www.asap.org>.

National Institute for Neurological Disorders and Stroke. P.O. Box 5801, Bethesda, MD 20824. (301) 496-5761 or (800) 352-9424. <http://www.ninds.nih.gov>.

Antonio Farina, MD, PhD

Systemic lupus erythematosus *see* **Lupus**

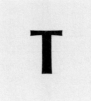

Tabes dorsalis

Definition

Tabes dorsalis is a late manifestation of untreated syphilis and is characterized by a triad of clinical symptoms namely gait unsteadiness, lightning pains and urinary incontinence. It occurs due to a slow and progressive degeneration of nerve cells and fibers in spinal cord. It is one of the forms of tertiary syphilis or neurosyphilis.

Description

The first description of the disorder was given by a French **neurologist**, Guillame Duchenne in 1858 who called it *l'ataxie locomotrice progressive* (progressive locomotor **ataxia**). But the word tabes dorsalis was coined in 1836 even before the actual cause was discovered. *Tabes* in Latin means "decay" or "shriveling"; *dorsalis* means "of the back." These indicate the location and type of damage occurring in the spinal cord. It is also called "spinal syphilis" or "syphilitic myelopathy."

Syphilis was widespread in the early part of the twentieth century but there has been a ten-fold decrease in incidence since then due to better screening measures and effective antibiotic therapy. Therefore classic, full blown forms of tabes dorsalis are seldom seen in the twenty-first century.

Demographics

The Center for Disease Control (CDC) reports the annual incidence of syphilis and from this, an estimate of the number of tabes dorsalis cases can be made. In 2001, there was around 2.2 per 100,000 population, or 7,000 new cases of syphilis reported. Three to seven percent of untreated patients develop neurosyphilis, of whom about 5% develop tabes dorsalis. Normally, fifteen or twenty years elapse after the initial syphilis infection, but this is shortened in patients with **AIDS**. Tabes dorsalis is more common in middle-aged males, homosexuals and inner city population in New York, San Francisco and the southern part of the United States.

Causes and symptoms

Syphilis is a sexually transmitted disease caused by a bacteria named *Treponema pallidum*. During initial infection, the bacteria spread through the blood stream into remote sites like the brain and spinal cord, but remain silent in these areas. If proper treatment is not instituted, neurological disorders arise about a decade later and is called neurosyphilis. Damage to the spinal cord substance due to syphilis is called tabes dorsalis.

Inflammation occurs in the dorsal columns of the spinal cord. These columns are in the portion of the spinal cord closest to the back and have nerve fibers that carry sensory information like deep **pain** and position sense (proprioception) from the legs and arms to the brain. As a result of this, the nerve fibers lose their insulation and start atrophying. The pathological process starts in the lowermost portion of the spinal cord that receives information from the legs and spreads upwards. The inflammation can also involve other nerves that control vision, hearing, eye movements, bladder and bowel.

In the twenty-first century, mostly atypical cases of tabes dorsalis are seen due to previous partial antibiotic treatment. Much of the description of the classic disease comes from scientific articles and patient reports more than fifty years ago. The earliest and probably the most troublesome symptom is pain. This is often described as "stabbing" or "lightning-like" and is quite intense. It appears very suddenly, usually in the legs, spreads rapidly to other parts of the body and then disappears quickly. Unfortunately, this cycle can repeat itself several times a day and for days together, making the patient's life miserable. They also experience uncomfortable abnormal sensations or "paresthesias," like tingling, burning, or coldness. Later the feet become progressively numb. "Visceral crisis" develops either spontaneously or after stress in about 15% of patients due to autonomic nerve dysfunction. These episodes are frightening and severe but rarely life threatening. They consist of excruciating abdominal pain and vomiting or vocal cord spasm or burning rectal pain.

A characteristic unsteady gait called "sensory ataxia" develops. Due to degeneration of nerves that carry position sense from the legs, patients are unable to judge the position of their feet in relation to the ground while walking. They become very unsteady especially while walking in a straight line, on uneven surfaces, or while turning suddenly. This becomes dramatically accentuated in the dark or while closing the eyes as visual compensation is removed. A person with tabes dorsalis walks stooped forward with a wide based "high-stepping" gait and eyes glued to the ground in order to prevent falling. With progression of the disease, they become unable to walk although muscle strength is intact.

Visual symptoms are quite common and include double vision, blurred vision, narrowed field of vision and finally blindness. The pupils are characteristically small and non-reactive to light and called "Argyll-Robertson" pupils. Urine overflow incontinence is very common as the bladder loses its muscular tone. Constipation, impotence, deafness, painless foot ulcers and painless hip and knee arthritis are other features. Decreased memory, disorientation, personality changes and sometimes frank psychiatric illness can also occur.

Diagnosis

Diagnosis is mainly clinical. Syphilis has often been called "the great mimicker" and requires an astute physician to diagnose. There are three steps in diagnosis.

First, the physician has to suspect the diagnosis. The classic signs seen in tabes dorsalis are a triad of 3A's; Argyll-Robertson pupil, areflexia (absent tendon reflexes), and ataxia. Poor visual acuity, asymmetrical eye movement, deafness, clumsy hand and leg movements are other tell-tale signs.

Secondly, it has to be differentiated from other disorders that can present similarly. This is done with the help of **CT scans**, **MRI** scans, spinal tap and certain screening blood tests. The most common screening blood test is called the Venereal Disease Research Laboratory (VDRL) test. This measures the level of certain antibodies that are elevated in the blood in syphilis. It reflects disease activity and therefore may be falsely negative in very late "burnt out" cases of tabes. On the other hand, it maybe falsely elevated in a host of other medical conditions. Therefore, it is a sensitive but not a very specific test. It is only a screening test and any positive result has to be confirmed with other blood tests. The cerebrospinal fluid (CSF) circulates around the brain and spinal cord and reflects underlying inflammation. In tabes, the white cell count and protein level in the CSF are elevated. A positive VDRL test in the CSF is a definitive diagnostic test for tabes dorsalis.

Thirdly, confirmatory tests should be done on the spinal fluid and blood. There are two confirmatory tests for syphilis, namely the Fluorescent Treponemal Antibody Absorption (FTA-ABS) and Micro Hemagglutination of Treponema Pallidum (MHA-TP). These detect very specific antibodies in the blood that are present when the person has syphilis and not otherwise. FTA-ABS in the CSF is a very sensitive test and a negative result virtually rules out tabes dorsalis. It is mandatory that all patients with syphilis undergo testing for HIV.

Elevated white cells and protein in the CSF with a positive CSF VDRL test in a person with appropriate clinical findings is diagnostic for tabes dorsalis.

Treatment team

The team consists of a neurologist, an internist, an infectious disease specialist, psychiatrist and sometimes a pain management specialist. They will closely interact with physical therapists and occupational therapists.

Treatment

Treatment is aimed at curing the infection and hopefully halting the progression of neurologic damage. Treatment is unfortunately limited in reversing the damage already done and the degree of recovery depends on the extent of damage when therapy is started. Appropriate treatment however does reduce future nerve damage, reduces symptoms and normalizes the CSF abnormalities.

The CDC of the United States Department of Health and Human Services has extensive guidelines for treatment of tabes. It recommends antibiotic treatment with intravenous aqueous crystalline penicillin G for two weeks. If the patient has penicillin allergy, he should be desensitized first before treatment. Otherwise, the antibiotic Ceftriaxone can be used as an alternative but the adequacy of this has not been fully approved by the CDC. Serum VDRL titers are checked every three months till they start declining. CSF is checked at six and twelve months and if still abnormal, rechecked at two years. Re-treatment is recommended if neurological damage progresses, if CSF white cell count does not normalize in six months, VDRL titers do not decline or show a four-fold increase and if the first course of treatment was suboptimal. Symptomatic analgesic treatment is given for pain. This can range from simple over the counter medications like aspirin or Tylenol or more potent analgesics like narcotics. Certain anti-seizure medications like Phenytoin, **Carbamazepine** and Valproic acid are efficacious in treating resistant pain. If

Key Terms

AIDS Acquired Immune Deficiency Syndrome is a sexually transmitted disease caused by the Human Immunodeficiency Virus (HIV). It weakens the immune system and makes a person susceptible to many infections and malignancies.

Ataxia Clumsiness or loss of co-ordination of the arms and legs due a variety of causes. It is a symptom of an underlying disease process of the nervous system.

Cerebrospinal fluid This is a colorless fluid that is produced in the brain and circulates around the brain and spinal cord in the subarachnoid space.

Dementia This denotes a chronic condition where there is loss of mental capacity due to an underlying organic cause. It may involve progressive deterioration of thinking, memory, behavior and personality.

Dorsal columns This refers to nerve fiber tracts that run in the portion of the spinal cord that is closest to the back. It carries sensory information like position sense and deep pain from the legs and arms to the brain.

Locomotor Means of or pertaining to movement or locomotion.

Myelopathy Disease of the spinal cord.

Neurosyphilis This is slowly progressive destruction of the brain and spinal cord due to untreated tertiary syphilis. It can be asymptomatic or cause different disorders like tabes dorsalis, general paresis and meningovascular syphilis.

Paresthesia Abnormal sensation of the body like numbness or prickling.

Proprioception The ability to sense the location and postion and orientation and movement of the body and its parts.

Syphilis Sexually transmitted disease caused by a corkscrew shaped bacterium called Treponema pallidum. It is characterized by three clinical stages namely primary, secondary and tertiary or late syphilis.

Tendon reflex This is a simple circuit that consists of a stimulus like a sharp tap delivered to a tendon and the response is one of the appropriate muscle contraction. It is used to test the integrity of the nervous system.

Spinal cord The part of the central nervous system that extends from the base of the skull and runs through the vertebral column in the back. It acts as a relay to convey information between the brain and the periphery.

patients become demented and have behavioral issues, anti-psychotic medications can be given.

Primary and secondary prevention of syphilis is important to prevent development of tabes dorsalis. Safe sex (using a condom) is a way of primary prevention. Screening, detection and treatment of early syphilis are measures of secondary prevention. Sexually active people should consult a physician about any rash or sore in the genital area. Those who have been treated for another sexually transmitted infection like gonorrhea, should be tested for syphilis and HIV. Persons who have been exposed sexually to another person who has syphilis of any stage should be clinically evaluated, undergo testing and even be presumptively treated in certain instances.

Recovery and rehabilitation

Assistance or supervision may be needed for self-care activities like eating, showering, dressing etc. Patients may require assistive devices like a cane, walker or a wheelchair to overcome gait difficulty. Diapers or urinary catheters are used for urinary incontinence. Surgery can help replace joints destroyed by arthritis. Patients need a good bowel regimen to avoid constipation, which can trigger a visceral crisis. Since this is a chronic illness, **respite** care should be provided for the caregivers.

Clinical trials

There is no trial open for tabes dorsalis, but there is an ongoing phase III multicenter randomized trial as of early 2004 funded by the National Institute of Allergy and Infectious Diseases (NIAID) for assessing the antibiotic Azithromycin given orally in treatment of primary, secondary or early latent syphilis. The NIAID and the National Institute of Neurological Diseases and Stroke (NINDS) are carrying out research to develop a non-invasive test for detecting syphilis and to develop a vaccine. The genome of *Treponema pallidum* has been sequenced through NIAID-funded research. This is a wealth of information that will hopefully lead to clues to better diagnose, treat and vaccinate against syphilis.

Prognosis

Tabes dorsalis is a chronic, annoying and incapacitating disease but is *per se* seldom fatal. If tabes dorsalis is diagnosed in its very early stages, fairly good recovery is possible. Pain is quite bothersome and has a serious impact on quality of life. Ataxia, **dementia** and blindness are incapacitating. Death usually occurs due to rupture of enlarged blood vessels and damage to heart valves, which occur as a part of tertiary syphilis. Rarely, a urinary infection will lead to sepsis and death.

Special concerns

Tabes dorsalis can affect thinking and memory and all patients must have **neuropsychological testing** for dementia. They will need to get legal advice for estate and financial planning and their wishes for future medical care.

Resources

BOOKS

Aminoff, Michael J., ed. *Neurology and General Medicine*, 3rd ed. New York: Churchill Livingstone, 2001.

Rowland, Lewis P., ed. *Merritt's Neurology*, 10th ed. Philadelphia: Lippincott Williams & Wilkins, 2000.

Victor, Maurice, and Allan H. Ropper, eds. *Principles of Neurology*, 7th ed. New York: McGraw-Hill, 2001.

PERIODICALS

Birnbaum, N. R., R. H. Goldschmidt, and W. O. Buffet. "Resolving the Common Clinical Dilemmas of Syphilis." *American Family Physician* 59 (April 1999): 2233–2240.

Estanislao, L. B, and A. R. Pachner. "Spirochetal Infection of the Nervous System." *Neurologic Clinics* 17 (November 1999): 783–800.

Golden, R. M., M. M. Christina, and K. K. Holmes. "Update on Syphilis: Resurgence of an Old Problem." *Journal of American Medical Association* 290 (September 2003): 1510–1514.

WEBSITES

Clinical Trials Website. <http://www.clinicaltrials.gov/>.

ORGANIZATIONS

Centers for Disease Control and Prevention. 1600 Clifton Road, Atlanta, GA 30333. (800) 232-3228. <http://www.cdc.gov>.

National Institute of Allergy and Infectious Diseases. 31 Center Drive, MSC 2520, Bethesda, MD 20892-2520. (301) 496-5717. <http://www.niaid.nih.gov>.

Chitra Venkatasubramanian, MBBS, MD

Tacrine *see* **Cholinesterase inhibitors**

Tarlov cysts *see* **Perineural cysts**

Tay-Sachs disease

Definition

Tay-Sachs disease is a genetic disorder caused by a missing enzyme that results in the accumulation of a fatty substance in the nervous system. This results in disability and death.

Description

Gangliosides are a fatty substance necessary for the proper development of the brain and nerve cells (nervous system). Under normal conditions, gangliosides are continuously broken down, so that an appropriate balance is maintained. In Tay-Sachs disease, the enzyme necessary for removing excess gangliosides is missing. This allows gangliosides to accumulate throughout the brain, and is responsible for the disability associated with the disease.

Tay-Sachs disease is particularly common among Jewish people of Eastern European and Russian (Ashkenazi) origin. About one out of every 3,600 babies born to Ashkenazi Jewish couples will have the disease. Tay-Sachs is also more common among certain French-Canadian and Cajun French families.

Causes and symptoms

Tay-Sachs is caused by a defective gene. Genes are located on chromosomes, and serve to direct specific development/processes within the body. The genetic defect in Tay-Sachs disease results in the lack of an enzyme, called hexosaminidase A. Without this enzyme, gangliosides cannot be degraded. They build up within the brain, interfering with nerve functioning. Because it is a recessive disorder, only people who receive two defective genes (one from the mother and one from the father) will actually have the disease. People who have only one defective gene and one normal gene are called carriers. They carry the defective gene and thus the possibility of passing the gene and/or the disease onto their offspring.

When a carrier and a non-carrier have children, none of their children will actually have Tay-Sachs. It is likely that 50% of their children will be carriers themselves. When two carriers have children, their children have a 25% chance of having normal genes, a 50% chance of being carriers of the defective genne, and a 25% chance of having two defective genes. The two defective genes cause the disease itself.

Classic Tay-Sachs disease strikes infants around the age of six months. Up until this age, the baby will appear to be developing normally. When Tay-Sachs begins to show itself, the baby will stop interacting with other people, and develop a staring gaze. Normal levels of noise will

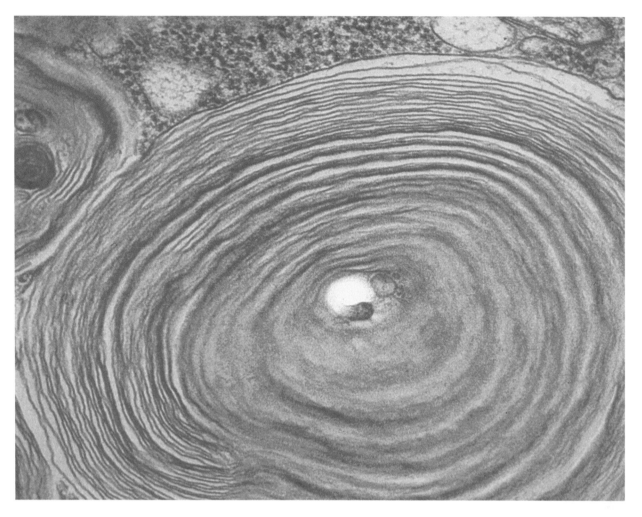

Scanning electron micrograph of cerebromacular degeneration as result of Tay-Sachs disease. *(Graph/Custom Medical Stock Photo. Reproduced by permission.)*

startle the baby to an abnormal degree. By about one year of age, the baby will have very weak, floppy muscles, and may be completely blind. The head will be quite large. Patients also present with loss of peripheral (side) vision, inability to breath and swallow, and paralysis as the disorder progresses. Seizures become a problem between ages one and two, and the baby usually dies by about age four.

A few variations from this classical progression of Tay-Sachs disease are possible:

• Juvenile hexosaminidase A deficiency. Symptoms appear between ages two and five; the disease progresses more slowly, with death by about 15 years.

• Chronic hexosaminidase A deficiency. Symptoms may begin around age five, or may not occur until age 20-30. The disease is milder. Speech becomes slurred. The individual may have difficulty walking due to weakness,

Key Terms

Ganglioside A fatty (lipid) substance found within the brain and nerve cells.

muscle cramps, and decreased coordination of movements. Some individuals develop mental illness. Many have changes in intellect, hearing, or vision.

Diagnosis

Examination of the eyes of a child with Tay-Sachs disease will reveal a very characteristic cherry-red spot at the back of the eye (in an area called the retina). Tests to determine the presence and quantity of hexosaminidase A can be performed on the blood, specially treated skin cells, or white blood cells. A carrier will have about half of the normal level of hexosaminidase A present, while a patient with the disease will have none.

Treatment

There is no treatment for Tay-Sachs disease.

Prognosis

Sadly, the prognosis for a child with classic Tay-Sachs disease is certain death. Because the chronic form of Tay-Sachs has been discovered recently, prognosis for this type of the disease is not completely known.

Prevention

Prevention involves identifying carriers of the disease and providing them with appropriate information concerning the chance of their offspring having Tay-Sachs disease. When the levels of hexosaminidase A are half the normal level a person is a carrier of the defective gene. Blood tests of carriers reveals reduction of Hexosaminidase A.

When a woman is already pregnant, tests can be performed on either the cells of the baby (amniocentesis) or the placenta (chorionic villus sampling) to determine whether the baby will have Tay-Sachs disease.

Resources

BOOKS

Behrman, Richard, ed. *Nelson Textbook of Pediatrics.* Philadelphia: W. B. Saunders, 1996.

PERIODICALS

Motulsky, Arno G. "Screening for Genetic Disease." *New England Journal of Medicine,* 336, no. 18 (May 1, 1997): 1314+.

Rosebush, Patricia I. "Late-Onset Tay-Sachs Disease Presenting as Catatonic Schizophrenia: Diagnostic and Treatment Issues." *Journal of the American Medical Association* 274, no. 22 (December 13, 1995): 1744.

ORGANIZATIONS

Late Onset Tay-Sachs Foundation. 1303 Paper Mill Road, Erdenheim, PA 19038. (800) 672-2022.

March of Dimes Birth Defects Foundation. National Office. 1275 Mamaroneck Avenue, White Plains, NY 10605. (888) 663-4637. resourcecenter@modimes.org. <http://www.modimes.org>.

National Tay-Sachs and Allied Diseases Association, Inc. 2001 Beacon Street, Suite 204, Brighton, MA 02146. (800) 906-8723. Fax: 617-277-0134. NTSAD-Boston@worldnet.att.net. <http://www.ntsad.org>.

Laith Farid Gulli, MD

Temporal arteritis

Definition

Temporal arteritis is a disease that causes inflammation and sometimes blockage of medium and large arteries in the head (often near the side of the head or temples).

Description

The mechanism responsible for temporal arteritis (also called giant cell arteritis) is complex and can affect medium and large size arteries, but commonly strikes the temporal artery causing temporal located **headaches**. In affected arteries there is an abnormal reaction that causes the infiltration of immune cells, such as lymphocytes, multinucleated giant cells, and plasma cells. Frequently the arteries in the head and neck are involved, but vasopathy can extend to the carotids and aorta. The abnormal mechanism is a cell-mediated immune response that is abnormally directed on an antigen (a foreign protein) near the elastic tissue component of an arterial wall. This immune response causes an infiltration of immune cells in an artery which could damage or even completely block the affected blood vessel. The exact cause of temporal arteritis (TA) is unknown. TA can be serious in cases where there is involvement of blood vessels that supply blood to the affected eye (i.e., posterior ciliary artery a branch of the ophthalmic artery) which can cause visual impairment.

Demographics

The disorder is more commonly observed in persons older than 50 years. TA occurs frequently with the occurrence ranging from 10 in 100,000 to 50 in 100,000. Internationally, there seems to be a higher incidence in countries higher in northern climates. The disorder occurs more frequently in Caucasian persons of northern European descent. TA rarely occurs in Blacks and Asians and it is four to six times more frequent in women than men. The mean age of onset is 70 years and the disorder is rarely seen in persons younger than 50 years. Long term survival is the same as for the general population. Visual loss is the most worrisome complication and can occur in over 50% of persons who are untreated, which could result in blindness for 20–50% of these patients.

Causes and symptoms

The cause of TA is not known. It is thought to be due to an immune cell response that attacks a foreign chemical (called an antigen) in the elastic layer of arteries in the head and neck.

In over 85% of affected persons, the most universal symptom is headache. The headache is severe and tends to be on one side (unilateral), and worsens at night. The **pain** tends to increase as days go by. Visual impairment may be the first presenting symptom since approximately 50% of patients complain of a sudden and painless visual loss. Loss of vision may be transient or permanent and blindness can occur if the condition is untreated.

In approximately 65% of persons, jaw claudication is prominent when chewing, swallowing or talking. Patients may have low grade fever and the effected arteries may be tender, warm, pulseless, dilated and thickened. Other symptoms that can occur include cough, anorexia, muscle aches, malaise, difficulty hearing, **fatigue**, fever/sweats and **depression**.

Diagnosis

Criteria for the diagnosis of TA were established in 1990 by the American College of Rheumatology. A diagnosis based on criteria for giant cell arteritis includes the presence of three of the following five items:

- new onset of headache or localized pain in the head region
- temporal artery tenderness to palpation
- development of symptoms in a person over 50 years of age
- lab result of over 50 for a special test called the Westergren Erythrocyte Sedimentation rate (WESR)
- decreased pulsations in head arteries, which cannot be attributed to arteriosclerotic disease of neck (cervical) arteries

A definitive diagnosis is made by the temporal artery **biopsy** which can be performed as an outpatient procedure (same day surgery).

Blood tests may reveal a high white blood cell count (leukocytosis), mild anemia or an increase in platelet cells (thrombocytosis), which are responsible for blood coagulation. Approximately 50% of patients affected with temporal arteritis have abnormal liver function tests. Chest radiograph may be useful to detect involvement of a chest (thoracic) artery. Ocular pneumoplethysmography can help make the diagnosis of temporal arteritis. Multiple biopsies may be indicated if initial findings are negative, but the suspicion for this diagnosis remains high.

Treatment team

The condition can be diagnosed by a primary care provider. Consultations may be indicated with an ophthalmologist (if there are visual complications). Generally an internist or rheumatologist directs the general care for systemic symptoms.

Treatment

Oral steroids are effective treatment for TA. Treatment is critical and important to avoid vision loss. Treatment should be initiated based on clinical suspicion and should not be delayed for biopsy results. The use of steroid or prednisone can be initially given at a dose of 60 to 100 mg per day. The dose can be tapered down in an individualized manner at a rate of approximately 10% per week, while concurrently taking into account symptomatic state and lab result improvement.

Recovery and rehabilitation

Most patients can be treated on an outpatient basis, with steroids, and symptoms usually begin to resolve within one to three days. Patients may require oral steroid medication for up to one year, depending on individual response. Nonsteroidal anti-inflammatory drugs may provide some pain relief.

Clinical trials

A clinical trial sponsored by the Cleveland Clinic Foundation Hospital and the National Institute of Health concerning the treatment of TA. The study is a multi-institutional project which includes medical centers within the United States and in several countries overseas. Full details can be obtained from the website: <http://www.clinicaltrials.gov>.

Prognosis

The condition is self-limiting and can last up to two years. Treatment with corticosteroids produces relief of symptoms and can help with visual impairment.

Special concerns

A diagnosis of TA can be missed. The disorder should be suspected in older patients with a high erythrocyte sedimentation rate (ESR), even if other evidence is absent.

Resources

BOOKS

Goetz, Christopher G., et al., eds. *Textbook of Clinical Neurology.* 1st ed. Philadelphia: W. B. Saunders Company, 1999.

Goldman, Lee, et al. *Cecil's Textbook of Medicine.* 21st ed. Philadelphia: W. B. Saunders Company, 2000.

Noble, John., et al., eds. *Textbook of Primary Care Medicine.* 3rd ed. St. Louis: Mosby, Inc., 2001.

WEBSITES

American Heart Association. <http://www.americanheart.org>.

ORGANIZATIONS

National Heart, Lung, and Blood Institute, Building 31, Room 5A52. 31 Center Drive MSC 2486, Bethesda, MD 20892. (301) 592-8573; Fax: (301) 592-8563. nhlbiinfo@nhlbi.nih.gov. <http://www.nhlbi.nih.gov>.

Laith Farid Gulli, MD
Robert Ramirez, DO
Alfredo Mori, MBBS

Temporal lobe epilepsy

Definition

Temporal lobe **epilepsy** (TLE) is a term that refers to a condition where **seizures** are generated in the portion of the brain called the temporal lobe. Either the right or the left temporal lobe can be involved, and in rare cases both temporal lobes can be involved in a particular individual.

Description

Under the broad category of TLE, there are a number of specific types. In mesial TLE (MTLE), there are characteristic abnormalities in the mesial aspect of the temporal lobe. This variably involves sclerosis (scarring), loss of nerve cells in the hippocampus and mossy cell fiber sprouting. Of course, there are other different pathologies that can be seen in the temporal lobe including tumors, **stroke, multiple sclerosis** plaques, and tubers (as seen in **tuberous sclerosis**). Another type of TLE is lateral TLE. This is where the seizures originate in the lateral portion of the particular temporal lobe. Again, various pathologies can be found such as cortical malformations and stroke. However, imaging studies, such as **magnetic resonance imaging (MRI)**, often may not show any obvious lesions or abnormalities. As more information is gathered regarding the genetics that may be involved in some cases, the classification of TLE will likely change.

Demographics

TLE, as a whole, constitutes a common type of epilepsy. The exact incidence is not clear but it is suspected to make up a significant proportion of medication-resistant epilepsy. Approximately 30% (of the 2.7 million cases of epilepsy in the United States) do not adequately respond to medications. Up to a half of these may be due to TLE. One of the risk factors that may predispose children to, in particular, mesial TLE is complicated or prolonged febrile convulsions before the age of five years. Mesial TLE can also run in some families.

Causes and symptoms

The abnormalities most associated with mesial TLE are sclerosis (scarring) of the hippocampus, neuronal cell loss in the hippocampal area, and inappropriate sprouting (growth) of mossy cell fibers. The cause of these variable pathological findings is still being studied. There is some evidence that mesial TLE may be a progressive condition where seizures become more resistant to medications over time. Likely, seizures over time play a role in the changes seen in the mesial temporal lobe. Likewise, the mesial temporal abnormalities contribute to the epileptogenicity (seizure potential) of that region. Although these pathologies are the most common findings in cases of mesial TLE, other lesions can be the suspected cause of epilepsy such as stroke, multiple sclerosis plaques, tumors, and cortical malformations. Lateral TLE can also be affected by strokes, cortical malformations, multiple sclerosis plaques, etc., and be the cause of seizures from this area. In the rare condition of benign familial TLE the cause is genetic and runs in families. Exactly how any of the previously mentioned abnormalities actually cause groups of neurons to generate seizure activity is complex and not fully understood. Because there can be different lesions, there can also be different mechanisms of generating a seizure. The temporal lobe epilepsies should not be considered as diseases. Rather, they are syndromes (groups of physical signs and symptoms) with many causes.

The age of onset of TLE is highly variable depending on the cause. In mesial TLE, seizure can begin as early as childhood or even later in adulthood. There is a characteristic remission that can occur during childhood, lasting a few years, but then seizures resume in adulthood.

The seizures that occur in TLE are simple partial seizures or complex partial seizures. Uncommonly, a generalized tonic-clonic seizure may occur. The simple partial seizures can take the form of auras. Although these are viewed as seizure warnings, they are actually minor seizures that do not affect consciousness. The most common aura is a visceral sensation. This can take the form of a rising feeling in stomach. Other kinds of auras can be déjà vu (a sense of familiarity) or *jamais vu* (the opposite of déjà vu, a sense of unfamiliarity or uniqueness); distortion of perceptions of size, or movement (vertigo); or olfactory (odors) distortions and buzzing sounds depending on what portion of the temporal lobe is involved. Emotional auras can also occur; fear, for example. Still other auras are too difficult for patients to describe. All these minor seizures are usually not serious unless they are occurring frequently and are disturbing to the person.

Seizures that affect or alter consciousness are present in the majority of people with TLE. These complex partial seizures variably involve cessation of activity, a certain degree of starring off, lip smacking or other oral movements. Moreover, the arm contralateral (opposite) the temporal lobe displays a posturing action. The arm ipsilateral (same side) as the affected temporal lobe has automatisms (semi-purposeful motions). During this phase of the seizure, the person has little to no awareness of the environment and will virtually be unresponsive to those around him or her. The aura plus the complex-partial-seizure phase typically lasts less than two to three minutes. Then there is a variable period of confusion lasting longer. If the seizure involves primarily the dominant (usually left) hemisphere (where language is processed) then a so-called post-ictal (after seizure) **aphasia** (loss of language) can occur and last several minutes. All these behavioral features can help decide which hemisphere, if not temporal lobe, is involved.

Diagnosis

The diagnosis of TLE can be made by a careful history (of an accurate description of the seizures) coupled with abnormalities on high resolution magnetic resonance imaging (MRI) of the brain and electroencephalogram (EEG). Current MRIs are sensitive, but subtle lesions such as mesial temporal sclerosis can be missed either by routine MRIs or inexperienced radiologists. The routine EEG (usually 30 minutes of testing) can be normal between seizures but may sometimes show occasional characteristic wave patterns in the temporal regions suggesting the location of seizure generation. Long term monitoring with EEG/closed circuit T.V. (LTME) is extremely helpful to determining which temporal lobe is abnormal.

Treatment

The treatment goal of any epilepsy is freedom from seizures with no side-effects of medications. Although this is the goal, it is frequently not attained. There may be a highly variable response to medications. There are over 20 seizure medications available. It is important to understand, however, that if a trial of up to three different well-chosen medications alone or in combination fail to control seizures, then the likelihood that some other medication will work is slim. Therefore, the general concept is that not all medications and combinations need to be tried to know if an epilepsy will be resistant. A timely referral to a comprehensive epilepsy center should be done to explore other treatment options, such as surgery. In mesial TLE, medications frequently fail to adequately control the seizures. Fortunately, this particular epilepsy is most responsive to surgical treatment. Brain surgery should not be viewed as "a last resort" when pharmacoresistant epilepsies are considered. With modern screening methods and neurosurgical technique, complications are rare. The surgery for mesial TLE offers up to an 80% chance of cure. The surgery involves the removal of a portion of the affected temporal lobe. On the other hand, seizures that are generated from other areas of the temporal lobe are more complicated.

Recovery and rehabilitation

Recovery and rehabilitation are a consideration if epilepsy surgery is performed. If a partial temporal lobectomy has been done, the patient remains in the hospital for several days. Post-operatively, there can be headaches and nausea that are managed with medications and resolved in one to three days. Complications of surgery are rare but include infection (managed with antibiotics) and bleeding (which, if severe, may require a transfusion). Neurological deficits are uncommon; when they are present they are usually mild. This includes a limited visual field deficit, contralateral (opposite to surgical side) weakness or speech difficulty. When neurological complications occur, they usually improve with time and are not disabling.

Clinical trials

Currently there is a multicenter randomized controlled trial (Early Randomized Surgical Epilepsy Trial called ERSET) comparing epilepsy surgery and optimal **pharmacotherapy** in patients 12 years and older with mesial TLE within two years of determination of pharmacoresistance. The official website is <http://www.erset.org>. Information is also available from the National Institute of Neurological Disorders and Stroke <http://www.ninds.nih.gov> regarding other funded studies under the general heading of epilepsy.

Prognosis

The prognosis for TLE varies considerably depending on the type of TLE. Although medications should be tried initially, mesial TLE and many of the lateral TLEs are often resistant. Timely referral to an epilepsy center that can determine the nature of the seizure disorder and offer other kinds of treatment approaches should be undertaken. Epilepsy surgery for mesial TLE offers up to an 80% chance of sustained seizure freedom and the possibility of discontinuing medications.

Special concerns

Long-standing, poorly controlled epilepsy has a number of psychosocial ramifications. These can include (but are not limited to) memory difficulty, reduced self-esteem, **depression**, reduced ability for gainful employment, and greater difficulty with interpersonal relationships. These issues may be underestimated in the setting of treating the seizure disorder. Recognizing the psychosocial well-being of the patient will greatly help in improving quality of life.

Resources

BOOKS

Browne, T. R., and G. L. Holmes. *Handbook of Epilepsy,* 2nd edition. Lippincott Williams & Wilkins, 2000.

Devinski, O. *A Guide to Understanding and Living with Epilepsy.* F. A. Davis Company, 1994.

Engel, Jr. J., and T. A. Pedley. *Epilepsy: A Comprehensive Textbook.* 3 volumes. Lippincott-Raven, 1998.

Wyllie, E. *The Treatment of Epilepsy: Principles and Practice,* 3rd Edition. Lippincott Williams & Wilkins, 2001

PERIODICALS

Kwan, P., and M. J. Brodie. "Early Identification of Refractory Epilepsy." *New England Journal of Medicine* 342 (2000): 314–319.

Wiebe, S., Blume, W. T., and J. P. Girvin. "A Randomized, Controlled Trial of Surgery for Temporal-lobe Epilepsy." *New England Journal of Medicine* 345, no. 5 (August 2, 2001): 311–89.

ORGANIZATIONS

American Epilepsy Society. 342 North Main Street, West Hartford, CT 06117-2507. (860) 586-7505. <http://www.aesnet.org>.

Epilepsy Foundation of America. 4351 Garden City Drive, Landover, MD 20785-7223. (800) 332-1000. <http://www.epilepsyfoundation.org>.

International League Against Epilepsy. Avenue Marcel Thiry 204, B-1200, Brussels, Belgium. + 32 (0) 2 774 9547; Fax: + 32 (0) 2 774 9690. <http://www.epilepsy.org>.

Roy Sucholeiki, MD

Tension headache *see* **Headache**

Tethered spinal cord syndrome

Definition

Tethered spinal cord syndrome (TSCS), also known as occult spinal dysraphism sequence, is a congenital condition that causes the spinal cord, before or after birth, to become attached to the spinal column at some point along its length, most often in the lower (lumbar) portion. TSCS is related to **spina bifida**, since both disorders arise from a failure of the neural tube to close completely during embryonic development. There are differing forms and degrees of severity of TSCS, including tight filum terminale, lipomeningomyelocele, split cord malformations, and dermal sinus tracts.

Description

The normal spinal cord, a cable of nerves, extends vertically from the base of the brain to the lumbar region, or lower back, contained within the hollow cylinder formed by the bony vertebrae and soft tissues of the spinal column. The spinal cord hangs freely within the spinal column, cushioned by cerebrospinal fluid, and is attached at its lower end to a strand of elastic tissue, the filum terminale, which is in turn attached to the lower end of the spinal column and which secures the lower end of the cord but allows it to be stretched without injury. Beyond the lower end of the cord proper, the major afferent and efferent nerves for the muscles of the legs, lower bowel, and bladder, the cauda equina, continue down the spinal canal and branch to those areas.

TSCS is initiated by incomplete closure, during embryonic development, of the neural tube, the early embryonic foundation of the spinal cord and column, resulting in malformations of the spinal column and cord. One disorder brought about by the malformation is spina bifida, in which the spine is open on its dorsal surface, somewhere along its length. Spina bifida can range in severity from not being visible externally, or spina bifida occulta, to a visible, open cavity with major impairment of the spinal cord at and below that spot. Among these extremes, tethered spinal cord may occur in the invisible forms, or spina bifida occulta.

In cases of relatively mild spina bifida that result in TSCS, the flaw occurs most often along the lower (lumbar) portion of the spinal column and cord. Cases of tethered cord in the cervical and thoracic regions of the spinal column are known but are extremely rare.

The developmental flaw causes soft tissues of the spinal column to grow into the hollow containing the spinal cord and to attach to the spinal cord, anchoring it at

Key Terms

Neural tube   A hollow column of ectodermal tissue that forms in early embryonic development and goes on to become the spinal cord and spinal column.

Spina bifida   A defect in the spinal column, brought about by incomplete closure of the developing neural tube, in which the column is cleft on its dorsal side.

Spina bifida occulta   A relatively mild form of spina bifida in which the defect is not visible from the surface.

Filum terminale   The strand of elastic, fibrous tissue that secures the lower end of the spinal cord.

that spot. Since the spinal cord grows more slowly than the spinal column, a tethered spinal cord becomes stretched and stressed over time, causing neurological damage in the cord and the nerves of the cauda equina that results in physical problems that manifest in a range of diagnostic symptoms and signs. Bending or stretching movements of the body put additional tension on the tethered cord.

As the cord is stretched, circulation of blood to the lower portion and cauda equina may be reduced as the blood vessels there are compressed by the tension in the cord. This in turn results in hypoxia, or loss of oxygen, delivered in the blood to that part of the cord, eventually causing damage and loss of function in the neurons.

If left untreated, the stress induced in the tethered cord can cause permanent damage and malfunction to the nerves and muscles that control movements of the legs, feet, bowel and bladder. Severe consequences can be deformed feet and legs, paralysis and incontinence.

Other forms of tethered cord include tight filum terminale syndrome, in which malformations in the embryonic neural tube at its lowermost point result in a defective filum terminale, the normally flexible anchor of the cord's lower end. A defective filum terminale is short and fibrous, with reduced elasticity or none, thus tethering the spinal cord at its lower end.

A lipomeningomyelocele is an abnormal growth of fatty tissue at the base of the developing spinal cord that entangles the lower end of the cord and thus tethers it.

In diastematomyelia, or split cord syndrome, an abnormal growth of bony or fibrous tissue forms a spur within the spinal canal, parting longitudinally (not severing) the nerves of the spinal cord, which rejoin into a single tract below the spur. The spinal cord can become tethered at the location of the split.

A dermal sinus tract is a canal lined with epithelial (skin) tissue, one end of which shows as an opening in the lumbar skin, the other end connecting with the tissues of the spinal cord or canal, or with adjacent tissues. Tumors form in the internal end of the sinus in about half of all cases, the tumors often bringing about spinal cord tethering.

TSCS may also develop following surgery for spina bifida, when scar tissue resulting from surgery grows and snags the spinal cord, thus tethering it.

Demographics

TSCS is a relatively rare disorder. Its exact frequency is unknown, mostly because of a general lack of research on the disorder, and because the mildest forms may never be detected. TSCS in all forms affect both sexes and all races and ethnic groups.

Causes and symptoms

Congenital TSCS is initiated by incomplete closure of the neural tube during embryonic development. During the eighteenth to twenty-second day of embryonic development, the beginning structure of the neural tube, which will become the spinal column and cord, is formed by ectodermal tissue on the back of the embryo that forms a groove, which deepens and forms into a hollow tube, still open dorsally along its length. The tube begins to close itself, starting in the thoracic region, then moving on toward the head and lumbar regions. During the twenty-eighth to forty-eighth day of development, ectodermal tissue in the tail area of the embryo forms a separate, short length of neural tube, the conus medullaris, whose anterior end meets and fuses with the main neural tube while the posterior forms the filum terminale. The conus medullaris also produces the cauda equinae nerves.

Symptoms of TSCS may be visible at birth or appear later, even in adulthood, but most often in childhood. The symptoms may be visible or behavioral. Various visible signs on the skin of the lower back, along and near the spinal cord, are:

• lipomas, or fatty tumors below the skin

• hairy patches

• spots of increased pigmentation

• dimples that may indicate dermal sinus tracts

- skin lesions
- skin tags or outgrowths
- angiomas, or port-wine stains
    Behavioral symptoms manifest as:
- chronic lower back pains
- progressive scoliosis, or curvature of the spine
- foot deformities
- numbness and loss of sensation in the legs or feet
- awkward gait and stumbling
- weakness in legs or feet
- unequal growth in the legs or feet
- progressive loss of control over bladder and bowel functions (incontinence)
- urinary tract infections

Diagnosis

The initial indicators of TSCS are the physical and behavioral ones listed above. A newborn that carries any of the symptomatic skin defects should be diagnosed further for possible TSCS. Among the behavioral signs, a child will likely complain to parents of lower back pains, while other behavioral symptoms will become obvious to parents. An adult who shows any of the physical or behavioral symptoms should bring these to the attention of his family physician, who should suspect TSCS as the cause. Symptoms, physical or behavioral, may not appear until many years after birth, including well into adulthood, depending on the time of tethering, degree of stretching of the spinal cord, and severity of damage to the nerves of the cord.

The next steps in diagnosis of TSCS are taking x-ray images of the spine to detect bone abnormalities, followed by the application of diagnostic neuro-imaging by means of **MRI (magnetic resonance imaging)** to produce three-dimensional images of the spinal column and spinal cord. Since a defect in the spinal cord or column makes it likely that there are other defects in the cord, column, or brain, an entire imaging of the brain and spinal column are recommended. **Electromyography** (EMG) can be used to check for or assess damage to nerve conduction in the spinal cord and the nerves of the cauda equinae. Ultrasound imaging can be used to monitor unborn infants for evidence of TSCS, should there be a reason to suspect it.

Since the muscles of the bladder are often affected by TSCS, urodynamics testing is recommended to discover the extent of the damage.

Treatment team

A family doctor is probably the person most likely to first link symptoms in a child or adult to TSCS, when parents bring in a child for a routine health check or because

of the physical and behavioral signs and problems. Following the tentative diagnosis, the patient will be sent to neurologists, MRI imaging technicians, EMG technicians, urologists, surgeons and neurophysiologists if surgery is called for, and the personnel monitoring recovery.

Treatment

TSCS is corrected by surgery to detach the cord at its place of tethering. Follow-up examinations are necessary because the freed spinal cord sometimes becomes re-tethered to growing scar tissue.

In the case of tight filum terminale, the filum terminale is severed, allowing the cord to float freely.

Surgery for TSCS generally takes four to six hours, and is conducted according to the form of TSCS in the patient. The spinal column is opened from behind to reach the site of tethering. Neurophysiologists are present to monitor spinal cord and nerve functioning to reduce the risk of damage to nerves and other tissues.

Recovery and rehabilitation

The degree of recovery is based on the amount of damage induced by the TSCS and the success of the surgery. Nearly all patients improve or at least show no worsening of signs. A successful operation leaves 2% or less possibility of the symptoms getting worse, and a 50% likelihood of sensation and movement problems becoming normal. **Back pain** usually is reduced or eliminated and strength to the lower part of the body improves. On the other hand, bladder dysfunction usually does not improve.

Ongoing monitoring of a patient following surgery for TSCS is required, in case the spinal cord should retether.

Prognosis

The prognosis for tethered spine syndrome is favorable, since skin symptoms may be visible at birth or later, allowing early detection and treatment, while behavioral symptoms manifest slowly enough for diagnosis and treatment before the condition becomes severe.

Special concerns

Spinal surgery is always risky because of possible damage to the nerves of the spinal cord. The patient may also have to deal with permanent damage caused by TSCS that surgery cannot improve.

Resources
BOOKS

Parker, James N. and Philip M. Parker. *The Official Patient's Sourcebook on Tethered Spinal Cord Syndrome (Revised* and Updated). ICON Health Publications, San Diego, CA, 2002.

Weinstein, Stuart L. *Pediatric Spine Surgery.* Philadelphia: Lippincott Williams & Wilkins Publishers, 2001

PERIODICALS

Baskaya, M. K., J. A. Menendez, and B. K. Willis. "Late presentation of tethered spinal cord in a 73-year-old patient." *Journal of the American Geriatric Society* 49, no. 5 (May 2000): 682–683.

Ratliff, J., P. S. Mahoney, and D. G. Kline. "Tethered cord syndrome in adults." *Southern Medical Journal* 92, no. 12 (December 1999): 1199–1203.

Witkamp, T. D., W. P. Vandertop, F. J. Beek, et al. "Medullary cone movement in subjects with a normal spinal cord and in patients with a tethered spinal cord." *Radiology* 220, no. 1 (July 2001): 208–212.

WEBSITES

NINDS Tethered Spinal Cord Syndrome Information Page. National Institute of Neurological Disorders and Stroke. <http://www.ninds.nih.gov/health_and_medical/ disorders/tethered_cord.htm>.

ORGANIZATIONS

National Organization for Rare Disorders (NORD). P.O. Box 1968 (55 Kenosia Avenue), Danbury, CT 06813-1968. 203-744-0100 or 800-999-NORD (6673); Fax: 203-798-2291. orphan@rarediseases.org. <http://www.rare diseases.org>.

Spina Bifida Association of America. 4590 MacArthur Blvd. NW, Suite 250, Washington, DC 20007-4266. 202-944-3285 or 800-621-3141; Fax: 202-944-3295. sbaa@sbaa.org. <http://www.sbaa.org>.

Kevin Fitzgerald

Third nerve palsy

Definition

Third nerve palsy describes a condition involving the third cranial nerve (also called the oculomotor nerve), which is responsible for innervating some of the muscles responsible for eye movement.

Description

Third nerve palsy results in an inability to move the eye normally in all directions. Injury to the third nerve can occur anywhere along its path, from where it originates within the brain to where it innervates the muscles that move the eyeball. Third nerve palsy prevents the proper functioning of the medial, superior, and inferior recti, and inferior oblique muscles. As a result, the eye cannot move up, down, or in. When at rest, the eye tends to look down and to the side, due to an inequality of muscle functioning.

The muscle responsible for keeping the upper eyelid open (levator palpebrae superioris) is also affected, resulting in a drooping upper eyelid (ptosis).

Causes and symptoms

A wide variety of conditions can result in third nerve palsy, including pressure and damage from tumors; blocked arteries or **aneurysms** leading to oxygen deprivation of nerves; meningitis; vascular complications of diabetes or high blood pressure; complications of migraine headaches; traumatic injury; birth injury; congenital defects; and conditions that strip nerve fibers of their myelin coating, resulting in slowed nervous transmission.

Some patients have severe **pain** and double vision (diplopia), in addition to problems moving their eyes normally. The affected eye tends to move down and out, due to an inequality in muscle functioning. The eye cannot move up, down, or in. In some cases, the pupil remains fixed in a dilated state. The upper eyelid is droopy (ptosis). The eyeball itself may actually be slightly displaced, pushed more forward than normal (proptosis).

Additionally, after the acute phase of third nerve palsy, as the nerve attempts to regenerate, a phenomenon called oculomotor synkinesis may take place. In this associated condition, nerve sprouts accidentally misdirect nerve transmission, so that efforts to utilize certain muscle groups accidentally prompt the functioning of other muscle groups. Therefore, attempts to accomplish certain muscular tasks actually result in different muscular tasks occurring. For example, as an individual with oculomotor synkinesis attempts to look down, the eyelid may raise up; when attempting to look up, the eye instead moves towards the midline; when attempting to look towards the midline, the pupil constricts.

Diagnosis

Eye muscle dysfunction is usually revealed during the course of a basic physical examination, which should always include testing of eye movements and examination of the pupils. **MRI**, **CT**, or **angiography** (a dye test that lights up the arteries throughout the brain, allowing the arteries to be better visualized on CT or MRI) may reveal the underlying cause of third nerve palsy.

Treatment team

Ophthalmologists and neurologists may work together to care for patients with third nerve palsy. In addition, physicians who manage diabetes, high blood pressure, or other underlying causative conditions will be involved in the patient's care.

Treatment

Steroids may treat pain and double vision. Special lenses with prisms may improve diplopia. Surgery on the eye muscles or eyelid may be necessary in some cases, although most clinicians recommend waiting six months from onset so that the patient's condition stabilizes.

Prognosis

In individuals who have no pupil involvement, and whose third nerve palsy is due to complications of diabetes or high blood pressure, symptoms may actually resolve within three to six months of onset. Other patients have a variable outcome, depending on the underlying condition responsible for the third nerve palsy.

Resources

BOOKS

Donahue, Sean P. "Nuclear and Fascicular Disorders of Eye Movement." In *Opthalmology*, edited by Myron Yanoff, et al. St. Louis: Mosby, 2003.

Goodwin, James. "Cranial Nerves III, IV, and VI: The Oculomotor System." In *Textbook of Clinical Neurology*, edited by Christopher G. Goetz. Philadelphia: W. B. Saunders Company, 2003.

Noble, John, et al., eds. *Noble: Textbook of Primary Care Medicine*. St. Louis: W. B. Saunders Company, 2001.

Rosalyn Carson-DeWitt, MD

Thoracic radiculopathy *see* **Radiculopathy**

Thoracic outlet syndrome

Definition

Thoracic outlet syndrome refers to a condition that results in compression of neurovascular anatomical structures at the superior aperture of the chest (thorax).

Description

Thoracic outlet syndrome (TOS) refers to compression of nerves and blood vessels in the upper portion of the thorax. Neurologic symptoms occur in 95% of affected persons. The cause and treatment of TOS is controversial. In 95% of cases the brachial plexus is involved. The lower two nerves (C8 and T1) are most commonly affected in 90% of persons, following the ulnar nerve distribution. Blood vessels can also be affected. The subclavian vein is involved in 40% of cases and the subclavian artery in 1%

of cases. The second most common nerve root involvement occurs in brachial plexus nerves C5, C6, and C7, and symptoms, if these nerves are affected, can be referred to upper back, upper chest, ear, neck, and outer arm that follows a radial nerve distribution.

Demographics

Reports concerning demographic information are controversial and range from three per 1,000 to 80 per 1,000 people. Overall the disorder is three times more common in women than men, with the exception of nervous system involvement which is more common in males. Some reports indicate that TOS is nine times more common in females than males. In the United States the incidence of vascular or neurogenic TOS is considered rare with only one new case per million population for the neurogenic TOS. The usual age of onset is from the second to eighth decade, with a peak age of onset in the fourth decade. Arterial involvement (arterial thoracic outlet syndrome) has no specific gender predilection.

Causes and symptoms

There are three major causes of TOS which include anatomic causes, trauma/repetitive activities, and neurovascular (nerve and blood vessels) entrapment in the chest. Certain anatomic abnormalities of the muscles in the neck and first rib (and a vertebral disk, C7) can cause compression of nerves and arteries. Anatomic abnormalities account for the majority of cases of neurologic and arterial thoracic outlet syndrome. Trauma such as hyperextension injury from motor vehicle accident or effort vein thrombosis (spontaneous thrombosis of the axillary veins following vigorous arm extension) may cause thoracic outlet syndrome. Repetitive activities similar to those of musicians are especially susceptible if they maintain the shoulder in abduction or extension positions for long periods. Nerves and blood vessels can be compressed anatomically in the costoclavicular space between the first rib and the head of the clavicle.

Neurologic **pain** can occur on either sides of the forearm, upper back and upper chest, neck and ear. Pain is especially evident on the ring and small finger. Patients often experience nocturnal paresthesias, awakening with numbness or pain (dysesthesia). There is often a loss of dexterity, cold intolerance and **headache**. Venous involvement causes pain, edema (swelling), cyanosis (bluish discoloration of the skin due to lack of oxygen), and distended superficial veins of the shoulder and chest. Arterial involvement causes pain and claudication, pallor, pulselessness, lower blood pressure in affected arm, and embolization (infarcts) of hand and finger. Patients usually have a subtle weakness of affected limb.

Key Terms

Brachial plexus A group of lower neck and upper back spinal nerves supplying the arm, forearm and hand.

Claudication Cramping or pain in a leg caused by poor blood circulation. This condition is frequently caused by hardening of the arteries (atherosclerosis). Intermittent claudication occurs only at certain times, usually after exercise, and is relieved by rest.

Clavicle Also called the collarbone. Bone that articulates with the shoulder and the breastbone.

Embolization A technique to stop or prevent hemorrhage by introducing a foreign mass, such as an air-filled membrane (balloon), into a blood vessel to block the flow of blood. This term also refers to an

alternative to splenectomy that involves injecting silicone or a similar substances into the splenic artery to shrink the size of the spleen.

Hyperextension Extension of a limb or body part beyond the normal limit.

Ischemia A decrease in the blood supply to an area of the body caused by obstruction or constriction of blood vessels.

Thrombosis The formation of a blood clot in a vein or artery that may obstruct local blood flow or may dislodge, travel downstream, and obstruct blood flow at a remote location. The clot or thrombus may lead to infarction, or death of tissue, due to a blocked blood supply.

Diagnosis

Chest x ray may reveal an anatomic abnormality. Color flow duplex scanning (ultrasound analysis) is indicated for suspected case of vascular thoracic outlet syndrome. If symptoms suggest arterial involvement an arteriogram may be indicated as well as venography (in suspected cases of venous involvement). Nerve conduction evaluation by nerve root stimulation is the best approach to diagnose neurologic thoracic outlet syndrome.

Treatment team

The treatment team usually consists of appropriate specialists which depend on the presentation. Specialists that can be consulted include a **neurologist**, vascular surgeon or orthopedic surgeon. Physical medicine physicians are required for outpatient workup and evaluation.

Treatment

Neurologic TOS requires outpatient referral and conservative outpatient physiotherapy. Vascular thoracic outlet syndrome requires more urgent care that typically includes immediate heparinization, vascular surgery consultation, color flow (ultrasound), duplex scanning and **angiography** or venography. Neurologic thoracic outlet syndrome patients may also require surgery if conservative medical therapy fails for more than four months. However, surgical results are not encouraging since a study demonstrated that 60% of postsurgical patients were still work disabled one year after surgery. Outpatient medications can include Coumadin (a blood thinner or anticoagulant), analgesics or short-term antidepressants if there is protracted pain.

Recovery and rehabilitation

Recovery includes stress avoidance and work simplification and modifications on the job site. Recommendations include avoidance of sustained muscular contraction and repetitive or overhead work. **Exercise** programs may help with chronic pain. Exercises are recommended to maximize the potential outlet space through special stretching and strengthening maneuvers of the shoulder. These exercise can include maneuvers such as bilateral (both sides) shoulder retraction while standing or lying prone, standing corner pushups, hand circles and cervical and lumbar spine extension. Outpatient management typically includes occupational/physical therapy, and manipluation. Inpatient treatment is not indicated unless the patient is a surgical candidate.

Clinical trials

There are projects funded by the National Institute of Neurological Diseases and Stroke <http://www.ninds.nih.gov> concerning pain and pain management. The projects forcus on seeking new treatments for nerve damage and pain.

Prognosis

Neurologic TOS is not progressive and but requires treatment. Arterial or venous thoracic outlet syndrome respond well to adequate treatment and the results are generally good. Some patients can develop chronic pain (neurologic type) or thrombosis (venous and arterial thoracic outlet syndrome). Other complications that can develop include loss of functional ability of arms, neurologic deficit, **depression**, and ischemia.

Special concerns

Pregnancy can cause an increase in TOS symptoms, because of increased body size and displacement of the abdomen. Increased breast size common during and after pregnancy can displace the shoulder girdle and cause postural changes that can precipitate symptoms. Patients should be educated concerning precipitating factors of TOS, which can decrease the likihood of recurrence.

Resources

BOOKS

Goetz, Christopher G., et al., eds. *Textbook of Clinical Neurology*, 1st ed. Philadelphia: W. B. Saunders Company, 1999.

Marx, John A., et al., eds. *Rosen's Emergency Medicine: Concepts and Clinical Practice*, 5th ed. St. Louis: Mosby, Inc., 2002.

Townsend, Courtney M. *Sabiston Textbook of Surgery*, 16th ed. W. B. Saunders Company, 2001.

WEBSITES

National Rehabilitation Information Center. <http://www.naric.com>.

ORGANIZATIONS

American Chronic Pain Association. P.O.Box 850, Rocklin, CA 95677-0850. (916) 632-0922 or (800) 533-3231; Fax: (916) 632-3208. ACPA@pacbell.net. <http://www.theacpa.org>.

Laith Farid Gulli, MD
Nicole Mallory, MS, PA-C
Alfredo Mori, MBBS

Thyrotoxic myopathy

Definition

Thyrotoxic **myopathy** is a neuromuscular disorder that occurs due to overproduction of thyroid hormone and is characterized by excessive fatigability, muscle wasting and weakness. It mainly affects muscles of the shoulder, hips and hands. The adverse effects of thyroid hormone on the structure and function of muscles gives rise to this myopathy. Although diagnosis can be tricky, this disorder is reversible with appropriate treatment.

Description

Thyrotoxic myopathy is known by several other names like hyperthyroid myopathy, Graves and Basedow's myopathy or Basedow paraplegia. It was first recognized in the early nineteenth century by Graves and Von Basedow as occurring infrequently in severe hyperthyroidism. In the middle of the twentieth century, researchers found that up to 80% of hyperthyroid patients manifested at least some degree of muscle weakness and this was confirmed on electromyographic studies.

Myopathy or muscle disease is categorized based on the underlying cause, inheritance pattern, etc. One of the broader categories is endocrine myopathies, which occur when there is an abnormal level of endocrine hormones in the body. The thyroid gland produces the hormone thyroxine which regulates maturation of the nervous system, growth and metabolism. Of all the endocrine myopathies, the myopathy due to dysfunction of the thyroid gland is the most common.

Demographics

Although some degree of muscle weakness is common in most hyperthyroid patients, it is still a rare disorder overall and there are no accurate estimates of incidence. In a series of hyperthyroid patients studied by Ruurd Duyff in 2000, 67% had symptoms attributable to myopathy. From a series of over 100 hyperthyroid patients studied by Ramsay in 1974 and Puvanendran *et al* in 1979, it was found that only 33–64% percent of patients complained of weakness but 61–82% actually had demonstrable weakness on examination. Although hyperthyroidism is more common among women, symptomatic myopathy is more common among middle aged hyperthyroid men. Unlike the classic myopathy, **periodic paralysis**, which is an unusual neuromuscular complication of hyperthyroidism, is seen among young Asian males.

Causes and symptoms

Much research has been done to elucidate how thyroxine affects muscle function. Muscle is made up of thousands of individual muscle fibers and myofibrils. The latter have myofilaments that are composed of contractile proteins called actin and myosin. In order for a muscle to contract, a command originates from the brain, travels along the spinal cord and then the nerve to terminate on the muscle. This impulse is then transmitted via a complicated process to the myofilaments that contract and relax appropriately. Adenosine triphosphate (ATP) is a chemical that supplies the necessary energy for contraction. Calcium which is released during contraction is taken up to cause muscle relaxation. Muscle fibers are of two types, slow and fast twitch. The slow or type 1 fibers are needed for sustained effort like standing and are more responsive to thyroxine. The fast type 2 fibers are needed for short rapid bursts like sprinting.

In hyperthyroidism, there is an accelerated production of ATP and reuptake of calcium. This leads to very rapid contraction and relaxation. When this occurs repetitively, the structure and mechanics of the slow fiber is changed to that of a fast fiber. Hyperthyroidism increases the body's basal metabolic rate and much of this energy is inefficiently used for muscle contraction. In turn, the muscles lose their endurance, **fatigue** easily, and become weak and wasted.

Hyperthyroidism can occur due to several causes. Of these, only two are commonly associated with myopathy. One of them is multinodular goiter, when the thyroid gland becomes studded with nodules, enlarges and overproduces thyroxine. The other is Graves disease, where the body launches an autoimmune attack on the thyroid gland and causes it to produce excess thyroxine.

A hyperthyroid person who has muscle weakness may or may not have other recognizable manifestations of hyperthyroidism. Myopathy can sometimes be the first presentation of the underlying hyperthyroid state. There are several types depending on the rapidity of symptom development and patterns of muscle involvement.

CHRONIC THYROTOXIC MYOPATHY The symptom onset is very insidious, so much so that patients very often do not notice the wasting or weakness. An average of six months elapses before the diagnosis is made, as the symptoms are subtle and the progress is very gradual. As mentioned earlier, only around 30% of patients complain of neuromuscular symptoms whereas around 80% show muscle weakness on testing. Patients complain of low **exercise** tolerance, easy fatigability, difficulty in doing certain tasks, muscle stiffness, muscle twitching and sometimes muscle wasting. Shoulder, hand and then pelvic muscles are affected and tasks like climbing stairs, getting up from a low chair or lifting arms above the shoulders become strenuous. Due to the weakness, movements become clumsy and effortful. The degree of wasting varies among individuals. It is usually mild to moderate but on occasions can be so severe that the scapulae look "winged." Despite a remarkable degree of wasting and weakness, patients remain ambulatory. If the myopathy progresses untreated, then facial muscles, swallowing, and respiratory muscles are involved with resultant difficulty swallowing and breathing. Muscles that control eye movement can also be affected, leading to double vision and squint.

ACUTE THYROTOXIC MYOPATHY This was first described by Laurent in 1944 and is a much rarer form than the chronic myopathy. It is rapidly progressive with profound muscle weakness developing over a few days. Muscle **pain**, cramps and muscle breakdown develop and lead to rhabdomyolysis. Patients are confused, have very weak respiratory muscles, and develop severe respiratory failure necessitating artificial ventilation.

OCULAR MYOPATHY This is also called "dysthyroid opthalmopathy" or "exopthalmic opthalmoplegia." It is more common in females, can be unilateral and may or

may not be associated with chronic thyrotoxic myopathy. It can occur even after treatment for hyperthyroidism. The eye muscles become swollen and weak due to inflammation from an autoimmune attack. Eyes are bulging, the cornea is inflamed and eye movements are restricted especially in the horizontal direction. In severe cases, the cornea is ulcerated and blindness occurs. It progresses over six to 18 months and longer delays in treatment result in severe residual deficit.

THYROTOXIC PERIODIC PARALYSIS This is very rare and occurs mostly in young adult males of Asian ancestry around the third decade. It is characterized by sudden episodes of muscle weakness involving the trunk and limb muscles, developing over few minutes to hours and lasting for hours to a couple of days. It is due to altered muscle membrane excitability secondary to low potassium levels. Although it is reversible spontaneously or with administration of potassium, death can occur due to cardiac arrhythmias.

Diagnosis

The diagnosis is clinical and is usually made by a **neurologist** who has expertise in neuromuscular disorders. There should be a high index of clinical suspicion as the pattern of muscle weakness is nonspecific and often patients do not know that they are hyperthyroid. The combination of symptoms in a severe case of hyperthyroid myopathy, like muscle wasting, difficulty swallowing and muscle twitching can lead to a mistaken diagnosis of Lou-Gehrig's disease (ALS). A classic picture is that of a patient, who despite a ravenous appetite has significant muscle wasting, weakness and brisk tendon reflexes. Associated hyperthyroid features like enlarged thyroid gland, tremor, bulging eyes, and a fast heart rate may be seen.

Blood tests show an elevated thyroxine level. In Graves disease, antibodies against the thyroid gland are present. Levels of creatine phosphokinase (CPK), a muscle enzyme is normal except when there is acute muscle breakdown. **Electromyography** is a technique used to diagnose myopathies, by studying the response of muscle contraction to an electrical stimulus. In hyperthyroid myopathy, this may be normal or show a "polyphasic" or "myopathic" response. Muscle **biopsy** again may be normal or show some degenerating fibers in a non-specific pattern. **CT scans** or **MRI** scans can be used to see the swollen eye muscles.

Treatment team

Treatment for hyperthyroid myopathy involves the interaction between a neuromuscular specialist, endocrinologist, a surgeon, and an ophthalmologist. Physiatrists and

Key Terms

Amyotrophic lateral sclerosis ALS, also called Lou Gehrig's disease, is a progressive neuromuscular condition due to degeneration of the motor nerve cells and fiber tracts in the spinal cord. The cause is not yet well defined. It leads to progressive weakening of the limb muscles and that of swallowing and breathing. ALS leads to death within a couple of years of onset.

Autoimmune An immune response by the body against its own tissues or cells.

Contracture Loss of range of motion at a joint due to abnormal shortening of soft tissues around the joint.

Creatine phosphokinase A muscle enzyme present in various skeletal muscles and the heart which is released due to any type of muscle injury. This can be measured in the blood.

Electromyography Technique used to measure the function of muscles by studying their contraction response to an electrical stimulus. A needle is inserted into the muscle, an electrical stimulus is given, and the resulting contraction is recorded from which normal and abnormal patterns can be interpreted.

Euthyroid State of normal function of the thyroid gland.

Goiter A swelling or enlargement of the thyroid gland.

Hormone Chemical substance produced by certain endocrine glands that are released into the bloodstream where they control and regulate functioning of several other tissues.

Hyperthyroid State of excess thyroid hormone in the body.

Myofilament Ultrastructural microscopic unit of a muscle that is made up of proteins that contract.

Myopathy Disease of muscle.

Opthalmoplegia Paralysis of the muscles that control eye movements.

Paraplegia Paralysis of the legs and lower part of the body.

Rhabdomyolysis Breakdown of muscle fibers resulting in release of muscle contents into the blood.

Thyroxine Hormone produced by the thyroid gland.

physical and occupational therapists are also part of the team helping in rehabilitation.

Treatment

Hyperthyroid myopathy is fortunately reversible provided the underlying hyperthyroidism is corrected and a normal thyroid state (euthyroidism) is restored. This can be done with medications, **radiation**, or surgery. Treatment is also aimed at symptomatic relief, prevention, and treatment of complications.

Medications

Beta-blockers are used to block the effects of adrenaline on peripheral tissues, as adrenergic systems are unregulated in hyperthyroidism. This affords symptomatic but temporary relief. Definitive treatment however aims at reducing the output of thyroxine from the thyroid gland. Propylthiouracil and methimazole are medications that inhibit production and release of thyroxine and also block tissue effects of thyroxine. Radiation in the form of oral radio-iodine therapy destroys the overactive thyroid gland. Steroids, other anti-inflammatory medications, or radiation is used to treat the ocular myopathy. Artificial tears and lubricating ointments are used to prevent

corneal ulceration. Potassium chloride given intravenously will reverse the thyrotoxic periodic paralysis.

Surgical treatment

Surgical removal of portions of the enlarged and unsightly thyroid gland can be done to restore euthyroid state. In severe cases of ocular myopathy, surgical widening of the walls of the orbit is done to allow the eyes to decompress. Corneal grafting can be done to treat corneal ulceration.

Recovery and rehabilitation

When proper treatment is given, full recovery of the myopathy is possible and complications can be avoided. Physical therapists can help in devising muscle strengthening exercises and in preventing muscle contractures. Protective eye glasses and eye patches are used to prevent corneal exposure and ulceration.

Clinical trials

There were no **clinical trials** ongoing as of early 2004, mainly because there is an effective treatment already available.

Prognosis

Prognosis is quite good. In two to four months after euthryoid state is achieved, muscle weakness improves. But it may take up to a year for muscle bulk to return. Respiratory failure is very rare. Patients have a normal life expectancy and lead normal lives if properly and promptly treated.

Resources

BOOKS

Aminoff, Michael J., editor. "Thyroid disorders and the nervous system." *Neurology and General Medicine.* Philadelphia: Churchill Livingstone, 2001.

Victor, Maurice, and Allan H. Ropper, eds. "Electrophysiologic Testing and Laboratory aids in the diagnosis of neuromuscular disease." *Principles of Neurology.* New York: McGraw-Hill, 2001.

Victor, Maurice, and Allan H. Ropper, eds. "Principles of Clinical Myology: Diagnosis and Classification of Muscle Diseases-General Considerations." *Principles of Neurology.* New York: McGraw-Hill, 2001.

Victor, Maurice, and Allan H. Ropper, eds. "The Metabolic and Toxic Myopathies." *Principles of Neurology.* New York: McGraw-Hill, 2001.

PERIODICALS

Alshekhlee, A., H. J. Kaminski, and R. L. Ruff. "Neuromuscular manifestations of endocrine disorders." *Neurologic Clinics* 20 (February 2002): 35–58.

Horak, H., and R. Pourmand. "Endocrine myopathies." *Neurologic Clinics* 18 (February 2000): 203–213.

Klein, I., and K. Ojamaa. "Thyroid (neuro)myopathy." *The Lancet* 356 (August 2000): 614.

WEBSITES

National Institutes of Neurological Disorders and Stroke (NINDS). *Thyrotoxic Myopathy Information Page.* <http://www.ninds.nih.gov/health_and_medical/disorders/thyrotoxic_myopathy.htm.>.

ORGANIZATIONS

Muscular Dystrophy Association. 3300 East Sunrise Drive, Tucson, AZ 85718-3208. (520) 529-2000 or (800) 572-1717; Fax: (520) 529-5300. mda@mdusa.org. <http://www.mdusa.org>.

National Institute of Health Neurological Institute. P.O. Box 5801, Bethesda, MD 20824. (301) 496-5751 or (800) 352-9424. <http://www.ninds.nih.gov/>.

Chitra Venkatasubramanian, MBBS, MD

▌Tiagabine

Definition

Tiagabine is an anticonvulsant medication indicated for the control of **seizures** in the treatment of **epilepsy**. Epilepsy is a neurological disorder in which excessive surges of electrical energy are emitted in the brain, causing seizures.

Purpose

Tiagabine decreases abnormal electrical activity within the brain that may trigger seizures. Although tiagabine controls some types of seizures associated with epilepsy, especially partial seizures, there is no known cure for the disorder.

Description

In the United States, tiagabine is sold under the brand name Gabitril. While the exact mechanism by which tiagabine reduces seizures is unknown, the drug boosts the levels of GABA, a neurotransmitter, in the brain. **Neurotransmitters** such as GABA are naturally occurring chemicals that transmit messages from one neuron (nerve cell) to another. When one neuron releases GABA, it normally binds to the next neuron, transmitting information and preventing the transmission of extra electrical activity. When levels of GABA are reduced, there may not be enough GABA to sufficiently bond to the neuron, leading to extra electrical activity in the brain and seizures. Tiagabine works to block GABA from being re-absorbed too quickly into the tissues, thereby increasing the amount available to bind to neurons.

Recommended dosage

Tiagabine is taken by mouth in tablet form and is prescribed by physicians in varying dosages.

Beginning a course of treatment with tiagabine requires a gradual dose-increasing regimen. Adults and teenagers 16 years or older typical take 4 mg a day at the beginning of treatment. The prescribing physician may raise a patient's daily dosage gradually over the course of several weeks. The usual dose is not greater than 56 mg per day. The full benefits of tiagabine may not be realized until after several weeks of therapy.

A person should not take a double dose of tiagabine. If a daily dose is missed, the next dose should be taken as soon as possible. However, if it is almost time for the next dose, the missed dose is skipped.

When discontinuing treatment including tiagabine, physicians typically direct patients to gradually reduce their daily dosages. Stopping the medicine suddenly may cause seizures to return or occur more frequently.

Precautions

A physician should be consulted before taking tiagabine with certain non-prescription medications. Patients should avoid alcohol and CNS depressants (medicines that can make one drowsy or less alert, such as

Key Terms

Epilepsy A disorder associated with disturbed electrical discharges in the central nervous system that cause seizures.

Partial seizure An episode of abnormal activity in a localized (specific) part of the brain, causing temporary changes in attention and muscle movement.

Neurotransmitter A chemical that is released during a nerve impulse that transmits information from one nerve cell to another.

antihistimines, sleep medications, and some **pain** medications) while taking tiagabine. Tiagabine can exacerbate (potentiate) the side effects of alcohol and other medications.

Tiagabine may not be suitable for persons with a history of liver or kidney disease, mental illness, high blood presure, angina (chest pain), irregular heartbeats, or other heart problems. Before beginning treatment with tiagabine, patients should notify their physician if they consume a large amount of alcohol, have a history of drug use, are pregnant, or plan to become pregnant. Physicians often advise the use of effective birth control while taking tiagabine. Studies in animals indicate that tiagabine may cause birth defects. Patients who become pregnant while taking tiagabine should contact their physician immediately.

Side effects

Patients and their physicians should weigh the risks and benefits of tiagabine before beginning treatment. Tiagabine is usually well-tolerated, but may case a variety of usually mild side effects. Dizziness, nausea and drowsiness are the most frequently reported side effects of tiagabine. Other possible side effects include:

• trouble sleeping

• fever

• **headache**

• unusual tiredness or weakness

• **tremors**

• abdominal pain

• increased appetite

• vomiting, diarrhea or constipation

• heartburn or indigestion

• aching joints and muscles or chills

• unpleasant taste in mouth or dry mouth

• tingling or prickly feeling on the skin

Many of these side effects disappear or occur less frequently during treatment as the body adjusts to the medication. However, if any symptoms persist or become too uncomfortable, the prescribing physician should be notified.

Other, uncommon side effects of tiagabine can be serious. A patient taking tiagabine who experiencs any of the following symptoms should contact their physician:

• rash or bluish patches on the skin

• mood or mental changes

• shakiness or unsteady walking

• excessive anxiety

• difficulty with memory

• double vision

• numbness in a limb.

• unsteadiness or clumsiness

• speech or language problems

• difficulty breathing

• chest pain

• irregular heartbeat

• faintness or loss of consciousness

• persistent severe headaches

• persistent fever or pain

Interactions

Tiagabine may have negative interactions with some antihistimines, antidepressants, antibiotics, and monoamine oxidase inhibitors (MAOIs). Other medications such as **diazepam** (Valium), **phenobarbital** (Luminal, Solfoton), nefazodone, metronidazole, **acetazolamide** (Diamox), phenytoin (Dilantin), **primidone**, and propranolol (Inderal) may also adversely react with triagabine. Tiagabine should be used with other other seizure prevention medications only if advised by a physician.

Many **anticonvulsants** may decrease the effectiveness of some forms of oral contraceptives (birth control pills).

Resources

BOOKS

Weaver, Donald F. *Epilepsy and Seizures: Everything You Need to Know.* Richmond Hill, Ontario: Firefly Books, 2001.

OTHER

"Tiagabine." *Medline Plus.* National Library of Medicine. (March 20, 2004). <http://www.nlm.nih.gov/medlineplus/druginfo/uspdi/203392.html>.

ORGANIZATIONS

American Epilepsy Society. 342 North Main Street, West Hartford, CT 06117-2507. <http://www.aesnet.org>.

Epilepsy Foundation. 4351 Garden City Drive, Landover, MD 20785-7223. (800) 332-1000. <http://www.epilepsy foundation.org>.

Adrienne Wilmoth Lerner

Tic douloureux *see* **Trigeminal neuralgia**

Tinnitus *see* **Hearing disorders**

Todd's paralysis

Definition

Todd's paralysis is a brief period of paralysis that occurs in the aftermath of a seizure.

Description

The period of time directly following a seizure is called the "postictal state." During this time period, the individual's brain is still recovering from the major changes brought on by the seizure. Drowsiness and confusion are very common symptoms of the postictal state. In some cases, the symptoms are even more pronounced and dramatic, and may even involve severe weakness or paralysis of a limb or one side of the body (hemiparesis), odd sensations such as numbness, or pronounced vision changes or blindness.

Demographics

Todd's paralysis usually strikes individuals who have **epilepsy** (recurrent **seizures**), although it may occur after any seizure.

Causes and symptoms

A seizure is an episode of abnormal electrical activity in a particular part of the brain. There are many kinds of seizures, and they may affect any specific part of the brain, or may spread to affect a wider distribution of the brain. The behavior of an individual suffering from a seizure may range from a simple, brief staring episode to complete loss of consciousness, with involuntary jerking of the muscles. The aftermath of a seizure is referred to as the postictal state. During the postictal period, although the seizure itself has ended, the brain is still recovering from the abnormal electrical discharges that precipitated the seizure activity. During this time period, the individual may be drowsy, less responsive than normal, or confused. Todd's paralysis is thought to occur due to

depressed activity in the area of the brain that underwent the seizure.

The symptoms of Todd's paralysis depend on the area of the brain where the seizure took place. For example, if the seizure occurred in the motor cortex (that part of the brain responsible for purposeful movement of the muscles), Todd's paralysis may result in hemiparesis, an inability to move the muscles of one-half of the body. Because the occipital lobe (the lower back part of the brain) is responsible for vision, an occipital lobe seizure may result in visual change or outright blindness during the postictal phase. In fact, tracking the specific symptoms of Todd's paralysis may actually help the physician diagnose the specific area of the brain in which an individual's seizures are occurring.

The symptoms of Todd's paralysis are often gone within minutes or hours of their onset. In some, more rare cases, the symptoms may last as long as 48 hours. Ultimately, however, full function is restored.

Diagnosis

Diagnosis of Todd's paralysis is crucial, because the symptoms can closely resemble those of a **stroke** (injury to the brain due to oxygen deprivation after bleeding or a blockage of an artery). It is important to distinguish between Todd's paralysis and a stroke, because the treatments are quite different.

Generally, Todd's paralysis can be easily diagnosed when it occurs in the aftermath of a documented seizure. The quick resolution of symptoms is another clue pointing to Todd's paralysis. When the diagnosis is unclear, however, tests may be run, including an electroencephalogram or EEG (a test that records information about the brain's electrical activity) or **MRI**. In the case of a seizure, the EEG may be abnormal; in the event of a stroke, the MRI may show an area of damage.

Treatment team

Todd's paralysis, like seizures and epilepsy, is usually treated by a **neurologist**.

Treatment

There is no specific treatment necessary for Todd's paralysis. The symptoms should fully resolve within minutes to hours or days.

Recovery and rehabilitation

Because of the quick and complete resolution of symptoms of Todd's paralysis, no rehabilitation is necessary.

Key Terms

Epilepsy   A condition in which an individual has recurrent seizures.

Hemiparesis   Severe weakness or paralysis affecting one side of the body.

Postictal   The time period immediately following a seizure.

Seizure   An episode of abnormal electrical activity in the brain.

Prognosis

The prognosis of Todd's paralysis is excellent, with full recovery to be anticipated.

Resources

BOOKS

Pedley, Timothy A. "The Epilepsies." *Cecil Textbook of Internal Medicine*, edited by Lee Goldman, et al. Philadelphia: W.B. Saunders Company, 2000.

Pollack, Charles V., and Emily S. Pollack. "Seizures." *Rosen's Emergency Medicine: Concepts and Clinical Practice*, 5th ed., edited by Lee Goldman, et al. St. Louis: Mosby, Inc., 2002.

PERIODICALS

Binder, D.K. "A history of Todd and his paralysis." *Neurosurgery* 54 (2) (February 2004) 486–487.

Iriarte, J. "Ictal paralysis mimicking Todd's phenomenon" *Neurology* 59 (3) (August 2002) 464–465.

Kellinghaus, Christoph; Kotagal, Prakash" Lateralizing value of Todd's palsy in patients with epilepsy" *Neurology* 62 (2) (January 27, 2004) 289–291.

Urrestarazu, E. "Postictal paralysis during video-EEG monitoring studies" *Review of Neurology* 35 (5) (September 1, 2002) 486–487.

WEBSITES

National Institute of Neurological Disorders and Stroke (NINDS). *Todd's Paralysis Fact Sheet.* Bethesda, MD: NINDS, 2003. <http://www.ninds.nih.gov>.

Rosalyn Carson-DeWitt, MD

▌Topiramate

Definition

Topiramate is an anticonvulsant indicated for the control of **seizures** in the treatment of **epilepsy** (a neurological dysfunction in which excessive surges of electrical energy are emitted in the brain) and **Lennox-Gastaut syndrome** (a disorder which causes seizures and developmental delays).

In psychiatry, topiramate may also be used in the treatment of bipolar **affective disorders**.

Purpose

Topiramate is thought to decrease and balance the abnormal electrical activity within the brain that may trigger seizures. While topiramate controls some types of seizures associated with epilepsy, there is no known cure for the disorder.

In patients with bipolar disorders, topiramate stabilizes mood without producing a euphoric feeling or inducing manic episodes.

Description

In the United States, topiramate is sold under the brand name Topamax.

Topiramate is most commonly prescribed to treat patients who do not respond to other anticonvulsant medications, or is part of a combination of anticonvulsant medications used to treat intractable seizures. Although the precise mechanisms by which it exerts its therapeutic effects in epilepsy and other seizure disorders are unknown, topiramate has three specific seizure-reducing actions:

- topiramate decreases nerve-cell excitation by blocking targeted **neurotransmitters** from binding to certain receptors in the brain.

- topiramate blocks sodium channels in nerve cells, thus decreasing excessive nerve-cell firing.

- topiramate increases the availability of GABA, (gamma-aminobutyric acid), a neurotransmitter that inhibits nerve-cell excitation in the brain.

Recommended dosage

Topiramate is taken by mouth in tablet or sprinkle form. Topiramate is available in strengths of 25 mg, 100 mg, and 200 mg tablets, along with 15 mg and 25 mg sprinkle capsules. Patients usually take topiramate twice daily. Typical total daily doses are usually between 200 milligrams (mg) to 400 mg for treatment of seizure disorders. For the treatment of bipolar disorders, dosages vary.

Beginning a course of treatment which includes topiramate requires a gradual dose-increasing regimen. The prescribing physician determines the proper beginning dosage and may raise a patient's daily dosage gradually over the course of several weeks. It may take several weeks to realize the full seizure-reducing benefits of topiramate.

Key Terms

Bipolar affective disorder A psychiatric disorder marked by alternating episodes of mania and depression. Also called bipolar illness, manic-depressive illness.

Epilepsy A disorder associated with disturbed electrical discharges in the central nervous system that cause seizures.

Lennox-Gastaut syndrome A severe form of epilepsy in children, resulting in intractable (difficult to control) seizures and developmental delays.

Seizure A convulsion, or uncontrolled discharge of nerve cells that may spread to other cells throughout the brain.

A double dose of topiramate should not be taken to make up for a missed or forgotten dose. If a daily dose is missed, it should be taken as soon as possible. However, if it is almost time for the next dose, the missed dose is skipped. When discontinuing treatment with topiramate, physicians typically direct patients to gradually taper their daily dosages. Stopping the medicine suddenly may cause seizures to return or occur more frequently.

In the treatment of bipolar disorders, persons should not stop taking topiramate without consulting the prescribing physician. Stopping the medicine suddenly may cause seizures, or severely and suddenly alter a patient's mood.

Precautions

Topiramate is not habit-forming. A physician should be consulted before combining topiramate with certain non-prescription medications. Patients should avoid alcohol and CNS depressants (medicines that can make one drowsy or less alert, such as antihistimines, sleep medications, and some **pain** medications) while taking topiramate. Because topiramate may cause drowsiness, persons should not drive or operate heavy machinery until they know how they will react to the drug.

Persons taking topiramate, particularly those with predisposing factors, should maintain an adequate fluid intake in order to minimize the risk of kidney stone formation. Approximately 1.5% of people taking topiramate develop kidney stones.

Topiramate may not be suitable for persons with a history of liver or kidney disease, mental illness, high blood presure, angina (chest pain), irregular heartbeats, or other heart problems. Before beginning treatment with topiramate, patients should notify their physician if they consume a large amount of alcohol, have a history of drug use, are pregnant or planning on becoming pregnant.

Topiramate may inhibit perspiration, causing body temperature to increase. Persons taking topiramate are at a greater risk for heat **stroke**, and should use caution during strenuous **exercise**, prolonged exposure during hot weather, and while using saunas or hot tubs.

Topiramate may cause birth defects. Use effective birth control while taking topiramate. Patients who become pregnant while taking topiramate should contact their physician immediately.

Side effects

Patients and their physicians should weigh the risks and benefits of topiramate before beginning treatment. Topiramate is usually well tolerated, but may cause a variety of usually mild side effects. **Dizziness** and drowsiness are the most frequently reported side effects of topiramate. Other possible side effects include:

• double vision

• tingling or prickly feeling of the extremeties

• language problems described as "trouble finding the right word"

• loss of appetite and nervousness (in children)

Many of these side effects disappear or occur less frequently during treatment as the body adjusts to the medication. However, if any symptoms persist or become too uncomfortable, the prescribing physician should be consulted.

Other, uncommon side effects of topiramate can lead to serious complications. A person taking topiramate who experiences any of the following symptoms should immediately contact their physician:

• blurred vision and eye pain

• extreme mood or mental changes

• shakiness or unsteady walking

• kidney stones

• difficulty breathing

• chest pain

• irregular heartbeat

• faintness or loss of consciousness

Interactions

Topiramate may have negative interactions with some antihistimines, antidepressants, antibiotics, and monoamine oxidase inhibitors (MAOIs). Other medications such as **diazepam** (Valium), **phenobarbital** (Luminal, Solfoton), nefazodone, metronidazole, **acetazolamide** (Diamox), lanoxin (Digoxin, Digitek), phenytoin (Dilantin), **primidone**, and propranolol (Inderal) may also need to be adjusted and closely monitored if taken with topiramate. Topiramate, like many other anticonvulsant medications, may decrease the effectiveness of oral contraceptives (birth control pills).

Resources

BOOKS

Devinsky, Orrin. *Epilepsy: Patient and Family Guide,* 2nd. ed. Philadelphia: F. A. Davis Co., 2001.

Weaver, Donald F. *Epilepsy and Seizures: Everything You Need to Know.* Toronto: Firefly Books, 2001.

OTHER

Ortho-McNeil Pharmaceuticals. "Information for People Taking TOPAMAX®." *Topamax.* (April 4, 2004). <http://www.topamax.com/patients/index.htm>.

"Topiramate." *Medline Plus.* National Library of Medicine. (April 4, 2004). <http://www.nlm.nih.gov/medlineplus/druginfo/medmaster/a697012.html>.

ORGANIZATIONS

American Epilepsy Society. 342 North Main Street, West Hartford, CT 06117-2507. <http://www.aesnet.org>.

Epilepsy Foundation. 4351 Garden City Drive, Landover, MD 20785-7223. (800) 332-1000. <http://www.epilepsyfoundation.org>.

Adrienne Wilmoth Lerner

Tourette syndrome

Definition

Tourette syndrome (TS) is an inherited neurological disorder that typically appears in childhood. The main features of TS are repeated movements and vocalizations called tics. TS can also be associated with behavioral and developmental problems.

Description

Tourette syndrome is a variable disorder with onset in childhood. Though symptoms can appear anywhere between the ages of two and 18, typical onset is around age six or seven. Tics, which may be motor or vocal, tend to wax and wane (increase and decrease) in severity over time. Facial tics, such as rapid blinking or mouth twitches, are the most common initial sign of TS. Other early symptoms include involuntary sounds such as throat clearing and sniffing, or tics of the limbs. Symptoms usually intensify during teenage years and diminish in late adolescence or early adulthood. Patients may also develop co-occurring behavioral disorders, namely obsessive-compulsive disorder (OCD), **attention deficit hyperactivity disorder** (ADHD) or attention deficit disorder (ADD), poor impulse control, and/or sleep disorders. Though some children have learning disabilities, intelligence is not impaired. TS is not degenerative and life span is normal.

Tourette syndrome is classified by the *Diagnostic and Statistical Manual of Mental Disorders*, Fourth Edition Text Revision (DSM-IV-TR) as a "Tic Disorder." The *International Classification of Disease and Related Health Problems*, Tenth Revision (ICD-10) calls TS a "combined vocal and multiple motor tic disorder (de la Tourette's syndrome)." A French **neurologist**, Jean Marc Itard, described the first known case of Tourette syndrome in the 1825. He had recorded the ticcing and cursing behavior of an aristocratic woman, Madame de Dampierre. The disorder is named for another French physician, Georges Gilles de la Tourette, who reported a series of cases in 1885, the primary example of which was the marquise. Tourette syndrome may also be referred to as Gilles de la Tourette syndrome (GTS).

Demographics

Tourette syndrome occurs worldwide, in people of all racial and ethnic groups. It is thought that approximately 200,000 people in the United States have TS. About three-quarters of patients are males. Once thought to be a rare disorder, TS is one of the most common genetic conditions. Recent estimates of prevalence suggest that TS occurs in one in 1,000 to one in 100 male children. One report indicated that prevalence may be as high as 25% in children in special education classes.

Causes and symptoms

Genetic factors are believed to play a major role in the development of TS. Several chromosomal regions have been identified as possible locations of genes that confer susceptibility to TS. Some family studies have indicated that TS is inherited in an autosomal dominant manner. In an autosomal dominant condition, an individual has a 50% chance to pass the gene to his or her children. Not everyone who inherits a TS gene will show symptoms. Approximately 70% of females and 99% of males with a TS gene will express symptoms. An individual who inherits the TS gene may develop TS, a milder tic disorder, obsessive-compulsive disorder (OCD) without any tics, or no signs of TS. The gender of a person influences the expression (the disease symptoms and severity) of the TS gene; males are more likely to have TS or tics and females are more likely to have OCD. Approximately one in ten children who inherit the TS gene from a parent will show symptoms that are severe enough to warrant medical treatment.

Non-genetic factors are also believed to contribute to the development of TS. In about 10-15% of cases, TS is not genetic. Certain stressful processes during gestation (pregnancy) or at the time of birth may increase the chance for a person to develop TS. For example, it is known that when both twins have TS, the twin who weighed less at birth tends to have more severe tics. Other non-genetic factors that may predispose a person to TS include: severe psychological trauma, recurrent daily stresses, extreme emotional excitement, PANDAS (pediatric autoimmune neuropsychiatric disorder with streptococcal infection), drug abuse, and certain co-existing medical or psychiatric conditions. In PANDAS, children experience an abrupt onset of TS symptoms and/or obsessive-compulsive symptoms following a strep throat infection.

It is thought that TS is the result of abnormal metabolism of a neurotransmitter (a chemical in the brain that carries signals from one nerve cell to another) called dopamine and possibly of other **neurotransmitters** including serotonin and norepinephrine. As of December 2003, the exact mechanisms by which the TS gene or genes lead to disease symptoms were unresolved. It is hoped that locating the gene or genes responsible for TS will improve understanding of how TS develops and eventually will lead to more effective treatments.

Tics seen in patients with TS can range in intensity, frequency, duration, type and complexity. Although there is wide range of severity observed in TS, the majority of cases are mild. A minority of patients has symptoms that are severe enough to interfere with daily functioning. In the most severe cases, patients experience numerous debilitating tics during all waking hours. Tics usually occur in "bouts" with many tics over a short interval of time. Many patients experience waxing and waning (fluctuations in severity) of their tics over the course of weeks or months. Tics can be made worse by stress or **fatigue** and tend to improve when the individual is absorbed in an activity or task that requires concentration. Although the tics associated with TS are involuntary (not deliberate), people with TS can sometimes control their tics for a period of time ranging from minutes to hours. However the tic must eventually be expressed and will come out. Coprolalia, a sensationalized type of tic in which people make obscene or socially inappropriate comments, is present in less than 15% of TS patients.

Tics are classified as either simple or complex. Simple tics are sudden, repetitive movements that involve a limited number of muscle groups. Simple motor tics are fast and without purpose. They can cause both emotional and physical **pain** (such as head jerking or jaw snapping). Simple vocal tics are meaningless sounds or noises. Complex tics are coordinated patterns of stepwise movements that involve multiple muscle groups. Complex motor tics

Key Terms

Biofeedback A training technique that enables an individual to gain some element of control over involuntary or automatic body functions.

Dyslexia A type of reading disorder often characterized by reversal of letters or words.

Gene A building block of inheritance, which contains the instructions for the production of a particular protein, and is made up of a molecular sequence found on a section of DNA. Each gene is found on a precise location on a chromosome.

appear slower and more deliberate than simple motor tics. Complex vocal tics involve meaningful words, phrases or sentences.

SIMPLE MOTOR TICS

- blinking eyes
- jerking head
- shrugging shoulders
- facial grimacing
- rolling eyes up
- squinting
- smacking lips
- jaw snapping

SIMPLE VOCAL TICS

- throat clearing
- yelping
- sniffing
- tongue clicking
- grunting
- coughing
- spitting
- humming
- whistling

COMPLEX MOTOR TICS

- jumping
- touching other people or things
- smelling
- twirling about
- thrusting of arms, groin, or torso
- pinching

- fiddling with clothing
- self-injurious actions including hitting or biting oneself (rare)

COMPLEX VOCAL TICS

- uttering words or phrases out of context
- repeating words or sounds
- stuttering
- repeating others' words (echolalia)
- repeating one's own last word or sound (palilalia)
- talking to oneself
- muttering
- vocalizing socially unacceptable words (a rare tic called coprolalia)

Co-occurring disorders

In addition to tics, patients with TS can also have additional problems that include:

- Obsessive-compulsive disorder (OCD). OCD is a condition characterized by the presence of obsessions (persistent involuntary thoughts, images or impulses that are experienced as unwanted and bothersome) and compulsions (the actual behaviors that are performed over and over in response to the obsessions). Examples of obsessive-compulsive behavior include excessive hand washing and repeatedly checking to see that a door is locked. In patients with TS, onset of OCD usually occurs before puberty and it may lead to serious impairment. It is thought that some forms of OCD have the same etiology (cause) as TS. Obsessive-compulsive behaviors can negatively impact a child's performance at school if they are time-consuming or distracting.

- Attention deficit disorder with or without hyperactivity (ADHD or ADD). Attention deficit disorder may precede symptoms of TS. It is estimated that ADD or ADHD occurs in as many as 75% of individuals with TS. Children with ADHD can be fidgety, have a very short attention span, be impulsive, and have difficulty completing tasks. ADD is similar except without the high level of activity seen in ADHD.

- Learning disabilities. Approximately one-third of patients with TS have a learning disability. Learning disabilities found in TS include difficulties with reading, writing and mathematics, and visual and auditory perception problems. Children with TS can also have **dyslexia** and problems with retaining information. Some tics seen in TS such as repetitive eye-blinking or head-jerking can make it difficult for the student with TS to read and thus interfere with learning.

- Sleep disorders. Sleep problems such as difficulty falling asleep, waking early, sleepwalking, night terrors and enuresis (bed-wetting) are fairly common in TS. For example, in one study the percentage of different grades of TS patients having trouble getting to sleep ranged from about 45% to 65% as compared to 15% of controls.

- Problems with impulse control. Individuals with TS may display overly aggressive behavior, socially inappropriate acts, self-injurious behavior such as lip biting or banging one's head, and defiant behaviors.

Diagnosis

There is no specific lab test or other medical study that can establish the definitive diagnosis of TS. Usually, diagnosis is made through observation of an individual's symptoms and by assessment of family history. Some patients may undergo blood tests, imaging studies such as **magnetic resonance imaging (MRI)**, or an electroencephalogram (EEG) scan in order to rule out other possible explanations for the symptoms. The process of making a TS diagnosis usually involves monitoring symptoms over a period of several months. The family may be asked to keep records. This period of observation will help determine to what extent the child's symptoms are interfering with ability to function at home, school, and in the community. A neurological examination may be performed. Assessment of cognitive functioning and school performance may be recommended if the child is having difficulty in school.

The American Psychiatric Association published diagnostic criteria, listed below, is from the *Diagnostic and Statistical Manual of Mental Disorders*, Fourth Edition Text Revision (DSM-IV-TR). Another similar set of criteria exists in the *International Classification of Disease and Related Health Problems*, Tenth Revision (ICD-10). The ICD-10 criteria are not as strict about the age of onset as the DSM-IV-TR criteria.

Diagnostic and Statistical Manual of Mental Disorders, Fourth Edition Text Revision (DSM-IV-TR) criteria

- Both multiple motor and one or more vocal tics present at some time during the illness although not necessarily simultaneously.

- The occurrence of tics multiple times per day (usually in bouts), nearly every day or intermittently during a span of more than one year without a tic-free period of more than three consecutive months.

- The disturbance causes significant distress or impairment in social, occupational, or other important areas of functioning.

- Onset before age 18.

- The disturbance is not due to the direct physiological effects of a substance or a general medical condition.

Treatment team

Treatment of TS disorders requires a multidisciplinary approach. In addition to the patient's primary health care professionals, medical professionals involved in the care of patients with an MPS usually includes specialists in neurology, psychiatry, psychology, social work, genetics, and education. Tourette syndrome support groups may help families in coping with this condition.

Treatment

There is no cure for TS. Management of TS requires integration of behavioral, psychological and sometimes pharmacologic (medication) therapies. Occupational therapy may also be indicated for TS patients. The decision to treat an individual case of TS depends on the degree to which the symptoms interfere with that person's ability to function. Treatment is crucial in helping the affected child avoid **depression**, social isolation, and strained family relationships. In general, pharamacologic therapy is reserved for patients with severe symptoms. Education about the condition and reassurance are key components of any treatment program.

Behavior therapy

Various types of behavior therapy may benefit patients with TS. Using a technique known as habit-reversal training, individuals with severe tics are taught how to substitute one tic for another that is more socially acceptable. Also, since stress can exacerbate tics, individuals with TS may find that relaxation techniques and biofeedback can help alleviate stress reactions and reduce tics. Behavior modification may be necessary for children with poor impulse control.

Psychological therapy

Psychological counseling may help individuals with TS to cope with the social and emotional problems that occur as a result of their symptoms. Depression and self-esteem problems are common among persons with TS. Counseling is especially important for children with TS as they approach adolescence, a time in which tics tend to get worse. Affected children and their parents may also benefit from family therapy. Severe or frequent tics and the presence of co-occurring problems such as ADHD and OCD can negatively impact quality of life for people with TS, especially if family support is inadequate. Parents may have difficulty accepting a diagnosis and in deciding which how best to handle unwanted behaviors. The goal of family therapy is to educate family members about the disorder and to find ways to handle those symptoms that have a negative impact on family members.

Pharmacologic therapy

No single or combination (more than one) drug therapy offers complete cessation of symptoms without adverse effects.

Pharmacologic treatment of TS (alone, without OCD or ADHD) usually begins with a trial of clonidine. If clonidine is unsuccessful, treatment moves to one of the dopamine receptor antagonists. Haloperidol, a dopamine receptor antagonist, has been the main drug used in TS treatment since the 1960s. It has been reported that over 80% of patients show improvement of tics with this therapy. A similar drug known as pimozide has also been used as an anti-tic drug since the 1980s. Due to adverse effects associated with haloperidol and pimozide, other dopamine receptor antagonists, including risperidone, sulpiride (not available in North America as of 2003), and olanzipine have gradually displaced haloperidol and pimozide as the main drug therapies for tics. Newer drugs, ziprasidone and quetiapine, may also be effective; as of 2003, evidence regarding their efficacy was preliminary. For those individuals who are unable to tolerate the above medications, treatment with a related medication, tetrabenazine, may be recommended. Drug therapy with a dopamine agonist may be attempted if none of the above drugs are effective. There are preliminary reports of positive therapeutic effects with other treatments including nicotine, tetrahydrocannbinol (marijuana), baclofen, and **botulinum toxin** injection yet confirmation of safety and efficacy of these treatments awaits further study.

Clomipramine or one of the selective serotonin uptake inhibitors (SSRIs) are the first choice for treatment of OCD. Examples of SSRI's in use for OCD treatment include fluoxetine, fluvoxamine, sertraline, paroxetine, and citalopram. For those TS patients with OCD who do not respond to SSRIs alone, addition of a dopamine receptor antagonist such as haloperidol, pimozide, risperidine, or olanzipine may be indicated. New therapies under investigation for the treatment of OCD as of 2003 included neurosurgery, **deep brain stimulation** (DBS), transcranial magnetic stimulation (TMS), and injection with botulinum toxin.

Methylphenidate and dextroamphetamine, medications known as psychostimulants, have been shown to be safe and effective in the treatment of ADHD in TS patients. There has been controversy over the use of psychostimulants to treat ADHD due to concerns about worsening of tics. Results from a randomized, placebo-controlled clinical trial reported in 2002 indicated that methylphenidate and another drug, clonidine, do not adversely affect tics. The researchers also found that a combination of the drugs is more effective than either drug alone.

Recovery and rehabilitation

Children with TS may require academic and occupational interventions. For some TS students, modifying the school environment can help to minimize stress. For the student with vocal tics, untimed exams in a private room and permission to leave the classroom when tics become problematic may help. Children with auditory processing difficulties and fine motor skill problems may benefit from occupational therapy. For example, the use of tape recorders, typewriters, or computers may be recommended to help with reading and writing. Occupational therapy can also help with poor handwriting, a common problem in children with TS. Some students with TS may be eligible for an Individual Education Plan (IEP). An IEP provides a framework from which administrators, teachers, and parents can meet the educational needs of a child with TS. Depending upon severity of TS symptoms and the degree of learning difficulties, some children with TS may be best served by special education classes or a private educational setting.

Clinical trials

As of December 2003, thirteen **clinical trials** were actively recruiting patients with Tourette syndrome. The National Institute of Neurological Disorders and Stroke (NINDS) in Bethesda, Maryland, were sponsoring the following trials. Information on these trials can be found at <http://www.clinicaltrials.gov> or by contacting the Patient Recruitment and Public Liaison Office at 1-800-411-1222 or at prpl@mail.cc.nih.gov.

• Magnetic Resonance Spectroscopy (MRS) to Evaluate Tourette's Syndrome. This study will use **magnetic resonance imaging** (**MRI**) and magnetic resonance spectroscopy (MRS) of the brain to try to gain a better understanding of the disease process in Tourette's syndrome. More information can be found at the National Institutes of Health (NIH) web link, <http://clinicalstudies.info.nih.gov/detail/A_2002-N-0128.html>.

• Study of Tics in Patients with Tourette's Syndrome and Chronic Motor Tic Disorder. This study will investigate which areas of the brain are primarily involved in and responsible for tics in patients with Tourette's syndrome and chronic motor tic disorder. More information can be found at the National Institutes of Health (NIH) web link, <http://clinicalstudies.info.nih.gov/detail/A_2002-N-0175.html>.

• Study of GABA-A receptors in the Generation of Tics in Patients with Tourette's Syndrome. This study will investigate how the brain generates tics in patients with Tourette's syndrome and which areas of the brain are primarily affected. More information can be found at the National Institutes of Health (NIH) web link, <http://clinicalstudies.info.nih.gov/detail/A_2002-N-0181.html>

• Brain Dynamics Involved in Generating Tics and Controlling Voluntary Movement. This study will use **electroencephalography** (EEG) and **electromyography** (EMG) to examine how the brain generates tics and controls voluntary movement in patients with Tourette's syndrome and chronic motor tic disorder. More information can be found at the National Institutes of Health (NIH) web link, <http://clinicalstudies.info.nih.gov/detail/A_2003-N-0126.html>.

• Brain Activation in Vocal and Motor Tics. This study will investigate the brain areas that are activated by vocal and motor tics in patients with Tourette's syndrome and other tic disorders. More information can be found at the National Institutes of Health (NIH) web link, <http://clinicalstudies.info.nih.gov/detail/A_2002-N-0027.html>.

The following trials were being sponsored by the National Center for Research Resources (NCRR) and coordinated by the Yale University School of Medicine in New Haven, Connecticut. Information on these trials can be found at <http://www.clinicaltrials.gov> or by contacting the study chair, James F. Leckman at 203-785-7971.

• Study of the Neurobiology of Tourette Syndrome and Related Disorders. This study will investigate the pathobiology of Tourette syndrome and related disorders by measuring various compounds of interest in cerebrospinal fluid, plasma, and urine of patients with Tourette syndrome, obsessive compulsive disorder, and/or chronic tics; determine the pattern of familial aggregation of Tourette syndrome and obsessive compulsive disorder by systematic assessment of all first-degree family members of patients selected for cerebrospinal fluid studies; and establish the neurochemical and neuropeptide profile associated with the range of expression of the putative Tourette gene expression in adult and adolescent patients.

• Developmental Phenomenology of Obsessive Compulsive Disorder and Tourette Syndrome in Children and Adolescents. This study will characterize the natural history, associated features, and severity of symptoms of obsessive compulsive disorder and Tourette syndrome in children and adolescents, and identify factors that influence the clinical course and prognosis of these patients.

The National Institute of Mental Health (NIMH) in Bethesda, Maryland, was sponsoring the following trials. Information on these trials can be found at <http://www.clinicaltrials.gov>.

• Brain Tissue Collection for Neuropathological Studies. This study will collect and study the brain tissue of deceased individuals to learn more about the nervous system and mental disorders. More information can be found at the National Institutes of Health (NIH) web page for this study at <http://clinicalstudies.info.nih.gov/detail/A_1990-M-0142.html> or by contacting Joel E. Kleinman, MD at (301) 402-7909 or kleinmaj@intra.nimh.nih.gov.

- Evaluation and Follow-up of Individuals with Obsessive-Compulsive Disorder and Related Conditions. This study will aim to better understand the long-term progress of people with obsessive-compulsive disorder (OCD) and related conditions such as anorexia nervosa, Tourette syndrome, and trichotillomania. More information can be found at the National Institutes of Health (NIH) web page for this study at <http://clinicalstudies.info.nih.gov/detail/A_2000-M-0067.html> or by contacting the patient recruitment and public liaison office at (800) 411-1222 or prpl@mail.cc.nih.gov.

- Brain Imaging of Childhood Onset Psychiatric Disorders, Endocrine Disorders, and Healthy Children. This study will use MRIs to assess **brain anatomy** and function in normal volunteers and patients with a variety of childhood onset psychiatric disorders. More information can be found at the National Institutes of Health (NIH) web page for this study at <http://clinicalstudies.info.nih.gov/detail/A_1989-M-0006.html> or by contacting the patient recruitment and public liaison office at (800) 411-1222 or prpl@mail.cc.nih.gov.

- Treatment of Obsessive-Compulsive Disorder. This study aims to find the best treatment for TS-spectrum obsessive-compulsive disorder (OCD), which includes symptoms of TS, e.g., repeated and involuntary body movements (tics). More information can be found by contacting the University of Florida at clintrls@psych.med.ufl.edu; the study chair, Wayne Goodman, MD at (877) 788-3994 or wkgood@psychiatry.ufl.edu; or Candy Hill at (352) 392-3681 or chill@psychiatry.ufl.edu.

- Genetics of Obsessive-Compulsive Disorder. This study to identify genes that affect susceptibility to obsessive-compulsive disorder (OCD). More information can be found at the National Institutes of Health (NIH) web page for this study at <http://clinicalstudies.info.nih.gov/detail/A_1996-M-0124.html> or by contacting Diane M. Kazuba at (301) 496-8977 or kazubad@intra.nimh.nih.gov.

- Central Mechanisms in Speech Motor Control Studied with H215O PET. This study will use radioactive water (H215O) and **Positron Emission Tomography** (PET scan) to measure blood flow to different areas of the brain in order to better understand the mechanisms involved in speech motor control, and is sponsored by the National Institute on Deafness and Other Communication Disorders (NIDCD) in Bethesda, Maryland. More information can be found at the National Institutes of Health (NIH) web page for this study at <http://clinicalstudies.info.nih.gov/detail/A_1992-DC-0178.html> or

by contacting the patient recruitment and public liaison office at 1-800-411-1222 or prpl@mail.cc.nih.gov.

Prognosis

The majority of cases of TS are mild and as such they do not require medical attention. Most affected individuals show improvement of symptoms in late adolescence or early adulthood and up to one-third of people will experience remission of tic in adult years. In fewer than 10% of patients, tics become more severe in adulthood. TS is not a degenerative disease and patients can anticipate a normal life span.

Special concerns

All students with TS need an educational environment that is supportive and flexible. Children with TS frequently have problems in school because they are teased by peers and misunderstood by teachers. It is important to educate the students, the teachers, and other school personnel who come in contact with the child with TS about the disorder.

Resources

BOOKS

American Psychiatric Association. *Diagnostic and Statistical Manual of Mental Disorders, 4th edition, text revision (DSM-IV-TR).* Washington, DC: American Psychiatric Association, 2000.

Comings, D. E. *Search for the Tourette Syndrome and Human Behavior Genes.* Duarte, CA: Hope Press, 1996.

Kurlan, R. *Handbook of Tourette Syndrome and Related Tic and Behavioral Disorders.* Rochester, NY: Marcel Dekker, 2003.

Leckman, J. F. and D. J. Cohen *Tourette's Syndrome—Tics, Obsessions, Compulsions: Developmental Psychopathology and Clinical Care,* reprint ed. John Wiley and Sons, 2001.

Robertson, M. M., and S. Baron-Cohen. *Tourette Syndrome: The Facts,* 1st ed. London: Oxford Press, 1998.

PERIODICALS

Jankovic, J. "Tourette's Syndrome." *New England Journal of Medicine* 345 (October 2001): 1184–1192.

Leckman, J. F. "Tourette's Syndrome." *Lancet* 360 (November 2002): 1577–1586.

Miguel, E. C., R. G. Shavitt, Y. A. Ferraro, S. A. Brotto, and J. B. Diniz. "How to Treat OCD in Patients with Tourette Syndrome." *Journal of Psychosomatic Research* 55 (July 2003): 49–57.

Pauls, D.L. "An Update on the Genetics of Gilles de la Tourette Syndrome." *Journal of Psychosomatic Research* 55 (July 2003): 7–12.

Robertson, M. M. "Diagnosing Tourette Syndrome: Is It a Common Disorder." *Journal of Psychosomatic Research* 55 (July 2003): 3–6.

Sandor, P. "Pharmacologic Management of Tics in Patients with TS." *Journal of Psychosomatic Research* 55 (July 2003): 419–48.

WEBSITES

The National Institute of Neurological Disorders and Stroke (NINDS). *Tourette Syndrome Information Page.* <http://www.ninds.nih.gov/health_and_medical/disorders/tourette.htm>.

Tourette's Disorder Home Page. <http://www.tourettes-disor-der.com//home.html>.

ORGANIZATIONS

National Tourette Syndrome Association, Inc. 42-40 Bell Boulevard, Bayside, New York 11361-2820. (718) 224-2999 or (888) 4-TOURET (486-8738); Fax: (718) 279-9596. ts@tsa-usa.org. <http://www.tsa-usa.org>.

Tourette Syndrome Foundation of Canada. #206, 194 Jarvis Street, Toronto, Ontario M5B 2B7, Canada. (416) 861-8398 or (800) 361-3120; Fax: (416) 861-2472. tsfc@tourette.ca. <http://www.tourette.ca/index.shtml>.

Dawn J. Cardeiro, MS, CGC

Transient global amnesia

Definition

Transient global amnesia (TGA) is a temporary short-term memory loss that may result from the deactivation of the brain's temporal lobes and/or thalamus (the part of the brain that serves as a center for the relay of sensory information). Usually occurring in otherwise healthy persons, TGA triggers memory loss from external stresses such as strenuous exertion, high levels of anxiety, sexual intercourse, immersion in water, and other similar conditions. The event may also be triggered by a condition called the Valsalva maneuver. During this maneuver, a person performs the "breathe-in-bear-down" movement that is automatically performed during strenuous **exercise**. It is thought that this maneuver temporarily siphons blood from the temporal lobes of the brain. The temporal lobes are where the memories are stored. This loss of blood may induce the loss of memory by persons experiencing TGA. While this hypothesis is still under review, it has been accepted as a logical explanation for a condition that currently has no generally accepted causal explanation.

Description

Transient global amnesia was first identified and described around 1960. Since that time, there have been extensive writings and studies about the condition, but its etiology (causation) is still not clearly known or understood.

TGA affects memory function. People experiencing TGA can register information and there is no loss of social skills and sense of identity, but their ability to retain information is severely impaired. One of the puzzling associations with TGA is that many people who experience this disorder are also migraine **headache** sufferers. However, there is no report of a migraine prior to onset, nor is there any reported nausea, sensitivity to light or sound, or headache.

Demographics

There are no race or inherited conditions associated with TGA. Men experience the condition more often than women. In addition, the occurrence of this type of amnesia rarely happens before middle age, with about 12 out of 100,000 people ever experiencing the condition before age 50. The most likely ages in which to experience TGA are the 50s and 60s. About 3% of people who experience one episode of TGA will experience another episode sometime during their lifetime, but it is very rare for a person to experience more than three episodes of TGA.

The reason people in their 50s and 60s are more likely to experience TGA is not understood. No definitive links to any particular pathology or reaction to medication have been discovered. It is an elusive medical experience. For example, the connection of TGA with exposure to cold water cannot be explained in any convincing way. However, the condition has, as one of its major triggers, the exposure to cold water as in swimming, or prolonged exposure to cold rain or snow.

Causes and symptoms

The causes of this disorder are not yet fully understood. The hypotheses that the event is triggered by a temporary loss of blood to certain regions of the brain are most popular. In some cases, there is evidence of small strokes and local evidence of minor depressions on the surface of the brain. A well-accepted hypothesis suggests that blood is reduced to the temporal region of the brain during Valsalva, or weight-bearing movement.

People who have experienced TGA are also screened for current use of medications. Some drug interactions have been known to cause other types of amnesia, although not the type associated with TGA.

Another suggestion as a cause for TGA is that venous congestion (congested blood flow in the veins) inhibits blood flow to the thalamic or temporal regions of the brain. The support for this hypothesis is that increases in sympathetic nervous system activity and/or pressure within the thorax may exert pressure on the jugular veins. This, in turn, may disrupt arterial blood flow within the brain, resulting in ischemia (lack of oxygen) to memory

Key Terms

Amnesia   A general medical term for loss of memory that is not due to ordinary forgetfulness. Amnesia can be caused by head injuries, brain disease, or epilepsy, as well as by dissociation. Includes: 1) Anterograde amnesia: inability to retain the memory of events occurring after the time of the injury or disease which brought about the amnesic state. 2) Retrograde amnesia: inability to recall the memory of events which occurred prior to the time of the injury or disease which brought about the amnesic state.

Anterograde amnesia   Amnesia for events that occurred after a physical injury or emotional trauma but before the present moment.

Retrograde amnesia   Amnesia for events that occurred before a traumatic injury.

Valsalva maneuver   A strain against a closed airway combined with muscle tightening, such as happens when a person holds his or her breath and tries to move a heavy object. Most people perform this maneuver several times a day without adverse consequences, but it can be dangerous for anyone with cardiovascular disease. Pilots perform this maneuver to prevent black-outs during high-performance flying.

centers or other areas of the brain. While the common precipitating factors have been discussed, why these events might trigger a TGA episode are not well understood.

Diagnosis

TGA is sometimes a difficult condition to diagnose. It is extremely helpful for an observer to contribute information to the physician. Some of the criteria for identifying the event are the impairment of memory, both newly learned and past. There is no loss of consciousness or personal identity. There must be no recent experience of head trauma. Patients must not be epileptics nor can they have experienced any form of a seizure in the last two years.

The episode usually lasts for only a few hours and is usually completely resolved by the end of 24 hours. However, rare cases have been documented in which the patient experiences the amnesia for up to a month.

Anterograde amnesia, which sometimes also follows head trauma, is a component of TGA. With the anterograde types of amnesia, the person experiences a memory

loss of recent experiences, however, long-term memory persists. Persons with anterograde amnesia often ask questions and, after receiving a response, immediately ask the same question again. Physicians examining a person with amnesia will rule out retrograde amnesia, which is not a part of TGA. Retrograde amnesia is somewhat the opposite of anterograde amnesia, whereby the affected person can remember events that occur after the head trauma, but not before.

With TGA, a person experiences temporary confusion and lack of memory. The person is disoriented and confused, but no loss of personal identity occurs and long-term memories are intact. The person may be frightened and sometimes mildly delusional, but this passes soon and the incidence of recurrence is rare.

The initial kinds of tests a physician will request are those that rule out infection, **stroke**, brain injury, and other physiological conditions.

Blood tests such as a CBC with differential help to rule out infection. Another test often performed is running an electrolyte panel. Eletrolytes are common salt minerals such as potassium, calcium, magnesium, etc. Most professional and amateur athletes are aware of how important proper electrolyte balances are for proper body functioning. A lowering of electrolytes may cause some of the symptoms described by a person experiencing TGA. Other types of blood tests, including the search for clotting potentials, are often performed. To determine whether the patient may be prone to blood clotting, a physician may request a pothrombin time (PT) and activated partial thromboplastin time (aPTT). Quick clotting times could indicate a propensity towards thrombosis (blood clotting), which could lead to stroke.

Part of the diagnosis involves conducting several types of imaging tests. The uses of **positron emission tomography (PET)** and diffusion-weighted **magnetic resonance imaging** (MRI-DWI) have shown a small degree of ischemia (lack of blood flow) to certain areas of the brain with TGA. However, these same tests have shown conflicting results in other patients. No definitive tests have been suggested to diagnose the condition.

Treatment team

Initially, most persons with TGA receive care from a physician in a hospital emergency department. A **neurologist** usually provides diagnosis and treatment. Both physicians usually order tests to differentiate TGA from other acute neurological events such as a stroke. As there is really no specific treatment for TGA, diagnosis and reassurance by a physician are important for a person experiencing TGA, as well as for family members.

Treatment

After ruling out trauma to the brain from accident, disease, or stroke, most people who have experienced TGA receive very little treatment because the condition is benign. A follow-up appointment with the neurologist is usually recommended.

Recovery and rehabilitation

Expected average times for recovery are within hours. A TGA patient rarely experiences the symptoms any longer than 24 hours. For most people, the condition lasts only 4–8 hours. Many people even report a shorter duration of one or two hours of disorientation and confusion. They may become frightened, but this is often alleviated with diagnosis and an explanation of the condition.

Prognosis

The prognosis for TGA patients is excellent. There are no debilitating side effects or any permanent loss of memory. TGA does not portend a serious stroke or similar condition involving the circulatory system. This is one of the reasons that TGA is such a perplexing syndrome for researchers; it is impossible to predict who will experience it. Because repeat occurrences are rare, numerous re-evaluations by a physician are usually not necessary.

Special concerns

It is important for people to be aware of the possibility of TGA. Seeking medical help, personal protection, and reassurance are the beneficial to offer someone displaying TGA symptoms.

Resources

BOOKS

Adams, R. D., M. Victor, and A. H. Ropper. "Transient Global Amnesia." In *Principles of Neurology.* New York: McGraw-Hill, 1997.

PERIODICALS

Simons, Jon S. and John R. Hodges. "Previous Cases: Transient Global Amnesia." *Neurocases* (2000): 6, 211–230.

OTHER

Tuen, Charles. Neuroland. *Transient Global Amnesia.* January 4, 2004 (March 24, 2004). <http://neuroland.com/sands/tga.htm>.

ORGANIZATIONS

National Institute for Neurological Disorders and Stroke. P.O. Box 5801, Bethesda, MD 20824. (301) 496-5761 or (800) 352-9424. <http://www.ninds.nih.gov>.

Brook Ellen Hall

Transient ischemic attack

Definition

A transient ischemic attack (TIA), or "mini-stroke," is a neurologic episode resembling a **stroke** but resolving completely within a short period of time. By definition, symptoms of TIA resolve within 24 hours, and symptoms lasting longer than that are termed a stroke. A TIA is caused by brief interruption of the blood supply to a specific brain region, and it may warn of impending stroke.

Description

Symptoms of TIA begin suddenly and are similar to those of stroke, but leave no residual damage. By definition, symptoms of TIA resolve within 24 hours, but typically they last less than five minutes, or about one minute on average.

The symptoms of TIA vary depending on what part of the brain is affected. Anterior circulation TIAs interrupt the blood supply to most of the front part of the brain known as the cerebrum, including the frontal, parietal, and temporal lobes.

Symptoms suggesting anterior circulation TIAs may include difficulty speaking or understanding speech. Blindness in one eye suggests amaurosis fugax, a type of TIA caused by decreased blood flow through the carotid artery. This large artery in the neck supplies blood to the optic nerve responsible for vision in the eye on the same side as the artery.

Posterior circulation TIAs involve the blood supply to the back part of the brain, including the occipital lobe, **cerebellum**, and brainstem. Symptoms suggesting posterior circulation TIAs include loss of consciousness, **dizziness**, ringing in the ears, and loss of coordination. Because nerve pathways involved in motor function and sensation pass through multiple brain regions, symptoms of weakness and numbness may occur with either anterior or posterior circulation TIAs.

Demographics

Every year in the United States, approximately 50,000 individuals experience a TIA, and about one-third of these patients will go on to have a stroke at some point in the future.

TIAs rarely affect persons younger than 60 years of age. For individuals 50 to 59 years of age, the incidence of TIA is estimated to be four to eight episodes per 1,000 persons per year.

In addition to advancing age, other factors increasing risk of TIA are a history of TIA or stroke in a family member, and black race, thought to be in part because of the higher rates of high blood pressure and diabetes in this group. Although the risk of TIA in older men and women is approximately equal, younger men have a slightly higher risk of stroke than do women of the same age.

In a study from the Mayo Clinic reported in *Stroke* in 1998, the incidence of TIA in Rochester, Minnesota, from 1985 to 1989 was 16 cases per year per 100,000 people aged 45 to 54 years. After adjusting for age and sex, the incidence rate for any TIA was 68 per 100,000 people. These rates had not changed significantly from those determined during the years 1960 to 1972, suggesting no improvement in risk factors predisposing to TIA during the intervening time period.

In that study, about three-fifths of TIAs affected the anterior circulation, about one-fifth were amaurosis fugax, and the remaining one-fifth affected the posterior circulation. The incidence rate of TIA was 41% of the rate of stroke incidence, and it was higher than had been previously reported for other sites throughout the world.

Causes and symptoms

The symptoms of a TIA occur when there is temporary blockage of an artery supplying part of the brain, causing ischemia, or not enough blood supply to provide the brain with the oxygen and nutrients it needs to function properly. The ischemia does not last long enough to cause permanent damage as would occur with a stroke. When the arterial blockage is reversed, the symptoms of the TIA go away.

The underlying causes of the arterial blockage are the same for both TIAs and strokes. The most common cause is a buildup of atherosclerotic plaques, or fatty deposits containing cholesterol, in the wall of the artery.

Damage to the arterial lining may cause platelets to stick together around the injured area as a normal part of the clotting and healing process. When cholesterol and other fats are deposited in this area, a plaque forms within the lining of the artery and narrows the channel through which blood passes. This causes blood flow to slow down and become irregular, which increases the natural tendency of blood to clot.

If a thrombus, or clot, forms at the site of the plaque, it may block the blood vessel at that location. Pieces of the plaque or thrombus may break off and travel downstream to progressively narrower arteries, forming an embolus that can temporarily block these arteries and cause a TIA until it dissolves or is dislodged. In a similar fashion, an embolus moving to the brain from the heart or elsewhere in the body can also cause a TIA.

Diseases that increase the tendency of blood to clot may cause TIAs. These include cancer, disorders of blood clotting, sickle cell anemia, and hyperviscosity syndromes in which the blood is very thick.

Injury to or inflammation of blood vessels may cause them to narrow or to go into spasm. Inflammation affecting the blood vessels is called arteritis, with specific examples including fibromuscular dysplasia, polyarteritis, granulomatous angiitis, systemic **lupus** erythematosus, and syphilis.

In patients with atherosclerotic plaques, conditions which can increase the risk of TIA include low blood pressure, high blood pressure, heart disease, migraine headaches, smoking, diabetes, and increasing age.

The symptoms of TIA come on suddenly and can be the same as those of a stroke, except that they disappear rapidly, always within 24 hours and usually within five minutes, without leaving any permanent brain injury.

Because it is impossible to tell until the symptoms are over whether they were related to a TIA or a stroke, it is crucial to take these symptoms as a serious warning and to seek immediate medical attention. If the blood flow to part of the brain is interrupted for a sufficient length of time, nerve cells supplied by the affected blood vessel may die. Any delay in starting stroke treatment can result in additional irreversible brain damage or even death.

Symptoms of either TIA or stroke vary depending on what brain region is affected. Numbness, weakness, or a heavy sensation on one side of the face, arm, and/or leg usually represents an anterior circulation stroke or TIA, whereas these symptoms on both sides suggest posterior circulation stroke or TIA.

Confusion, garbled speech, or other difficulty in talking or in understanding speech may occur with decreased anterior circulation affecting the left half of the brain (in right-handed individuals). Difficulty with vision in one eye, often described as a curtain descending over the eye, is a classic symptom of amaurosis fugax. On the other hand, decreased vision involving both eyes usually indicates a posterior circulation disturbance.

Other symptoms of posterior circulation stroke or TIA may include loss of consciousness, dizziness, loss of balance and coordination, and vertigo (a sensation that the person or the room is moving). A sudden, severe **headache** with no known cause may occur with any stroke or TIA.

Diagnosis

The characteristic history or description of a TIA, with its sudden onset, rapid resolution, and typical symptoms, aid the doctor in diagnosis. Risk factors for atherosclerosis, such as smoking, heart disease, high blood pressure, and family history of heart disease or stroke also suggest the diagnosis of TIA. The specific symptoms associated with the TIA will help the physician determine which portion of the brain and which blood vessels were involved.

By the time the person who had a TIA reaches medical attention, the neurological examination is usually normal, although there may be subtle signs related to previous strokes.

The general physical examination may indicate evidence of atherosclerotic plaques, such as a bruit or abnormal sound heard with the stethoscope placed over the carotid artery in the neck. Although an audible bruit may be present in the early stages of arterial narrowing when blood flow is turbulent, the sound may disappear when blood flow decreases further. Looking at the back of the eye through an instrument called an ophthalmoscope, the doctor may see cholesterol emboli in the tiny arteries of the retina.

Carotid **ultrasonography** helps determine if there is narrowing, also known as stenosis, or plaque formation in the carotid arteries. In this painless and harmless test, a transducer sends high-frequency sound waves into the neck, and deflections of these waves are analyzed as images on a screen.

Computed tomography (**CT**) scanning creates cross-sectional x-ray images of the brain. The CT may show strokes, but often fails to give sufficiently detailed views of the blood vessels. To improve blood vessel visualization, computerized tomography **angiography** (CTA) scanning uses injection of a contrast dye into a blood vessel.

Magnetic resonance imaging (MRI) uses a strong magnetic field to align water molecules in the brain, giving highly detailed cross-sectional images that are very good at detecting small strokes. Magnetic resonance angiography (MRA) uses similar technology to study the arteries in the neck and brain.

The clearest way to see the structure, course, and diameter of brain arteries is with arteriography. Unfortunately, this test is associated with a low rate of serious complications including bleeding, stroke, and even death. Therefore, it should be performed only if the results would change patient management, for example in guiding the decision of whether surgery is needed.

In this test, a radiologist inserts a thin catheter, or flexible tube, through a small groin incision into the large femoral artery supplying the leg. Using x-ray guidance, the radiologist threads the catheter through the major arteries and into the carotid or vertebral artery. An injection of contrast dye through the catheter then allows x-ray images of the arteries in the anterior or posterior circulation.

If the heart is thought to be the source of emboli causing the TIA, testing may include an electrocardiogram and

Holter monitoring to detect any changes in heart rhythm, or arrhythmias, occurring during the course of a normal day's activities. After the technician attaches electrodes to the patient's chest, the patient can go home overnight with a portable tape recorder. The recordings are later analyzed for arrthymias, during which emboli might tend to leave the heart and cause TIAs.

Transesophageal echocardiography (TEE) allows clear, detailed ultrasound images of blood clots within the heart which could act as a source of emboli, but which might be missed by traditional echocardiography. During this test, the doctor passes a flexible probe containing a transducer into the esophagus, which is located directly behind the heart.

Other tests may determine if there are any underlying conditions causing TIA, including blood tests for arteritis, sickle cell anemia, diabetes, and hyperviscosity syndromes. Certain procedures may help to rule out other disorders that may cause symptoms resembling those of TIA.

For example, an electroencephalogram (EEG) may determine if there is abnormal electrical activity of the brain diagnostic of a **seizure** disorder, because the symptoms associated with some seizures may resemble those of a TIA. Other conditions that may be confused with TIA include **fainting** or migraine headache.

A study reported in the October 2003 issue of *Clinical Chemistry* describes a blood test which may help to diagnose TIA and to rule out bleeding into the brain, or intracerebral hemorrhage, which can sometimes be confused with TIA. The test analyzes antibodies to specialized receptors involved in communication between nerve cells. These N-methyl-D-aspartate receptor antibodies are thought to be key markers of nerve cell damage caused by lack of blood flow to the brain.

Treatment team

Because time is so critical in preventing damage from acute stroke, and because it is impossible to tell right away whether symptoms of brain ischemia are caused by TIA or acute stroke, the treatment team begins with those who are first aware of the symptoms.

The patient and their family must take these symptoms as a serious warning of impending neurologic disaster and seek immediate medical attention by calling 911, rather than by hoping the symptoms will go away. Public awareness of stroke symptoms and their significance is therefore just as important as knowing that crushing chest **pain** needs to be evaluated right away in the emergency room to rule out or to treat heart attack.

The emergency medical technician, internist, **neurologist**, cardiologist, and diagnostic technicians all play an important role in TIA management. At stroke centers

Key Terms

Amaurosis fugax A type of TIA caused by decreased blood flow through the carotid artery, characterized by blindness or decreased vision in one eye.

Anterior circulation The blood supply to most of the front part of the brain known as the cerebrum, including the frontal, parietal, and temporal lobes.

Antiplatelet agents Drugs that reduce the tendency of platelets to clump together, used to reduce the risk of TIA or stroke.

Atherosclerotic plaques Fatty deposits containing cholesterol that build up in the wall of arteries, causing narrowing and increased risk of TIA.

Atrial fibrillation A condition in which part of the heart is enlarged and beats irregularly, which may cause emboli to travel to the brain.

Bruit An abnormal sound heard with the stethoscope placed over the carotid artery in the neck, suggesting decreased blood flow through the vessel.

Carotid angioplasty (stenting) Surgery for carotid artery stenosis using a balloon-like device to open the clogged artery, followed by placing a stent, or small wire tube, within the artery to keep it open.

Carotid artery A large artery in the neck supplying blood to the brain.

Carotid endarterectomy Surgery for carotid artery stenosis in which the atherosclerotic plaques are removed through a neck incision.

Carotid ultrasonography A painless and harmless test using high-frequency sound waves to determine if there is narrowing or plaque formation in the carotid arteries.

Embolus A fragment of plaque or thrombus that breaks off from its original location and travels downstream to progressively narrower arteries, where it may block the vessel.

Ischemia Reduced blood supply to the brain, preventing it from getting the oxygen and nutrients it needs to function properly.

Posterior circulation The blood supply to the back part of the brain, including the occipital lobe, cerebellum, and brainstem.

Stenosis Narrowing of an artery which reduces blood flow through the vessel.

Thrombus A blood clot, which may form at the site of an atherosclerotic plaque and block the artery.

Transesophageal echocardiography (TEE) A test using sound waves to reveal blood clots or other abnormalities within the heart that might be missed by traditional echocardiography.

and larger hospitals, members of a specialized stroke team designated for rapid response may be the first health care professionals to see the patient with TIA.

Other providers who may become involved in helping the patient reduce their risk factors for TIA and stroke may include nutritionists, dieticians, and nurses specializing in lifestyle counseling for issues such as quitting smoking.

Neurosurgeons or vascular surgeons will become involved in management of the patient with carotid artery stenosis if surgery is needed to restore blood flow or to bypass the obstruction.

Treatment

Ideally, patients with symptoms suggesting TIA or acute stroke should be evaluated within 60 minutes. Even if the symptoms resolve by the time the patient reaches the emergency room, prompt evaluation is needed to identify the specific cause of the TIA and to begin appropriate treatment.

Patients who have had a TIA within 48 hours are usually admitted to the hospital for observation, diagnostic testing, and treatment planning in a controlled situation, in case the TIA recurs or a stroke develops. If there are any medical conditions causing the TIA, such as sickle cell anemia or arteritis, these should be treated.

Drugs that reduce the tendency of platelets to clump together, known as antiplatelet agents, may reduce the risk of future TIA or stroke. Within this drug class, aspirin is the most often prescribed, least expensive, and safest treatment in terms of possible side effects. Although the optimal dose of aspirin to prevent stroke and TIA has long been debated, there may not be a clear dose-response relationship.

Other antiplatelet agents include dipyridamole; Aggrenox, which is a combination of low-dose aspirin and dipyridamole; clopidogrel (Plavix), which may be given alone or together with aspirin; and ticlopidine (Ticlid).

If the medical evaluation reveals a condition called atrial fibrillation, in which part of the heart is enlarged and beats irregularly, causing emboli to travel to the brain, blood thinners or anticoagulants may be prescribed. These drugs inhibit proteins involved in blood clotting but do not affect platelet function.

Warfarin (Coumadin) is the best known drug of this class for long-term use, whereas heparin is typically given only for a limited period, usually while the patient is still in the hospital. Because anticoagulants reduce blood clotting and hence TIAs, they can also cause serious bleeding. Drug levels must therefore be monitored with blood tests usually done at least once weekly.

Atrial fibrillation or other conditions in which the heart beats erratically, known as arrythmias, may be treated with antiarrhythmic agents that stabilize electrical impulses in the heart to allow a more regular heart beat.

A vital part of TIA treatment is to reduce treatable risk factors for stroke, including cardiovascular disease, smoking, diabetes, hyperlipidemia, and obesity. Heart disease caused by previous heart attack, abnormalities of the heart valve, and arrythmias may prevent the heart from pumping blood efficiently.

Cigarette smoking increases blood clotting and accelerates development of atherosclerotic plaques. Nicotine makes the heart work harder by increasing heart rate and blood pressure, and carbon monoxide in cigarette smoke decreases the amount of oxygen reaching the brain.

In a similar fashion to smoking, diabetes makes atherosclerosis worse and speeds its progression, as do high blood levels of low-density lipoprotein (LDL) cholesterol and low levels of high-density lipoprotein (HDL) cholesterol.

Increased homocysteine level is another risk factor for atherosclerosis that may be treatable. This amino acid occurs naturally in the blood, but in high concentrations it can cause arterial walls to become thicker and scarred, increasing the chances of plaque formation.

Supplementing the diet with B complex vitamins including B6, B12, and folic acid reduces blood levels of homocysteine and may protect against heart disease, but it is not yet known whether this will reduce stroke risk.

High blood pressure, heart disease, diabetes, and undesirable cholesterol levels may require treatment with specific drugs, or they may be controlled by lifestyle changes alone.

Whether or not medications are needed, lifestyle changes should include stopping smoking, weight control, avoiding heavy drinking, and eating a balanced diet low in saturated fats, salt, and sugar and high in vegetables, fruits, and fiber. Nutritional or lifestyle counseling, structured **exercise** programs, and/or support groups may help patients achieve these goals.

If carotid artery testing reveals moderate or severe narrowing or stenosis, surgery may be indicated to improve blood flow and prevent future stroke or TIA. Usually, there is a reduction in artery diameter of more than 70% before surgery is considered. The portion of the artery downstream from the site of blockage also needs to be relatively free of narrowing or obstruction for surgery to be successful.

Carotid endarterectomy involves opening the artery through a neck incision, removing atherosclerotic plaques, then closing the artery. In some cases, carotid angioplasty or stenting may be a viable alternative. Using a balloon-like device, the surgeon opens the clogged artery and then places a stent, or small wire tube, within the artery to keep it open.

According to a study by the Carotid Endarterectomy Trialists' Collaboration, published in the November 2003 issue of *Stroke,* blood pressure control needs to be more closely regulated in patients with **carotid stenosis** than in other patients. Overly aggressive reduction of blood pressure in these patients may actually decrease blood flow through the obstructed artery.

Clinical trials

The National Institutes of Neurological Disorder and Stroke (NINDS) is the primary sponsor of research on stroke and TIA in the United States, including patient studies and laboratory research into the biological mechanisms of strokes.

The NINDS is recruiting patients for a study evaluating whether a specific type of carotid artery surgery can reduce subsequent stroke risk in high-risk patients who have recently suffered from stroke or TIA. The surgical procedure, known as extracranial-intracranial bypass surgery, involves removing an artery from the scalp, making a small hole in the skull, and then connecting the scalp artery to a brain artery within the skull. By circumventing the carotid artery obstruction in the neck, the rationale is to provide more blood flow to the brain. Contact information is William J. Powers, MD, 314-362-3317 or wjp@npg.wustl.edu.

Another study for which the NINDS is recruiting patients is the "Aspirin or Warfarin to Prevent Stroke" study, designed to determine whether aspirin or warfarin is more effective in preventing stroke in patients with narrowing of one of the arteries in the brain. Contact information is Harriet Howlett Smith, RN, 1-404-778-3153 or hhowlet@emory.edu.

The pharmaceutical company AstraZeneca is currently recruiting patients for a study testing the safety and effectiveness of their drug NXY-059 when given within six hours of limb weakness suggesting TIA or acute stroke. Contact information is the AstraZeneca Information Center, 800-236-9933.

Prognosis

A single TIA is by definition very brief, and recovery is complete, but that good outcome should not lull the patient into a false sense of security. After a first TIA, additional episodes may occur later on the same day or at some point in the future. Ironically, patients who recover substantially within 24 hours of acute brain ischemia may be at greater risk of subsequent neurological deterioration than those who take longer to recover, according to a report in the October 2003 issue of the *Annals of Neurology.*

TIAs are an ominous sign of increased risk for debilitating stroke. Although most strokes are not preceded by TIAs, approximately one-third of patients who have a TIA will have an acute, major stroke days, weeks, or even months later. About half of the time, the stroke occurs within one year of the TIA. Stroke risk is higher in a person who has had one or more TIAs than in someone of the same age and sex who has never suffered a TIA.

Even among patients given antiplatelet agents or anticoagulants after a TIA or stroke, 10% will have a stroke within 90 days. Stroke can have devastating consequences, as it is the third leading cause of death and the primary cause of disability in the United States.

Besides recurrent TIA and stroke, complications of TIA may include injury from falls, if the patient becomes weak or loses balance with the TIA, or bleeding from anticoagulant drugs used to treat the TIA.

Although a single episode of TIA is not fatal, the TIA reflects generalized atherosclerosis. The leading cause of death after a TIA is coronary artery disease causing a heart attack. For that reason, a patient with TIA should have a heart evaluation to determine cardiovascular risk and decide on management of potential coronary artery disease.

Special concerns

Preventing TIA is a worthwhile goal, especially since the same strategies will help prevent heart disease, stroke, high blood pressure, and diabetes. Healthy lifestyle, regular medical checkups, stopping smoking, avoiding alcohol and illegal drugs, regular exercise, and nutritionally sound diet all have additional benefits beyond their effects on cardiovascular and stroke risk.

When the symptoms of TIA strike, it is no time to be brave or stoic. It is a medical emergency demanding that 911 or other local emergency number be called immediately. Even if the symptoms resolve, they are an urgent warning that must not be ignored, and require immediate attention to prevent stroke. Having a TIA may in some ways be a blessing in disguise if the warning is heeded, as most patients who suffer a stroke do so without this warning sign.

Because the symptoms of TIA cannot be distinguished from those of acute stroke, these symptoms must be aggressively treated as soon as possible. Research suggests that emergency care of stroke within the first three to six hours of the first symptom may greatly reduce the disabling, long-term effects of stroke. Sadly, the average time elapsed between experiencing the first symptoms of stroke and seeking medical attention is 13 hours, and 42% of patients wait as long as 24 hours. Recognizing the symptoms of stroke and obtaining immediate emergency care can prevent disability and even death.

Resources
PERIODICALS
Adams, Harold P. Jr., Robert J. Adams, Thomas Brott, et al. "Guidelines for the Early Management of Patients with Ischemic Stroke." *Stroke* 34 (2003): 1056-1083.

Brown, R. D. Jr., G. W. Petty, W. M. O'Fallon, et al. "Incidence of Transient Ischemic Attack in Rochester, Minnesota, 1985-1989." *Stroke* 29, no. 10 (October 1998): 2109-13.

Dambinova, S. A., G. A. Khounteev, G. A. Izykenova, et al. "Blood Test Detecting Autoantibodies to N-Methyl-D-Aspartate Neuroreceptors for Evaluation of Patients with Transient Ischemic Attack and Stroke." *Clinical Chemistry* 49, no. 10 (October 2003): 1752-62.

Goldstein, Larry B., Robert Adams, Kyra Becker, et al. "Primary Prevention of Ischemic Stroke." *Circulation* 32 (2001): 280-299.

Johnson, E. S., S. F. Lanes, C. E. Wentworth, et al. "A Metaregression Analysis of the Dose-Response Effect of Aspirin on Stroke." *Archives of Internal Medicine* 159 (June 14, 1999): 1248-53.

Johnston, S. C., E. C. Leira, M. D. Hansen, and H. P. Adams Jr. "Early Recovery After Cerebral Ischemia Risk of Subsequent Neurological Deterioration." *Annals of Neurology* 54, no. 4 (October 2003): 439-44.

Rothwell, P. M., S. C. Howard, and J. D. Spence. "Relationship Between Blood Pressure and Stroke Risk in Patients with Symptomatic Carotid Occlusive Disease." *Stroke* 34, no. 11 (November 2003): 2583-90.

Scott, P. A., and R. Silbergleit. "Misdiagnosis of Stroke in Tissue Plasminogen Activator-Treated Patients: Characteristics and Outcomes." *Annals of Emergency Medicine* 42, no. 5 (November 2003): 611-18.

WEBSITES
American Heart Association. <http://www.americanheart.org>.
Clinical Trials. <http://www.clinicaltrials.gov/ct/action/GetStudy>.
eMedicine. <http://www.emedicine.com/emerg/byname/transient-ischemic-attack.htm>.
Mayo Clinic. <http://www.mayoclinic.com/invoke.cfm?id=DS00220>.

National Institute of Neurological Disorders and Stroke. NIH
   Neurological Institute. <http://www.ninds.nih.gov/
   health_and_medical/disorders/tia_doc.htm>.
National Stroke Association. <http://www.stroke.org>.
U.S. National Library of Medicine. <http://www.nlm.nih.gov/
   medlineplus/transientischemicattack.html>.

Laurie Barclay

Transmissible spongiform encephalopathies
   see **Prion diseases**

Transverse myelitis

Definition

Transverse myelitis is an inflammation of the full
width of the spinal cord that disrupts communication to
the muscles, resulting in **pain**, weakness, and muscle
paralysis.

Description

The symptoms of transverse myelitis are due to damage and/or destruction of the myelin sheath, the fatty white
covering of nerve fibers that serves both to insulate the
nerve fibers and to speed nervous conduction along them.
Areas of missing myelin and areas of scarring along the
affected nerves result in slowed or disrupted nervous conduction and muscle dysfunction.

Transverse myelitis may have a gradual onset or a remarkably quick onset. Symptoms of transverse myelitis
may reach their peak within 24 hours of onset for some patients (considered the hyperacute form of the condition).
Other patients experience a more gradual increase in symptom severity, with peak deficits occurring days (acute form
of transverse myelitis) to weeks (subacute form of transverse myelitis) after the initial symptoms first presented.
Patients with the quicker onset form and who experience
more severe initial symptoms tend to have more complications and a greater likelihood of permanent disability.

Transverse myelitis often occurs in people who are recovering from a recent viral illness, including chickenpox,
herpes simplex, cytomegalovirus, Epstein-Barr, influenza,
and measles. When this association is present, the condition often follows the more sudden hyperacute course.

Demographics

In the United States, there are only about 4.6 cases of
transverse myelitis per million people per year. In the
Unites States, about 1,400 people a year develop transverse myelitis; about 33,000 people in the United States
have disabilities due to transverse myelitis. Individuals of

all ages can be affected; reports have been made of patients ranging from the age of six months to 88 years. The
peak ages appear to be 10-19 years and 30-39 years.

About 30-60% of all cases of transverse myelitis
occur in individuals who have just recovered (within the
previous 8 weeks) from a relatively minor viral infection.
Recent vaccination is another risk factor for transverse
myelitis. Other individuals at higher risk for transverse
myelitis include patients with preexisting autoimmune diseases (such as **multiple sclerosis**, systemic **lupus** erythematosus, or Devic's disease); patients with recent histories
of infections such as **Lyme disease**, tuberculosis, or
syphilis; and intravenous drug abusers who inject heroine
and/or amphetamines.

Causes and symptoms

Although the specific mechanism of transverse
myelitis has not been delineated, the basic cause is thought
to be an autoimmune response. Under normal conditions,
the immune system reacts to the presence of a viral or bacterial illness by producing a variety of immune cells designed to attack the invading viruses or bacteria.
Unfortunately, in the case of transverse myelitis, the immune cells mistake the body's own tissues as foreign, and
attack those tissues as well. These errant immune cells are
called autoantibodies; that is, antibodies that actually attack the body's own tissues.

Symptoms of transverse myelitis can develop over
several hours, days, or weeks. The types of symptoms and
their severity are dependent on the area of the spinal cord
affected. When the transverse myelitis occurs in the neck,
the arms and legs will be affected; when the transverse
myelitis occurs lower in the back, only the legs will be
affected.

Symptoms of transverse myelitis often begin with
back pain, **headache**, achy muscles, flu-like symptoms,
and stiff neck. Over hours or days, symptoms expand to include loss of sensation, numbness, dysesthesia (sensations
of burning, lightning flashes of pain, prickly pinpoints),
muscle weakness, partial or complete paralysis, and impaired bladder and bowel function. Symptoms of weakness and then paralysis usually begin in the feet, ascending
over time to the legs, and then to the trunk and arms when
the lesion is in the neck. Symptoms are bilateral, meaning
that they affect both sides of the body simultaneously.
Over time, muscles become increasingly tight and spastic,
further limiting mobility. When the muscles of respiration
are affected, breathing can be compromised.

Diagnosis

Diagnosis involves meeting specific symptom criteria, as well as demonstrating spinal cord involvement with
MRI scanning and examination of cerebrospinal fluid.

Key Terms

Myelin The fatty white substance that wraps around nerve fibers, providing insulation and speeding electrical conduction of nerve impulses along the fibers.

Symptom criteria include the evolution of symptoms peaking over four hours to 21 days, with symptoms clearly traceable to spinal cord dysfunction, and including muscle weakness or paralysis and sensory defects such as numbness occurring on both sides of the body. The presence of a spinal cord tumor or another condition that is exerting pressure on the spinal cord, vitamin B12 deficiency, or a history of **radiation** therapy to or cyclophosphamide injection into the spinal cord excludes the possibility of a diagnosis of transverse myelitis.

Treatment team

The mainstay of the treatment team for patients with transverse myelitis will be a **neurologist**. A rheumatologist, specializing in autoimmune illness, may also be consulted. In order to regain maximum function, a physiatrist (a physician specializing in rehabilitation medicine) may be required, as well as the services of both physical and occupational therapists.

Treatment

Treatment is aimed at calming the immune response that caused the **spinal cord injury** in the first place. To this end, high doses of intravenous and then oral steroids are the first-line treatments for transverse myelitis. In severe cases of transverse myelitis, the very potent immunosupressant cyclophosphamide may be administered. In patients with moderately severe transverse myelitis unimproved by five to seven days of steroid treatment, a procedure called plasma exchange may be utilized. This procedure involves removing blood from the patient, and separating it into the blood cells and the plasma (fluid). The blood cells are then mixed into a synthetic plasma replacement solution and returned to the patient. Because the immune cells are in the plasma, this effectively removes the damaging immune cells from the body, hopefully quelling the myelin destruction.

Treatments to reverse the process involved in transverse myelitis should be attempted for about six months from the onset of the condition. After that point, treatment efforts should be shifted to effective rehabilitation.

Pain and other **dysesthesias** (uncomfortable sensations, such as burning, pins-and-needles, or electric shock sensations) are treated with a variety of medications, such as **gabapentin**, **carbamazepine**, nortriptyline, or tramadol. Another treatment for pain and dysesthesias is transcutaneous electrical nerve stimulation, called TENS therapy. This involves the use of a device that stimulates the painful area with a small electrical pulse, which seems to disrupt the painful sensation.

Because constipation and urinary retention are frequent problems in the patient with transverse myelitis, medications may be necessary to treat these problems. Oxybutinin, hyoscyamine, tolterodine, and propantheline can treat some of the bladder problems common to transverse myelitis patients. When urinary retention is an issue, sacral nerve stimulation may help the patient avoid repeated bladder catheterizations. Dulcolax, senekot, and bisacodyl can help improve constipation.

Tight, spastic muscles may improve with baclofen, tizanidine, or **diazepam**. When these medications are given orally, they sometimes result in untenable side effects.

Recovery and rehabilitation

Rehabilitation has both short- and long-term components. Even in the earliest stages of the condition, passive exercises should be performed. Passive exercises involve a physical therapist putting a particular muscle group or joint through range of motion and strengthening **exercise**, even when the patient cannot assist in its movement. During the recovery phase, the patient should be given progressive exercises to improve strength and range of motion, and to attempt to regain mobility. Physical therapists can also be helpful with pain management, using such techniques as heat and/or cold application, nerve stimulation, ultrasound, and massage. Physical therapy may also be helpful to retrain muscles necessary for improved bladder and bowel control and relief of constipation and urinary retention. Occupational therapists can help the patient relearn old skills for accomplishing the activities of daily living, or strategize new techniques that take into account the patient's disabilities.

Braces or assistive devices such as walkers, wheelchairs, crutches, or canes may be necessary during rehabilitation or permanently.

Prognosis

The area on the spinal cord affected by transverse myelitis will determine the individual's level of functioning. The higher-up the lesion, the greater the disability. High cervical lesions will require complete care; as lesions drop lower and lower in the cervical, thoracic, or lumbar region, the chance to participate in self-care or even to ambulate increases.

Recovery from transverse myelitis seems to follow the law of thirds: about a third of all patients make a full recovery from their level of functioning at the condition's peak, a third make a partial recovery, and a third make no recovery at all. Most patients make a good or even a complete recovery within one to three months of the onset of their symptoms. Patients who have not begun to improve by month three after symptom onset usually will not accomplish a complete recovery from their disability. Factors that do not bode well include abrupt onset of symptoms, prominent pain upon onset, and severe disability and deficit at the peak of the condition.

Resources

BOOKS

Aminoff, Michael J. "Inflammatory disorders affecting the spinal cord." In *Cecil Textbook of Internal Medicine*, edited by Lee Goldman, et al. Philadelphia: W. B. Saunders Company, 2000.

Schneider, Deborah Ross. "Transverse Myelitis." In *Essentials of Physical Medicine and Rehabilitation*, 1st ed., edited by Walter R. Frontera. Philadelphia: Hanley and Belfus, 2002.

PERIODICALS

Transverse Myelitis Consortium Working Group. "Proposed diagnostic criteria and nosology of acute transverse myelitis." In *Neurology* 59, no. 4 (27 August 2002): 499–505

WEBSITES

National Institute of Neurological Disorders and Stroke (NINDS). *NINDS Transverse Myelitis Information Page.* July 1, 2001 (June 10, 2004). <http://www.ninds.nih.gov/health_and_medical/disorders/transversemyelitis_doc.htm>.

ORGANIZATIONS

Transverse Myelitis Association. 1787 Sutter Parkway, Powell, OH 43065. (614) 766-1806. ssiegel@myelitis.org. <http://www.myelitis.org/index.html>.

The Johns Hopkins Transverse Myelitis Center. 600 N. Wolfe Street, Baltimore, MD 21287. (410) 502-7099; Fax: (410) 502-6736. dkerr@jhmi.edu. <http://www.hopkinsmedicine.org/jhtmc/>.

Rosalyn Carson-DeWitt, MD

▌Traumatic brain injury

Definition

Traumatic brain injury (TBI) is the result of physical trauma to the head causing damage to the brain. This damage can be focal, or restricted to a single area of the brain, or diffuse, affecting more than one region of the brain. By definition, TBI requires that there be a head injury, or any physical assault to the head leading to injury of the scalp, skull, or brain. However, not all head trauma is associated with TBI.

Description

TBI is sometimes known as acquired brain injury. The least severe and most common type of TBI is termed a concussion, which is technically defined as a brief loss of consciousness after a head injury without any physical evidence of damage on an imaging study such as a **CT** or **MRI** scan. In common parlance, concussion may refer to any minor injury to the head or brain.

Symptoms, complaints, and neurological or behavioral changes following TBI depend on the location(s) of the brain injury and on the total volume of injured brain. Usually, TBI causes focal brain injury involving a single area of the brain where the head is struck or where an object such as a bullet enters the brain. Although damage is typically worst at the point of direct impact or entry, TBI may also cause diffuse brain injury involving several other brain regions.

Closed head injury refers to TBI in which the head is hit by or strikes an object without breaking the skull. In a penetrating head injury, an object such as a bullet fractures the skull and enters brain tissue.

Diffuse brain damage associated with closed head injury may result from back-and-forth movement of the brain against the inside of the bony skull. This is sometimes called coup-contrecoup injury. "Coup," or French for "blow," refers to the brain injury directly under the point of maximum impact to the skull. "Contrecoup," or French for "against the blow," refers to the brain injury opposite the point of maximum impact.

For example, coup-contrecoup injury may occur in a rear-end collision, with high speed stops, or with violent shaking of a baby, because the brain and skull are of different densities, and therefore travel at different speeds. The impact of the collision causes the soft, gelatinous brain tissue to jar against bony prominences on the inside of the skull.

Because of the location of these prominences and the position of the brain within the skull, the frontal lobes (behind the forehead) and temporal lobes (underlying the temples) are most susceptible to this type of diffuse damage. These lobes house major brain centers involved in speech and language, so problems with communication skills often follow closed head injuries of this type.

Depending on which areas of the brain are injured, other symptoms of closed head injury may include difficulty with concentration, memory, thinking, swallowing, walking, balance, and coordination; weakness or paralysis; changes in sensation; and alteration of the sense of smell.

Consequences of TBI can be relatively subtle or completely devastating, related to the severity and mechanism of injury. Diffuse axonal injury, or shear injury, may follow contrecoup injury even if there is no damage to the skull or obvious bleeding into the brain tissue. In this type of injury, damage to the part of the nerve that communicates with other nerves degenerates and releases harmful substances that can damage neighboring nerves.

When the skull cracks or breaks, the resulting skull fracture can cause a contusion, or an area of bruising of brain tissue associated with swelling and blood leaking from broken blood vessels. A depressed skull fracture occurs when fragments of the broken skull sink down from the skull surface and press against the surface of the brain. In a penetrating skull fracture, bone fragments enter brain tissue. Either of these types of skull fracture can cause bruising of the brain tissue, called a contusion. Contrecoup injury can also lead to brain contusion.

If the physical trauma to the head ruptures a major blood vessel, the resulting bleeding into or around the brain is called a hematoma. Bleeding between the skull and the dura, the thick, outermost layer covering the brain, is termed an **epidural hematoma**. When blood collects in the space between the dura and the arachnoid membrane, a more fragile covering underlying the dura, it is known as a **subdural hematoma**. An intracerebral hematoma involves bleeding directly into the brain tissue.

All three types of hematomas can damage the brain by putting pressure on vital brain structures. Intracerebral hematomas can cause additional damage as toxic breakdown products of the blood harm brain cells, cause swelling, or interrupt the flow of cerebrospinal fluid around the brain.

Demographics

Estimates for the number of Americans living today who have had a TBI range from between 2.5 and 6.5 million, making it a major public health problem costing the United States more than $48 billion annually. A recent review suggests that the incidence of TBI in the United States is between 180 and 250 per 100,000 population per year, with even higher incidence in Europe and South Africa.

Although TBI can affect anyone at any age, certain age groups are more vulnerable because of lifestyle and other risk factors. Males ages 15 to 24, especially those in lower socioeconomic levels, are most likely to become involved in high-speed or other risky driving, as well as physical fights and criminal activity. These behaviors increase the likelihood of TBI associated with automobile and motorcycle accidents or with violent crimes.

Infants, children under five years of age, and adults 75 years and older are also at higher risk for TBI than the general population because they are most susceptible to falls around the home. Other factors predisposing the very young and the very old to TBI include physical abuse, such as violent shaking of an infant or toddler that can result in **shaken baby syndrome**.

Causes and symptoms

Accidents, especially motor vehicle accidents, are the major culprit implicated in TBI. Because accidents are the leading cause of death or disability in men under age 35, and because over 70% of accidents involve injuries of the head and/or spinal cord, this is not surprising. In fact, transportation accidents involving automobiles, motorcycles, bicycles, and pedestrians account for half of all TBIs and for the majority of TBIs in individuals under the age of 75. At least half of all TBIs are associated with alcohol use. Sports injuries cause about 3% of TBIs; other accidents leading to TBI may occur at home, at work, or outdoors.

In those age 75 and older, falls are responsible for most TBIs. Other situations leading to TBI at all ages include violence, implicated in about 20% of TBIs. Firearm assaults are involved in most violent causes of TBI in young adults, whereas child abuse is the most common violent cause in infants and toddlers. In the shaken baby syndrome, a baby is shaken with enough force to cause severe countrecoup injury.

The symptoms of TBI may occur immediately or they may develop slowly over several hours, especially if there is slow bleeding into the brain or gradual swelling. Depending on the cause, mechanism, and extent of injury, the severity of immediate symptoms of TBI can be mild, moderate, or severe, ranging from mild concussion to deep coma or even death.

With concussion, the injured person may experience a brief or transient loss of consciousness, much like **fainting** or passing out, or merely an alteration in consciousness described as "seeing stars" or feeling dazed or "out of it." On the other hand, coma refers to a profound or deep state of unconsciousness in which the individual does not respond to the environment in any meaningful way.

When a person with TBI regains consciousness, some symptoms are immediately apparent, while others are not noticed until several days or weeks later. Symptoms which may be obvious right away after mild TBI include **headache**, changes in vision such as blurred vision or tired eyes, nausea, **dizziness**, lightheadedness, ringing in the ears, bad taste in the mouth, or altered sense of smell which is usually experienced as loss of the sense of taste.

Approximately 40% of patients with TBI develop postconcussion syndrome within days to weeks, with symptoms including headache, dizziness or a sensation of spinning (vertigo), memory problems, trouble concentrating, sleep disturbances, restlessness, irritability, **depression**, and anxiety. This syndrome may persist for a few weeks, especially in patients with depression, anxiety, or other psychiatric symptoms before the TBI.

With more severe injuries, there may also be immediate numbness or weakness of one or more limbs, blindness, deafness, inability to speak or understand speech, slurred speech, lethargy with difficulty staying awake, persistent vomiting, loss of coordination, disorientation, or agitation. In addition to some of these symptoms, young children with moderate to severe TBI may also experience prolonged crying and refusal to nurse or eat.

While the injured person is preoccupied with headache or **pain** related to other physical trauma, symptoms such as difficulty in thinking or concentrating may not be evident. Often these more subtle symptoms may appear only when the individual attempts to return to work or to other mentally challenging situations. Similarly, personality changes, depression, irritability, and other emotional and behavioral problems may initially be attributed to coping with the stress of the injury, and they may not be fully appreciated until the individual is recuperating at home.

Seizures may occur soon after a TBI or may first appear up to a year later, especially when the damage involves the temporal lobes. Other symptoms which may appear immediately or which may be noticed only while the individual is returning to usual activities are confusion, **fatigue** or lethargy, altered sleep patterns, and trouble with memory, concentration, attention, and finding the right words or understanding speech.

Diagnosis

Recognizing a serious head injury, starting basic first aid, and seeking emergency medical care can help the injured person avoid disability or even death. When encountering a potential TBI, it is helpful to find out what happened from the injured person, from clues at the scene, and from any eyewitnesses. Because **spinal cord injury** often accompanies serious head trauma, it is prudent to assume that there is also injury to the spinal cord and to avoid moving the person until the paramedics arrive. Spinal cord injury is a challenging diagnosis; nearly one-tenth of spinal cord injuries accompanying TBI are missed initially.

Signs apparent to the observer that suggest serious head injury and mandate emergency treatment include shallow or erratic breathing or pulse; drop in blood pressure; broken bones or other obvious trauma to the skull or face such as bruising, swelling or bleeding; one pupil larger than the other; or clear or bloody fluid drainage from the nose, mouth, or ears.

Symptoms reported by the injured person that should also raise red flags include severe headache, stiff neck, vomiting, paralysis or inability to move one or more limbs, blindness, deafness, or inability to taste or smell. Other ominous developments may include initial improvement followed by worsening symptoms; deepening lethargy or unresponsiveness; personality change, irritability, or unusual behavior; or incoordination.

When emergency personnel arrive, they will stabilize the patient, evaluate the above signs and symptoms, and assess the nature and extent of other injuries, such as broken bones, spinal cord injury, or damage to other organ systems. Medical advances in early detection and treatment of associated injuries have improved the overall outcome in TBI. The initial evaluation measures vital signs such as temperature, blood pressure, pulse, and breathing rate, while the neurological examination assesses reflexes, level of consciousness, ability to move the limbs, and pupil size, symmetry, and response to light.

These neurological features are standardized using the Glasgow Coma Scale, a test scored from 1 to 15 points. Each of three measures (eye opening, best verbal response, and best motor response) is scored separately, and the combined score helps determine the severity of TBI. A total score of 3 to 8 reflects a severe TBI, 9 to 12 a moderate TBI, and 13 to 15 a mild TBI.

Imaging tests reveal the location and extent of brain injury and associated injuries and therefore help determine diagnosis and probable outcome. Sophisticated imaging tests can help differentiate the variety of unconscious states associated with TBI and can help determine their anatomical basis.

Until neck fractures or spinal instability have been ruled out with skull and neck x rays, and with head and neck computed tomography (CT) scan for more severe injuries, the patient should remain immobilized in a neck and back restraint.

By constructing a series of cross-sectional slices, or x ray images through the head and brain, the CT scan can diagnose bone fractures, bleeding, hematomas, contusions, swelling of brain tissue, and blockage of the **ventricular system** circulating cerebrospinal fluid around the brain. In later stages after the initial injury, it may also show shrinkage of brain volume in areas where neurons have died.

Using magnetic fields to detect subtle changes in brain tissue related to differences in water content, the magnetic resonance imaging (MRI) scan shows more detail than x rays or CT. However, it takes more time than the CT and is not as readily available, making it less suited for routine emergency imaging.

For patients with seizures or for those with more subtle episodic symptoms thought possibly to be seizures, the

Key Terms

Cerebrospinal fluid (CSF) A protective fluid surrounding and protecting the brain and spinal cord.

Closed head injury TBI in which the head strikes or is struck by an object without breaking the skull.

Coma A decreased level of consciousness with deep unresponsiveness.

Computed tomography (CT) scan A neuroimaging test that generates a series of cross-sectional x rays of the head and brain.

Concussion Injury to the brain causing a sudden, temporary impairment of brain function.

Contrecoup An injury to the brain opposite the point of direct impact.

Contusion A focal area of swollen and bleeding brain tissue.

Dementia pugilistica "Punch-drunk" syndrome of brain damage caused by repeated head trauma.

Depressed skull fracture A fracture in which fragments of broken skull press into brain tissue.

Diffuse axonal injury (shear injury) Traumatic damage to individual nerve cells resulting in breakdown of overall communication between nerve cells in the brain.

Epidural hematoma Bleeding into the area between the skull and the dura, the tough, outermost brain covering.

Glasgow coma scale A measure of level of consciousness and neurological functioning after TBI.

Hematoma Bleeding into or around the brain caused by trauma to a blood vessel in the head.

Intracerebral hematoma Bleeding within the brain caused by trauma to a blood vessel.

Increased intracranial pressure Increased pressure in the brain following TBI.

Magnetic resonance imaging (MRI) A noninvasive neuroimaging test using magnetic fields to visualize water shifts in brain tissue.

Penetrating head injury TBI in which an object pierces the skull and enters brain tissue.

Post-concussion syndrome A complex of symptoms including headache following mild TBI.

Post-traumatic amnesia (PTA) Difficulty forming new memories after TBI.

Post-traumatic dementia Persistent mental deterioration following TBI.

Post-traumatic epilepsy Seizures occurring more than one week after TBI.

Shaken baby syndrome A severe form of TBI resulting from shaking an infant or small child forcibly enough to cause the brain to jar against the skull.

Subdural hematoma Bleeding between the dura and the underlying brain covering.

Ventriculostomy Surgery that drains cerebrospinal fluid from the brain to treat hydrocephalus or increased intracranial pressure.

electroencephalogram (EEG) may reveal abnormalities in the electrical activity of the brain or brain waves. Other diagnostic techniques that may be helpful include cerebral **angiography**, transcranial Doppler ultrasound, and single photon emission computed tomography (SPECT).

Treatment team

The first responder at the scene of TBI is usually a paramedic or emergency medical technician (EMT). In the emergency department, a trauma specialist may determine the extent of associated injuries. The **neurologist** is usually the primary treating physician assessing and managing the symptoms and consequences of TBI. Diagnostic technicians involved in TBI management include radiological and EEG technicians and audiologists who assess hearing.

If surgery is needed to remove blood clots or to insert a shunt to relieve increased pressure within the skull, a neurosurgeon is needed. After surgery, or for any patient with loss of consciousness, intensive care is managed by a specialized treatment team including neurologists, neurosurgeons, intensivists, respiratory therapists, and specialized nurses and technicians.

After the physical condition has stabilized, a speech therapist and/or **neuropsychologist** may evaluate swallowing, cognitive, and behavioral abilities and carry out appropriate rehabilitation. Other specialized therapists include the occupational therapist, who addresses sensory deficits, hand movements, and the ability to perform activities of daily living such as dressing; and the physical therapist who directs **exercise** and other programs to rehabilitate weakness annd loss of coordination. Vocational planners, psychologists, and psychiatrists may help the individual with TBI cope with returning to society and to gainful employment.

Treatment

Although no specific treatment may be needed for a mild head injury, it is crucial to watch the person closely for any developing symptoms over the next 24 hours. Acetaminophen or ibuprofen, available over the counter, may be used for mild headache. However, aspirin should not be given because it can increase the risk of bleeding.

If the person is sleeping, he should be awakened every two to three hours to determine alertness and orientation to name, time, and place. Immediate medical help is needed if the person becomes unusually drowsy or disoriented, develops a severe headache or stiff neck, vomits, loses consciousness, or behaves abnormally.

Treatment for moderate or severe TBI should begin as soon as possible by calling 911 and beginning emergency care until the EMT team arrives. This includes stabilizing the head and neck by placing the hands on both sides of the person's head to keep the head in line with the spine and prevent movement which could worsen spinal cord injury. Bleeding should be controlled by firmly pressing a clean cloth over the wound unless a skull fracture is suspected, in which case it should be covered with sterile gauze dressing without applying pressure. If the person is vomiting, the head, neck, and body should be rolled to the side as one unit to prevent choking without further injuring the spine.

Although the initial brain damage caused by trauma is often irreversible, the goal is to stabilize the patient and prevent further injury. To achieve these goals, the treatment team must insure adequate oxygen supply to the brain and the rest of the body, maintain blood flow to the brain, control blood pressure, stabilize the airway, assist in breathing or perform CPR if necessary, and treat associated injuries.

About half of severely head-injured patients require neurosurgery for hematomas or contusions. Swelling of the injured brain may cause increased pressure within the closed skull cavity, known as increased intracranial pressure (ICP). ICP can be measured with a intraventricular probe or catheter inserted through the skull into the fluid-filled chambers (ventricles) within the brain. Placement of the ICP catheter is usually guided by CT scan. If ICP is elevated, ventriculostomy may be needed. This procedure drains cerebrospinal fluid from the brain and reduces ICP. Drugs that may decrease ICP include mannitol and barbiturates.

A recent review suggests that using intraventricular catheters coated with antibiotics reduces the risk for infection. Keeping the patient's body temperature low (hypothermia) also improves outcome after moderate to severe TBI. Increasing the level of oxygen in the blood beyond normal concentrations is also being explored as a treatment option for improving brain metabolism in TBI. Large, multicenter trials of these and other treatments, such as early surgery to relieve increased ICP, are still needed, and the quest continues for a therapy that could prevent nerve cell death in TBI.

Although some patients need medication for psychiatric and physical problems resulting from the TBI, prescribing drugs may be problematic because TBI patients are more sensitive to side effects.

Both in the immediate and later stages of TBI, rehabilitation is vital to optimal recovery of ability to function at home and in society. The Consensus Development Conference on Rehabilitation of Persons with TBI, held by the National Institutes of Health in 1998, recommended individualized rehabilitation based on specific strengths and abilities.

Problems with orientation, thinking, and communication should be addressed early, often during the hospital stay. The focus is typically on improving alertness, attention, orientation, speech understanding, and swallowing problems.

As the patient improves, rehabilitation should be modified accordingly. The panel suggested that physical therapy, occupational therapy, speech/language therapy, physiatry (physical medicine), psychology/psychiatry, and social support should all play a role in TBI rehabilitation. Appropriate settings for rehabilitation may include the home, the hospital outpatient department, inpatient rehabilitation centers, comprehensive day programs, supportive living programs, independent living centers, and school-based programs. Families should become involved in rehabilitation, in modifying the home environment if needed, and in psychotherapy or counseling as indicated.

Clinical trials

The National Institute of Neurological Disorders and Stroke (NINDS) supports research on the biological mechanisms of brain injury, strategies to limit brain damage following head trauma, and treatments of TBI that may improve long-term recovery. Research areas include mechanisms of diffuse axonal injury; the role of calcium entry into damaged nerves causing cell death and brain swelling; the toxic effects of glutamate and other nerve chemicals causing excessive nerve excitability; natural processes of brain repair after TBI; the therapeutic use of cyclosporin A or hypothermia to decrease cell death and nerve swelling; and the use of stem cells to repair or replace damaged brain tissue.

NINDS-supported clinical research focuses on enhancing the ability of the brain to adapt to deficits after TBI; improving rehabilitation programs for TBI-related disabilities; and developing treatments for use in the first hours after TBI. Early treatments being investigated include hypothermia for severe TBI in children, magnesium sulfate to protect nerve cells after TBI, and lowering ICP and increasing blood flow to the brain.

To address the specific problems in thinking and communication following TBI, the NINDS is designing new evaluation tools for children, developing computer programs to help rehabilitate children with TBI, and determining the effects of various medications on recovery of speech, language, and cognitive abilities.

The NINDS website (www.clinicaltrials.gov/ct/action/GetStudy) lists specific contact information for ongoing trials. These include hypothermia to treat severe brain injury, open to subjects age 16 to 45 years with non-penetrating brain injury with a post-resuscitation Glasgow Coma Score less than 8 (contact Emmy R. Miller, PhD, RN, 713-500-6145).

The Prospective Memory in Children with Traumatic Brain Injury study is open to children age 12-18 years, with a post-resuscitation Glasgow Coma Scale score of either 13 to 15 or 3 to 8. Contact information is Stephen R. McCauley, PhD, 713-798-7479, mccauley@bcm.tmc.edu.

The Measuring Head Impacts in Sports study will test a new device to measure the speed of head impact in football players. The study is open to college football players, age 18–24 years. Contact information is Rick Greenwald, PhD, RGreenwald@simbex.com.

A trial sponsored by Avanir Pharmaceuticals will be testing the safety of the drug AVP-923 in the treatment of uncontrolled laughter and crying associated with TBI as well as with other conditions. Study subjects must be age 18–75 years without any history of major psychiatric disturbance. Contact information varies by state and is available on the website; for Arizona it is Louis DiCave, 602-406-6292, ldicave@chw.edu.

Prognosis

Although the symptoms of minor head injuries often resolve on their own, more than 500,000 head injuries each year are severe enough to require hospitalization; 200,000 are fatal; and 200,000 require institutionalization or other close supervision. Each year in the United States, head injury causes one million head-injured people to be treated in hospital emergency rooms, 270,000 to have moderate or severe TBI, 70,000 to die, and 60,000 to develop **epilepsy**.

Outcome varies with cause: 91% of TBIs caused by firearms, two-thirds of which may represent suicide attempts, are fatal, compared with only 11% of TBIs from falls. Low Glasgow Coma Scale scores predict a worse outcome from TBI than do high scores.

The Swedish Council on Technology Assessment in Health Care concluded that of 1,000 patients arriving at the hospital with mild head injury, one will die, nine will require surgery or other intervention, and about 80 will have abnormal findings on brain CT and will probably need to be hospitalized.

Immediate complications of TBI may include seizures, enlargement of the fluid-filled chambers within the brain (**hydrocephalus** or post-traumatic ventricular enlargement), leaks of cerebrospinal fluid, infection, injury to blood vessels or to the nerves supplying the head and neck, pain, bed sores, failure of multiple organ systems, and trauma to other areas of the body.

About one-quarter of patients with brain contusions or hematomas and about half of those with penetrating head injuries develop seizures within the first 24 hours of the injury. Those that do are at increased risk of seizures occurring within one week after TBI.

Hydrocephalus usually occurs within the first year of TBI, and it is associated with deteriorating neurological outcome, impaired consciousness, behavioral changes, poor coordination or balance, loss of bowel and bladder control, or signs of increased ICP.

Long-term survivors of TBI may suffer from persistent problems with behavior, thinking, and communication disabilities, as well as epilepsy; loss of sensation, hearing, vision, taste, or smell; ringing in the ears (tinnitus), coordination problems, and/or paralysis. Recovery from cognitive deficits is most dramatic within the first six months after TBI, and less apparent subsequently.

Memory loss is especially common in severely head-injured patients, with loss of some specific memories and partial inability to form or store new memories. Anterograde post-traumatic amnesia refers to impaired memory of events that occurred after TBI, while retrograde post-traumatic amnesia refers to impaired memory of events that occurred before the TBI.

Personality changes and behavioral problems may include depression, anxiety, irritability, anger, apathy, paranoia, frustration, agitation, mood swings, aggression, impulsive behaviors or "acting out," social inappropriateness, temper tantrums, difficulty accepting responsibility, and alcohol or drug abuse.

Following TBI, patients may be at increased risk of other long-term problems such as **Parkinson's disease**, **Alzheimer's disease**, "punch-drunk" syndrome (**dementia** pugilistica), and post-traumatic dementia.

Because of all the above problems, some patients may have difficulty returning to work following TBI, as well as problems with school, driving, sports, housework, and social relationships.

Special concerns

Unlike most other devastating neurological diseases, TBI can be prevented. Practical measures to decrease risk include wearing seatbelts, using child safety seats, wearing helmets for biking and other sports, safely storing firearms and bullets; using step-stools, grab bars, handrails, window guards, and other safety devices; making playground surfaces from shock-absorbing material; and not drinking and driving.

Because TBI follows trauma, it is often associated with injuries to other parts of the body, which require immediate and specialized care. Complications may include lung or heart dysfunction following blunt chest trauma, limb fractures, gastrointestinal dysfunction, fluid and hormonal imbalances, nerve injuries, deep vein thrombosis, excessive blood clotting, and infections.

Resources

PERIODICALS

Arzaga, D., V. Shaw, and A. T. Vasile. "Dual Diagnoses: The Person with a Spinal Cord Injury and a Concomitant Brain Injury." *Spinal Cord Injury Nursing* 20, no. 2 (Summer 2003): 86-92.

Bruns, J. Jr, and W. A. Hauser. "The Epidemiology of Traumatic Brain Injury: A Review." *Epilepsia* 44, Supplement 10 (2003): 2-10.

Chisholm, J., and B. Bruce. "Unintentional Traumatic Brain Injury in Children: The Lived Experience." *Axone* 23, no. 1 (September 2001): 12-17.

Geijerstam, J. L., and M. Britton. "Mild Head Injury— Mortality and Complication Rate: Meta-analysis of Findings in a Systematic Literature Review." *Acta Neurochirugica (Wien)* 145, no. 10 (October 2003): 843-50.

Gunnarsson, T., and M. G. Fehlings. "Acute Neurosurgical Management of Traumatic Brain Injury and Spinal Cord Injury." *Current Opinion in Neurology* 16, no. 6 (December 2003): 717-23.

Krotz, M., U. Linsenmaier, K. G. Kanz, K. J. Pfeifer, W. Mutschler, and M. Reiser. "Evaluation of Minimally Invasive Percutaneous CT-Controlled Ventriculostomy in Patients with Severe Head Trauma." *European Radiology* (November 6, 2003).

Reitan, R. M., and D. Wolfson. "The Two Faces of Mild Head Injury." *Archives of Clinical Neuropsychology* 14, no. 2 (February 1999): 191-202.

WEBSITES

National Institute of Neurological Disorders and Stroke. NIH Neurological Institute. <http://www.ninds.nih.gov/health_and_medical/pubs/TBI.htm#research>.

National Institute on Deafness and Other Communication Disorders. National Institutes of Health. <http://www.nidcd.nih.gov/health/voice/tbrain.asp>.

U.S. National Library of Medicine. <http://www.nlm.nih.gov/medlineplus/ency/articl/000028.htm>.

Clinical Trials. <http://www.clinicaltrials.gov/ct/action/GetStudy>.

Laurie Barclay

Tremors

Definition

Tremor is an unintentional (involuntary) rhythmical alternating movement that may affect the muscles of any part of the body. Tremor is caused by the rapid alternating contraction and relaxation of muscles and is a common symptom of diseases of the nervous system (neurologic disease).

Description

Occasional tremor is felt by almost everyone, usually as a result of fear or excitement. However, uncontrollable tremor or shaking is a common symptom of disorders that destroy nerve tissue such as **Parkinson's disease** or **multiple sclerosis**. Tremor may also occur after **stroke** or **head injury**. Other tremor appears without any underlying illness.

Causes and symptoms

Tremor may be a symptom of an underlying disease, and it may be caused by drugs. It may also exist as the only symptom (essential tremor).

Underlying disease

Some types of tremor are signs of an underlying condition. About a million and a half Americans have Parkinson's disease, a disease that destroys nerve cells. Severe shaking is the most apparent symptom of Parkinson's disease. This coarse tremor features four to five muscle movements per second. These movements are evident at rest but decline or disappear during movement.

Other disorders that cause tremor are **multiple sclerosis**, Wilson's disease, mercury **poisoning**, thyrotoxicosis, and **liver encephalopathy**.

A tremor that gets worse during body movement is called an intention tremor. This type of tremor is a sign

Key Terms

Computed tomography (CT) scan An imaging technique in which cross-sectional x rays of the body are compiled to create a three-dimensional image of the body's internal structures.

Essential tremor An uncontrollable (involuntary) shaking of the hands, head, and face. Also called familial tremor because it is a sometimes inherited, it can begin in the teens or in middle age. The exact cause is not known.

Fetal tissue transplantation A method of treating Parkinson's and other neurological diseases by grafting brain cells from human fetuses onto the affected area of the human brain. Human adults cannot grow new brain cells but developing fetuses can. Grafting fetal tissue stimulates the growth of new brain cells in affected adult brains.

Intention tremor A rhythmic purposeless shaking of the muscles that begins with purposeful (voluntary) movement. This tremor does not affect muscles that are resting.

Liver encephalopathy A condition in which the brain is affected by a buildup of toxic substances that would normally be removed by the liver. The condition occurs when the liver is too severely damaged to cleanse the blood effectively.

Multiple sclerosis A degenerative nervous system disorder in which the protective covering of the nerves in the brain are damaged, leading to tremor and paralysis.

Magnetic resonance imaging (MRI) An imaging technique that uses a large circular magnet and radio waves to generate signals from atoms in the body. These signals are used to construct images of internal structures.

Pallidotomy A surgical procedure that destroys a small part of a tiny structure within the brain called the globus pallidus internus. This structure is part of the basal ganglia, a part of the brain involved in the control of willed (voluntary) movement of the muscles.

Parkinson's disease A slowly progressive disease of that destroys nerve cells. Parkinson's is characterized by shaking in resting muscles, a stooping posture, slurred speech, muscular stiffness, and weakness.

Thalamotomy A surgical procedure that destroys part of a large oval area of gray matter within the brain that acts as a relay center for nerve impulses. The thalamus is an essential part of the nerve pathway that controls intentional movement. By destroying tissue at a particular spot on the thalamus, the surgeon can interrupt the nerve signals that cause tremor.

Thalamus A large oval area of gray matter within the brain that relays nerve impulses from the basal ganglia to the cerebellum, both parts of the brain that control and regulate muscle movement.

Thyrotoxicosis An excess of thyroid hormones in the blood causing a variety of symptoms that include rapid heart beat, sweating, anxiety, and tremor.

Tremor control therapy A method for controlling tremor by self-administered shocks to the part of the brain that controls intentional movement (thalamus). An electrode attached to an insulated lead wire is implanted in the brain; the battery power source is implanted under the skin of the chest, and an extension wire is tunneled under the skin to connect the battery to the lead. The patient turns on the power source to deliver the electrical impulse and interrupt the tremor.

Wilson's disease An inborn defect of copper metabolism in which free copper may be deposited in a variety of areas of the body. Deposits in the brain can cause tremor and other symptoms of Parkinson's disease.

---

that something is amiss in the **cerebellum**, a region of the brain concerned chiefly with movement, balance, and coordination.

Essential tremor

Many people have what is called essential tremor, in which the tremor is the only symptom. This type of shaking affects between three and four million Americans.

The cause of essential tremor is not known, although it is an inherited problem in more than half of all cases. The genetic condition has an autosomal dominant inheritance pattern, which means that any children of an affected parent will have a 50% chance of developing the condition.

Essential tremor most often appears when the hands are being used, whereas a person with Parkinson's disease will most often have a tremor while walking or while the hands are resting. People with essential tremor will usually have shaking head and hands, but the tremor may involve other parts of the body. The shaking often begins in the dominant hand and may spread to the other hand, interfering with eating and writing. Some people also develop a quavering voice.

Essential tremor affects men and women equally. The shaking often appears at about age 45, although the disorder may actually begin in adolescence or early adulthood. Essential tremor that begins very late in life is sometimes called senile tremor.

Drugs and tremor

Several different classes of drugs can cause tremor as a side effect. These drugs include amphetamines, antidepressants drugs, antipsychotic drugs, caffeine, and lithium. Tremor also may be a sign of withdrawal from alcohol or street drugs.

Diagnosis

Close attention to where and how the tremor appears can help provide a correct diagnosis of the cause of the shaking. The source of the tremor can be diagnosed when the underlying condition is found. Diagnostic techniques that make images of the brain, such as computed tomography scan (**CT scan**) or **magnetic resonance imaging** (**MRI**), may help form a diagnosis of multiple sclerosis or other tremor caused by disorders of the **central nervous system**. Blood tests can rule out metabolic causes such as thyroid disease. A family history can help determine whether the tremor is inherited.

Treatment

Neither tremor nor most of its underlying causes can be cured. Most people with essential tremor respond to drug treatment, which may include propranolol, **primidone**, or a benzodiazepine. People with Parkinson's disease may respond to levodopa or other **antiparkinson drugs**.

Research has shown that about 70% of patients treated with **botulinum toxin** A (Botox) have some improvement in tremor of the head, hand, and voice. Botulinum is derived from the bacterium *Clostridium botulinum*. This bacterium causes **botulism**, a form of **food poisoning**. It is poisonous because it weakens muscles. A very weak solution of the toxin is used in cases of tremor and **paralysis** to force the muscles to relax. However, some patients experience unpleasant side effects with this drug and cannot tolerate effective doses. For other patients, the drug becomes less effective over time. About half of patients don't get relief of tremor from medications at all.

Tremor control therapy

Tremor control therapy is a type of treatment using mild electrical pulses to stimulate the brain. These pulses block the brain signals that trigger tremor. In this technique, the surgeon implants an electrode into a large oval area of gray matter within the brain that acts as a relay center for nerve impulses and is involved in generating movement (thalamus). The electrode is attached to an insulated wire that runs through the brain and exits the skull where it is attached to an extension wire. The extension is connected to a generator similar to a heart pacemaker. The generator is implanted under the skin in the chest, and the extension is tunneled under the skin from the skull to the generator. The patient can control his or her tremor by turning the generator on with a hand-held magnet to deliver an electronic pulse to the brain.

Some patients experience complete relief with this technique, but for others it is of no benefit at all. About 5% of patients experience complications from the surgical procedure, including bleeding in the brain. The procedure causes some discomfort, because patients must be awake while the implant is placed. Batteries must be replaced by surgical procedure every three to five years.

Other surgical treatments

A patient with extremely disabling tremor may find relief with a surgical technique called thalamotomy, in which the surgeon destroys part of the thalamus. However, the procedure is complicated by numbness, balance problems, or speech problems in a significant number of cases.

Pallidotomy is another type of surgical procedure sometimes used to decrease tremors from Parkinson's disease. In this technique, the surgeon destroys part of a small structure within the brain called the globus pallidus internus. The globus is part of the basal ganglia, another part of the brain that helps control movement. This surgical technique also carries the risk of disabling permanent side effects.

Fetal tissue transplantation (also called a nigral implant) is a controversial experimental method to treat Parkinson's disease symptoms. This method implants fetal brain tissue into the patient's brain to replace malfunctioning nerves. Unresolved issues include how to harvest the fetal tissue and the moral implications behind using such tissue, the danger of tissue rejection, and how much tissue may be required. Although initial studies using this technique looked promising, there has been difficulty in consistently reproducing positive results.

Small amounts of alcohol may temporarily (sometimes dramatically) ease the shaking. Some experts recommend a small amount of alcohol (especially before dinner). The possible benefits, of course, must be weighed against the risks of alcohol abuse.

Prognosis

Essential tremor and the tremor caused by neurologic disease (including Parkinson's disease) slowly get worse and can interfere with a person's daily life. While the condition is not life-threatening, it can severely disrupt a person's everyday experiences.

Prevention

Essential tremor and tremor caused by a disease of the central nervous system cannot be prevented. Avoiding use of stimulant drugs such as **caffeine** and amphetamines can prevent tremor that occurs as a side effect of drug use.

Resources

BOOKS

Greenberg, David A., et al. *Clinical Neurology.* 2nd ed. Norwalk, CT: Appleton & Lange, 1993.

Weiner, William J., and Christopher Goetz. "Essential Tremor." In *Neurology for the Non-Neurologist.* Philadelphia: J. B. Lippincott, 1994.

ORGANIZATIONS

American Academy of Neurology. 1080 Montreal Ave., St. Paul, MN 55116. (612) 695-1940. <http://www.aan.com>.

American Parkinson Disease Association. 60 Bay Street, Suite 401, Staten Island, NY 10301. (800) 223-2732. <http://www.apdaparkinson.org>.

International Tremor Foundation. 7046 West 105th St., Overland Park, KS 66212. (913) 341-3880.

National Parkinson Foundation. 1501 N.W. 9th Ave., Miami, FL 33136-1494. (800) 327-4545. <http://www.parkinson.org>.

Carol A. Turkington

❙ Trigeminal neuralgia

Definition

Trigeminal neuralgia is a disorder of the trigeminal nerve that causes severe facial **pain**. It is also known as tic douloureux, Fothergill syndrome, or Fothergill's syndrome.

Description

Trigeminal neuralgia is a rare disorder of the sensory fibers of the trigeminal nerve (fifth cranial nerve), which innervate the face and jaw. The neuralgia is accompanied by severe, stabbing pains in the jaw or face, usually on one side of the jaw or cheek, which usually last for some seconds. The pain before treatment is severe; however, trigeminal neuralgia as such is not a life-threatening condition. As there are actually two trigeminal nerves, one for each side of the face, trigeminal neuralgia often affects only one side of the face, depending on which of the two trigeminal nerves is affected.

Demographics

There have been no systematic studies of the prevalence of trigeminal neuralgia, but one widely quoted estimate published in 1968 states that its prevalence is approximately 15.5 per 100,000 persons in the United States. Other sources state that the annual incidence is four to five per 100,000 persons, which would imply a higher prevalence (prevalence is the number of cases in a population at a given time; incidence is the number of new cases per year). In any case, the disorder is rare. Onset is after the age of 40 in 90% of patients. Trigeminal neuralgia is slightly more common among women than men.

Causes and symptoms

A number of theories have been advanced to explain trigeminal neuralgia, but none explains all the features of the disorder. The trigeminal nerve is made up of a set of branches radiating from a bulblike ganglion (nerve center) just above the joint of the jaw. These branches divide and subdivide to innervate the jaw, nose, cheek, eye, and forehead. Sensation is conveyed from the surfaces of these parts to the upper spinal cord and then to the brain; motor commands are conveyed along parallel fibers from the brain to the muscles of the jaw. The sensory fibers of the trigeminal nerve are specialized for the conveyance of cutaneous (skin) sensation, including pain.

In trigeminal neuralgia, the pain-conducting fibers of the trigeminal nerve are somehow stimulated, perhaps self-stimulated, to send a flood of impulses to the brain. Many physicians assume that compression of the trigeminal nerve near the spinal cord by an enlarged loop of the carotid artery or a nearby vein triggers this flood of impulses. Compression is thought to cause trigeminal neuralgia when it occurs at the root entry zone, a .19–.39 in (0.5–1.0 cm) length of nerve where the type of myelination changes over from peripheral to central. Pressure on this area may cause demyelination, which in turn may cause abnormal, spontaneous electrical impulses (pain).

Compression is apparently the cause in some cases of trigeminal neuralgia, but not in others. Other theories focus on complex feedback mechanisms involving the subnucleus caudalis in the brain. **Multiple sclerosis**, which demyelinates nerve fibers, is associated with a higher rate of trigeminal neuralgia. Brain tumors can also be correlated with the occurrence of trigeminal neuralgia. Ultimately, however, the exact mechanisms of trigeminal neuralgia remain a mystery.

Trigeminal neuralgia was first described by the Arab physician Jurjani in the eleventh century. Jurjani was also

Key Terms

Anticonvulsant Class of medications usually prescribed to prevent seizures.

Demyelination Destruction or loss of the myelin (a fatty substance) sheath that surrounds and insulates the axons of nerve cells and is necessary for the proper conduction of neural impulses.

Neuralgia Pain along the pathway of a nerve.

Trigeminal nerve The main sensory nerve of the face and motor nerve for chewing muscles.

the first physician to advance the vascular compression theory of trigeminal neuralgia. French physician Nicolaus André gave a thorough description of trigeminal neuralgia in 1756 and coined the term tic douloureux. English physician John Fothergill also described the syndrome in the middle 1700s, and the disorder has sometimes been called after him. Knowledge of trigeminal neuralgia slowly grew during the twentieth century. In the 1960s, effective treatment with drugs and surgery began to be available.

The pains of trigeminal neuralgia have several distinct characteristics, including:

- They are paroxysmal, pains that start and end suddenly, with painless intervals between.

- They are usually extremely intense.

- They are restricted to areas innervated by the trigeminal nerve.

- As seen on autopsy, nothing is visibly wrong with the trigeminal nerve.

- About 50% of patients have trigger zones, areas where slight stimulation or irritation can bring on an episode of pain. Painful stimulation of the trigger zones is actually less effective than light stimulation in triggering an attack.

- The disorder comes and goes in an unpredictable way; some patients show a correlation of attack frequency or severity with stress or menstrual cycle.

Stimulation of the face, lips, or gums, such as talking, eating, shaving, tooth-brushing, touch, or even a current of air, may trigger the severe knifelike or shocklike pain of trigeminal neuralgia, often described as excruciating. Trigger zones may be a few square millimeters in size, or large and diffuse. The pain usually starts in the trigger zone, but may start elsewhere. Approximately 17% of patients experience dull, aching pain for days to years before the onset of paroxysmal pain; this has been termed pre-trigeminal neuralgia.

The pain of trigeminal neuralgia is severe enough that patients often modify their behaviors to avoid it. They may suffer severe weight loss from inability to eat, become unwilling to talk or smile, and cease to practice oral hygiene. Trigeminal neuralgia tends to worsen with time, so that a patient whose pain is initially well-controlled with medication may eventually require surgery.

Diagnosis

Trigeminal neuralgia is a possible diagnosis for any patient presenting with severe, stabbing, paroxysmal pain in the jaw or face. However, the most common causes of facial pain are dental problems and diseases of the mouth. Trigeminal neuralgia must also be differentiated from migraine headaches and from other cranial neuralgias (i.e., neuralgias affecting cranial nerves other than the trigeminal). Many persons with trigeminal neuralgia see multiple physicians before getting a correct diagnosis, and may have multiple dental procedures performed in an effort to relieve the pain.

There is no definitive, single test for trigeminal neuralgia. Imaging studies such as computed tomography (**CT**) scans or **magnetic resonance imaging (MRI)** may help to rule out other possible causes of pain and to indicate trigeminal neuralgia. High-definition MRI **angiography** of the trigeminal nerve and brain stem is often able to spot compression of the trigeminal nerve by an artery or vein. Trial and error also has its place in the diagnostic process; the physician may initially give the patient **carbamazepine** (an anticonvulsant) to see if this diminishes the pain. If so, this is positive evidence for the diagnosis of trigeminal neuralgia.

Treatment team

Many different sorts of health care professionals may be consulted by patients with trigeminal neuralgia, including dentists, neurologists, neurosurgeons, oral surgeons, and ear, nose, and throat surgeons. A referral to a **neurologist** should always be sought, as trigeminal neuralgia is essentially a neurological problem.

Treatment

Treatment is primarily with drugs or surgery. Drugs are often preferred because of their lower risk, but may have intolerable side effects such as nausea or **ataxia** (loss of muscle coordination). The two most effective drugs are carbamazepine (an anticonvulsant often used in treating **epilepsy**), used for trigeminal neuralgia since 1962, and **gabapentin**. Drugs are prescribed initially in low doses and increased until an effective level is found. Other drugs in use for trigeminal neuralgia are phenytoin, baclofen, clonazepam, **lamotrigine topiramate**, and trileptal.

Carbamazepine, which inhibits the activity of sodium channels in the cell membranes of neurons (thereby reducing their excitability), is deemed the most effective medication for trigeminal neuralgia. Unfortunately, it has many side effects, including vertigo (**dizziness**), ataxia, and sedation (mental dullness). This may make it harder to treat elderly patients, who are more likely to have trigeminal neuralgia. Carbamazepine provides complete or partial relief for as many as 70% of patients. Phenytoin is also a sodium channel blocker, and also has adverse side effects, including hirsutism (increased facial hair), coarsening of facial features, and ataxia.

For patients whose pain does not respond adequately to medication, or who cannot tolerate the medication itself due to side effects, surgery is considered. Approximately 50% of trigeminal neuralgia patients eventually undergo surgery of some kind for their condition. The most common procedure is microvascular decompression, also known as the Jannetta procedure after its inventor. This involves surgery to separate the vein or artery compressing the trigeminal nerve. Teflon or polivinyl alcohol foam is inserted to cushion the trigeminal nerve against the vein or artery. This procedure is often effective, but some physicians argue that since other procedures that disturb or injure the trigeminal nerve are also effective, the benefit of microvascular decompression surgery is not relief of compression but disturbance of the trigeminal nerve, causing nonspecific nerve injury that leads to a change in neural activity.

Other surgical procedures are performed, some of which focus on destroying the pain-carrying fibers of the trigeminal nerve. The most high-tech and least invasive procedure is gamma-ray knife surgery, which uses approximately 200 convergent beams of gamma rays to deliver a high (and highly localized) **radiation** dose to the trigeminal nerve root. Almost 80% of patients undergoing this procedure experience significant relief with this procedure, although about 10% develop facial paresthesias (odd, non-painful sensations not triggered by any external stimulus).

Clinical trials

As of mid-2004, one clinical trial related to trigeminal neuralgia was recruiting patients. This study, titled "Randomized Study of L-Baclofen in Patients with Refractory Trigeminal Neuralgia," was being carried out at the University of Pennsylvania, Pittsburgh, and was sponsored by the FDA Office of Orphan Products Development (dedicated to promoting the development of treatments for diseases too rare to be considered profitable by pharmaceutical companies). Its goal is to test the effectiveness and safety of the drug L-baclofen in patients with refractory (treatment-resistant) trigeminal neuralgia. The contact is Michael J. Soso at the University of Pittsburgh School of Medicine, Pittsburgh, Pennsylvania, 15261, telephone (412) 648-1239. Forms of baclofen have been used for the treatment of trigeminal neuralgia since 1980.

Prognosis

Trigeminal neuralgia is not life threatening. It tends, however, to worsen with time, and many patients who initially were successfully treated with medication must eventually resort to surgery. Some doctors advocate surgery such as microvascular decompression early in the course of the syndrome to forestall the demyelination damage. However, there is still much controversy and uncertainty about the causes of trigeminal neuralgia and the mechanism of benefit even in those treatments that provide relief for many patients.

Resources

BOOKS

Fromm, Gerhard H., and Barry J. Sessle, eds. *Trigeminal Neuralgia: Current Concepts Regarding Pathogenesis and Treatment.* Stoneham, MA: Butterworth-Heinemann, 1991.

Zakrzewska, Joanna M., and P. N. Patsalos. *Trigeminal Neuralgia.* London: Cambridge Press, 1995.

PERIODICALS

Brown, Cassi. "Surgical Treatment of Trigeminal Neuralgia." *AORN Journal* (November 1, 2003).

Mosiman, Wendy. "Taking the Sting out of Trigeminal Neuralgia." *Nursing* (March 1, 2001).

OTHER

Komi, Suzan, and Abraham Totah. "Understanding Trigeminal Neuralgia." *eMedicine.* April 30, 2004 (May 27, 2004). <http://www.emedicine.com/med/topic2899.htm>.

ORGANIZATIONS

Trigeminal Neuralgia Association. 2801 SW Archer Road, Gainesville, FL 32608. (352) 376-9955; Fax: (352) 376-8688. tnanational@tna-support.org. <http://www.tna-support.org/>.

Larry Gilman

Tropical spastic paraparesis

Definition

Tropical spastic paraparesis (TSP) is a slowly progressive spastic paraparesis caused by the human T-cell lymphotropic virus-1 (HTLV-1), with an insidious onset in adulthood. It has been found all around the world (except in the poles), mainly in tropical and subtropical regions.

Description

For several decades the term tropical spastic paraparesis (TSP) was used to describe a chronic and progressive clinical syndrome that affected adults living in equatorial areas of the world. Neurological and modern epidemiological studies found that in some individuals no one cause could explain the progressive weakness, sensory disturbance, and sphincter dysfunction that affected individuals with TSP. During the mid-1980s, an important association was established between the first human HTLV-1 virus and idiopathic TSP. Since then, this condition has been named HTLV-1 associated myelopathy/tropical spastic paraparesis or HAM/TSP and scientists now understand that it is a condition caused by a retrovirus that results in immune dysfunction. The main neurological features of HAM/TSP consist of **spasticity** and hyperreflexia (increased reflex action) of the lower extremities, urinary bladder disturbance, lower-extremity muscle weakness, sensory disturbances, and loss of coordination. Patients with HAM/TSP may also exhibit arthritis, lung changes, and inflammation of the skin.

Co-factors that may play a role in transmitting the disorder include being a recipient of transfusion blood products, breast-feeding from an infected mother, intravenous drug use, or being the sexual partner of an infected individual for several years.

Demographics

Sporadic cases of TSP have been reported in the United States, mostly in immigrants from countries where this disease is endemic (naturally occurring). In the United States, the lifetime risk of an HTLV-1-infected person developing TSP/HAM has been calculated to be 1.7–7%, similar to that reported for United Kingdom, Africa, and the Caribbean.

The international incidence is difficult to estimate because of the insidious nature of this disease. HAM/TSP is common in regions of endemic HTLV-1, such as the Caribbean, equatorial Africa, Seychelles, southern Japan, and South America. However, it also has been reported from non-endemic areas, such as Europe and the United States. The prevalence in southern Japan is in the range of 8.6–128 per 100,000 inhabitants. An estimated 10–20 million individuals worldwide are carriers of HTLV-1.

HAM/TSP generally affects women more than men, with a female-to-male ratio of 3:1. This disease may occur at any age, with a peak in the third or fourth decade.

Causes and symptoms

The cause of HAM/TSP is still a matter of debate. Whereas only a small proportion of HTLV-1-infected individuals develop HAM/TSP, the mechanisms responsible

---

Key Terms

Paraparesis Weakness of the legs.

Retrovirus An RNA virus containing an enzyme that allows the viruses' genetic information to become part of the genetic information of the host cell as the virus replicates.

Spastic Involving uncontrollable, jerky contractions of the muscles.

---

for the progression of an HTLV-1 carrier state to clinical disease are not clear. However, three hypotheses are considered by scientists as the most likely cause of TSP: direct toxicity, autoimmunity, and bystander damage. The direct toxicity theory of HAM/TSP pathogenesis suggests that HTLV-1-infected cells are directly damaged by certain white blood cells. The autoimmunity theory postulates that the immune system attacks cells that react to HTLV-1 infected cells. In the bystander damage hypothesis, circulating antivirus-specific cells migrating through the **central nervous system** produce damage to nearby cells that is directed against the infected cells.

Symptoms may begin years after infection. In response to the infection, the body's immune response may injure nerve tissue, causing symptoms including:

- spasms and loss of feeling or unpleasant sensations in the lower extremities, accompanied by weakness
- decreased sense of touch in mid-body areas
- a vibration sensation, especially in the lower extremities, resulting from spinal cord or peripheral nerve involvement
- low lumbar **pain** with irradiation to the legs
- increased reflexes of the upper extremities
- increased urinary frequency and associated increased incidence of urinary tract infection

Less frequently observed symptoms include **tremors** in the upper extremities, optical nerve atrophy, deafness, abnormal eye movements, cranial nerve deficits, and absent or diminished ankle jerk reflex.

Diagnosis

During the clinical examination, it is important to exclude other disorders causing progressive spasticity and weakness in the legs. Diagnosis of HAM/TSP criteria typically involve documenting the following:

- absence of a history of difficulty walking or running during school age

- within two years of onset: increased urinary frequency, nocturia, or retention, with or without impotence; leg cramps or low **back pain**; symmetric weakness of the lower extremities

- within six months of onset: complaints of numbness or **dysesthesias** of the legs or feet

- a clinical examination documenting increased reflexes; spasticity of both legs, abnormal gait (manner of walking), and absence of normal sensory level

Laboratory diagnosis using ELISA (enzyme-linked immunosorbent assay) detects the presence of antibodies against HTLV-1, confirmed by the western blot assay. Electrodiagnostic studies and **magnetic resonance imaging** may also be helpful to show evidence of active denervation, associated with HTLV-1.

Treatment team

Persons with TPS have multiple needs and the team should include a **neurologist** and a physical therapist. An occupational therapist can prescribe exercises designed to develop fine coordination or compensate for tremor or weakness, or suggest assistive devices. More advanced patients require continual nursing assistance.

Treatment

The US Food and Drug Administration (FDA) has not officially approved any drug for the specific treatment of HAM/TSP in the United States. Many patients benefit from oral prednisolone or equivalent glucocorticoid therapy. A response rate of up to 91% has been reported in less advanced cases. Oral treatment with methylprednisolone may produce excellent to moderate responses in around 70% of patients. Plasmapheresis, interferon, oral azathiaprine, danazol, and vitamin C have been tried and also show transient effects. None of these treatments has been systematically studied in a controlled clinical trial. **Antiviral drugs** like AZT would be expected to help in reducing viral replication and associated direct cell injury.

Patients with HAM/TSP sometimes report neuropathic pain. Useful drugs include antiepileptics (e.g., **carbamazepine**, phenytoin, **gabapentin**, **topiramate**), baclofen, and tricyclic antidepressants. The dosages used usually are well below those used in the treatment of **epilepsy**. Physical therapy is commonly used in combination with medication for nerve pain.

Recovery and rehabilitation

The goal of a rehabilitation program for a person affected with HAM/TSP is to restore functions essential to daily living in individuals who have lost these capacities through injury or illness. Most rehabilitation programs are comprehensive in nature and have several different aspects.

Physical therapy is designed to help restore and maintain useful movements or functions and prevent complications such as frozen joints, contractures, or bedsores. Examples of physical therapy include:

- stretching and range of motion exercises

- exercises to develop trunk control and upper arm muscles

- training in walking and appropriate use of assistive devices, such as ambulatory aids, braces, and wheelchairs

- training in how to get from one spot to another, such as from the bed to a wheelchair or from a wheelchair to the car

- training in how to fall safely in order to cause the least possible damage

Occupational therapy focuses on specific activities of daily living that primarily involve the arms and hands. Examples include grooming, dressing, eating, handwriting, and driving.

Some rehabilitation centers have innovative programs designed to help people compensate for loss of memory or slowed learning ability. Rehabilitation may be carried out in a residential or an outpatient setting.

Clinical trials

In 2004 there were some open **clinical trials** for the study and treatment of TSP, including:

- "Evaluation of Patients with HAM/TSP," "Phase I/II Study of HTLV-I-Associated Myelopathy/Tropical Spastic Paraparesis (HAM/TSP) Using the Humanized MiK-beta-1 Monoclonal Antibody," and "Assessment of Patients with Multiple Sclerosis," sponsored by National Institute of Neurological Disorders and Stroke (NINDS).

- "Phase I Study of T Cell Large Granular Lymphocytic Leukemia in Humanized MiK-Beta-1 Monoclonal Antibody Directed Toward the IL-2R/IL-15R Subunit (CD122)," sponsored by National Cancer Institute (NCI).

Further updated information on these clinical trials can be found at the National Institutes of Health website for clinical trials at <www.clinicaltrials.gov>.

Prognosis

HAM/TSP is usually a progressive neurological disorder, but it is rarely fatal. Most patients live for several decades after the diagnosis. Their prognosis improves if they take steps to prevent urinary tract infection and skin sore formation, and if they enroll in physical and occupational therapy programs.

Special concerns

An important component in the care of patients with TSP is the prevention of infections with the HTLV-1 virus. Several studies indicate that transmission of the HTLV-1 virus occurs through sexual or other intimate contact, intrauterine exposure, newborn exposure via breast milk, sharing of needles by drug abusers, and blood transfusion from infected persons. Transfusion of HTLV-1 antibody-positive blood causes infection in about 60% of recipients. Breastfeeding is contraindicated for mothers who are carriers of HTLV-1.

Resources

BOOKS

Parker, James N., and Philip M. Parker. *The Official Patient's Sourcebook on Tropical Spastic Paraparesis.* San Diego: Icon Group International, 2002.

PERIODICALS

Mora, Carlos A., et al. "Human T-lymphotropic Virus Type I-associated Myelopathy/Tropical Spastic Paraparesis: Therapeutic Approach." *Current Treatment Options in Infectious Diseases* 5 (2003): 443–455.

OTHER

"NINDS Tropical Spastic Paraparesis Information Page." *National Institute of Neurological Disorders and Stroke.* (April 20, 2004). <http://www.ninds.nih.gov/health_and_medical/disorders/tropical_spastic_paraparesis.htm>.
"Tropical spastic paraparesis." *Dr. Joseph F. Smith Medical Library.* Thompson Corporation. (April 20, 2004). <http://www.chclibrary.org/micromed/00069230.html>.

ORGANIZATIONS

National Organization for Rare Disorders (NORD). P.O. Box 1968 (55 Kenosia Avenue), Danbury, CT 06813-1968. (203) 744-0100 or (800) 999-NORD (6673); Fax: (203) 798-2291. orphan@rarediseases.org. <http://www.rarediseases.org>.
National Institute of Allergy and Infectious Diseases (NIAID). 31 Center Drive, Rm. 7A50 MSC 2520, Bethesda, MD 20892-2520. (301) 496-5717. <http://www.niaid.nih.gov>.

Francisco de Paula Careta
Iuri Drumond Louro

Tuberous sclerosis

Definition

Tuberous sclerosis (TS) is a hereditary neurological condition that affects all ages. The name arises from the potato stem-shaped growths that occur in the brain, also known as tubers. These growths often involve overgrowth of nerves or the connective tissue within them, which is described by the term sclerosis.

Description

TS is also known by the names tuberous sclerosis complex and Bourneville's disease. Neurological symptoms may include tubers and other non-cancerous growths in the brain, cancerous brain tumors, **seizures**, and **mental retardation** or developmental delay.

Nearly everyone with TS has some symptoms affecting their skin. These include light-colored patches called ash-leaf spots, acne-type growths on the face, nail beds, and the body, and shagreen patches. Other common symptoms of TS are kidney cysts, kidney growths, and heart tumors that may develop at a very young age or even before birth.

Demographics

According to the National Institute of Neurological Disorders and Stroke (NINDS), TS affects about 1 in 6,000 newborns. As many as 25,000 to 45,000 people in the United States and 1-2 million people worldwide have the disorder. Its true incidence may be higher because mildly affected individuals may not come to medical attention. TS has been reported in all ethnic groups and races with equal frequency.

Two genes for TS have been identified, and males and females are equally affected with the condition. About one third of people with TS have an affected parent as well.

Causes and symptoms

Always known to be hereditary, mutations in two different genes are now known to cause TS. These genes are TSC1 and TSC2, and were discovered in 1993 and 1997 on chromosomes 16 and 9 respectively. TS is inherited in an autosomal dominant manner, meaning that an affected individual has a 50/50 chance to pass a disease-causing mutation to his or her children, regardless of their gender. As a result, strong family histories of TS are common.

TSC1 and TSC2 normally code for specific proteins, hamartin and tuberin, which are felt to be necessary for neurological functioning. Reduced amounts of these proteins in the brains of people with TS may contribute to the neurological complications associated with the condition.

The most common neurological symptoms in TS include seizures, learning and behavioral problems, and **hydrocephalus**. Seizures affect about 85% of people at some point in their lives. They can begin in very early childhood as **infantile spasms**, sometimes with hypsarrhythmia. The presence of these spasms at an early age often means more significant learning problems and more significant **epilepsy** later on.

Key Terms

Aneurysm   Increased size of a blood vessel like an artery, which may burst open.

Angiofibroma   Non-cancerous growth of the skin, which is often reddish in color and filled with blood vessels.

Angiomyolipoma   Non-cancerous growth in the kidney, most often found in tuberous sclerosis.

Computed tomography (CT) scan   Three-dimensional internal image of the body, created by combining x ray images from different planes using a computer program.

"Confetti" skin lesions   Small changes in the skin color and texture, which may be as small as pieces of confetti.

Connective tissue   Supportive tissue in the body that joins structures together, lending strength and elasticity.

Cyst   Sac of tissue filled with fluid, gas, or semi-solid material.

Echocardiogram   Ultrasound of the heart, which shows heart structure in detail.

Electrocardiogram   Test that shows a heart's rhythm by studying its electrical current patterns.

Electroencephalogram (EEG)   Test that shows a brain's electrical wave activity patterns.

Gingival fibroma   Small non-cancerous growth on the toe- or fingernail beds.

Hamartoma   Abnormal growth that may resemble cancer, but is not cancerous.

Hydrocephalus   A state when fluid builds up in the brain, which may cause increased internal pressure and enlarged head size.

Hypomelanotic macule   Skin patch that is lighter in color than the area around it.

Hypsarrhythmia   Typical brain wave activity found in infantile spasms.

Lymphangioleimyoma   Non-cancerous growth in the lung, typical of tuberous sclerosis.

Magnetic resonance imaging (MRI) scan   Three-dimensional internal image of the body, created using magnetic waves.

Mutation   A change in the order of deoxyribonucleic acid (DNA) bases that make up genes, akin to a misspelling.

Periungual fibroma   Small non-cancerous growth on the toe- or fingernail beds.

Plaque   Another term to describe angiofibromas on the forehead.

Polyp   Piece of skin that pouches outward.

Renal cell carcinoma   A type of kidney cancer.

Retinal achromic patch   Small area of the retina that is lighter than the area around it.

Rhabdomyoma   Non-cancerous growth in the heart muscle.

Sequencing   Genetic testing in which the entire sequence of deoxyribonucleic acid (DNA) bases that make up a gene is studied, in an effort to find a mutation.

Shagreen patches   Patches of skin with the consistency of an orange peel.

Skin tag   Abnormal outward pouching of skin, with a varying size.

Spasms   Sudden involuntary muscle movement or contraction.

Subependymal giant cell astrocytoma   Specific type of cancerous brain tumor found in tuberous sclerosis.

Tubers   Firm growths in the brain, named for their resemblance in shape to potato stems.

Ultrasound   Two-dimensional internal image of the body, created using sound waves.

Vascular   Related to the blood vessels.

White matter radial migration line   White lines seen on a brain scan, signifying abnormal movement of neurons (brain cells) at that area.

Woods lamp   Lamp that uses ultraviolet light, making subtle skin changes more obvious.

Learning problems are not a certainty with TS; about 50% of people with the condition are known to have developmental delay or mental retardation. People with TS have an increased chance to develop certain behavioral disorders. **Autism** is seen in about 25–50% of people with

TS, and this is felt to have a major influence on an individual's daily functioning. Parents of children with TS often raise concerns about autism or autistic-type characteristics, because this has a significant impact on routine activities like attending school. Though scientific studies

Close-up of light-brown skin with a lighter patch in the center, known as an ash-leaf spot. Nearly everyone with tuberous sclerosis has some symptoms affecting the skin. *(© LI Inc./Custom Medical Stock Photo. Reproduced by permission.)*

have been done to find exact neurological causes for autism in TS, none has provided consistent results.

A unique brain finding in TS is the cortical tuber, which is seen in about 90% of people with the condition. The number and size of tubers in a person can correlate with the degree of learning problems and seizures they may experience. Other brain findings in TS include subependymal hamartomas. Some of these may grow in childhood and block the normal flow of spinal fluid, causing hydrocephalus. Brain tumors like subependymal giant cell astrocytomas are a cause of health complications and death in TS.

Since skin changes are so common in TS, they can be some of the first signs of the condition that are noticed. Ash-leaf spots are the most common skin finding, followed by facial angiofibromas. These angiofibromas may cause slight disfigurement, but more often are a cosmetic concern. Darkened skin patches called cafe-au-lait spots may also occur, along with skin tags. Fortunately, none of the skin symptoms usually cause serious medical complications.

Kidney disease can be a serious medical concern in TS; it is the most frequent cause of death in people with TS older than 30 years. The most common renal finding is the angiomyolipoma, which is more commonly found in women at a younger age. Though these growths are noncancerous, they can enlarge and disturb normal kidney function. Kidney cysts may occur, again more commonly in younger women. These cysts may be numerous and similarly disrupt normal kidney function as a result. Renal cell carcinoma can be a further symptom of TS, and kidney transplants may be necessary for any significant renal complication.

Cardiac rhabdomyomas are typically seen in early childhood, but occasionally may even be seen on a prenatal ultrasound. Most rhabdomyomas disappear with age, remaining stable and causing no symptoms; others may cause heart rhythm problems. Vascular disease may also be a part of TS, with some people having **aneurysms** of the abdomen and other areas of the body.

Lung problems are a part of TS, and affect women more often. Lymphangioleimyomas of the lung are common and affect about 1-4% of people with TS by interfering with normal lung function. Hormones may be a factor because pregnancy, menstruation, and estrogen have been associated with a worsening of these symptoms in some women. Interestingly, pulmonary problems have been associated with a milder case of TS, often with fewer learning problems and seizures.

Other symptoms of TS include growths on the retinas called hamartomas, which are not usually problematic. There have been no typical ages in which eye involvement occurs in TS.

Diagnosis

Up until the discovery of TSC1 and TSC2, the diagnosis of TS was made on a clinical basis. Criteria for clinical diagnosis were updated in 1998 at the Tuberous Sclerosis Complex Consensus Conference.

Revised diagnostic criteria for tuberous sclerosis complex (TSC)

The major features include:

- facial angiofibromas or forehead plaque
- non-traumatic ungual or periungual fibroma
- hypomelanotic macules (more than three)
- shagreen patch
- multiple retinal nodular hamartomas
- cortical tuber
- subependymal nodule
- subependymal giant cell astrocytoma
- cardiac rhabdomyoma, single or multiple
- lymphangioleimyomatosis
- renal angiomyolipoma

The minor features include:

- multiple randomly distributed pits in dental enamel

- hamartomatous rectal polyps
- bone cysts
- cerebral white matter radial migration lines
- gingival fibromas
- non-renal hamartoma
- retinal achromic patch
- "confetti" skin lesions
- multiple renal cysts

Definite TSC: Either two major features, or one major feature plus two minor features. Probable TSC: One major plus one minor feature. Possible TSC: Either one major feature, or two or more minor features.

Most brain findings in TS can be identified with **magnetic resonance imaging (MRI)** or computed tomography (**CT**) scans. Seizures can be documented from electroencephalogram (EEG) monitoring. Skin changes are often found by using a Woods lamp, which makes them more obvious during a physical examination. Routine ultrasounds of the kidney often find and help monitor cysts and angiomylipomas. Cardiac involvement may be seen as early as a prenatal ultrasound, or with an echocardiogram in early life. Electrocardiograms may be necessary to help detect heart rhythm problems. For women in particular, a CT scan of the chest is important to detect lung lymphangiomyomatosis. For all, an ophthalmology examination is important to detect retinal involvement.

Genetic testing is available for TS via gene sequencing. It is useful for confirming a clinical diagnosis, prenatal diagnosis, or family testing when there is an identified TSC mutation in the family. Sequencing of the TSC1 and TSC2 genes is not perfect; it detects about 80% of people with TS. An informative test result is one that identifies a known mutation in either gene, and this confirms that the person has TS. A negative test result does not identify a mutation in either gene. This either means that the tested individual does not have TS, or has a mutation that cannot be found through testing and truly has the diagnosis.

Treatment team

Treatment for people with TS is usually very specific to the person, since symptoms vary greatly. The typical treatment team for someone with TS may include a **neurologist**, neurosurgeon, medical geneticist, genetic counselor, dermatologist, cardiologist, pulmonologist, nephrologist, ophthalmologist, social worker, and a primary care provider. Often times there are pediatric specialists in these fields who aid in the care for children. Care providers in pediatric development are particularly important, such as speech-language therapists and pediatric neuropsychologists.

Treatment

There is no cure for tuberous sclerosis. Therefore, treatment is based upon symptoms.

Seizures may be treated with various anti-epilepsy medications. Those with significant seizures may be tried on a ketogenic diet, which consists of frequent meals of high-fat foods. While challenging, the ketogenic diet yields good results in some cases.

Learning or behavioral problems are often serious issues, but awareness and developmental interventions often help families with TS. Pediatricians who have an interest in child development are a good resource, particularly if a child with TS is showing signs of autism.

Hydrocephalus can be serious and even lead to learning problems if left untreated, so surgery to drain accumulated fluid in the brain may be necessary. While most growths in the brain are non-cancerous, brain tumors are typically treated as they would be in someone without TS.

Since most skin complications of TS cause no medical problems, treatment is not often necessary. Some angiofibromas, particularly on the face, may be problematic and require removal. Laser treatments may also be effective to reduce the appearance of some skin changes.

Many kidney growths cause no health problem in TS, but some individuals may have kidney cysts similar to those found in polycystic kidney disease (Type 1). In these cases, kidney function may be disturbed and the person might need a kidney transplant after some time. Those with renal cell carcinoma would be treated as anyone with this complication.

Most rhabdomyomas cause no problems, but some may need surgery to keep their hearts working well. Surgery may also be required for someone with a severe heart rhythm problem.

People with lung function problems may need to be treated with medications, hormone therapy, or surgery if necessary.

Visual complaints are not as common for people with TS, since retinal growths do not usually cause symptoms. In rarer cases, vision may be disturbed and treated like someone without TS.

Clinical trials

As of early 2004, there were two clinical studies recruiting subjects in the United States. Both were at the National Heart, Lung, and Blood Institute (NHLBI) at the National Institutes of Health in Bethesda, Maryland. One study was studying skin tumors in people with TS, and the other was studying disease progression in people with TS who have lymphangioleimyomatosis. More information about these trials can be found at www.clinicaltrials.gov.

Prognosis

Prognosis for someone with tuberous sclerosis is highly dependent upon symptoms they experience. Those who die may do so as a result of significant neurological, pulmonary or cardiac complications. People with TS often have routine medical appointments dealing with symptoms as they arise.

Many people with TS survive into adulthood, and studies are attempting to learn more about long-term prognosis as people with TS age. It is challenging to gain this information because older people with milder forms of TS may not present for medical care frequently, or may not even know they have the condition.

Resources

BOOKS

Curatolo, Paolo, Peter G. Procopis, Isabelle Rapin, and John Stobo Prichard. *Tuberous Sclerosis Complex: From Basic Science to Clinical Phenotypes.* Mac Keith Publishers, 2003.

Gomez, Manuel Rodriguez, Julian R. Sampson, and Vicky Holets Whittemore. *Tuberous Sclerosis Complex,* 3rd ed. Oxford University Press, 1999.

Parker, James N., and Philip M. Parker. *The Official Patient's Sourcebook on Tuberous Sclerosis: A Revised and Updated Directory for the Internet Age.* Icon Health Publishers, 2002.

PERIODICALS

Curatolo, Paolo, Magda Verdecchia, and Roberta Bombardieri. "Tuberous sclerosis complex: a review of neurological aspects." *European Journal of Paediatric Neurology* 6 (2002): 15-23.

Franz, David Neal. "Diagnosis and Management of Tuberous Sclerosis Complex." *Seminars in Pediatric Neurology* 5, no. 4 (December 1998): 253-268.

Lendvay, Thomas S., and Fray F. Marshall. "The Tuberous Sclerosis Complex and its Highly Variable Manifestations." *Clinical Urology* 169, no. 5 (May 2003): 1635-1642.

McClintock, William M. "Neurologic Manifestations of Tuberous Sclerosis Complex." *Current Neurology and Neuroscience Reports* 2 (2002): 158-163.

Sparagana, Steven P., and E. Steve Roach. "Tuberous sclerosis complex." *Current Opinion in Neurology* 13 (2000): 115-119.

Walz, Nicolay Chertkoff, Anna Weber Byars, John C. Egelhoff, and David Neal Franz. "Supratentorial Tuber Location and Autism in Tuberous Sclerosis Complex." *Journal of Child Neurology* 17, no. 11 (November 2002): 830-832.

WEBSITES

GeneTests/GeneReviews. <http://www.genetests.org>.

National Institute of Neurological Disorders and Stroke. <http://www.ninds.nih.gov/index.htm>.

Online Mendelian Inheritance in Man. <http://www.ncbi.nlm.nih.gov/omim/>.

Tuberous Sclerosis International (Worldwide Organisation of Tuberous Sclerosis Associations). <http://www.stsn.nl/tsi/tsi.htm>.

ORGANIZATIONS

Tuberous Sclerosis Alliance. 801 Roeder Road, Suite 750, Silver Spring, MD 20910. 301-562-9890 or 800-225-6872; Fax: 301-562-9870. ntsa@ntsa.org. <http://www.tsalliance.org>.

The Tuberous Sclerosis Association, U.K. Janet Medcalf, P.O. Box 9644, Bromsgrove, England B61 OFP. +44 (0)1527 871898; Fax: +44 (0)1527 579452. <http://www.tuberous-sclerosis.org>.

The Australasian Tuberous Sclerosis Association. 5 Parer Avenue, Condell Park, Australia NSW 200. 1300 733 435 (Australia only). atss@netspace.net.au. <http://atss.customer.netspace.net.au/index.htm>.

Deepti Babu, MS, CGC

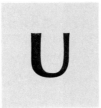

U

Ulnar neuropathy

Definition

Ulnar neuropathy is an inflammation or compression of the ulnar nerve, resulting in paresthesia (numbness, tingling, and **pain**) in the outer side of the arm and hand near the little finger.

Description

The ulnar nerve transmits impulses to muscles in the forearm and hand. The nerve is responsible for the proper sensing of touch, texture, and temperature throughout the fourth and fifth digits of the hand, the palm, and the underside of the forearm. Ulnar neuropathy arises most commonly because of damage to the nerve as it passes through the wrist. The elbow is also a frequent site of nerve damage. Ulnar neuropathy is variously known as bicycler's neuropathy, cubital tunnel syndrome, Guyon or Guyon's canal syndrome, and tardy ulnar palsy.

Demographics

Ulnar neuropathy that originates at the elbow is very common. Estimates are that 40% of Americans experience some form of this neuropathy at some point in their lives. While the ulnar nerve is structurally identical in men and women, men tend to develop ulnar neuropathy more than women. This is because men generally do not have as much fat overlaying the elbow, and so the underlying nerve can be more susceptible to irritation and damage.

The onset of ulnar neuropathy can occur slowly. As a result, many of those who are affected are middle-aged or older adults. Demographic risk factors include a family history of diabetes, alcoholism, and presence of human immunodeficiency virus. Because leaning on the elbows can trigger ulnar neuropathy, people such as telephone operators, receptionists, and those who operate computers for extended periods of time are at risk for developing the disorder.

Causes and symptoms

Ulnar neuropathy is caused by nerve damage. The nature of the nerve damage is varied, and can result from inflammation or compression. Nerve damage at the elbow can result from compression of the nerve when sensation is obliterated during general anesthesia. As well, a blow to the elbow or even too much leaning on the elbow can be damaging, as can diseases (rheumatoid arthritis) and metabolic disturbances (diabetes). Even malnutrition can be a factor, as protective fatty deposits and muscle mass waste away. Damage to the nerve at the wrist can be caused by a blow, tumors, and impinging of an artery.

The nerve damage that results in ulnar neuropathy can involve the main body of the nerve, the branching region at the end of the nerve known as the axon (which is involved in the movement of the nerve impulse to the adjacent nerve), and the protective myelin coating around the nerve. When the main body of the nerve is involved, the problem is usually a block in the passage of the impulse down the nerve. Axon damage typically decreases the movement of the nerve impulse away from the nerve or the wavelength of the impulse. As a result, the impulse may not reach the adjacent nerve, or may not be recognized by the receptors of that adjacent nerve. Finally, damage to the myelin sheath (demyelination) also impedes the movement of signal down the body of the nerve.

Depending on the site of the neuropathy and whether the neuropathy arises suddenly (acute) or has been present for a long time (chronic), various symptoms can arise. Acute and chronic ulnar neuropathy of the elbow is always associated with numbness and weakness. Pain is present almost 40% of the time in the acute form of the disorder and almost 80% of the time in the chronic disorder. When the ulnar neuropathy involves the wrist, weakness is ever-present in a main muscle controlling wrist movement, generalized weakness in the absence of pain in 50% of those afflicted, and finger numbness occurs in about 25% of cases.

Other physical signs include the adoption of a clawed shape by the hand and the inability of the entire thumb to move to the forefinger in a single motion.

Diagnosis

Typically, the development of weakness in the elbow or wrist is the sign that alerts a clinician to the possibility of ulnar neuropathy. Follow-up tests can include ultrasound or **magnetic resonance imaging** to visualize cysts or structural abnormalities. The functioning of the nerve can be assessed in a nerve conduction test. Laboratory analyses of blood can be done to detect the presence of diabetes or infections that can damage nerves (such as **Lyme disease**, human immunodeficiency virus, or hepatitis viruses).

Treatment team

Treatment can involve the family physician, family members, neurosurgeons, hand surgeon, pain specialist, and physical and occupational therapists. Therapists can often provide exercises that assist in maximizing muscular strength and orthotic devices to maintain proper positioning during repetitive or stressful movements, thereby reducing inflammation.

Treatment

Treatment can consist of the use of nonsteroidal anti-inflammatory drugs to control swelling around the nerve. The use of splints or cushions can ease the discomfort and the stress on the ulnar nerve. For some, surgery is a useful option, when relief can be gained by removal of a cyst or correction of damage caused by a blow.

Recovery and rehabilitation

Sports and other normal activity can be resumed when the person is able to perform normal hand-gripping tasks such as opening a jar, forcefully grip a tennis racquet or bicycle handlebars, or work at a keyboard without pain or tingling in the elbow or hand. Braces and other orthotic devices, if worn consistently, often prevent reoccurrence of ulnar neuropathy.

Prognosis

If nerve damage has been caused by a blow or by trauma such as putting too much pressure on the elbow or wrist, recovery can be complete.

Key Terms

Axon The long, slender part of a nerve cell that carries electrochemical signals to another nerve cell.

Electromyogram Often done after a nerve conduction velocity test, an electromyogram (EMG) is a diagnostic used test to evaluate nerve and muscle function.

Myelin sheath Insulating layer around some nerves that speeds the conduction of nerve signals.

Nerve impulse The electrochemical signal carried by an axon from one neuron to another neuron.

Neuron A nerve cell.

Orthotic device Devices made of plastic, leather, or metal which provide stability at the joints or passively stretch the muscles.

Paresthesia Abnormal physical sensations such as numbness, burning, prickling, or tingling.

Resources

PERIODICALS

Hochman, M. G., and J. L. Zilberfarb. "Nerves in a pinch: imaging of nerve compression syndromes." *Radiology Clinics of North America* (January 2004): 221–245.

Kern, R. Z. "The electrodiagnosis of ulnar nerve entrapment at the elbow." *Canadian Journal of Neurological Science* (November 2003): 314–319.

OTHER

"Ulnar Neuropathy." *emedicine.com.* <http://www.emedicine.com/neuro/topic387.htm> (May 5, 2004).

ORGANIZATIONS

National Institute for Neurological Diseases and Stroke. P.O. Box 5801, Bethesda, MD 20824. (301) 496-5751 or (800) 352-9424. <http://www.ninds/nih.gov>.

National Chronic Pain Outreach Organization (NCPOA). P.O. Box 274, Millboro, VA 24460. (540) 862-9437; Fax: (540) 862-9485. ncpoa@cfw.org. <http://www.chronicpain.org>.

National Institute of Arthritis and Musculoskeletal and Skin Diseases (NIAMS). 31 Centre Dr., Rm. 4Co2 MSC 2350, Bethesda, MD 20892-2350. (301) 496-8190 or (877) 226-4267. info@mail.nih.gov. <http://www.niams.nih.gov>.

American Chronic Pain Association (ACPA). P.O. Box 850, Rocklin, CA 95677-0850. (916) 632-0922 or (800) 533-3231; Fax: (916) 632-3208. ACPA@pacbell.net. <http://www.theacpa.org>.

Brian Douglas Hoyle, PhD

Ultrasonography

Definition

Ultrasonography is a diagnostic technique that involves directing high frequency sound waves at tissues in the body to generate images of anatomical structures. Ultrasonography is also called sonography, diagnostic sonography, and echocardiography when it is used to image the heart.

Purpose

Ultrasonography has a variety of uses in medical diagnostics. It is most well suited for imaging soft tissues that are solid and uniform or filled with fluid. It does not perform well when imaging calcified objects such as bone or objects filled with air like the bowel. Some of the more common uses for ultrasonography include imaging fetus development during pregnancy, diagnosing gallbladder disease and some forms of cancer, and evaluating abnormalities in the scrotum and prostate, heart, and thyroid gland. Ultrasound can also be used to perform breast exams. A technique called Doppler imaging ultrasonography can also be used to view the movement of blood through blood vessels and to guide needles through anatomical structures for obtaining specimens for **biopsy**. Three-dimensional ultrasounds provide detailed images of fetuses in the uterus.

The majority of ultrasonic exams are performed externally by running a transducer over the surface of the skin. Usually a gel is applied to the skin on which the transducer will glide during the exam. The gel helps prevent the formation of air pockets between the transducer and the skin that interfere with the ultrasonic signal. Some ultrasound diagnostic tests require the insertion of a probe into a body orifice. For example, during a transesophageal echocardiogram a specialized transducer is placed in the esophagus to better image the heart. Transrectal exams require a transducer to be inserted into a man's rectum to obtain images of the prostate. Transvaginal ultrasounds are used to provide images of a woman's ovaries and uterus or of a fetus during the early weeks of pregnancy.

Ultrasound is generally a painless procedure. Some discomfort may be felt when the transducer is pressed against the skin or when the transducer is inserted in the body. Most ultrasonic procedures take less than half of an hour.

Cranial ultrasound

Cranial ultrasonography is most often used in infants to diagnose problems with the brain and the ventricles in the brain through which cerebrospinal fluid (the clear fluid that circulates through the brain and spinal cord) flows. These abnormalities are often associated with premature birth. Because ultrasound waves are poorly conducted through bones, cranial ultrasonography must be performed on infants before the fontanel (gaps between the bones of the cranium) have closed. Cranial ultrasonography is also performed on adults during brain surgery to help identify the location of brain tumors. In adults, the skull must be surgically opened in order to use ultrasonography.

In infants, cranial ultrasonography is most often used to diagnose two complications. Intraventricular hemorrhage (IVH) occurs when there is bleeding in the brain. This occurs more commonly in premature babies and is likely to happen within the first week of the infant's life. **Periventricular leukomalacia** (PVL) occurs when the tissue around the ventricles in the brain is damaged. This complication can occur within several weeks of birth. Both IVH and PVL are associated with mental disabilities and developmental delays. Cranial ultrasonography can also be used to evaluate brain abnormalities in babies, such as congenital **hydrocephalus** or tumors, or to detect infection.

Description

Ultrasonography relies on sound waves to create an image of the soft tissues in the body. Sound waves are a form of energy called longitudinal pressure waves that result when molecules are pushed together and then become rarified (less dense). The molecules through which the wave passes are not transported by the wave; rather, they vibrate back and forth around a neutral position. The number of times that a molecule moves through a compression and rarification cycle in one second is called the frequency of the wave. The unit of the frequency of a sound wave is the Hertz (Hz). Frequencies between about 20 Hz and 20,000 Hz are audible to the human ear and the greater the frequency, the higher a sound wave sounds. Frequencies above 20,000 Hz are called ultrasonic and the human ear cannot detect these sound waves. The frequencies of sound waves used in ultrasonography are between about one million and 15 million Hz (or one and 15 MHz).

An ultrasound machine typically consists of four parts: the transducer, which allows for the movement of the ultrasound machine over the body; the electronic signal processing unit, which controls the power to the transducer; the display unit, which is usually a computer screen; and a device for storing the images, which is usually a videotape or a camera.

The transducer is the most technologically interesting part of the ultrasonography machine. It is usually a handheld device that can be pushed against the skin or inserted into an orifice. The transducer is made up of a plastic or ceramic material that has piezoelectric properties. This means that it is capable of generating and detecting ultrasound waves. If pulses of electric current are applied to the surface of a transducer, the piezoelectric surface will change in thickness in response to the pulses. This change in thickness causes a change in pressure in the molecules surrounding the piezoelectric surface, generating sound waves. If the pulses occur between one and 15 million times a second, then the result is a sound wave with an ultrasonic frequency. Similarly, the piezoelectric surface acts as a receptor for return waves. When sound waves collide with the piezoelectric surface, they cause a change in its thickness. This change in thickness is converted to a change in the electric current in the transducer, which is then interpreted as various shades of gray and used to form an image on the display unit. The electronics of the transducer are constructed so that ultrasound beams are generated, followed by a pause during which the return waves are detected; this cycle continues during the entire diagnostic procedure.

An ultrasonic wave that is directed out of the transducer and into tissues of the body has one of four outcomes: it can be absorbed by the material, in which case the transducer will receive no return signal; it can be reflected back to the transducer, in which case the transducer will receive a strong return signal; it can be refracted so that it changes direction and only a part of the signal will return to the transducer; finally, the wave can be scattered, greatly reducing the signal received by the transducer. At various tissue interfaces, different amounts of the wave energy are returned to the transducer as a result of various combinations of absorption, reflection, refraction, and scattering. For example, at a fat-muscle interface, about 1% of the incident wave is returned to the transducer, while at a bone-muscle interface, about 40% of the incident wave is returned. At any interface that involves air, such as a gas bubble in the bowel, nearly 100% of the incident wave will be returned to the transducer. Similarly, bones and other calcified objects like kidney stones and gallstones result in very high reflection of the incident wave. Because air acts as such a strong reflector of an ultrasonic wave, gel or some other lubricant is usually placed between the transducer and the skin during an ultrasonic exam.

Some ultrasonic machines take advantage of the Doppler effect in order to display color images of the flow of blood or other fluids. When an ultrasound wave is directed at a stationary object, the return wave will remain the same frequency as the incident wave, although it will be attenuated depending upon the structures with which it interacts. On the other hand, when an ultrasound wave is directed at a moving object, the return wave will have a different frequency than the incident wave depending on whether the moving object is in the same direction as, or in the opposite direction from, the incident wave. This

Key Terms

Sound waves Changes in air pressure that produce an oscillating wave that transmits sound.

Ultrasound High frequency sound waves directed at tissues in the body to generate images of anatomical structures.

change in frequency can be interpreted, for example, as the speed of blood flow within a vessel.

The recent development of color Doppler sonography (CDS) has improved several diagnostic exams. In this technique, a black and white image of the anatomical structures resulting from traditional ultrasonography is overlaid with a color image showing the flow of a fluid within the tissues generated from a Doppler ultrasonograph. CDS has proven extremely useful for evaluating the blood flow to the placenta and uterus during pregnancy. It has also been used to quantify the blood flow to various tumors; malignant tumors tend to have greater rates of blood flow and longer residence times than benign ones.

Several other new technologies associated with ultrasonography are becoming available as diagnostic tools. Some physicians are using ultrasonography in conjunction with contrast agents that provide better resolution of internal structures. This is particularly useful for visualizing the heart and kidneys more effectively. Harmonic imaging is a technique that is used to improve the signal-to-noise ratio of an ultrasonic image. It is based on the idea that the tissues of the body resonate harmonically, similar to a musical instrument. Therefore, taking advantage of sound waves at two and three times the frequency of the incident wave should provide additional information about the internal structures of the body. For example, if the incident wave of the transducer is 4 MHz, then using return waves that are 8 MHz should improve the resolution of the image. Finally, three-dimensional sonography is available on some machines. In some cases, the three-dimensional image is reconstructed from several sweeps of the transducer at different levels through the body. In others, two transducers that are oriented perpendicular to each other are used to build a three-dimensional image. This technology has been used most frequently to visualize fetuses in the uterus.

Preparation

Preparation for ultrasonography differs depending on the type of exam being performed. For some exams, no preparation is necessary. For others, fasting and abstaining from drinking for up to 12 hours prior to the exam is required. Some exams, like the transabdominal ultrasound, require that the patient have a full bladder because the ultrasonic waves are best transmitted through fluid. If a biopsy is required, antibiotics may be administered prior to the test. The physician or technician performing the exam usually provides instructions on proper preparation prior to the exam.

Risks

Because ultrasonography uses high frequency sound waves, and not x rays or other forms of **radiation**, there are very few risks associated with its use. Sound waves are either reflected back to the transducer, or the tissues of the body absorb them and they dissipate as heat. There may be a slight increase in heat in the body as a result, but no negative effects of this heat have been documented.

Normal results

Results of ultrasonic tests are usually sent to a physician and possibly to a radiologist. They are usually made available to the patient within one to two days.

Resources

BOOKS

Fleischer, Arthur C., et al. *Sonography in Obstetrics and Gynecology: Principles and Practice*, 6th ed. New York: McGraw-Hill Companies, Inc. 2001.

Fleischer, Arthur C., and Donna M. Kepple. *Diagnostic Sonography: Principles and Clinical Applications*, 2nd ed. Philadelphia: W. B. Saunders Company, 1995.

OTHER

"Ultrasound Imaging." *The Mayo Clinic.* January 3, 2004 (April 4, 2004). <http://www.mayoclinic.com/ invoke.cfm?objectid=2F0F9036-342F-4723-9DDBAB9FAEA73A77>.

Moyer, Paula. "3-D Ultrasound: Do You Really Need It?" *WebMDHealth.* February 2, 2004 (April 4, 2004). <http://my.webmd.com/content/article/21/1728_ 55256.htm?lastselectedguid={5FE84E90-BC77-4056-A91C-9531713CA348}>.

"Ultrasound." *Medline Plus National Library of Medicine.* December 3, 2003 (April 4, 2004). <http://www.nlm.nih.gov/medlineplus/tutorials/ ultrasound/rd209101.html>.

Juli M. Berwald, PhD

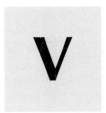

Valproic acid and divalproex sodium

Definition

Valproic acid is an anticonvulsant used to control **seizures** in the treatment of **epilepsy**, a neurological dysfunction in which excessive surges of electrical energy are emitted in the brain.

Valproic acid is closely related to divalproex sodium and valproate sodium. While these drugs are primarily used in the treatment of epilepsy, divalproex sodium is also indicated for the treatment of manic episodes (abnormally and persistently elevated mood) associated with bipolar disorder.

Purpose

Valproic acid is thought to depress activity in certain areas of the brain, suppressing the irregular firing of neurons to prevent seizures. Divalproex sodium is a stable coordination compound formed with valproic acid.

While valproic acid and divalproex sodium control the seizures associated with epilepsy, there is no known cure for the disease.

Description

In the United States, valproic acid and divalproex sodium are sold under the brand names Depekene and Depakote. Valproic acid is available in tablet and syrup form. Divalproex sodium is available in tablet, injection, or in sprinkle form.

Recommended dosage

Valproic acid usually requires two to four oral doses each day. The typical total daily dose is initiated at 15mg per kilogram (2.2 pounds) of body weight, and is increased in weekly intervals by 5–10 mg per kilogram of body weight until seizures are controlled. The frequency

of adverse effects may increase with increasing doses, therefore, changes in dosage are made gradually. It may require several weeks of dosage titration (adjustment for maximum benefit and minimum risk) to realize the full benefits of valproic acid or divalproex sodium.

Persons should not take a double dose of anticonvulsant medications. If a daily dose is missed, it should be taken as soon as possible. However, if it is almost time for the next dose, the missed dose should be skipped.

When discontinuing treatment including valproic acid or divalproex sodium, physicians typically direct patients to gradually reduce their daily dosages. Stopping the medicine suddenly may cause seizures to occur or become more frequent.

Precautions

Persons should avoid alcohol while taking valproic acid or divalproex sodium. It can exacerbate (heighten) the side effects of alcohol and other medications. A physician should also be consulted before taking valproic acid or divalproex sodium with certain non-prescription medications, such as medicines for asthma, appetite control, coughs, colds, sinus problems, allergies, and hay fever.

Valproic acid and divalproex sodium may not be suitable for persons with a history of liver or kidney disease, mental illness, high blood presure, angina (chest **pain**), irregular heartbeats, or other heart problems. Valproic acid and divalproex sodium may cause liver damage (hepatotoxicity), though the risk is low in adults. The prescribing physician may order routine blood tests to screen for liver damage.

Before beginning treatment with valproic acid or divalproex sodium, patients should notify their physician if they consume a large amount of alcohol, have a history of drug use, are pregnant, or plan to become pregnant.

Valproic acid and divalproex sodium may cause birth defects, and have been linked to an increased risk of **spina**

bifida. Physicians often counsel their patients to use effective birth control while taking either of these medications. Unlike many other anti-convulsant medications, valproic acid will not decrease the effectiveness of oral contraceptives (birth control pills). Patients who become pregnant while taking valproic acid or divalproex sodium should contact their physician immediately.

Side effects

Research indicates that valproic acid and divalproex sodium are generally well tolerated. In certain individuals and especially children under two years of age, however, valproic acid may cause severe damage to the liver or pancreas. It is important to keep all appointments with the physician and laboratory to monitor the body's response to valproic acid. Temporary nausea, vomiting, stomach cramps, weight gain, temporary hair loss, shaking, and an irregular menstrual cycle are the most frequently reported side effects of valproic acid and divalproex sodium. Other possible side effects include:

- nervousness
- anxiety
- difficulty with memory
- double vision
- loss of appetite
- restlessness
- sleepiness or sleeplessness
- unusual drowsiness
- diarrhea or constipation
- heartburn or indigestion
- aching joints and muscles or chills
- unpleasant taste in mouth or dry mouth
- tingling or prickly feeling on the skin

Many of these side effects disappear or occur less frequently during treatment as the body adjusts to the medication.

Other, uncommon side effects of valproic acid and divalproex sodium can be potentially serious. A patient taking valproic acid who experiencs any of the following symptoms should contact their physician:

- jaundice (yellow tone to skin and eyes)
- facial swelling
- persistent fatigue
- rash
- mood or mental changes
- **depression**
- persistent trembling of the arms and hands
- restlessness

Key Terms

Bi-polar disorder A mood disorder characterized by periods of excessive excitability and energy alternating with periods of depression and lack of energy.

Epilepsy A disorder associated with disturbed electrical discharges in the central nervous system that cause seizures.

Hepatotoxicity Damaging or destructive to the liver.

Seizure A convulsion, or uncontrolled discharge of nerve cells that may spread to other cells throughout the brain.

Spina bifida A birth defect in which the neural tube fails to close during fetal development and a portion of the spinal cord and nerves fail to develop properly.

- excessive sleeplessness
- hallucinations
- difficulty breathing
- chest pain
- irregular heartbeat
- faintness
- persistent, severe **headaches**
- persistent fever or pain.

Interactions

Valproic acid and divalproex sodium may have negative interactions with some antacids, tricyclic antidepressants, antibiotics, monoamine oxidase inhibitors (MAOIs), and asprin and other non-steroidal anti-inflammatories (NSAIDs). Other medications such as **Diazepam** (Valium), **phenobarbital** (Luminal, Solfoton), nefazodone, metronidazole, **acetazolamide** (Diamox), phenytoin (Dilantin), **primidone**, propranolol (Inderal), and warfarin may also adversely react with volparic acid.

Volparic acid and divalproex sodium may react adversely with other **anticonvulsants** and anti-epilepsy drugs (AEDs). They should be used with other other seizure prevention medications only if advised by a physician.

Resources

BOOKS

Weaver, Donald F. *Epilepsy and Seizures: Everything You Need to Know*. Richmond Hill, Ontario: Firefly Books, 2001.

OTHER

American Society of Health-System Pharmacists, Inc. "Valproic acid." *Medline Plus.* <http://www.nlm.nih.gov/medlineplus/druginfo/medmaster/a682412.html> (March 20, 2004).

"Introduction to valproic acid." *Epilepsy.com.* The Epilepsy Project. <http://www.epilepsy.com/medications/b_valproicacid_intro.html> (March 20, 2004).

ORGANIZATIONS

American Epilepsy Society. 342 North Main Street, West Hartford, CT 06117-2507. <http://www.aesnet.org>.

Epilepsy Foundation. 4351 Garden City Drive, Landover, MD 20785-7223. (800) 332-1000. <http://www.epilepsyfoundation.org>.

Adrienne Wilmoth Lerner

Vasculitic neuropathy

Definition

Vasculitic neuropathy refers to damage to the peripheral nerves (the nerves that are located outside of the brain and spinal cord) as a consequence of **vasculitis** (a condition characterized by inflammation and destruction of blood vessels).

Description

Vasculitis refers to a number of conditions that cause inflammation in the blood vessels of the body. This inflammation can prevent sufficient blood flow from reaching various organs and tissues of the body. Because adequate blood flow is required to provide the organs and tissues with oxygen, vasculitis causes damage to oxygen-deprived organs and tissues. When peripheral nerves are oxygen-deprived due to vasculitis, vasculitic neuropathy ensues.

Peripheral neuropathy can occur as the only symptom of vasculitis, or it can be part of a symptom complex.

Demographics

About 60-70% of all patients with vasculitis will experience peripheral neuropathy. In fact, about 34% of all patients with vasculitis will manifest peripheral neuropathy as the sole manifestation of their vasculitis. The average age of an individual with vasculitic neuropathy is 62.

Causes and symptoms

Vasculitic neuropathy can accompany a number of types of vasculitis, including polyarteritis nodosa, Churg-Strauss syndrome, Wegener's granulomatosis, Sjogren's syndrome, rheumatoid vasculitis, and vasculitis due to infections (such as **Lyme disease**, hepatitis, or HIV). Vasculitis occurs when the body's immune system accidentally misidentifies markers on the blood vessel walls as foreign. The immune system then begins to produce immune cells that attack and destroy the blood vessels. As the blood vessels become inflamed, blood flow through them is diminished, resulting in oxygen deprivation of the organs or tissues they normally serve. When the oxygen-deprived tissues are nerve cells, vasculitic neuropathy results.

Most people with vasculitic neuropathy notice **pain** and then weakness in a random, nonsymmetric distribution throughout their limbs; a smaller number (about one-third of all sufferers) notice pain and weakness that progress in a symmetric fashion, beginning with the feet or hands and progressing up the limbs. The pain of vasculitic neuropathy can include shooting, sharp pain, tingling, numbness, burning, and stinging. Some patients with vasculitic neuropathy will also experience fever, decreased appetite, weight loss, rash, **fatigue**, joint pain, and kidney problems.

Diagnosis

Examining a sample of an affected nerve cell (**biopsy**) will allow the diagnosis to be made. The biopsy will demonstrate the inflammation and destruction of blood vessel walls characteristic of vasculitis. Electrodiagnostic studies use needle electrodes to stimulate affected nerves or muscles, in order to demonstrate a slow or abnormal response.

Treatment team

Vasculitic neuropathy may be treated by a **neurologist** or a rheumatologist. Physical and occupational therapists can help optimize recovery of function.

Treatment

Treatment for vasculitic neuropathy involves medications that decrease inflammation and suppress the activity of the immune system. Such medications include corticosteroids and cyclophosphamide. Physical and occupational therapy can help restore functioning and can provide strategies to help overcome any permanent disabilities caused by the vasculitic neuropathy.

Prognosis

Once treatment for vasculitic neuropathy has been initiated, symptom progression should halt, and the condition should stabilize. Some improvement in already established

Key Terms

Neuropathy A disease of the nervous system.

Peripheral nerves Nerves outside of those in the brain and spinal cord.

Vasculitis A condition in which inflammation of the blood vessels deprives organs and tissues of oxygen, resulting in damage.

symptoms is possible; pain may decrease, and some degree of weakness may improve, although recovery of function is usually very slow and only partial.

Resources

BOOKS

Chalk, Colin. "Peripheral Neuropathies." In *Conn's Current Therapy 2004*, 56th ed., edited by Shaun Ruddy, et al. Elsevier, 2004.

Griffin, John W. "Immune-Mediated Neuropathies." In *Cecil Textbook of Internal Medicine*, edited by Lee Goldman, et al. Philadelphia: W. B. Saunders Company, 2000.

PERIODICALS

Griffin, John W. "Vasculitic Neuropathies." *Rheumatic Diseases Clinics of North America* 27 (November 2001): 751–760.

Nadeau, S. E. "Neurologic Manifestations of Systemic Vasculitis." *Neurologic Clinics* 20, no. 1 (February 2002): 123–150.

Pascuzzi, Robert M. "Peripheral Neuropathies in Clinical Practice." *Medical Clinics of North America* 87 (May 2003): 697–724.

Rosalyn Carson-DeWitt, MD

Vasculitis

Definition

Vasculitis refers to a condition that causes inflammation of blood vessels (arteries, capillaries, and/or veins). When the blood vessels become inflamed, scarring, thickening of the vessel walls, and narrowing of the vessel caliber decrease the amount of blood flow through the blood vessels. When there is less blood flow, the organs or tissues that should be receiving blood flow are deprived of oxygen, causing damage to them. Because blood vessels anywhere in the body can be affected by vasculitis, organs and tissues anywhere in the body can be damaged by its

consequences. Vasculitis can occur very focally (in a relatively small, circumscribed area) or diffusely (a widespread network of blood vessels are inflamed).

Description

Vasculitis describes a large number of conditions. Vasculitis can be primary (the vessel inflammation occurs spontaneously, with no other associated disease process) or secondary (the vessel inflammation occurs due to some other preexisting disease). Secondary vasculitis can be a manifestation of a large number of disease processes, including a variety of connective tissue or autoimmune diseases such as rheumatoid arthritis, systemic **lupus** erythematosus, Raynaud's phenomenon, Sjogren's syndrome, sclerodactyly, **polymyositis**, and **dermatomyositis**, as well as sarcoidosis, malignancy, hepatitis B and hepatitis C infections, allergic reactions to antibiotics and/or diuretics, and severe bacterial infections such as endocarditis, pneumonia, meningitis, gonorrhea, or syphilis.

Normally, inflammation is an immune system response to the presence of either an injury or an infection with an invading organism such as a virus, bacteria, or fungi. When faced with either of these threats, the immune system produces a variety of cells and chemicals that cause blood vessels in the injured or infected area to dilate and then become leaky. Fluid, protein, and blood cells leak out of the blood vessels and into the surrounding tissues, causing swelling. The affected area turns red, warm, and painful.

Inflammation causes a cascade of effects, both in the tissues adjacent to the initial area of inflammation and at distant sites throughout the body. Locally, the process of inflammation causes various chemicals of inflammation to leak out into the neighboring tissues, prompting the same cycle of vessel dilatation and leakiness, resulting in swelling of those neighboring tissues. Chemicals of inflammation traveling through the bloodstream can precipitate the cycle of inflammation in tissues and/or organs at a distance from the initial site of inflammation.

In vasculitis, the inflammation response has gone awry: it may be kicked off initially by the presence of an invader such as vasculitis secondary to a severe bacterial infection; it may be part of an overall immune system over-reactiveness as occurs when vasculitis occurs secondary to an autoimmune disease such as systemic lupus erythematosus and rheumatoid arthritis; or it may erupt spontaneously as in cases of primary vasculitis. The end results, however, are inflammation and destruction of blood vessel walls, blood clot blockages within blood vessels, **aneurysms** (weakened bulging areas of blood vessel walls which can rupture, causing catastrophic bleeding),

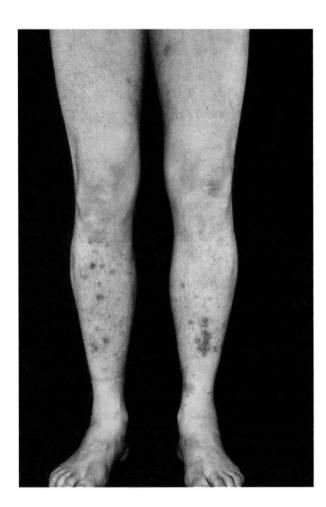

Some symptoms of vasculitis. *(Custom Medical Stock Photo. Reproduced by permission.)*

Demographics

Each type of vasculitis has its own primary demographic. Those that tend to strike older individuals include polyarteritis nodosa, giant cell or temporal arteritis, and Wegener's granulomatosis. Takayasu's arteritis tends to strike individuals in middle age. Henoch-Schonlein pupura and Kawaskai disease tend to strike children.

Causes and symptoms

Some researchers believe that vasculitis is prompted by the deposition of antibody-antigen complexes along the inside of blood vessel walls. Antibodies are immune cells that recognize and attach to specific markers (antigens) on foreign cells such as bacteria, viruses, and fungi. The presence of antibody-antigen complexes serves to jumpstart the immune cell response, prompting it to produce a variety of other cells and chemicals in an effort to rid the body of a foreign invader. Sometimes, however, the body accidentally produces antibodies that accidentally identify antigens on the body's own cells as foreign. When these antibodies bind to the body's antigens, the same immune response is provoked, but instead of being directed against a foreign invader, it is directed against the body itself.

Some researchers believe that the immune system is prompted into action by the presence of an actual threat (in the case of secondary vasculitis due to a bacterial infection), or is already overreacting (in the case of secondary vasculitis due to a preexisting autoimmune disease), or spontaneously swings into an overreactive state (in the case of primary vasculitis).

Symptoms of vasculitis depend on the specific organs or tissues affected. Affected body systems and potential symptoms include:

• Skin. Vasculitis of the skin may lead to a variety of rashes, bumps, bruises, or areas of subtle bleeding such

and oxygen deprivation of the affected organs and/or tissues, leading to damage and destruction of various tissue or organs throughout the body.

A variety of classification systems have been developed to describe and organize the various types of vasculitis. These include systems that are based on the specific organs affected, and systems that are based on the size and type of vessels affected, and the kinds of microscopic, cellular changes seen within those vessels. One of the most popular systems for classification of vasculitis is called the Chapel Hill system, named for the creators at the University of North Carolina-Chapel Hill. This system divides the types of vasculitis into three categories: large-vessel vasculitis (including giant cell or **temporal arteritis** and Takayasu's arteritis); medium-vessel vasculitis (including polyarteritis nodosa and Kawasaki's disease); and small-vessel vasculitis (including Wegener's granulomatosis, Churg-Strauss syndrome, microsopic polynagiitis, Henoch-Schonlein purpura, essential cryoglobulinemic vasculitis, and cutaneous leukocytoclastic angiitis).

as petechia (tiny red dots), pupura (larger reddish purple spots), or ecchymoses (large, complexly colored areas of bruising). When areas of skin are completely deprived of any blood flow, and therefore of any oxygen delivery, the skin may die and turn black (gangrene).

- Joints. Vasculitis-induced arthritis occurs when the lining of the joints is affected by vasculitis, causing swelling, **pain**, decreased range of motion, and reduced functioning.

- Brain and nervous system. When vasculitis affects the nervous system, a variety of symptoms may result. Vasculitis of blood vessels in the brain can lead to headaches, confusion, personality changes, **seizures**, and coma. Depending on the area of the brain affected, other senses may suffer, including vision, hearing, and/or balance. Vasculitis of the nerves that provide sensation to the arms or legs can lead to pain and paresthesias (odd sensations of tingling, burning, pinpricks, lightning-flashes of pain, or numbness). A **stroke** occurs when an area of the brain tissue is completely deprived of oxygen, causing severe damage or destruction. The results of a stroke may be temporary or permanent, and the specific types of potential disability depend on what functions are normally controlled by the area of brain injured by the stroke.

- Gastrointestinal system. Any part of the gastrointestinal system can be affected by vasculitis, including the liver. Symptoms referable to the gastrointestinal system include pain, diarrhea, constipation, and vomiting. When blood flow is cut off to an area of the intestine, that area will become gangrenous or necrotic and die. This is a medical emergency.

- Heart. Vasculitis of the coronary arteries, which normally feed the heart muscle, can result in weakening of the heart muscle with compensatory enlargement, heart attack, or myocardial infarction. When the walls of the arteries or the aorta undergo serious destruction due to vasculitis, weakened bulges called aneurysms may develop. If these aneurysms rupture, hemorrhage may occur.

- Lungs. Vasculitis of the complex network of blood vessels throughout the lungs can result in severe shortness of breath, cough, chest pain, and wheezing.

- Kidneys. When the kidney or renal arteries are damaged by vasculitis, high blood pressure results. The kidneys may fall behind in their normal role of filtering the blood, and kidney or renal failure may occur.

Diagnosis

Initial attempts to diagnosis vasculitis will depend on the area of the body affected and the kinds of symptoms exhibited. Blood tests that can demonstrate the presence of a strong inflammatory process include erythrocyte sedimentation rate, C-reactive protein, increased white blood cell count, and a variety of tests that can identify the presence of immune complexes or antibodies circulating within the blood. A variety of imaging techniques may reveal blood vessel inflammation, including ultrasound, echocardiography, computed tomography (**CT**), and **magnetic resonance imaging (MRI)** scanning. When the kidneys are involved, urine tests may reveal abnormalities. An x-ray procedure called **angiography** involves the injection of dye into a major artery to allow the detection of inflammation in the walls of blood vessels. Biopsies (tissue samples) may be taken from the blood vessels that serve affected organs or tissues to look for the presence of inflammation or scarring.

Treatment team

While rheumatologists specialize in the treatment of various autoimmune diseases (including various forms of vasculitis), patients may also be treated by specialists who concentrate on diseases that affect specific organs or tissues. For example, a patient may need to consult a cardiologist if the heart is affected; a nephrologist if the kidneys are affected; a **neurologist** if the nervous system is affected; a pulmonologist if the lungs are affected; a gastroenterologist if the gastrointestinal tract is affected; an ophthomologist if the eyes are affected; an otorhinolaryngologist if the ear, nose, and/or throat are affected; or a dermatologist if the skin is affected.

Treatment

Medications that calm the immune system and decrease inflammation are the mainstay of treatment for the various types of vasculitis. These include nonsteroidal anti-inflammatory medications (such as ibuprofen or aspirin) and corticosteroids (such as prednisone). More severe cases of vasculitis may require potent immunosuppressant drugs (such as cyclophosphamide or azathioprine).

Prognosis

The prognosis of vasculitis depends on the specific organ system affected and the severity of the particular case. In general, most people who receive appropriate treatment have a good recovery from vasculitis. However, when the disease causes kidney failure or affects the heart, the prognosis may be worse. Basic prognosis statistics of treated vasculitis include:

- Polyarteritis nodosa: about 90% of cases go into long-term remission.

- Hypersensitivity vasculitis: Most people recover completely, even without treatment.

- Giant cell arteritis: May require one to two years of steroid treatment, but most people recover completely.

• Wegener's granulomatosis: With treatment, 90% can expect symptom relief, and 75% go into complete remission.

• Takayasu's arteritis: 90% survive, with some spontaneous remission.

• Kawasaki disease: Under 3% of patients suffer fatal complications; most children recover uneventfully.

Resources

BOOKS

Fauci, Anthony S. "The Vasculitis Syndromes." In *Harrison's Principles of Internal Medicine*, edited by Eugene Braunwald, et al. New York: McGraw-Hill Professional, 2001.

Cercomb, Clare T. "Systemic Lupus Erythematosus and the Vasculitides." In *Rosen's Emergency Medicine: Concepts and Clinical Practice*, 5th ed., edited by Lee Goldman, et al. St. Louis: Mosby, Inc., 2002.

Sergent, John S. "Vasculitic Syndromes." In *Kelley's Textbook of Rheumatology*, edited by Shaun Ruddy, et al. Philadelphia: W. B. Saunders Company, 2001.

PERIODICALS

González-Gay, M. A. "Epidemiology of the Vasculitides." *Rheumatic Disease Clinics of North America* 27, no. 4 (1 November 2001): 729–749.

Langford, C. A. "Vasculitis." *Journal of Allergy and Clinical Immunology* 111, no. 2 (1 February 2003): 602–612.

Naides, Stanley. "Known Infectious Causes of Vasculitis in Man." *Cleveland Clinic Journal of Medicine* 69, no. 2.

ORGANIZATIONS

Johns Hopkins Vasculitis Center. Bayview Medical Center, 5501 Hopkins Bayview Circle, JHAAC, Room 1B.1A, Baltimore, MD 21224. (410) 550-6825. <http://vasculitis.med.jhu.edu/index.html>.

Rosalyn Carson-DeWitt, MD

Ventilatory assistance devices

Definition

Ventilatory assistance devices are mechanical devices that help a person breathe by replacing some or all of the muscular effort required to inflate the lungs.

Description

Ventilation is the process of inflating and deflating the lungs in order to breathe. Normally, a person uses several sets of muscles to accomplish this—the diaphragm at the base of the lungs, the muscles between the ribs (intercostals), and, to a small extent, the muscles of the lower neck and shoulder area. When these muscles are weakened through disease or injury, the ability to ventilate is impaired. As a result, a person cannot get sufficient oxygen

into, and carbon dioxide out of, the lungs in order to maintain appropriate levels in the blood. In addition, weakened ventilation muscles also impair the ability to cough, which is an essential part of clearing lung secretions and preventing infection.

Ventilatory assistance devices may be needed due to:

• muscular dystrophies (progressive muscle weakening disorders)

• amyotrophic lateral sclerosis (ALS), a progressive disease causing muscle weakness

• polio

• high **spinal cord injury** (injury to the spinal cord in the neck)

• Guillain-Barré syndrome (a rapidly progressive but reversible loss of muscle control)

• myasthenia gravis, acute crisis (MG is a muscle-weakening disease, in which patients may experience a "crisis" of rapid and dangerous loss of muscle strength)

• head trauma

• botulism (poisoning by **botulinum toxin**, usually from improperly preserved food)

• tetanus (poisoning by tetanus bacteria, usually by a deep puncture wound)

Nighttime ventilators are also used for people with obstructive **sleep apnea**. This is a condition in which breathing is impaired during sleep by obstructions in the airway, most often extra tissue at the rear of the throat.

Ventilatory assistance is not the same as supplying extra oxygen, as is done for people whose lungs are damaged. The person who needs ventilatory assistance generally has normal gas exchange capacity, and simply needs help moving air in and out. Supplemental oxygen can worsen the situation in such cases, as it may depress the normal signals from the brain to stimulate breathing.

Ventilators

A ventilator is a machine that uses a tube to blow air into, and suck it out of, the body. The ventilator may be designed to deliver air at a set volume (volume ventilator) or at a set pressure (pressure ventilator).

Volume ventilator settings may be adjusted to deliver a variable volume of air depending on the patient's needs, and can either cycle automatically or be initiated by the patient's voluntary efforts.

Pressure ventilators come in two major styles. Continuous positive airway pressure (CPAP) delivers air at a steady pressure, which assists the patient while breathing in (inspiration) and resists breathing out (expiration). The purpose of CPAP is not to completely inflate the lungs, but rather to maintain an open airway. This makes it most appropriate for use in sleep apnea, in which a patient's airway closes frequently during sleep. In contrast, bi-level positive airway pressure (BiPAP) delivers a higher pressure on inspiration in order to allow the patient to completely inflate the lungs, and then switches to a low pressure on expiration, to allow easy exhalation. BiPAP is a common choice for patients with neuromuscular disease, whose respiratory muscles are weakened.

There are other rarer devices in use, which surround a patient's chest cavity and abdomen with a rigid shell, and change the pressure within. By lowering the pressure, air rushes into the lungs. The "iron lung" is one such device; smaller and more portable "cuirasses" are occasionally used to similar effect.

Interfaces

The air from a ventilator is delivered to the patient either through a face mask or directly into the lungs through a tracheostomy (trach) tube. Each has its advantages and disadvantages.

A tracheostomy is an opening in the airway in the middle of the throat through which a tube is inserted to deliver air. The properly chosen trach tube will fit comfortably. A widespread misunderstanding about tracheostomy ventilation is that it prevents talking, but this does not have to be so. Trach tubes are available that do not interfere with speech, and patients contemplating tracheostomy should ensure that their respiratory specialist is familiar with them. Trach tubes may provide the patient a greater sense of security and, unlike a face mask, it can easily be hidden from view with a well-placed scarf. Trach tubes do require daily lung hygiene, either by the patient or by a trained caregiver. This involves suctioning out secretions from the lungs, which tend to be increased due to the presence of the tube.

Face masks fit snugly over the mouth and nose, and are held on with a strap. Finding the right mask takes some time, but a well-fitting mask is comfortable and easy to tolerate for many hours per day. The mask usually must be removed to talk, but this does not present a problem for many patients who retain some use of their hands. The mask may also be used at night.

Other noninvasive interfaces are also available, including mouthpieces and "nasal pillows" that fit into one or the other orifice and are smaller than masks. These methods are usually chosen for patients who need fewer hours per day of ventilatory assistance.

Coughing

Patients with weakened respiratory muscles may be even more in need of cough assistance than they are of ventilatory assistance. Cough assistance may be delivered manually by a caregiver or by a machine (the in-exsufflator or cough assist) that is designed to inflate the lungs and then rapidly withdraw air, as occurs in a normal cough. This clears secretions that would otherwise accumulate and provide a locus for infection, as well as interfere with gas exchange.

Resources

BOOKS

Bach, J. R. *Noninvasive Mechanical Ventilation.* Philadelphia: Hanley & Belfus, 2002.

Kinnear, W. J. M. *Assisted Ventilation at Home: A Practical Guide.* Oxford: Oxford Medical Publications, 1994.

OTHERS

Robinson, R. "Breathe Easy." *Quest Magazine* 5, no. 5 (October 1998) (April 18, 2004). <http://www.mdausa.org/publications/Quest/q55breathe.html>.

Robinson, R. "A Breath of Fresh Air." *Quest Magazine* 5, no. 6 (October 1998) (April 18, 2004). <http://www.mdausa.org/publications/Quest/q56freshair.html>.

WEBSITES

Muscular Dystrophy Association. <http://www.mdausa.org> (April 18, 2004).

Richard Robinson

Ventricular shunt

Definition

A ventricular shunt is a tube that is surgically placed in one of the fluid-filled chambers inside the brain (ventricles). The fluid around the brain and the spinal column is called cerebrospinal fluid (CSF). When infection or disease causes an excess of CSF in the ventricles, the shunt is placed to drain it and thereby relieve excess pressure.

Purpose

A ventricular shunt relieves **hydrocephalus**, a condition in which there is an increased volume of CSF within the ventricles. In hydrocephalus, pressure from the CSF usually increases. It may be caused by a tumor of the brain or of the membranes covering the brain (**meninges**), infection of or bleeding into the CSF, or inborn malformations of the brain. Symptoms of hydrocephalus may include **headache**, personality disturbances and loss of intellectual abilities (**dementia**), problems in walking, irritability, vomiting, abnormal eye movements, or a low level of consciousness.

Normal pressure hydrocephalus (a condition in which the volume of CSF increases without an increase in pressure) is associated with progressive dementia, problems walking, and loss of bladder control (urinary incontinence). Even though CSF is not thought to be under increased pressure in this condition, it may also be treated by ventricular shunting.

Demographics

The congenital form of hydrocephalus is believed to occur at an incidence of approximately one to four out of every 1,000 births. The incidence of acquired hydrocephalus is not exactly known. The peak ages for the development of hydrocephalus are in infancy, between four and eight years, and in early adulthood. Normal pressure hydrocephalus generally occurs in patients over the age of 60.

Description

The ventricular shunt tube is placed to drain fluid from the **ventricular system** in the brain to the cavity of the abdomen or to the large vein in the neck (jugular vein). Therefore, surgical procedures must be done both in the brain and at the drainage site. The tubing contains valves to ensure that fluid can only flow out of the brain and not back into it. The valve can be set at a desired pressure to allow CSF to escape whenever the pressure level is exceeded. In some cases where only brief drainage is needed, the shunt tube may simply drain to the outside.

A small reservoir may be attached to the tubing and placed under the scalp. This reservoir allows samples of CSF to be removed with a syringe to check the pressure. Fluid from the reservoir can also be examined for bacteria, cancer cells, blood, or protein, depending on the cause of hydrocephalus. The reservoir may also be used to inject antibiotics for CSF infection or chemotherapy medication for meningeal tumors.

Diagnosis/Preparation

The diagnosis of hydrocephalus should be confirmed by diagnostic imaging techniques such as computed tomography scan (**CT scan**) or **magnetic resonance imaging (MRI)** before the shunting procedure is performed. These techniques will also show any associated brain abnormalities. CSF should be examined if infection or tumor

Key Terms

Cerebrospinal fluid   Fluid bathing the brain and spinal cord.

Computed tomography (CT) scan   An imaging technique in which cross-sectional x rays of the body are compiled to create a three-dimensional image of the body's internal structures.

Dementia   Progressive loss of mental abilities.

Magnetic resonance imaging (MRI)   An imaging technique that uses a large circular magnet and radio waves to generate signals from atoms in the body. These signals are used to construct images of internal structures.

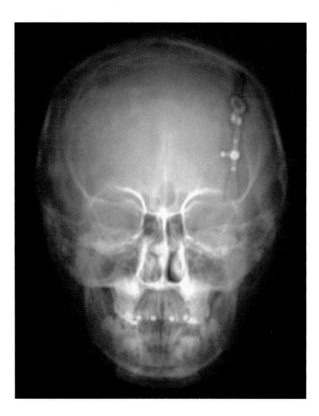

A digitally enhanced x ray of the skull of a nine-year-old boy showing the shunt that was placed into the ventricle of the brain. *(Scott Camazine / Photo Researchers, Inc.)*

of the meninges is suspected. Patients with dementia or **mental retardation** should undergo **neuropsychological testing** to establish a baseline psychological profile before the shunting procedure.

As with any surgical procedure, the surgeon must know about any medications or health problems that may increase the patient's risk. Because infections are both common and serious, antibiotics are often given before and after surgery.

Aftercare

To avoid infections at the shunt site, the area should be kept clean. The physician should periodically check CSF to be sure there is no infection or bleeding into the shunt. CSF pressure should be checked to be sure the shunt is operating properly. The eyes should be examined regularly because shunt failure may damage the nerve to the eyes (optic nerve). If not treated promptly, damage to the optic nerve causes irreversible loss of vision.

Risks

Serious and long-term complications of ventricular shunting are bleeding under the outermost covering of the brain (**subdural hematoma**), infection, **stroke**, and shunt failure. When a shunt drains to the abdomen (ventriculoperitoneal shunt), fluid may accumulate in the abdomen or abdominal organs may be injured. If CSF pressure is lowered too much, patients may have severe headaches, often with nausea and vomiting, whenever they sit up or stand.

Normal results

After shunting, the ventricles get smaller within three or four days. This shrinkage occurs even when hydrocephalus has been present for a year or more. Clinically detectable signs of improvement occur within a few weeks. The cause of hydrocephalus, duration of hydrocephalus before shunting, and associated brain abnormalities affect the outcome.

Of patients with normal pressure hydrocephalus who are treated with shunting, 25–80% experience long-term improvement. Normal pressure hydrocephalus is more likely to improve when it is caused by infection of or bleeding into the CSF than when it occurs without an underlying cause.

Morbidity and mortality rates

Complications of shunting occur in 30% of cases, but only 5% are serious. Infections occur in 5–10% of patients, and as many as 80% of shunts develop a mechanical problem at some point and need to be replaced.

Alternatives

In some cases of hydrocephalus, certain drugs may be administered to temporarily decrease the amount of CSF until surgery can be performed. In patients with hydrocephalus caused by a tumor, removal of the tumor often cures the buildup of CSF. Approximately 25% of patients respond to therapies other than shunt placement.

Patients with normal pressure hydrocephalus may experience a temporary improvement in walking and mental abilities upon the temporary drainage of a moderate amount of CSF. This improvement may be an indication that shunting will improve their condition.

Resources

BOOKS

Aldrich, E. Francois, Lawrence S. Chin, Arthur J. DiPatri, and Howard M. Eisenberg. "Hydrocephalus." *Sabiston Textbook of Surgery*, edited by Courtney M. Townsend Jr. 16th ed. Philadelphia: W. B. Saunders Company, 2001.

Golden, Jeffery A., and Carsten G. Bonnemann. "Hydrocephalus." *Textbook of Clinical Neurology*, edited by Christopher G. Goetz and Eric J. Pappert. Philadelphia: W. B. Saunders Company, 1999.

PERIODICALS

Hamid, Rukaiya K. A., and Philippa Newfield. "Pediatric Neuroanesthesia: Hydrocephalus." *Anesthesiology Clinics of North America* 19, no. 2 (June 1, 2001): 207–18.

ORGANIZATIONS

American Academy of Neurology. 1080 Montreal Ave., St. Paul, MN 55116. (800) 879-1960. (March 2, 2004). <http://www.aan.com>.

OTHER

Hord, Eugenia-Daniela. "Hydrocephalus." *eMedicine*, January 14, 2002 [cited March 2, 2004]. <http://www.emedicine.com/neuro/topic161.htm>.

Dalvi, Arif. "Normal Pressure Hydrocephalus." *eMedicine*, January 14, 2002 [cited March 2, 2004]. <http://www.emedicine.com/neuro/topic277.htm>.

Sgouros, Spyros. "Management of Spina Bifida, Hydrocephalus, and Shunts." *eMedicine*, May 14, 2003. [cited March 2, 2004]. <http://www.emedicine.com/ped/topic2976.htm>.

Laurie Barclay, MD
Stephanie Dionne Sherk

Ventricular system

Definition

A ventricle is an internal cavity of the brain. Within the normal human brain, there is a connecting system of ventricles, commonly referred to as the ventricular system, which is filled with cerebrospinal fluid (CSF). The ventricular system within the brain develops from the cavity of the neural tube in the embryo.

Description

The ventricular system is composed of two lateral ventricles and two midline ventricles, referred to as the third and fourth ventricles. The chambers are connected to allow the flow of cerebrospinal fluid via two interventricular foramen (referred to as the foramen of Monro) and the cerebral aqueduct (referred to as the aqueduct of Sylvius).

The chambers of the ventricular system are lined or covered with ependymal cells and are continuous with the central canal enclosed within the spinal cord. Ependymal cells also line the central canal of the spinal cord.

Basic anatomy
The lateral ventricles

The lateral ventricles are separated by the septum pellucidum and do not communicate directly (i.e., do not allow the flow of cerebrospinal fluid) with each other. Cerebrospinal fluid within the individual lateral ventricles must flow to the third ventricle via the interventricular foramen associated with each lateral ventricle.

Lateral ventricles themselves are descriptively divided into a body with anterior, posterior, and inferior horns.

The third ventricle

The third ventricle is a narrow cavity or cleft located between the two thalami. The third ventricle also contains two saclike recesses called the anterior supraoptic recess and the infundibular recess. The massa intermedia, the neural tissue that connects both halves of the thalamus in some brains, runs through the third ventricle. Posteriorly, the third ventricle communicates with the fourth ventricle via the cerebral aqueduct, a narrow channel that allows the flow of cerebrospinal fluid from the third to the fourth ventricle. There is no choroids plexus within the cerebral aqueduct.

The fourth ventricle

The fourth ventricle is a wide and flattened space located just anterior to the **cerebellum** and posterior to the upper, or superior, half of the medulla oblongata and the pons. The fourth ventricle also has two lateral saclike pouches that are called the lateral recesses. The fourth ventricle is continuous with the upper (superior) terminal end of the central canal of the spinal cord. The fourth ventricle also connects with the subarachnoid space via three small foramina: the two foramina of Luschka (one in each of the lateral recesses) and the foramen of Magendie.

The subarachnoid space continues as the space between the arachnoid matter and the pia mater (meningal

tissues that surround the brain and spinal cord) and is filled with CSF. The subarachnoid space also surrounds cranial and spinal nerves.

CSF flow and blockage of the ventricular system

The normal flow of cerebrospinal fluid—produced from brain surface tissue and the choroids plexuses within the ventricles—is from the two lateral ventricles through their respective interventricular foramina into the third ventricle. Then the CSF flows from the third ventricle through the cerebral aqueduct into the fourth ventricle and from there it can flow into the subarachnoid space where it is reabsorbed into the bloodstream.

Swellings or structures within the ventricular system may be due to congenital defect, trauma, or tumor.

If there is a blockage of the ventricular system the flow of CSF is interrupted. If, for example, there is a blockage within the cerebral aqueduct, the normal flow of fluid formed in the lateral ventricles and the third ventricle is interrupted, and the lateral ventricles and third ventricle begin to swell with cerebrospinal fluid. The swelling or enlargement is termed **hydrocephalus**. Hydrocephalus can also result from the formation of CSF (as can occur with a tumor in one of the choroid plexuses) that exceeds the amount that can flow through the ventricular system, or from a downstream-diminished capacity to absorb cerebrospinal fluid.

A tumor in one of the interventricular foramen connecting a lateral ventricle to the third ventricle obstructs the flow of cerebrospinal fluid from the same side lateral ventricle and results in an asymmetrical swelling of the blocked lateral ventricle.

Blockage of the flow of CSF through the foramen connecting the fourth ventricle to the subarachnoid space usually produces asymmetrical swelling or dilation of the entire ventricular system. The entire ventricular system can also swell in cases of meningitis in which the flow of cerebrospinal fluid over the outer surface of the brain is obstructed.

Resources
BOOKS

Bear, M., et al. *Neuroscience: Exploring the Brain.* Baltimore: Williams & Wilkins, 1996.

Goetz, C. G., et al. *Textbook of Clinical Neurology.* Philadelphia: W.B. Saunders Company, 1999.

WEBSITES

"Development of the Ventricular System." *Temple University Department of Neuroanatomy.* May 10, 2004 (May 27,

Key Terms

Ventricle In neurology, a fluid-filled chamber or cavity within the brain.

2004). <http://courses.temple.edu/neuroanatomy/lab/embryo/ventlate.htm>.

Paul Arthur

Vertebrobasilar disease

Definition

Vertebrobasilar disease describes a broad spectrum of vascular abnormalities in the arterial supply to the brain stem.

Description

The vertebrobasilar circulation (VC, also called the posterior circulation) consists of the arterial supply to the brain stem, **cerebellum**, and occipital cortex. The vertebral arteries arise from the subclavian arteries in the neck. In the brain, the vertebral arteries lie deep in the base of the brain and unite in an area called the medullopontine junction to form the basilar artery. The basilar artery branches again to form the posterior cerebral arteries. Any interruption in blood flow in the VC may cause a broad spectrum of symptoms determined by the specific arterial branch or branches involved, and the degree of occlusion inside the blood vessels. The brain stem is a major area of neurologic activity since this area contains cranial nerves, neurosensory tracts, and the reticular activating system (RAS). Problems in blood flow to the VC result in several overlapping clinical syndromes.

Demographics

In the United States, approximately 25% of strokes and TIAs (transient ischemic attacks or "mini" strokes) occur in the vertebrobasilar circulation. Research with **magnetic resonance imaging (MRI)** studies estimates that 40% of patients with vertebrobasilar TIAs (transient ischemic attacks) have brain stem infarction. The disease affects men twice as often as women. Vertebrobasilar ischemic disease occurs in late life, usually between 70–80 years of age. The incidence (number of new cases) is 20–30 cases per 1,000 for persons over age 75. In the United States, the death rate for **stroke** is higher among

blacks than whites. A severe form of the disorder, called basilar artery syndrome, caused by complete obstruction of the vertebrobasilar circulation (inside the brain) is fatal in 75–85% of cases. Approximately 50% of persons who have infarctions in the vertebrobasilar area report TIA events within days or months prior to onset of permanent deficit.

Causes and symptoms

The cause of vertebrobasilar disease (VD) is atherosclerosis that affects the vertebrobasilar (posterior) circulation at intracranial (inside the cranium and includes the basilar artery) sites and extracranial (outside the cranium and includes the vertebral artery) sites. Partial or complete occlusion can occur in major arteries or smaller arterial branches. The cause of VD is atherosclerosis and vertebrobasilar insufficiency in the brain caused by blockage (occlusion), and is more common among patients with cardiovascular risk factors that typically include obesity, smoking, use of oral contraceptives, advanced age, diabetes mellitus, hypertension (high blood pressure). and dyslipidemias (abnormalities that cause an increase in lipids in the blood). Other causes of vertebrobasilar disease can include destruction to arteries such as fibrotic changes in the muscular layer of arteries (a condition called fibromuscular dysplasia) and arterial dissection or **aneurysms**.

The symptoms of TIA have a short duration and usually last approximately eight minutes. Vertigo is the hallmark symptom of vertebrobasilar insufficiency. Other symptoms include visual defects (diplopia), syncope (drop attacks), dysphagia (difficulty swallowing), **dysarthria**, hoarseness, and facial numbness, or paresthesias. Patients with early stage vertebrobasilar insufficiency have transient episodes of neurologic symptoms. Persons with more advanced disease to the vertebrobasilar circulation may have eye deficits, limb **ataxia**, loss of taste, limb/trunk dysesthesia, nystagmus, and deficit in temperature/pain perception.

Diagnosis

Neuroimaging studies are the primary diagnostic tool necessary to confirm vertebrobasilar disease. Other tests are also indicated and include analysis of blood, electrolytes, glucose, urinalysis, thyroid function tests, and erythrocyte sedimentation rate (a special blood test that rules out other possible disorders). Computed tomography (**CT**) **scans** help to detect mass defects and MRIs can help visualize smaller areas of ischemia. Ultrasound studies can help assess and monitor vertebrobasilar patency (the degree of occlusion).

Key Terms

Cranial nerves The set of twelve nerves found on each side of the head and neck that control the sensory and muscle functions of the eyes, nose, tongue, face, and throat.

Dysarthria Slurred speech.

Hydrocephalus An abnormal accumulation of cerebrospinal fluid within the brain. This accumulation can be harmful by pressing on brain structures, and damaging them.

Infarction Death of tissue due to inadequate blood supply.

Nystagmus An involuntary, rhythmic movement of the eyes.

Paresthesia An abnormal sensation often described as burning, tickling, tingling, or "pins and needles."

Reticular activating system A network of structures, including the brain stem, medulla, thalamus, and nerve pathways, which function together to produce and maintain arousal.

Transient ischemic attack (TIA) A brief interruption of the blood supply to part of the brain that causes a temporary impairment of vision, speech, or movement. Usually, the episode lasts for just a few moments, but it may be a warning sign for a full-scale stroke.

Treatment team

A **neurologist** is typically required as the specialist coordinator of treatment. A neurosurgeon is used for surgical evacuation of hemorrhages complicated by **hydrocephalus**. An interventional neuroradiologist may be required to provide thrombolytic agents (chemicals that dissolve clots) by intra-arterial infusion delivery (injecting a chemical directly in an artery located in the brain using TV monitor-guided imagery).

Treatment

Treatment can be either supportive or interventional if arterial patency is an option. Emergency treatment for a bleeding patient includes airway preservation, control of blood pressure, and assessment of neurologic and mental status, intravenous fluid management, prevention of vomiting, and antiplatelet agents to prevent arterial occlusion. Additionally, a stroke patient may require treatment for

hypertension if present, and mouth feedings should be avoided since the patient may be unable to swallow or chew. Antiplatelet medication is the first line treatment for vertebrobasilar disease, however, the usefulness is unclear. Anticoagulants (heparin) and antiplatelets (aspirin and ticlopidine) are typically given to prevent recurrent or ongoing occlusion (caused by blood clots) of the posterior (vertebrobasilar) circulation.

Recovery and rehabilitation

Recovery is variable depending on the degree of occlusion in the vertebrobasilar circulation. Persons with the severe form, basilar artery occlusion, often die in 75–85% of cases. Rehabilitation depends on the extent of damage and the deficits caused by permanent injury in the brain.

Clinical trials

Research in this area is diversified and abundant. Currently, the National Institute of Neurological Disorders and Stroke (NINDS) is investigating molecular mechanisms associated with neuronal injury. Research concerning the genetics of stroke and **gene therapy** is ongoing in experimental models. New research in high resolution neuroimaging techniques, and rehabilitation have demonstrated compensatory mechanisms (re-circuitry of neurons) as a result of stroke. Further information can be found at <http://www.clinicaltrials.gov>. or <http://www.ninds.nih.gov>.

Prognosis

Vertebrobasilar TIAs have a favorable outcome since the chance for complete stroke is minimal. Collateral circulation from smaller blood vessels may help to improve the outcome.

Special concerns

Clinicians must be vigilant to be suspicious of vertebrobasilar insufficiency in elderly patients who suffer from vertigo. Hemorrhage has to be ruled out before blood thinner (anticoagulation) treatment is initiated. Additionally, it is important to take special precautions when feeding persons with brain stem infarction, because patients can develop problems with normal swallowing mechanisms that can cause aspiration pneumonia (caused by food lodged in the lungs).

Resources
BOOKS

Goldman, Lee, et al. *Cecil's Textbook of Medicine*, 21st edition. Philadelphia: W. B. Saunders Company, 2000.

Noble, John, et al. *Textbook of Primary Care Medicine*, 3rd edition. St. Louis: Mosby, Inc., 2001.

WEBSITES

Henry Ford Hospital *Vertebrobasilar Circulatory Disorders.* (April 27, 2004). <http://www.henryfordhealth.org/12470.cfm>.

ORGANIZATIONS

National Stroke Association. 9707 E. Easter Lane, Englewood, CO 80112. (303) 649-9299 or (800) STROKES; Fax: (303) 649-1328. <http://www.stroke.org>.

Laith Farid Gulli, MD
Alfredo Mori, MBBS
Nicole Mallory, MS,PA-C

Vertigo *see* **Dizziness**

▌ Vestibular schwannoma

Definition

A vestibular schwannoma is a type of benign (non-cancerous) tumor that affects the eighth cranial nerve.

Description

The eighth cranial nerve is involved in both hearing (the auditory or acoustic component of the nerve) and balance (the vestibular component of the nerve). Like all cranial nerves, the eighth cranial nerve (also called the acoustic or auditory nerve) is paired, meaning that there is one on each side of the body. Each eighth cranial nerve runs from the inner ear to the brain, passing through a bony canal called the internal auditory canal. This canal is shared with the seventh cranial nerve, the facial nerve.

Like many nerve fibers, the eighth cranial nerve is wrapped in a sheath composed of specialized Schwann cells that serve to speed the transmission of information along the nerve. When the Schwann cells grow in an uncontrolled fashion, they can develop into a tumor, called schwannoma or neuroma. Although a vestibular schwannoma is not malignant (cancerous), it can still result in serious symptoms caused by pressure on the eighth cranial nerve or on surrounding tissues or the adjacent facial nerve. Most cases of vestibular schwannoma are unilateral; that is, only one of the two eighth cranial nerves is affected.

Demographics

About 100,000 people in the United States develop vestibular schwannoma. Most people who develop a vestibular schwannoma are between the ages of 30 and 50; children rarely develop vestibular schwannoma. Women are slightly more likely than men to develop a vestibular schwannoma.

There is an increased risk of developing a vestibular schwannoma in individuals who have a disease called **neurofibromatosis**. In these cases, the tumors tend to develop on both sides (bilaterally). In fact, about 10% of all cases of vestibular schwannoma occur in individuals who have neurofibromatosis. People with neurofibromatosis who develop vestibular schwannoma may do so at a younger age, sometimes in their teens or early adulthood.

Causes and symptoms

No one knows exactly why some people develop a vestibular schwannoma. Most seem to occur sporadically, with no identifiable cause. There is an increased risk of developing a vestibular schwannoma in individuals with neurofibromatosis, and some research has suggested that individuals who are chronically exposed to loud noise may have an increased risk of developing a vestibular schwannoma.

The initial symptoms of vestibular schwannoma are caused by pressure on the eighth cranial nerve, and include gradually progressive one-sided hearing loss, buzzing in the ears (tinnitus), **dizziness**, and difficulty with balance. In particular, the hearing impairment greatly affects the ability to understand speech (speech discrimination). When the vestibular schwannoma puts pressure on the seventh cranial nerve, **pain** and numbness in the face may develop. Eventually, the facial muscles may become paralyzed. The individual may also experience difficulty chewing and/or swallowing, ear pain, and **headache**. When left untreated, hearing impairment may eventually lead to complete deafness in the affected ear. If the tumor begins to encroach on other brain tissues, the person may experience nausea, vomiting, fever, vision changes, and difficulty walking.

Diagnosis

A careful neurologic examination will reveal the deficits that are characteristic of vestibular schwannoma. Computed tomography (**CT**) or **magnetic resonance imagaing (MRI)** scan may help pinpoint the tumor. Audiometry and brain stem auditory evoked potential tests are performed to establish the degree of hearing deficit prior to treatment. Audiometry assesses hearing acuity by evaluating the ability to hear various volumes and tones. A brain stem auditory evoked potential test evaluates brain wave responses to clicking sounds, in order to assess the functioning of the auditory (hearing) pathways in the brain.

Key Terms

Acuity Sharpness.

Acoustic A term that refers to hearing.

Auditory A term that refers to hearing.

Benign Nonmalignant; not cancer.

Bilateral Occurring on both sides of the body.

Cranial nerve One of 12 pairs of nerves that leave the brain stem.

Neurofibromatosis Also called von Reclinghausen's disease; a disease in which tumors grow on nerve cells throughout the body.

Schwann cell A type of supportive cell in the nervous system that compose the myelin sheath around nerve fibers.

Unilateral Occurring on only one side of the body.

Vestibular A term that refers to the organs of balance.

Treatment team

When an individual is suspected of having a vestibular schwannoma, an otorhinolaryngologist and/or **neurologist** may be consulted to arrive at a diagnosis. An otorhinolaryngologist will be called upon if surgery is required.

Treatment

Surgery is nearly always necessary to treat vestibular schwannoma. There are several different types of surgery that are used to remove a vestibular schwannoma, classified by the anatomical pathway used to reach the tumor (called the "approach"). The surgeon will choose the approach based on tumor size, preoperative hearing acuity, and the patient's ability to tolerate surgical risk. In some cases, it is not possible to remove the entire vestibular schwannoma without considerable risk of damage to adjacent structures. In these cases, only part of the vestibular schwannoma may be removed, and the rest may be left in place (called "partial resection").

When a patient is medically frail, the surgeon may choose to simply monitor the growth of the vestibular schwannoma, delaying surgery until it becomes absolutely necessary. Occasionally, very small vestibular schwannoma may be treated with **radiation** therapy; when partial resection is necessary, surgery may be followed by radiation treatment.

Newer treatment techniques are called stereotactic radiosurgery or gamma knife surgery. Three-dimensional imaging allows the exact location of the tumor to be defined. The patient's head is held in a frame that allows high-dose radiation to be delivered from multiple angles directly at the tumor site.

Recovery and rehabilitation

In patients for whom the hearing impairment is not total, a hearing aid may be helpful. In patients who have completely lost hearing in one ear, a system called contralateral routing of sound (CROS) sends sound from the deaf ear through a microphone to the hearing ear, improving overall hearing acuity.

Prognosis

Without treatment, vestibular schwannoma will nearly always result in permanent deafness. Although surgery carries a high risk of hearing loss and facial nerve impairment, about 66% of patients who have small- to medium-sized vestibular schwannoma will have improved hearing acuity following surgery.

Resources

BOOKS

Janus, Todd J., and W. K. Alfred Yung. "Primary Neurological Tumors." *Textbook of Clinical Neurology*, edited by Christopher G. Goetz. Philadelphia: W. B. Saunders Company, 2003.

Ng, James J. "Acoustic Neuroma." *Ferri's Clinical Advisor: Instant Diagnosis and Treatment*, edited by Fred F. Ferri. St. Louis: Mosby, 2004.

Sagar, Stephen M., and Mark A. Israel. "Primary and Metastatic Tumors of the Nervous System." *Harrison's Principles of Internal Medicine*, edited by Eugene Braunwald, et al. New York: McGraw-Hill Professional, 2001.

Seidman, Michael D., George T. Simpson, and Mumtaz J. Khan. "Common Problems of the Ear." *Noble: Textbook of Primary Care Medicine*, edited by John Noble, et al. St. Louis: W. B. Saunders Company, 2001.

PERIODICALS

Ho, S. Y. "Acoustic Neuroma: Assessment and Management." *Otolaryngology Clinics of North America* 35, no. 2 (1 April 2002): 393–404.

ORGANIZATIONS

National Institute on Deafness and Other Communication Disorders, National Institutes of Health. 31 Center Drive, MSC 2320, Bethesda, MD 20892-2320. (301) 496-7243; Fax: (301) 402-0018. nidcdinfo@nidcd.nih.gov. <http://www.nidcd.nih.gov/health/hearing/acoustic_neuroma.asp>.

Acoustic Neuroma Association. 600 Peachtree Pkwy, Suite 108, Cumming, GA 30041-6899. (770) 205-8211; Fax: (770) 205-0239. ANAUSA@aol.com. <http://anausa.org/>.

Rosalyn Carson-DeWitt, MD

Visual disturbances

Definition

Visual disturbances are abnormalities of sight. Visual disturbances associated with neurological disorders often include double vision (diplopia), moving or blurred vision due to nystagmus (involuntary rapid movements of the eyes), reduced visual acuity, reduced visual field, and partial or total loss of vision as in papilledema, a swelling of the optic disc, or in blindness. Visual disturbances are often symptoms of other disorders, in particular neurological disorders, but can also occur due to muscular disorders, vascular diseases, cancer, or trauma. Additionally, diseases such as diabetes and hyperthyroidism can contribute to the visual abnormalities. Some visual disturbances arise from congenital conditions that are often hereditary.

Description

Diplopia

Diplopia, or double vision, causes a person to see two objects instead of one. There are two main reasons for diplopia: one is a physical change in the lens, conjuctiva, or retinal surface; the second reason involves an inability of the brain to overlay the images seen with both eyes, which happens in a person with normal vision. The first type usually involves only one eye and is not corrected by covering of the eye. Scars or other physical defects in the eye cause the split of a single image, thus resulting in double vision. In contrast, the second type usually involves both eyes (binocular) and is corrected when one eye is covered. Binocular diplopia arises when the eye movement in one direction is prevented, and is often a congenital (present at birth) condition. Binocular diplopia is usually caused by misalignment of the eyes, which can be nerve or muscle related.

Abnormalities in eye movement can result from conditions such as cranial nerve paralysis (paresis), neuromuscular disease (e.g., **myasthenia gravis**), **multiple sclerosis**, infection, **stroke**, overactive thyroid (Grave's disease), or direct trauma to the eye. Diplopia can also be a result of a growing tumor, which presses on the nerves involved in eye movements.

The nerves involved in diplopia include three cranial nerves: the oculomotor nerve (third cranial nerve), the abducens nerve (sixth cranial nerve), and the trochlear nerve

Key Terms

Diplopia Also known as double vision, a visual disorder due to unequal action of the eye muscles causing two images of a single object to be seen.

Intracranial pressure The pressure inside the skull.

Nystagmus Involuntary rapid and repetitive movement of the eyes.

Optic nerve The bundle of nerve fibers that carry visual messages from the retina to the brain.

Optic neuritis Inflammation of the optic nerve.

(fourth cranial nerve). These three nerves direct the movements of six extraocular muscles. Four muscles are innervated by the third cranial nerve, and the other two are innervated exclusively by either the fourth or the sixth cranial nerve. This arrangement allows the physician to determine the cause of visual disturbances observed in a patient. Misalignment of the eyes can be in any direction: inward, outward, upward, downward, or a combination. Damage to the third cranial nerve can cause outward and downward turning of the affected eye and the inability to pass midline in either of the two directions. Fourth cranial nerve damage will result in vertical diplopia, which is compensated by head tilting. Head turning is used to compensate for sixth cranial nerve damage that prevents outward movement of the eye.

Nystagmus

A different type of visual disturbance, nystagmus, is caused by abnormal eye movements and often results in blurred vision. Normal control of the eye movements depends on the neuronal connections between the eyes, brain stem, and the **cerebellum**. Changes in the **central nervous system** or peripheral labyrinthine apparatus can cause the uncontrolled, repetitive eye movements known as nystagmus. There are many types and subtypes of nystagmus depending on the underlying cause and movement involved. The most common form involves a jerking motion from side to side (horizontal nystagmus). The rapid eye movements can also appear in a vertical direction, usually indicating a problem with the central nervous system. Rotary movements are also sometimes observed in nystagmus.

Although nystagmus by itself does not cause loss of vision, it is often associated with poor vision. Nystagmus can develop in early childhood or in adulthood. Childhood nystagmus can be associated with eye defects (cataract or retinal disorders) or result from unknown causes (congenital idiopathic nystagmus). Most cases of congenital nystagmus are not caused by a disease process and are familial.

If nystagmus develops later in life, it can be a sign of a serious underlying problem such as stroke, multiple sclerosis, or complication from head trauma. The direction of the eye movement can help the physician to diagnose the underlying neurological problem. For example, in an unconscious person, vertical nystagmus can indicate brain stem damage. This illustrates that eye movements not only cause visual disturbances, but are also an important diagnostic tool to determine if the brain is still alive.

The presence of the occulocephalic reflex (doll's eye movements) in people with coma shows that the brain stem is intact. The physician turns the patient's head from side to side or left to right to elicit the reflex. When the reflex is present, the eyes appear to move freely in the opposite direction from the direction the head was turned, thus moving in relation to the head. When the eyes remain fixated, this suggests lack of cerebral activity. Another important diagnostic test is the cold caloric test. The cold caloric test traces the direction of nystagmus to assess the oculovestibular reflex. An unconscious person's ear is injected with cold water, causing slow horizontal movement of the eyes towards the stimulation, which is followed by a fast return of the eyes to the midline.

Blindness

Blindness is the partial or complete loss of vision. The leading causes of blindness are glaucoma, cataracts, and diabetic retinopathy. Blindness can also result from eye diseases, optic nerve disorders, or brain diseases involving visual pathways or the occipital lobe of the brain. The patterns of visual field reduction depend on the area that is being affected by disease. Damage to visual pathways as a result of macular degeneration, retinal detachment, or optic nerve atrophy can affect one or both eyes. In contrast, damage to the optic nerve chiasm or the pathway beyond it affects both eyes. There are many eye diseases that can cause visual abnormalities or/and blindness, including retinal detachment, cataracts, retinal disorders (often inherited), and macular degeneration.

Macular degeneration is the leading cause of blindness for those over age 55 in the United States. The macula is the central portion of the retina that records images and sends them from the eye to the brain via the optic nerve. If the macula deteriorates, the eye loses the ability to see in fine detail. The cause of macular degeneration is not fully understood, but risks for the disorder increase with age. Other abnormalities in the central retina can lead to blurry vision or can affect color perception. Color blindness can also originate from the lack of one or more type of cones, a type of light receptor on the eye. Total color blindness (monochromatic vision) is very rare; most commonly, varying levels of single color deficits are found among people with color blindness. Central vision can also be destroyed by small hemorrhages in the retina as a result of the aging process or diabetic retinopathy.

The neuronal diseases affecting the optic nerve and causing blindness can result from developmental abnormalities (hereditary or sporadic), abnormalities in the blood vessels causing an insufficient blood supply to the eyes or optic nerve, glaucoma, and demyelinating and inflammatory diseases such as multiple sclerosis, tumors, toxic agents, and trauma.

Optic nerve damage

Papilledema, the swelling of the optic nerve, can result from increased intracranial pressure or optic nerve deterioration (optic neuropathy). Inflammation, lack of adequate blood supply to the optic nerve, and certain diseases such as multiple sclerosis can cause the optic nerve to deteriorate. A brain tumor, bleeding or blood clots in the brain, brain swelling due to encephalitis or trauma, or a blockage in cerebrospinal fluid circulation can cause an increase in pressure inside the skull (intracranial pressure). The condition is often life threatening, and correct diagnosis of papilledema is important.

Papilledema arising from increased intracranial pressure is often accompanied by other symptoms, including diplopia, nausea, **headache**, and reduction of the visual field. When diagnosing papilledema, the physician looks for swelling of the optic disc (the area where the optic nerve enters the eye). The early signs include slight changes in appearance of the edge of neural tissue. Later, the disc rises from the retinal surface and can appear pale or can show signs of hemorrhages in severe cases. Persistent, chronic papilledema can cause atrophy of the optic nerve head and result in blindness.

The optic nerve can also be damaged by increased intraocular pressure (IOP) as in glaucoma. The pressure develops in aqueous area of the eye and is transmitted to the back of the eye, causing an initial reduction in peripheral vision and leading eventually to blindness. Glaucoma is often a complication arising from diabetes.

Additionally, optic neuritis, or inflammation of the optic nerve, can cause permanent loss of vision. Demyelinating diseases such as multiple sclerosis, systemic infections, diabetes, and hereditary factors can cause optic neuritis. Optic neuritis can also be a secondary complication of diseases such as meningitis, sinusitis, or tuberculosis, or reactions to toxins or trauma.

Other important causes of blindness are tumors affecting the optic chiasm (the area in the brain where the optic nerves cross) such as gliomas, cerebral tumors, and pituitary adenomas. In these cases, the transfer of visual stimuli through the optic nerve and visual pathways is directly affected and results in blindness.

Resources

BOOKS

Acheson, James, and Paul Riordan-Eva. *Fundamentals of Clinical Ophthalmology: Neuro-Ophthalmology.* London: BMJ Books, 1999.

Glaser, J. D. (ed). *Neuro-ophthalmology*, 3rd ed. Philadelphia: Lippincott Williams and Wilkins, 1999.

OTHER

"Double Vision (Diplopia)." *InteliHealth Inc.* February 28, 2004 (June 3, 2004). <http://www.intelihealth.com/IH/ihtIH/WSIHW000/9339/23796.html>.

"Understanding Nystagmus." *Royal National Institute of the Blind.* February 28, 2004 (June 3, 2004). <http://www.rnib.org.uk/xpedio/groups/public/documents/publicwebsite/public_rnib003659.hcsp>.

ORGANIZATIONS

National Eye Institute. 2020 Vision Place. Bethesda, MD 20892-3655. (301) 496-5248. <http://www.nei.nih.gov/>.

Agnieszka Maria Lichanska, PhD

Vitamine B12 deficiency *see*
Vitamin/nutritional deficiency

Vitamin/nutritional deficiency

Definition

Vitamins are substances that the human body requires but is unable to synthesize and therefore, must obtain externally. Deficiencies in three B vitamins, B1 or thiamine, B3 or niacin and B12 or cobalamin are known to cause neurological disorders. Thiamine deficiencies result in a disease called **beriberi**, which causes peripheral neurological dysfunction and cerebral neuropathy. Niacin deficiencies cause a wasting disease known as pellagra, which affects the skin, mucous membranes, gastrointestinal tract as well as the brain, spinal cord and peripheral nerves. Cobalamin deficiencies most often result in the disease pernicious anemia. Neurological symptoms of pernicious anemia include numbness in the extremities, impaired coordination and a ringing in the ears.

Description

Thiamine deficiency

Thiamine was the first water-soluble vitamin to be discovered, and is therefore, also known as vitamin B1.

Thiamine deficiency, or beriberi, manifests itself as both wet beriberi, which affects the cardiovascular system, and dry beriberi, which causes neurological dysfunction. People suffering from beriberi exhibit muscle atrophy or wasting (especially in the legs), edema (swelling), mental confusion, intestinal discomfort and an enlarged heart. Severe cases of dry beriberi may result in Wernicke-Korsakoff syndrome and acute cases of wet beriberi may cause shoshin beriberi. Both of these extreme forms of the disease are sometimes fatal. In most cases, administering thiamine successfully reverses symptoms associated with thiamine deficiencies.

Niacin deficiency

Niacin deficiency results in a disease called pellagra. The major symptoms of pellagra include dermatitis, **dementia** (loss of intellectual functions) and diarrhea. Pellagra means rough skin in Italian and it was named because of the characteristic roughened skin of people who have the disease. Skin lesions generally appear on both sides of the body (bilaterally) and are found in regions exposed to sunlight. The disease also affects mucous membranes of the mouth, vagina, and urethra. Gastrointestinal discomfort is an early symptom, followed by nausea, vomiting, and diarrhea, often bloody. Neurological dysfunctions associated with niacin deficiencies include memory loss, confusion and confabulation (imagined memory). Although treatment with niacin usually reverses all of the symptoms, untreated niacin deficiencies can result in multiple organ failure.

Vitamin B12 deficiency

Vitamin B12, also called cobalamin or cyanocobalamin, has the most complex chemical structure of all vitamins. It is unique in that it contains a cobalt atom embedded in a ring, similar to the iron atom in hemoglobin. The cobalt gives the molecule a dark red color. Vitamin B12 is found bound to animal protein and is very rare in vegetables. A deficiency of vitamin B12 results in a blood disorder, also called an anemia, which enlarges red blood cells so that the immune system destroys them at an increased rate. Because the blood cells are enlarged, the disease is characterized as a macrocytic anemia. Vitamin B12 functions in many important cellular processes including synthesis of red blood cells, DNA synthesis and the formation of the myelin sheath that acts as insulation around nerve cells. One of the most common causes of vitamin B12 deficiency is pernicious anemia. Pernicious anemia is caused by a lack of a glycoprotein called intrinsic factor that is required for absorption of vitamin B12. Intrinsic factor is secreted by the stomach, where it binds to the vitamin and transports it to the small intestine for absorption. Symptoms of vitamin B12 deficiency progress

Key Terms

Amino acid An organic compound composed of both an amino group and an acidic carboxyl group. Amino acids are the basic building blocks of proteins. There are 20 types of amino acids. Eight are "essential amino acids" that the body cannot make and must therefore be obtained from food.

Anemia A condition in which there is an abnormally low number of red blood cells in the bloodstream. It may be due to loss of blood, an increase in red blood cell destruction, or a decrease in red blood cell production. Major symptoms are paleness, shortness of breath, unusually fast or strong heart beats, and tiredness.

Vitamins Small compounds required for metabolism that must be supplied by diet, microorganisms in the gut (vitamin K), or sunlight (UV light converts pre-vitamin D to vitamin D).

from weakness and **fatigue** to neurological disorders including numbness in the extremities, poor coordination, and eventually, to hallucinations and psychosis. Vitamin B12 deficiencies are usually treated with intramuscular injections of vitamin B12 initially and oral vitamin B12 supplements on an ongoing basis.

Demographics
Thiamine deficiency

Thiamine deficiencies have no sex or racial predilection. Thiamine deficiency is more common in developing countries where poor nutrition occurs frequently, although no accurate statistics on its occurrence are available. In many of these countries, cassava or milled rice acts as a major staple of the diet. While cassava does contain some thiamine, it contains so much carbohydrate relative to the thiamine that eating cassava actually consumes thiamine. Most of the thiamine in rice is found in the husk. When the husk is removed from the rice during milling, the result is a diet staple that is an extremely poor source of thiamine.

Beriberi is often associated with alcoholism, likely because of low thiamine intake, impaired ability to absorb and store thiamine, and acceleration in the reduction of thiamine diphosphate. People who strictly follow fad diets, people undergoing starvation, and people receiving large amounts of intravenous fluids are all susceptible to beriberi. Some physical conditions such as hyperthyroidism, pregnancy, or severe illness may cause a person

to require more thiamine than normal and may put a person at risk for deficiency.

A form of beriberi specific to infants known as infantile beriberi can occur in babies between two and four months old that are fed only breast milk from mothers who are thiamine deficient.

Niacin deficiency

Pellagra is most common when maize is a major part of the diet. Although maize does contain niacin, it is not biologically available unless it is treated with basic compounds, such as lime. This process occurs in the making of tortillas, so populations in Mexico and Central America do not usually suffer from pellagra. Maize is also deficient in tryptophan, a precursor to niacin.

In the early 1900s, pellagra was epidemic in the southern United States because of the large amount of corn in the diet. After niacin was discovered to prevent pellagra in 1937, flour was fortified with niacin and reports of pellagra decreased dramatically. Currently, incidence rates of pellagra in the United States are unknown. People at risk for pellagra include alcoholics, people on fad diets, and people with gastrointestinal absorption dysfunction.

The group of people who most commonly suffer from pellagra live in the Deccan Plateau of India. Their diet is rich in millet or sorghum, which contains tryptophan, but also large concentrations of another amino acid, leucine. It is thought that leucine inhibits the conversion of tryptophan to niacin.

Vitamin B12 deficiency

Pernicious anemia is most common in patients of northern European descent and African Americans and less frequent in people of southern European descent and Asians. There is no sex predilection. Vitamin B12 deficiency occurs in 3–43% of people over the age of 65. A form of pernicious anemia is also found in children under the age of ten. It is more frequent in patients with other immune disorders such as Grave's disease or Crohn's disease. There is some evidence that relatives of people who have pernicious anemia are more likely to get the disorder, indicating some genetic component to the disease. Because vitamin B12 only occurs in animal proteins, vegetarians are susceptible to the disease and should take vitamin B12 supplements.

Causes and symptoms
Thiamine deficiency

Thiamine deficiencies are caused by an inadequate intake of thiamine. In most developed countries, getting enough thiamine is not a problem since it is found in all vegetables, especially the outer layer of grains. It is not present in refined sugars or fats and is not found in animal tissue. Diets rich in foods that contain thiaminases, enzymes that break down thiamine, such as milled rice, shrimp, mussels, clams, fresh fish and raw meat may be associated with thiamine deficiencies.

Thiamine is absorbed through the digestive tract by a combination of active and passive absorption. It is stored in the body as thiamine diphosphate, also called thiamine pyrophosphate, and thiamine triphosphate. Thiamine diphosphate is the active form and it is used as a coenzyme in several steps in cellular respiration. Thiamine may also have an important role in the function of nerve cells independent of cellular respiration. It is found in the cell membranes of nerve axons, and electrical stimulation of nerve cells causes a release of thiamine.

Early thiamine deficiency produces fatigue, abdominal **pain**, constipation, irritation, loss of memory, chest pain, anorexia and sleep disturbance. As the deficiency progresses, it can be classified as dry beriberi or wet beriberi depending on the activity of the patient. Many persons experience a mixture of the two types of beriberi, although pure forms do occur.

When caloric intake and physical activity are low, thiamine deficiency produces neurological dysfunction termed dry beriberi. Symptoms occur with equal intensity on both sides of the body and usually start in the legs. Impaired motor and reflex function coupled with pain, numbness and cramps are symptomatic of the disease. As the disease advances, ankle and knee jerk reactions will be lost, muscle tone in the calf and thigh will atrophy and eventually the patient will suffer from **foot drop** and toe drop. The arms may begin to show symptoms of neurological dysfunction after the legs are already symptomatic. Histological (tissue) tests may indicate patchy degradation of myelin in muscle tissues.

Wernicke-Korsadoff syndrome, also called cerebral beriberi, occurs in extreme cases of dry beriberi. The early stage is called Korsakoff's syndrome and it is characterized by confusion, the inability to learn, amnesia and telling stories that bear no relation to reality. Wernicke's **encephalopathy** follows with symptoms of vomiting, nystagmus (rapid horizontal or vertical eye movement), opthalmoplegia (inability to move the eye outwards) and ptosis (eyelid droop). If untreated, Wernicke's encephalopathy may progress to coma and, eventually death.

If a person has a high caloric intake and reasonable levels of activity, but has a diet with insufficient thiamine, myocardial dysfunction termed wet beriberi may result. This disease consists of vasodilatation and high cardiac output, retention of salt and water, and eventual damage to the heart muscle. A person suffering from wet beriberi will exhibit rapid heartbeat (tachycardia), swelling (edema), high blood pressure, and chest pain.

Shoshin beriberi is a more acute form of wet beriberi and it is characterized by damage to the heart muscle accompanied by anxiety and restlessness. If no treatment is received, the damage to the heart may be fatal.

Niacin deficiency

Niacin, also called vitamin B3, is a general term for two molecules: nicotinic acid and nicotinamine. Nicotinic acid is very easily converted into biologically important molecules including nicotinamide adenine dinucleotide (NAD or coenzyme I) and nicotinaminamide adenine dinucleotide phosphate (NADP or coenzyme II), both of which are crucial to oxidation-reduction reactions in cellular metabolism. These reactions play key roles in glycololysis, the generation of high-energy phosphate bonds, and metabolism of fatty acids, proteins, glycerol, and pyruvate. Because niacin plays such an important role in so many different cellular functions, the effect of niacin deficiencies on the body is extremely broad.

The amino acid, tryptophan is a precursor to niacin, and therefore, niacin deficiency can be averted if tryptophan is included in the diet. Some of the psychological symptoms of pellagra are thought to be related to decreased conversion rates of tryptophan to serotonin (a neurotransmitter) in the brain.

Causes of pellagra include diets that are deficient in niacin or its precursor, tryptophan. These diets often rely heavily on unprocessed maize. Other diets that may cause pellagra contain amino acid imbalances. For example, diets that rely on sorghum as a staple contain excessive amounts of the amino acid leucine, which interferes with tryptophan metabolism. Other causes of pellagra include alcoholism, fad diets, diabetes, cirrhosis of the liver, and digestive disorders that prevent proper absorption of niacin or tryptophan. One such disorder is called Hartnup disease, which is a congenital defect that interferes with tryptophan metabolism.

Symptoms of pellagra occur in the skin, in mucous membranes, the gastrointestinal tract, and the **central nervous system**. Skin symptoms are usually bilaterally symmetric. They include lesions characterized by redness and crusting, thickening of the skin and skin inelasticity. Secondary infections are common, especially after exposure to the sun. Mucus membranes are also affected by pellagra. Typically, the tongue becomes bright red first and then the mouth becomes sore, coupled with increased salivation and edema of the tongue. Eventually, ulcers may appear throughout the mouth. Gastrointestinal symptoms include burning of the mouth, esophagus and abdominal pain. Later symptoms include vomiting and diarrhea, often bloody.

The central nervous system is also affected by niacin deficiencies. Early symptoms include memory loss, disorientation, confusion, **hallucination**. More severe symptoms are characterized by loss of consciousness, rigidity in the extremities, and uncontrolled sucking and grasping.

Vitamin B12 deficiency

Vitamin B12 is required for the biochemical reaction that converts homocysteine to methionine, one of the essential amino acids required to synthesize proteins. Because vitamin B12 impairs DNA translation, cell division is slow, but the cytoplasm of the cell develops normally. This leads to enlarged cells, especially in cells that usually divide quickly, like red blood cells. In addition, there is usually a high ration of RNA to DNA in these cells. Enlarged red blood cells are more likely to be destroyed by the immune system in the bone marrow, causing a deficit of red blood cells in the blood. Methionine is also required to produce choline and choline-containing phospholipids. Choline and choline-containing phospholipids are a major component of cell membranes and acetocholine, which is crucial to nerve function.

Vitamin B12 requires several binding proteins in order to be absorbed properly. After ingestion into the stomach, it forms a complex with R binding protein, which moves into the small intestine. The stomach secretes another protein, intrinsic factor, which binds with vitamin B12 after R binding factor is digested in the small intestine. Intrinsic factor bound with vitamin B12 adheres to specialized receptors in the ileum, where it is brought inside of cells that line the intestinal wall. Vitamin B12 is then transferred to another protein, transcobalamin II, which circulates through the blood plasma to all parts of the body. Another protein, transcobalamin I, is found bound to vitamin B12; however its function is not well understood.

Because of the complexity of the steps required for vitamin B12 absorption, there are many different ways that deficiencies could arise. First, a person could have inadequate intake of vitamin B12. This is extremely rare, since it is found in most animal proteins, but it does occur in some strict vegetarians. If any of the proteins that usher vitamin B12 through the body are unavailable or damaged, vitamin B12 deficiencies could arise. The most common such problem is associated with inadequate production of intrinsic factor, which results in pernicious anemia. Inadequate production of intrinsic factor can occur because of atrophy (wasting) of the stomach lining, the removal of the part of the stomach that produces intrinsic factor, or in rare cases, because of a congenital defect. Rare cases of intestinal parasites such as a fish tapeworm and bacterial infections may also result in vitamin B12 deficiencies.

Finally, acid is often required to hydrolyze vitamin B12 from animal proteins in the stomach. If the stomach is not sufficiently acidic, for example in the presence of antacid medicines, quantities of vitamin B12 available for absorption may be deficient.

The liver stores large amounts of vitamin B12. It is estimated that if vitamin B12 uptake is suddenly stopped, it would take three to five years to completely deplete the stores in a typical adult. As a result, vitamin B12 deficiencies develop over many years. Initial symptoms include weakness, fatigue, lightheadedness, weight loss, diarrhea, abdominal pain, shortness of breath, sore mouth and loss of taste, and tingling in the fingers and toes.

As the disease progresses, neurological symptoms begin to appear. These include forgetfulness, **depression**, confusion, difficulty thinking, and impaired judgment. Eventually, a person with vitamin B12 deficiency will have numbness in the fingers and toes, impaired balance and poor coordination, ringing in the ears, changes in reflexes, hallucinations, and psychosis.

Diagnosis

Thiamine deficiency

A patient with bilateral symmetric neurological symptoms, especially in the lower extremities may be suffering from thiamine deficiency, especially if there is an indication that the diet may be poor. Some diseases with symptoms that are similar to beriberi include diabetes and alcoholism. Other neuropathies, such as **sciatica**, are often not symmetric and are not usually associated with beriberi.

Laboratory tests may show high concentrations of pyruvate and lactate in the blood and low concentrations of thiamine in the urine. Because the disease responds so well to thiamine, it is often used as a diagnostic tool. After administration of thiamine diphosphate, an increase in certain enzyme activity in red blood cells is an excellent indicator of thiamine deficiency.

Niacin deficiency

There are no diagnostic tests currently available to detect niacin deficiencies. Concentrations of niacin and tryptophan in the urine of patients suffering from pellagra are low, but not lower than other patients with malnutrition. Diagnosis must be made given a patient's symptoms and dietary history. Because replacement of niacin is so effective, it may be used as a diagnostic tool.

Vitamin B12 deficiency

A person suspected of suffering from vitamin B12 deficiency will be subjected to a physical examination along with blood tests. These blood tests will include a complete blood count (CBC). If blood analyses indicate that the red blood cells are enlarged, vitamin B12 deficiency may be diagnosed. Other disorders that exhibit enlarged red blood cells (macrocytes) include alcoholism, hypthyroidism, and other forms of anemia. White blood cells with segmented nuclei also indicate vitamin B12 deficiency. Other blood tests include a vitamin B12 test and folic acid tests. Low concentrations of both may indicate vitamin B12 deficiencies. Elevated levels of homocysteine, methylmalonic acid (MMA) or lactate dehydrogenase (LDH) indicate vitamin B12 deficiencies. Finally tests that indicate the presence of antibodies against intrinsic factor may indicate pernicious anemia.

Once a vitamin B12 deficiency has been established in a patient, the severity of the disease can be evaluated using a Schilling test. The patient is orally administered radioactive cobalamin and then an injection of unlabeled cobalamin is given intramuscularly. The ratio of radioactive to unlabeled cobalamin in the urine during the next 24 hours gives information on the absorption rate of cobalamin by the patient. If the rates are abnormal, pernicious anemia is diagnosed. As a final check, the patient is given cobalamin bound to intrinsic factor. With this, the patient's absorption rates should become normal if pernicious anemia is the cause of the symptoms.

Treatment
Thiamine deficiency

In most cases, rapid administration of intravenous thiamine will reduce symptoms of thiamine deficiency. Continued dosages of the vitamin should be continued for several weeks accompanied by a nutritious diet. Following recovery, a diet containing one to two times the recommended daily allowance of thiamine (1-1.5 mg per day) should be maintained. Shoshin beriberi requires cardiac support as well. Thiamine has not been found to be toxic for people with normal kidney function, even at high doses.

Niacin deficiency

Niacin deficiency can be treated effectively with replacement of niacin in the diet. In the case of Hartnup disease, large quantities of niacin may be required for effective reversal of symptoms.

Vitamin B12 deficiency

Vitamin B12 deficiency responds well to administration of cobalamin. Because absorption in the small intestine is often part of the problem, the best way to administer cobalamin is by intramuscular injection on a daily basis. After 6 weeks, the injections can be decreased to monthly for the rest of the patient's life. Usually, response to this treatment alleviates all symptoms of the disease. In severe cases, a blood transfusion may be needed and neurological conditions may not be completely reversed.

Resources
BOOKS

Garrison, Robert H., Jr. and Elizabeth Somer. *The Nutrition Desk Reference.* Keats Publishing, Inc., 1985.

Peckenpaugh, Nancy J. and Charlotte M. Poleman. *Nutrition: Essentials and Diet Therapy.* Philadelphia: W. B. Saunders Company, 1999.

OTHER

Lovinger, Sarah Pressman. "Beriberi" *MEDLINE plus.* National Library of Medicine. (February, 8 2004). <http://www.nlm.nih.gov/medlineplus/ency/article/000339.htm#Symptoms>.

"Niacin deficiency." *The Merck Manual.* (January 16, 2004). <http://www.merck.com/mrkshared/mmanual/section1/chapter3/3l.jsp>.

"Thiamine deficiency and dependency." *The Merk Manual.* (January 16, 2004). <http://www.merck.com/mrkshared/mmanual/section1/chapter3/3j.jsp>.

ORGANIZATIONS

NIH/National Digestive Diseases Information Clearinghouse. 2 Information Way, Bethesda, MD 20892-3570. (301) 654-3810 or (800) 891-5389; Fax: (301) 907-8906. nddic@info.niddk.nih.gov. <http://www.niddk.nih.gov>.

National Heart, Lung, and Blood Institute (NHLBI). P. O. Box 30105, Bethesda, MD 20824-0105. (301) 592-8573; Fax: (301) 592-8563. NHLBIinfo@rover.nhlbi.nih.gov. <http://www.nhlbi.nih.gov>.

Juli M. Berwald, PhD

von Economo disease *see* **Encephalitis lethargica**

von Recklinghausen disease *see* **Neurofibromatosis**

Von Hippel-Lindau disease
Definition

Von Hippel-Lindau disease (VHL) is a hereditary condition that involves cancer and can affect people of all ages. It was named after the physicians to first describe aspects of the condition in the early 1900s, German ophthalmologist Eugen von Hippel and Swedish pathologist Arvid Lindau. It was not until 1964 that the term von Hippel-Lindau disease was coined.

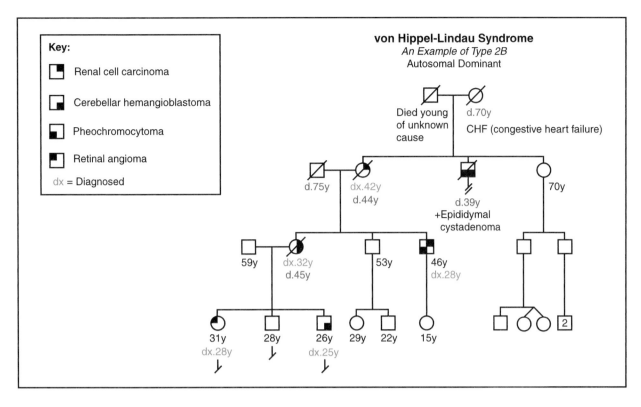

Key:
- ▢ Renal cell carcinoma
- ▢ Cerebellar hemangioblastoma
- ◨ Pheochromocytoma
- ◨ Retinal angioma
- dx = Diagnosed

von Hippel-Lindau Syndrome
An Example of Type 2B
Autosomal Dominant

Died young of unknown cause

d.70y
CHF (congestive heart failure)

d.75y
dx.42y d.44y

d.39y +Epididymal cystadenoma

70y

59y
dx.32y d.45y

53y

46y
dx.28y

31y dx.28y
28y
26y dx.25y
29y
22y
15y

2

See Symbol Guide for Pedigree Charts. *(Gale Group.)*

Description

VHL often involves symptoms in the **central nervous system** (CNS) and include hemangioblastomas of the **cerebellum**, spinal cord, brain stem, and nerve root. Retinal hemangioblastomas and endolymphatic sac tumors are CNS tumors that can also be seen. The kidneys, adrenal gland, pancreas, epididymis, and female broad ligaments may also be affected.

Behavioral and learning problems are not usually associated with VHL, but may be if the CNS tumors are quite significant. Symptoms of VHL do not usually cause concerns in very early childhood. However, VHL is a hereditary cancer syndrome for which screening is appropriate in late childhood and adolescence for those at risk.

Demographics

Studies from 1991 indicated an incidence of VHL of about one in 36,000 live births in eastern England. The condition affects people of all ethnic groups worldwide, with an equal proportion of males and females.

In 1993, the gene for VHL was identified. The majority of people with VHL also have an affected parent, but in about 20% of cases there is no known family history of VHL.

Causes and symptoms

Mutations in the VHL gene on chromosome 3 are now known to cause the condition. VHL is inherited in an autosomal dominant manner, meaning that an affected individual has a 50% chance to pass a disease-causing mutation to offspring, regardless of their gender.

VHL is a tumor-suppressor gene, or one whose normal function is to prevent cancer by controlling cell growth. Mutations in the VHL gene potentially cause uncontrolled cell growth in the gene, which is why a person with a VHL mutation is prone to developing cancer and other growths.

Hemangioblastomas of the CNS are the most common tumor in VHL; about 60–80% of people with VHL develop these tumors. The average age for CNS hemangioblastomas to develop is 33 years. The tubors are a frequent cause of death in people with VHL because they can disturb normal brain functioning. They can occur anywhere along the brain/spine areas, and swelling or cysts are often associated. The most common locations for CNS hemangioblastomas are in the spinal cord and cerebellum.

Symptoms from CNS hemangioblastomas depend on their size and exact location. Common symptoms include **headaches**, vomiting, gait disturbances, and **ataxia**, especially when the cerebellum is involved. Spinal hemangioblastomas often bring **pain**, but sensory and motor loss

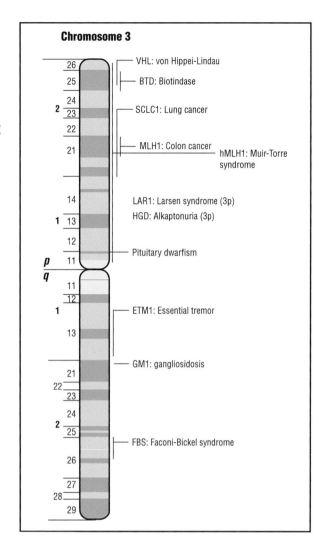

Chromosome 3

26 — VHL: von Hippei-Lindau
25 — BTD: Biotindase
24
2 23 — SCLC1: Lung cancer
22
21 — MLH1: Colon cancer — hMLH1: Muir-Torre syndrome
14 — LAR1: Larsen syndrome (3p)
1 13 — HGD: Alkaptonuria (3p)
12
p 11 — Pituitary dwarfism
q
11
12
1 — ETM1: Essential tremor
13
— GM1: gangliosidosis
21
22 23
24
2 25
— FBS: Faconi-Bickel syndrome
26
27
28
29

von Hippel-Lindau disease, on chromosome 3. *(Gale Group.)*

may develop only if the tumor is so large that it is pressing into the spinal cord. Some hemangioblastomas never cause symptoms, and are only seen with special imaging techniques.

Retinal hemangioblastomas are seen in as many as 60% of people, and many times may be the first sign of VHL. There may be multiple hemangioblastomas in one eye, or even in both eyes. The average age for these to develop is about 25 years, but some develop in people younger than 10 years of age. When in the early stages and quite small, retinal hemangioblastomas may not cause symptoms. As they progress, they can cause retinal detachment, with partial or total vision loss.

Endolymphatic sac tumors are seen in about 11% of people with VHL, but are very rare in the general population. The first sign of this form of tumor may be partial

hearing loss, which may progress to total hearing loss. Other symptoms can be tinnitus (buzzing in the ear), **dizziness**, and facial paresis. These tumors often erode or expand the inner bones of the ear, a major reason for the hearing loss.

Kidney involvement occurs in about 60% of people with VHL, which usually includes renal cell carcinoma and kidney cysts. The typical age that these symptoms develop is 39 years. One or both kidneys may be diseased, with multiple cysts or growths that may be seen in each kidney. Renal cell carcinoma is a major cause of death in VHL. Kidney disease may not cause symptoms, or may not cause a reduction in kidney function. In severe cases blood in the urine, a mass or pain may be felt in an affected person's side.

Adrenal gland pheochromocytomas occur in 10–20% of people with VHL; the average age of diagnosis is 30 years, though they have been seen in children under the age of 10. There may be a single tumor present, or multiple tumors. For people with a subset of VHL called type 2C, a pheochromocytoma is the only symptom they have. Five percent of all pheochromocytomas are cancerous, requiring treatment. Symptoms of pheochromocytomas may include intermittent or continuous high blood pressure, heart palpitations, a quickened heart rate, headaches, sweating episodes, nausea, and paleness of the skin. Pheochromocytomas may also cause the level of catecholamines to be elevated in urine.

Of all people with VHL, 35–70% have a pancreatic tumor, cyst, or cystadenoma. The masses often develop in the mid-30s, and are usually without symptoms. Pancreatic involvement is important to diagnose VHL, but is difficult to identify on its own because it may cause no medical problems.

Men with VHL have epididymal cystadenomas 25–60% of the time. There may be multiple masses, occurring in both sides. If occurring in both sides, in rare cases they may lead to infertility. Epididymal cystadenomas are non-cancerous and may show up in the teenage years. In women, a similar tumor to the epididymal cystadenoma in men is that of the broad ligaments. These are not very common, so the true frequency and age of development is unknown in VHL. They are non-cancerous and usually cause no specific symptoms.

Diagnosis

Until the discovery of the VHL gene, the diagnosis of the condition was made on a clinical basis. People with a family history of VHL need only have a CNS hemangioblastoma (including retinal), pheochromocytoma, or renal cell carcinoma to be given a diagnosis. Those without a family history must have two or more CNS hemangioblastomas, or one CNS and a visceral finding (with the exception of epididymal and renal cysts) to have a diagnosis.

There has been the creation of subtypes within VHL. Type 1 families are at a very low risk for pheochromocytomas, but have the typical risk for all other tumors that are seen. All type 2 families have a risk for pheochromocytomas; type 2A families have a low risk for renal cell carcinoma, while type 2B families have a high risk for it; type 2C families only have pheochromocytomas and no other signs of VHL.

Hemangioblastomas of the brain and spine are typically found through **magnetic resonance imaging (MRI)** scans. Those found in the retina can be seen by examination of the dilated eye by an ophthalmologist. Endolymphatic tumors may be visualized using computed tomography (**CT**) and **MRI** scans of the internal ear canals. Audiograms can also be done to identify and track hearing loss.

Renal and pancreatic involvement is often found through abdominal CT scans, MRI scans, or ultrasounds of the kidneys and pancreas. Pheochromocytomas can be seen on CT or MRI scans, and occasionally meta-iodobenzylguanidine (MIBG) scintigraphy is required to detect them. Epididymal cystadenomas are usually felt by a physical examination and confirmation through an ultrasound. Broad ligament cystadenomas can be diagnosed by CT scans or an ultrasound.

Genetic testing is available for VHL through gene sequencing and other methods. Testing is useful for confirming a clinical diagnosis or for family testing when there is an identified VHL mutation in the family. Analysis of the VHL gene is not perfect, but it detects about 90% of mutations that cause VHL. An informative test result is one that identifies a known mutation in the gene, and this confirms that the person has VHL. A negative test result means a mutation was not found in the gene. This either means that the tested individual does not have VHL, or instead has a mutation that cannot be found through testing but actually has the diagnosis.

Genetic testing for children at risk for VHL is recommended because some symptoms can show up in childhood. Earlier screening may reduce the chance of serious future complications. As with all genetic testing in people who have no symptoms, the risks, benefits, and limitations of testing should be discussed through proper genetic counseling.

Treatment team

Treatment for people with VHL is often specific to the person. A multi-disciplinary team and approach are essential. A treatment team for someone with VHL may include a **neurologist**, neurosurgeon, medical geneticist, genetic counselor, endocrinologist, pulmonologist, nephrologist, ophthalmologist, social worker, urologist, and a primary care provider. Often there are pediatric specialists in these fields who aid in the care for children. The key is good communication between the various specialists to coordinate medical care.

Treatment

There is no cure for von Hippel-Lindau disease. Treatment and management are often based on symptoms. Genetic testing has helped to identify individuals without symptoms, so medical screening may begin earlier than usual.

Most brain and spine hemangioblastomas can be treated by removal through surgery. **Radiation** therapy is sometimes used, if surgery is not possible. Growth patterns of these tumors can be unpredictable, so monitoring through regular imaging is important. Screening by MRI is recommended yearly, beginning at age 11.

Treatment for retinal tumors varies. Many tumors respond to laser therapy or cryotherapy. In rare cases, removal of the eye is needed to reduce severe pain or the risk for irreversible glaucoma. The key is early diagnosis and monitoring to prevent vision loss or blindness. For this reason, an ophthalmology exam is recommended first in infancy, and yearly thereafter.

Surgery may be quite successful for endolymphatic sac tumors, often preserving the hearing of a person with VHL. Radiation therapy is sometimes used for treatment, but its effectiveness is still unknown. CT and MRI scans of the internal ear canals and audiology exams are recommended if any typical symptoms develop.

Treatment for renal cell carcinoma often includes surgery, depending on the size of the affected area. Percutaneous ablation or cryoablation are experimental treatments that may work well because they are less invasive than other therapies. An abdominal ultrasound is first recommended at age eight, and then an MRI if necessary, and yearly thereafter. An abdominal CT scan is first recommended at age 18 or earlier if needed, and yearly thereafter.

Treatment for pheochromocytomas is most often by surgical removal, with an attempt to keep as much of the adrenal gland as possible. Medications such as corticosteroids are used as a treatment. Since pheochromocytomas can cause significant symptoms, it is important for the person with VHL to be screened prior to any surgery or delivery of a child. Blood or 24-hour checks of urine catecholamine and metanephrine levels are recommended beginning at age two, and yearly thereafter. They are also recommended if a person's blood pressure is raised.

Key Terms

Ataxia Uncoordinated muscular movement; often causes difficulty with walking and other voluntary movements.

Brain stem The entire unpaired subdivision of the brain (rhombencephalon, mesencephalon, and diencephalon).

Catecholamines Chemicals such as epinephrine, dopa, and norepinephrine; often at high levels in the urine if a pheochromocytoma is present.

Cerebellum Large area in the posterior of the brain (above the pons and below the cerebrum) responsible for functions like coordination.

Chemotherapy Chemical medical treatment often used for cancer.

Computed tomography (CT) scan Three-dimensional internal image of the body, created by combining x-ray images from different planes using a computer program.

Corticosteroids Steroid normally produced by the adrenal gland.

Cryoablation Using very cold temperatures to remove a foreign substance or body.

Cryotherapy Using very cold temperatures to treat a disease.

Cyst Sac of tissue filled with fluid, gas, or semi-solid material.

Cystadenoma Non-cancerous growth, in which fluid-filled, gas, or semi-solid areas may be present.

Endolymphatic sac tumor Growths that develop within inner ear structures called endolymph sacs.

Epididymis Male genital structure usually connected to the testis; an area where sperm collect.

Gait The way in which one walks.

Glaucoma Condition of the eye with increased internal pressure, often causing vision problems.

Hemangioblastoma Tumor often found in the brain, as in von Hippel-Lindau disease.

Magnetic resonance imaging (MRI) scan Three-dimensional internal image of the body, created using magnetic waves.

Meta-iodobenzylguanidine (MIBG) scintigraphy A procedure to look at the amount of a radioactive chemical, meta-iodobenzylguanidine, injected into the body to find growths like pheochromocytomas.

Metanephrine A byproduct of epinephrine, found elevated in urine if a pheochromocytoma is present.

Mutation A change in the order of deoxyribonucleic acid (DNA) bases that make up genes.

Nerve root Two groups of nerves that run from the spinal cord to join and form the spinal nerves.

Palpitation A heartbeat that is more pronounced, often felt physically.

Paresis Partial or total loss of movement or sensation.

Percutaneous ablation Attempting to remove a foreign body by a method just above the skin, like using an ointment.

Pheochromocytoma Non-cancerous growth in the adrenal gland.

Renal cell carcinoma A type of kidney cancer.

Retina Structure in the eye that receives and processes light.

Sequencing Genetic testing in which the entire sequence of deoxyribonucleic (DNA) bases that make up a gene is studied, in an effort to find a mutation.

Tinnitus Abnormal noises in the ear, like ringing.

Ultrasound Two-dimensional internal image of the body, created using sound waves.

Visceral Generally related to the digestive, respiratory, urogenital, or endocrine organs.

Surgery is the typical treatment for pancreatic growths and cysts, depending on their specific location and size. A goal is to keep as much of the pancreas as possible. If the tumors spread, chemotherapy is sometimes necessary. As with screening of the kidneys, abdominal ultrasounds are recommended beginning at age eight, and yearly thereafter; abdominal CT scans are recommended beginning at age 18, and yearly thereafter.

Both epididymal and broad ligament cystadenomas are non-cancerous and usually cause no symptoms. Therefore, treatment for both is only recommended if symptoms arise. There are no routine screening recommendations for either type. Ultrasounds can be used to find epididymal cystadenomas, and to monitor their growth over time. Ultrasounds or CT scans can be used to identify and monitor broad ligament cystadenomas.

Recovery and rehabilitation

Though VHL typically does not affect a person's thinking, learning, or behavior, the disease can have a significant impact on a person's life. Medical appointments can be frequent, and the pain from tumors may be considerable. Feelings of guilt associated with passing a disease-causing mutation to children have been reported in families. Professional therapy or family counseling may be helpful for some people.

Clinical trials

As of early 2004, there are several clinical studies studying various aspects of VHL. Many are currently recruiting subjects in the United States. Trials are being conducted at several institutions, including the National Cancer Institute and National Institute of Neurological Disorders and Stroke. Further information may be obtained at <http://www.clinicaltrials.gov>.

Prognosis

Prognosis for someone with von Hippel-Lindau disease is highly dependent on symptoms. Those people who die may do so as a result of significant complications with tumors. Renal cell carcinomas and CNS hemangioblastomas have been the greatest causes for death in people with VHL.

The outlook for people with VHL has improved significantly. Before the advent of comprehensive medical screening, the median survival of patients with the condition was less than 50 years of age. Genetic testing now helps identify people at risk before they even develop symptoms, so screening can begin as early as possible. This has helped to reduce the risk of complications and increase the quality of life for many. Medical screening may be further tailored to the individual as scientific studies identify medical complications associated with specific VHL mutations in families.

Resources

BOOKS

Parker, James N., and Philip M. Parker. *The Official Patient's Sourcebook on von Hippel-Lindau Disease: A Revised and Updated Directory for the Internet Age.* San Diego: Icon Health Publishers, 2002.

PERIODICALS

Couch, Vicki, Noralane M. Lindor, Pamela S. Karnes, and Virginia V. Michels. "Von Hippel-Lindau Disease." *Mayo Clinic Proceedings* (2000) 75: 265–272.

Hes, F. J., C. J. M Lips, and R. B. van der Luijt. "Molecular Genetic Aspects of von Hippel-Lindau (VHL) Disease and Criteria for DNA Analysis in Subjects at Risk." *The Netherlands Journal of Medicine* (2001) 59: 235–243.

Lonser, Russell R., et al. "Von Hippel-Lindau Disease." *The Lancet* 361 (June 14, 2003): 2059–2067.

WEBSITES

National Institute of Neurological Disorders and Stroke. (April 27, 2004). <http://www.ninds.nih.gov/index.htm>.

Online Mendelian Inheritance in Man. (April 27, 2004). <http://www.ncbi.nlm.nih.gov/omim/>.

ORGANIZATIONS

VHL Family Alliance. 171 Clinton Avenue, Brookline, MA 02455-5815. (617) 277-5667 or (800) 767-4VHL; Fax: (617) 734-8233. info@vhl.org. <http://www.vhl.org>.

Kidney Cancer Association. 1234 Sherman Avenue, Suite 203, Evanston, IL 60202-1375. (847) 332-1051 or (800) 850-9132; Fax: (847) 332-2978. office@kidneycancer association.org <http://www.kidneycancerassociation.org>.

Deepti Babu, MS, CGC

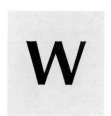

Walker *see* **Assistive mobile devices**

Wallenberg syndrome

Definition

Wallenberg syndrome is a type of brain stem **stroke** manifested by imbalance, vertigo, difficulty swallowing, hoarseness of voice, and sensory disturbance. It is caused by blockage in one of the arteries supplying the medulla and **cerebellum**.

Description

The first clinical description was given by Gaspard Viesseux in 1808 and published by Alexander John Gaspard Marcet in 1811. But it wasn't until 1895 that Adolf Wallenberg eloquently described the different symptoms and signs and confirmed the findings during autopsy. The syndrome is also known as lateral medullary infarct (LMI) or posterior inferior cerebellar artery syndrome (PICA).

It usually affects people over 40 years of age. They tend to have vascular risk factors such as hypertension, high cholesterol, and diabetes. Wallenberg syndrome can also occur in younger people, but the underlying causes are different.

Demographics

Wallenberg syndrome is rare, and accurate estimates about incidence are unavailable. In a large stroke registry in Sweden gathered by Norving and Cronquist in 1991, only about 2% of all strokes over a six-year period were caused by LMI.

Causes and symptoms

The stroke occurs in the medulla and cerebellum. The medulla controls such important functions as swallowing, speech articulation, taste, breathing, strength, and sensation. The cerebellum is important for coordination. The blood supply to these areas is via a pair of vertebral arteries and its branch, called the posterior inferior cerebellar artery (PICA).

Initially, the PICA was thought to be the blocked major artery, but this has been disproved from autopsy studies. In eight out of 10 cases, it is the vertebral artery that is occluded due to plaque buildup or because of a clot traveling from the heart. In younger patients, the vertebral artery dissection causes the infarct. The area of the stroke is only about 0.39 in (1 cm) vertically in the lateral part of the medulla and does not cross the midline.

Fully 50% of patients report transient neurological symptoms for several weeks preceding the stroke. During the first 48 hours after the stroke, the neurological deficit progresses and fluctuates. **Dizziness**, vertigo, facial **pain**, double vision, and difficulty walking are the most common initial symptoms. The facial pain can be quite bizarre with sharp jabs or jolts around the eye, ear, and forehead. Patients feel "seasick" or "off-balance" with nausea and vomiting. Objects appear double, tilted, or swaying. Along with gait imbalance, it becomes nearly impossible for the patient to walk despite good muscle strength. Other symptoms include hoarse voice, slurred speech, loss of taste, difficulty swallowing, hiccups, and altered sensation in the limbs of the opposite side.

The eye on the affected side has a droopy eyelid and a small pupil. The eyes jiggle when the person moves around; this is called nystagmus. There is decreased pain and temperature perception on the same side of the face. The limbs on the opposite side show decreased sensory perception. Voluntary movements of the arm on the affected side are clumsy. Gait is "drunken," and patients lurch and veer to one side.

Diagnosis

Accurate diagnosis usually requires the expertise of a **neurologist** or a stroke specialist. It is common for an inexperienced physician to dismiss the symptoms of nausea, vomiting, and vertigo as being caused by an ear infection or viral illness. Diagnosis requires a thorough

Key Terms

Brain stem The stalk-like portion of the brain that connects the cerebral hemispheres and the spinal cord. The brain stem receives sensory information and controls such vital functions as blood pressure and respiration.

Cerebellum Part of the brain that consists of two hemispheres, one on each side of the brain stem. It acts as a fine tuner for muscle tone, coordination of movement, posture, gait and skilled voluntary movement.

Dissection Tear in the wall of an artery that causes blood from inside the artery to leak into the wall and thereby narrows the lumen of the blood vessel.

Infarct Dead tissue resulting from lack of blood supply to brain; also called a stroke.

Medulla The lowermost portion of the brain stem that controls vital functions like respiration, blood pressure, swallowing, and heart rate.

Nystagmus Involuntary, uncontrollable, rapid, and repetitive movements of the eyeballs.

Stroke Also called as cerebrovascular accident (CVA) or cerebral infarction, it occurs when there is interruption of blood supply to a portion of the brain or spinal cord, resulting in damage or death of the tissue.

Vertigo Dizziness with a sense of spinning of self and/or surroundings with resultant loss of balance, nausea, and vomiting. Occurs due to a problem in the inner ears or the cerebellum and brain stem.

physical exam and neuroimaging. **CT scans** are insensitive and can detect only a large stroke or bleed in the cerebellum. **Magnetic resonance imaging (MRI)** scans are far superior, with the stroke showing up as a tiny bright spot in the medulla.

Treatment team

The team includes a neurologist or stroke specialist for initial diagnosis, workup, and medical management. Rehabilitation requires a physical therapist, occupational therapist, and speech therapist. Depending on whether complications arise, a neurosurgeon and a critical care physician may be involved.

Treatment

Treatment for Wallenberg syndrome is mostly symptomatic. The size of the underlying blocked artery is too small to allow any mechanical or chemical re-opening. Aim of treatment is to alleviate symptoms, modify underlying risk factors, and prevent complications and future strokes.

Medical therapy

Blood thinners like heparin are given intravenously in some patients for the first few days to stop further formation and propagation of the clot. Following that, the patient usually has to take other blood thinners such as aspirin for life. Medications are also used to control high blood pressure and cholesterol. Pain in Wallenberg syndrome can sometimes be quite severe and disabling. A variety of analgesics like Tylenol or narcotics are used. Some patients

need anti-seizure medications like **gabapentin** for pain management. Medications are also used for symptomatic treatment of vomiting and hiccups.

Surgical therapy

If the stroke is sufficiently large, the dead tissue swells up and can push the medulla downwards, impairing its vital functions and causing death. In this case, a neurosurgeon can remove a part of the skull to allow for the brain to swell.

Recovery and rehabilitation

Physical therapy focuses on improving balance and coordination. Assistive devices such as a cane, walker, or wheelchair may be used. Occupational therapy is used to help with daily activities like eating, which may be difficult due to clumsiness and incoordination. Speech training helps with articulation that has been impaired due to vocal cord paralysis. Special attention should be paid to food consistency to prevent aspiration. Initially, patients require pureed or semi-solid food. After initial treatment in the hospital, patients will need short-term placement in a nursing home or rehabilitation facility before going home. Modifications in living environment may include hand rails, non-slip rugs, etc.

Prognosis

Prognosis is usually quite encouraging both in the short and the long term. Nausea and vomiting disappear within a week. Clumsiness, difficulty swallowing, and gait imbalance improve over six months to a year. However, there is a 10% death rate due to complications like aspiration pneumonia, breathing difficulty, and cardiac arrhythmias.

Special concerns

Depression is very common among stroke survivors who face quite a challenge resulting from the abrupt change in lifestyle. They benefit from counseling, social support, and using antidepressant medications. There are several stroke support groups that help the patients and their families cope with the stroke and its aftermath.

Resources

BOOKS

"Vertebrobasilar Occlusive Disease." Chapter 11 in *Stroke— Pathophysiology, Diagnosis, and Management*, edited by Henry J. M. Barnett, OC, MD, FRCP; J. P. Mohr, MD; Bennett M. Stein, MD; and Frank M. Yatsu, MD. New York, NY: Churchill Livingstone, 1998.

"Medullary Infarcts and Hemorrhages." Chapter 41 in *Stroke Syndromes*, edited by Julien Bogousslavsky, MD, and Louis R. Caplan, MD. New York, NY: Cambridge University Press, 2001.

Parker, James N., MD, and Philip M. Parker, PhD, eds. *The Official Patient's Sourcebook on Wallenberg's Syndrome: A Revised and Updated Directory for the Internet Age*. San Diego, CA: ICON Health Publications, 2002.

PERIODICALS

Kim, J. S. "Pure Lateral Medullary Infarction: Clinical-radiological Correlation of 130 Acute, Consecutive Patients." *Brain* 126 (May 2003): 1864–1872

ORGANIZATIONS

National Stroke Association. 9707 East Easter Lane, Englewood, CO 80112. (303) 649-9299; Fax: (303) 649-1328. info@stroke.org. <http://www.stroke.org>.

American Stroke Association. 7272 Greenville Avenue, Dallas, TX 75231. (800) 242-8721 or (888) 4STROKE. <http://www.strokeassociation.org>.

National Rehabilitation Information Center. 4200 Forbes Blvd, Suite 202, Lanham, MD 20706-4829. (301) 562-2400 or (800) 346-2742; Fax: (301) 562-2401. naricinfo@heitech services.com. <http://www.naric.com>.

Chitra Venkatasubramanian, MBBS, MD

Werdnig-Hoffman disease *see* **Spinal muscular atrophy**

Wernicke-Korsakoff syndrome *see* **Beriberi**

West syndrome *see* **Infantile spasms**

▌West Nile virus infection

Definition

The West Nile virus is an arbovirus (meaning it is spread by mosquitos, ticks, or other arthropods) that can cause infections in animals and humans; in some cases, the infections can lead to fatal meningitis or encephalitis, which are inflammations of the spinal cord and brain. West Nile virus is considered a seasonal epidemic in North America, and it occurs mainly in the summer, but can continue into the fall. In many cases, it can be a serious illness that generally affects the **central nervous system**, leading to a variety of symptoms that differ from person to person. It is not contagious by touch, but can be spread by infected mosquitoes, transfusions, transplants, or from mother to child during pregnancy.

Description

West Nile virus infections usually begin with flu-like symptoms. Only approximately one in 150 people infected will develop severe symptoms, including **headaches**, neck stiffness, disorientation, **seizures**, fever, numbness, paralysis, and/or muscle weakness. In the worst cases, infection with West Nile virus can lead to death or permanent disability. These cases are usually due to either the age of the patient or the health status. Symptoms generally do not occur in healthy individuals.

Demographics

The West Nile virus has been observed mainly in temperate regions of Europe and North America, and has also been discovered to be the cause of human illness in the United States. The first known case in the United States was reported by the New York City Department of Health in late August 1999. Careful surveillance identified 59 patients who were hospitalized in New York City due to West Nile virus infections during August and September 1999. The median age of these patients was 71 years (range is five to 95). As of April 2004, only one case has been reported by the Centers for Disease Control. The West Nile virus has been observed in Africa, the Middle East, and west and central Asia. The first case was discovered in 1937 in an adult woman in the West Nile district of Uganda. The virus was characterized in Egypt during the 1950s.

An infection due to the West Nile virus does not produce symptoms in most people. In fact, only 20% of people who are infected will develop symptoms. Of these, the majority will recover and will not become infected again. The West Nile virus can infect males and females with equal frequency. There is no known predilection for people of specific ethnic backgrounds. People over 50 years old are at the highest risk of having serious illness associated with the infection. There is a very low risk of contracting this illness by medical procedures such as transplantation and blood transfusions. Although pregnancy and breast-feeding do not increase the risk of becoming infected with the virus, the risk to the fetus or nursing infant of an affected mother is currently being investigated. Horses, birds, and other animals have also been shown to be susceptible to viral infection.

Causes and symptoms

When a person is infected with West Nile virus, usually via a mosquito bite from a mosquito harboring the virus, it is unlikely that the individual will develop symptoms. Of the infected individuals that develop symptoms, there are either mild or severe clinical manifestations. The majority of infections are mild.

Characteristics of mild infections include:

- mild illness, including fever

- fever and symptoms persist no more than six days, usually lasting only three days

- symptoms usually develop three to 14 days after exposure, consistent with the incubation period

- illness can be sudden and accompanied by anorexia (loss of appetite), nausea, headaches, rash, muscle weakness, vomiting, and/or lymphadenopathy (swollen lymph glands)

Characteristics of severe infections include:

- Severe symptoms can result in neurological disease in approximately one in 150 cases, with the elderly at highest risk.

- Neurological symptoms include disorientation, seizures, and cranial nerve abnormalities.

- Symptoms include high fever, weakness, significant alterations in behavior, eye problems, and stomach problems.

- In rare cases, flaccid paralysis along with severe muscle weakness can occur.

- Illness can be sudden and accompanied by anorexia (loss of appetite), nausea, headaches, rash, muscle weakness, vomiting, and/or lymphadenopathy (swollen lymph glands).

Diagnosis

Diagnosis requires clinical observation by an experienced physician as well as positive results from specific laboratory tests. Factors that assist in the diagnosis are recent travel experiences, the season that the symptoms developed, the age of the patient, and whether there are

---

Key Terms

Arboviruses Viruses harbored by arthropods (mosquitoes and ticks) and transferred to humans by their bite. An arbovirus is the cause of West Nile infection.

Encephalitis Inflammation of the brain.

Flaccid paralysis Loss of muscle tone resulting from injury or disease of the nerves that innervate the muscles.

Lymphadenopathy Swelling of the lymph glands.

Meningitis Inflammation of the meninges, the membranes that surround the brain and spinal cord.

---

reports of other cases in the same geographical location that the patient was present during the time of exposure. Patients who have encephalitis, meningitis, or symptoms involving the central nervous system, which could lead a physician to suspect the West Nile virus, can be referred to health departments nationwide or the Centers for Disease Control (CDC) for testing. The CDC has confirmed all human cases.

The diagnostic test involves an assay that detects a virus-specific antibody (IgM) in the cerebral spinal fluid from patients. Blood can also be tested. If this test is negative, it is very unlikely that the infection is due to the West Nile virus; the other clinical explanations such as St. Louis encephalitis (SLE) should be considered. There is also a test that measures SLE virus-specific antibodies. Currently, there is a vaccination for horses, but not for humans.

Laboratory findings include normal to elevated white blood cell numbers with anemia (low red cell numbers). A deficiency of sodium in the blood (hyponatremia), which is usually associated with encephalitis, as well as normal glucose and a general increase in proteins can all be observed. A **magnetic resonance imaging (MRI)** scan can also be helpful, if specific areas of the brain show an abnormality, including the leptomeninges and/or the periventricular areas.

Treatment team

The treatment team might consist of the physician who initially sees the patient, usually a general practitioner, an infectious disease specialist, and **neurologist**. In severe cases, a complete medical team consisting of emergency room physicians and staff, nurses, and officers from the CDC might be necessary. Due to the risk of an epidemic, it is important for physicians to report these types of infections to the local health department.

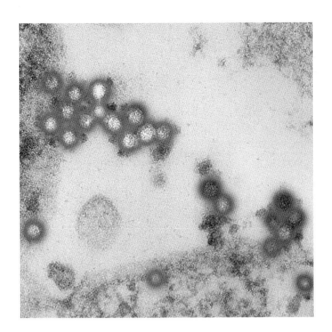

The West Nile virus. *(Scott Camazine/Photo Researchers, Inc.)*

Treatment

There is no cure for West Nile virus infection once the infection occurs. Treatment, therefore, is supportive and palliative. In the more severe cases, recurrent hospitalizations may necessitate life support services. The primary treatment is focused on lessening the symptoms and preventing secondary infections, which could include urinary tract infections and pneumonia in patients that develop severe illness. Intravenous fluids can be helpful during hospitalizations, along with airway management and good nursing care.

Recovery and rehabilitation

Most patients who develop symptoms recover from West Nile virus infections. The symptoms can be no worse than getting the flu. However, older patients and patients with health-related problems (particularly those that affect the immune system) have more difficulty recovering.

Clinical trials

The Warren G. Magnuson Clinical Center is currently recruiting participants for a clinical trial on the West Nile virus. The Patient Recruitment and Public Liaison Office's e-mail address is prpl@mail.cc.nih.gov.

The National Institutes of Health is conducting phase II **clinical trials** to investigate whether an experimental drug, Omr-IgG-am™IV, is a safe and effective treatment for West Nile virus-induced infections. This drug contains antibodies that help fight infection and is designed to target the West Nile virus. Another study by the same center has also been initiated to investigate the natural history of infection in patients with, or at risk of developing, West Nile virus-specific encephalitis or myelitis.

A third clinical trial sponsored by the National Institute of Allergy and Infectious Diseases (NIAID) in phase I and II is to test the tolerability of Omr-IgG-am, its efficacy as a vaccine, and its effectiveness in reducing morbidity and mortality (disability and death) in patients with a confirmed diagnosis of the West Nile virus disease. The contact is Walla Dempsey; the e-mail is wdempsey@niaid.nih.gov.

Finally, a clinical trial is ongoing to identify healthy individuals who might be eligible for a phase I vaccine clinical trial sponsored by the Vaccine Research Center at the National Institutes of Health. The Patient Recruitment and Public Liaison Office's e-mail address is prpl@mail.cc.nih.gov.

High doses of a drug called Ribavirin and another called interferon alpha-2b were found to be effective in research studies, but currently no controlled clinical trials in humans have been initiated for these or other types of medications in the therapeutic management of West Nile virus infections and encephalitis.

Prognosis

The prognosis for persons with West Nile virus infection is quite favorable in patients that are young and in otherwise good health. Older persons and patients with health complications can have a poorer prognosis. In rare cases, death is possible.

Special concerns

It is important to contact the local health department when finding dead birds or other animals that die suddenly of an unknown cause during suspected or confirmed local outbreaks of West Nile virus. Health officials monitor mosquito and bird populations to determine local risk for West Nile virus activity.

A person's exposure to mosquitoes and other insects that harbor arboviruses can be reduced by taking precautions when in a mosquito-prone area. Insect repellents containing DEET provide effective temporary protection from mosquito bites. Long sleeves and pants should be worn when outside during the evening hours of peak mosquito activity. When camping outside, intact mosquito netting over sleeping areas reduces the risk of mosquito bites. Communities also employ large-scale spraying of pesticides to reduce the population of mosquitoes, and encourage citizens to eliminate all standing water sources such as in bird baths, flower pots, and tires stored outside to eliminate possible breeding grounds for mosquitoes.

Resources

BOOKS

Despommier, Dickson. *West Nile Story.* New York: Apple Trees Productions, 2001.

White, Dennis J., and Dale L. Morse. *West Nile Virus: Detection, Surveillance, and Control.* New York: New York Academy of Sciences, 2002.

PERIODICALS

Nash, D., et al. "The Outbreak of West Nile Virus Infection in the New York City Area in 1999." *New England Journal of Medicine* 344, no. 24 (June 14, 2001): 1807–14.

OTHER

Bren, Linda. "West Nile Virus: Reducing the Risk." *U. S. Food and Drug Administration.* May 1, 2004 (June 3, 2004). <http://www.fda.gov/oc/opacom/hottopics/westnile.html>.

"West Nile Virus: Statistics, Surveillance, and Control." *United States Centers for Disease Control.* May 1, 2004 (June 3, 2004). <http://www.cdc.gov/ncidod/dvbid/westnile/surv&control.htm>.

"West Nile Virus." *United States Centers for Disease Control.* May 1, 2004 (June 3, 2004). <http://www.cdc.gov/ncidod/dvbid/westnile/>.

"What You Should Know About West Nile Virus." *American Veterinary Medical Association.* May 1, 2004 (June 3, 2004). <http://www.avma.org/communications/brochures/wnv/wnv_faq.asp>.

ORGANIZATIONS

Centers for Disease Control and Prevention (CDC) Division of Vector-Borne Infectious Diseases. P.O. Box 2087, Fort Collins, CO 80522. (800) 311-3435. dvbid@cdc.gov. <http://www.cdc.gov/ncidod/dvbid/index.htm>.

U. S. Food and Drug Administration. 5600 Fishers Lane, Rockville, MD 20857-0001. (888) INFO-FDA. <http://www.fda.gov/oc/opacom/hottopics/westnile.html>.

Bryan Richard Cobb, PhD

Wheelchair *see* **Assistive mobile devices**

Whiplash

Definition

Whiplash is an injury resulting from a sudden extension or flexion of the neck. Whiplash can also be termed neck sprain or neck strain or, more technically, cervical acceleration/deceleration trauma. It is most often associated with being struck from behind in a car, although it also occurs during contact sports, falls, or other physical activities. Whiplash may also cause damage to vertebrae, ligaments, cervical muscles, or nerve roots.

Description

Whiplash occurs when the body is struck, usually from behind, and the head travels backwards to catch up with the body. The neck will flex until either the facet joints in the back of the vertebrae or the anterior longitudinal ligament in the front of the vertebrae stop the motion.

The muscles that are most often injured during an impact that causes whiplash are the sternocleidomastoids and the longus colli. The sternocleidomastoids are the large straplike muscles running down the front of the neck that pop out when the jaw is flexed. They are used to turn and support the head. The longus colli is a muscle that runs directly in front of the spine is used to turn the head from side to side and to bend the neck forward. The longus colli muscle aids the sternocleidomastoids in holding up the head and moving the neck. Often, the lognus colli muscle is weakened during whiplash and the sternocleidomastoid muscles become overworked as they compensate.

The facet joints in the anterior of the neck may also be damaged during a whiplash injury. There are two facet joints on the back of each vertebra. They are about a centimeter in size and guide the movement of the spine. When the neck bends backward during a whiplash impact, the joints can be compressed and then swell in response. This can cause **pain**, both in the neck and can also refer pain to other parts of the body. For example, if the facet joints between the second and third cervical vertebrae are compressed, pain may be felt in the back of the head.

A whiplash impact can also damage the anterior longitudinal ligament, which is a tough band of tissue that runs down the front of the vertebral column and holds the vertebral bones together. In automobile accidents, this ligament is often overstretched or torn. If it is torn, it can lead to vertebral **disc herniation** or to excessive movement of the spinal column. Such movement can result in pain spasms in the neck, cracking and grinding in the neck, or even numbness in the hands and feet.

Whiplash can also result in a herniated vertebral disc. The vertebral bones are cushioned between vertebral discs that are made up of an interior gel-like substance surrounded by a tougher outer layer. If this outer layer becomes damaged, the disc may rupture and the gel-like interior will be compressed out. The ruptured disc can put pressure on adjacent nerve roots and cause tingling, numbness or burning.

Damage to the **central nervous system** or the **peripheral nervous system** may occur during a whiplash injury. Most of the damage to the nervous systems involves compression injuries during which pressure is applied to nervous tissues, although damage can also be caused by

Key Terms

Herniated disc   A blisterlike bulging or protrusion of the contents of the disk out through the fibers that normally hold them in place. It is also called a ruptured disk, slipped disk, or displaced disk.

Ligament   A type of tough, fibrous tissue that connects bones or cartilage and provides support and strength to joints.

Vertebrae   Singular, vertebra. The individual bones of the spinal column that are stacked on top of each other. There is a hole in the center of each bone, through which the spinal cord passes.

stretching or torquing (twisting) of nervous tissues. In severe cases, compression injuries can affect the brain resulting in subdural or extradural hematomas (pooling of blood between the brain and the skull). Symptoms of this complication include **anosmia** (loss of smell), double vision, brief loss of consciousness, confusion and loss of motor skills.

Compression, stretching, and torque injuries to the spinal cord may also occur during trauma associated with whiplash. The most frequently occurring is root syndrome. Nerve roots exit the spinal cord on both sides of the body between vertebrae. When the spaces between vertebrae, also called foramen, become compressed, the nerve roots can be compressed or damaged. This can result in slight numbness, burning or tingling in any of the parts of the body that the nerve enervates. In more severe car accidents, whiplash can cause more critical damage to the spinal cord resulting in major neurological dysfunction or paralysis below the location of the injury. The important variables controlling the severity of the symptoms appear to be the force and the direction of the impact on the spine. As the area impacted by the trauma increases due to increased force, a greater portion of the cord is involved resulting in greater neurological dysfunction.

The peripheral nervous system can also suffer damage in a whiplash injury. These nerves can be compressed in the vertebral foramen and can also be stretched or compressed by other anatomical structures along their path. Only a very small compression or stretching is required to interrupt blood flow to a nerve cell. For example, blood flow to a nerve cell can be completely stopped if the nerve cell is stretched to 15% more than its original length. Such trauma to a nerve cell can result in numbness or tingling in the region affected by the nerve, but usually not pain. It

is the irritation of the nerve following the trauma that causes pain in the peripheral nervous system.

Demographics

Anyone can suffer from whiplash, in particular people who drive in automobiles. Whiplash has been documented in people who are driving as slowly as five miles per hour. About 20% of people who are involved in rear-end accidents in cars suffer symptoms of whiplash. In the United States, it is estimated that about 1.8 million people are subject to chronic pain and disability after an automobile accident, the majority of whom suffer from neck pain.

Causes and symptoms

Symptoms of whiplash include neck pain and stiffness, shoulder pain and stiffness, lower **back pain**, **headaches** in the back of the head, pain, and/or tingling in the hand or arm, **dizziness**, ringing in the ears and blurred vision. Often the pain associated with whiplash worsens several days following the injury. Some people suffer cognitive or psychological symptoms including difficulty concentrating, difficulty sleeping, memory loss, **depression** and irritability.

Symptoms of whiplash appear to follow one of two courses. In most people, symptoms will slowly abate within approximately three months. In a smaller proportion of people who experience whiplash, the symptoms become chronic and disability may result.

Diagnosis

Orthopedists (physicians specializing in the bones and joints) use a variety of diagnostic tools to evaluate the extent of injury following whiplash. This usually begins with a history of the accident and the symptoms experienced. A physical examination allows the physician to evaluate the range of motion in the neck, locations of pain in the neck, arms and legs, and function of nerves. An x ray is almost always used to determine if any vertebrae have been damaged in the accident. However, because many of the injuries are to soft tissues, they are not well visualized using a standard x ray. The orthopedist may then recommend other diagnostic procedures that visualize these tissues more effectively. **Magnetic resonance imaging (MRI)** allows for visualization of the spinal cord and nerve roots that emerge between the vertebrae. A **computed tomography** study (**CT**) gives precise information about the bone and spinal canal using specialized x ray technology. Another technology called a myelogram combines x rays with an injection of dye into the spinal canal and allows for detailed visualization of the spinal canal and nerve roots. An electromyogram (EMG) may also be used to determine the health of nerves and muscles using electrical impulses.

Treatment

Treatment for whiplash includes a variety of techniques and medications including exercises, pain-relieving medications, traction, massage, heat and ice, and ultrasound, depending on the symptoms. Although a physician should evaluate people who suffer whiplash, most of the time whiplash can be treated using home treatments and extensive medical care is not prescribed.

Both heat and cold are useful for treatment of symptoms of whiplash. Initial treatment for whiplash usually includes cold packs of ice applied to the neck for the first 24 hours. Heat may then be used to relieve pain throughout the neck and shoulders either using heating pads or hot showers. Physical therapists can apply deep heat treatments using ultrasound equipment.

Medications are useful for relieving acute pain associated with whiplash. Non-steroidal anti-inflammatory medications can be very helpful in relieving pain. Antidepressants may be prescribed because they inhibit the transfer of nervous signals along pain pathways.

A soft cervical collar may provide some relief for symptoms of whiplash; however, most physicians recommend that the use of the collar be limited to two to three weeks. Using the cervical collar for long periods may cause muscle strength to decrease and inhibit muscle flexibility.

Physicians have found that movement is important in preventing chronic symptoms of whiplash. Many doctors assert that simple exercises such as walking, muscle strengthening, and range of motion exercises help improve symptoms more quickly than remaining sedentary. In 2000, a study reported in the journal *Spine* demonstrated that patients who frequently performed a set of exercises immediately following an injury that caused whiplash recovered faster than patients who exercised less. The more active group performed a set of repetitive motion exercises 10 times an hour beginning within 96 hours of injury, while the less active group performed exercises a few times a day beginning two weeks after the injury. Of the more active group, nearly 40% reported that they had no symptoms of whiplash six months following the accident, compared with only 5% of the less active group.

Traction, under the supervision of an orthopedic professional, removes the pressure from the neck, and some people report relief from pain for several hours to several days following treatments. Physical therapy and/or chiropractic adjustments are often prescribed to treat symptoms of whiplash. In rare cases, surgery is required to correct whiplash injuries.

Clinical trials

The National Institute of Arthritis and Musculoskeletal and Skin Diseases (NIAMS) conducting a study in 2004 focused on preventing acute pain, such as that associated with whiplash, from becoming chronic pain. Research suggests that the emotional response to an injury to the neck, particularly fear of reinjury, contributes significantly to the development of chronic pain from whiplash. The study focused on two anxiety-reducing treatments as a way to prevent such chronic pain from developing. The principal investigator on the two-year study is Dennis C. Turk, Ph.D. (telephone number: 206-543-3387, or email: wads@u.washington.edu). Information is available on the institute's website at <http://www.depts.washington.edu/wads>.

Resources

BOOKS

Foreman, Stephen M. and Arthur C. Croft. *Whiplash Injuries: The Cervical Acceleration/Deceleration Syndrome. Second Edition.* Philadelphia: Lippincott, Williams & Wilkins, 1995.

PERIODICALS

Cote, P., J. D. Cassidy, L. Carroll, et al. "A systematic review of the prognosis of acute whiplash and a new conceptual framework to synthesize the literature." *Spine* 26, no. 19 (2001): e445–e458.

Rosenfeld, M., R. Gunnarsson, and P. Borenstein. "Early Intervention in whiplash-associated disorders: A comparison of two treatment protocols." *Spine* 25, no. 14 (2000): 1882–1787.

OTHER

Centeno, Christopher J. "What is Whiplash?" *Whiplash 101.* (January 19, 2004). <http://www.whiplash101.com/default1.htm>.

Mayo Clinic Staff. "Neck Pain: Sometimes Serious." *The Mayo Clinic.* (February 07, 2002). <http://www.mayoclinic.com/invoke.cfm?id=HQ01111>.

"Neck Pain." *American Academy of Orthopaedic Surgeons.* 2000. (January 23, 2004). <http://orthoinfo.aaos.org/brochure/thr_report.cfm?thread_id=11&topcategory=neck>.

"Neck Sprain." *The America Academy of Orthopaedic Surgeons.* May 2000 (January 23, 2004). <http://orthoinfo.aaos.org/fact/thr_report.cfm?thread_id=141&topcategory=neck>.

"Whiplash." *The America Academy of Orthopaedic Surgeons.* October 2000 (January 23, 2004). <http://orthoinfo.aaos.org/fact/thr_report.cfm?Thread_ID=232&topcategory=Neck>.

"NINDS Whiplash Information Page." *National Institute of Neurological Disorders and Stroke.* July 1, 2001 (January 23, 2004). <http://www.ninds.nih.gov/health_and_medical/disorders/whiplash.htm?format=printable>.

ORGANIZATIONS

American Chronic Pain Association (ACPA). P.O. Box 850, Rocklin, CA 95677. (916) 632-0922 or (800) 533-3231; Fax: (916) 632-3208. ACPA@pacbell.net.

National Chronic Pain Outreach Association (NCPOA). P.O. Box 274, Millboro, VA 24460. (540) 862-9437; Fax: (540) 862-9485. ncpoa@cfw.com.

National Headache Foundation. 820 N. Orleans, Suite 217, Chicago, IL 60610. (773) 388-6399 or (888) NHF-5552; Fax: (773) 525-7357. info@headaches.org. <http://www.headaches.org>.

Juli M. Berwald, Ph.D.

Whipple's disease

Definition

Whipple's disease is a rare infectious disorder that can affect many areas of the body, including the gastro-intestinal and central nervous systems. Caused by the bacteria *Tropheryma whipplei,* it is typically diagnosed from malabsorption symptoms such as diarrhea and weight loss. If the **central nervous system** is infected, Whipple's disease can cause impairment of mental faculties and lead to **dementia**. It can be treated successfully with antibiotic therapy, but up to a third of patients suffer relapse.

Description

Whipple's disease, also known as intestinal lipodystrophy, was first reported in 1907 by George Hoyt Whipple (1878–1976). An autopsy on a thirty-seven year old male missionary revealed a granular accumulation of fatty acids in the walls of the small intestine and lymph nodes.

Historically, Whipple's disease has been considered an gastro-intestinal disorder, however, in the 1960s it was realized that other organs could be involved, with or without intestinal infection. It is now considered a systemic infection with a wide range of possible symptoms.

Demographics

The disorder typically affects middle-aged men of European descent. Most cases have been reported in North America and Europe. Many texts suggest the disorder affects eight times as many males as females, although there is some evidence to suggest the rate in females is rising.

The disease is extremely rare and no reliable estimate of incidence is known. Farmers and other rural people are most often diagnosed with Whipple's disease, but as yet, no specific environmental factors have been linked to the disorder.

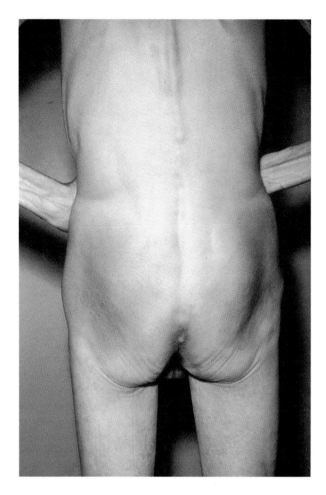

The effects of Whipple's disease. *(Phototake, Inc. All rights reserved.)*

Causes and symptoms

The bacterium that causes Whipple's disease was only successfully cultured in 1997. *Tropheryma whipplei* belongs to the high G+C phylum of gram-positive bacteria, and its genome was sequenced in 2003.

Whipple's disease has traditionally been regarded as a malabsorption disease of the small intestine, but in most cases the first symptoms are arthritic joints, which can precede the malabsorption symptoms of Whipple's disease by many years. Commonly, the disease progresses to the small intestine. Symptoms then include diarrhea, anemia, weight loss, and there is often fat present in the stool, all due to the bacteria disrupting absorption of fat and nutrients. If untreated, other malabsorption problems, such as reductions in the levels of calcium and magnesium, may result. Fever and night sweats are common, as well as general weakness. There are many further possible symptoms depending on the organs affected.

In cases where the central nervous system is affected, there may be a decrease in intellectual abilities, insomnia,

Key Terms

Ataxia Inability to coordinate muscle control resulting in irregularity of movements.

Malabsorption The inability to adequately or efficiently absorb nutrients from the intestinal tract.

Tinnitus Ringing sensation or other noise in the ears.

hearing loss or tinnitus (ringing in the ears), and uncontrolled muscle movements (**ataxia**) or eye movements. If untreated, the disorder can lead to dementia and progressive brain cell death, leading to coma and death over a period of months to years.

Diagnosis

Diagnosis of Whipple's disease is difficult, and is commonly suspected only if the patient presents with malabsorption symptoms. Then, a small-bowel **biopsy** can be made to locate the presence of the bacteria and confirm the diagnosis. However, symptoms can vary greatly depending on the areas of the body that are affected, and up to a third of sufferers do not present with malabsorption ailments.

Treatment team

Once diagnosed, the treatment of Whipple's disease is often straightforward, and can be monitored with minor hospital procedures. However, due to the rarity of the disease and the recent developments in studying the disorder it is recommended that contact be made with specialized centers of research or a **neurologist**.

Treatment

Whipple's disease generally responds well to antibiotic therapy. The recommended treatment is two weeks of intravenous antibiotics followed by a year or more of oral antibiotics. If the malabsorption symptoms are pronounced, the patient may require intravenous fluids and electrolytes, and other dietary supplements. A diet high in calories and protein is often recommended, and should be monitored by a physician.

Recovery and rehabilitation

When treated, symptoms such as diarrhea and fever can resolve within days, and most symptoms typically improve within a few weeks. In most cases, symptoms of the disorder are lessened or ameliorated by treatment. The progress of therapy can be checked by biopsy of the small intestine. In about one third of cases, the disease relapses and is more likely to affect the central nervous system than the initial infection. Periodic monitoring over several years, therefore, is essential to prevent neurological damage.

Clinical trials

Although as of early 2004, there were no ongoing **clinical trials** in the United States specific for Whipple's disease, the National Institute of Diabetes and Digestive and Kidney Diseases supports research for similar disorders.

Prognosis

If untreated, Whipple's disease can be fatal, but when treated with antibiotic therapy most patients experience rapid recovery and lasting remission. However, up to a third of patients may suffer a relapse.

Special concerns

Knowledge of Whipple's disease is rapidly evolving, and there have been many recent developments that may lead to new diagnostic options and new treatments in the near future.

Resources

PERIODICALS

Marth, Thomas, and Dider Raoult. "Whipple's disease," *Lancet* 361, no. 9353 (January 18, 2003): 239–247.

OTHER

"NINDS Whipple's Disease Information Page." National Institute of Neurological Disorders and Stroke. (March 10, 2004). <http://www.ninds.nih.gov/health_and_medical/disorders/whipples.htm>.

"Whipple's Disease." *National Digestive Diseases Information Clearinghouse.* (March 10, 2004). <http://digestive.niddk.nih.gov/ddiseases/pubs/whipple/index.htm>.

ORGANIZATIONS

National Organization for Rare Disorders (NORD). P.O. Box 1968 (55 Kenosia Avenue), Danbury, CT 06813-1968. (203) 744–0100 or (800) 999–NORD (6673); Fax: (203) 798–2291. orphan@rarediseases.org. <http://www.rarediseases.org>.

David Tulloch,

Williams syndrome

Definition

Williams syndrome, first described in 1961, is a rare genetic condition with a wide array of clinical features.

Description

Typical facial features seen in children with Williams syndrome include a wide mouth with full lips, a small chin, and a short, slightly upturned nose. Children with blue or green eyes often times show a starburst pattern in the colored part (iris) of the eyes. An unusual narrowing of the aorta called supravalvular aortic stenosis is often present, and hernias are often seen in the inguinal area of the abdomen. The blood vessels and abdominal wall often show weakness or altered development. Muscle tone is typically low, and children are often on the low end of birth weight, with relatively poor weight gain and growth in their early years.

Most children with Williams syndrome have a remarkable contrast between verbal abilities and spatial abilities. While overall intellectual performance on standardized IQ tests will be in the general range found in Down syndrome, children with Williams syndrome show a complex pattern of strengths and deficiencies that would not be evident by counting IQ points. Verbal abilities, for example, are exceptionally strong, and people with Williams syndrome tend to show very strong social skills relative to what one might anticipate based on IQ scores. Long-term memory is also generally excellent. Musical interest and ability are often strong. In contrast, fine motor skills often lag behind their IQ-matched peers, and, the sense of spatial relationships is very poor. If a therapist, for example, were to ask a child with Williams syndrome for a picture of a boy on a bike, the child might not be able to identify many of the parts of the picture. The parts will not likely be spaced in a way that makes much sense. However, if the therapist asks for a description of what it is like to ride a bike, the child will likely describe the sensation with a detailed and imaginative story.

For reasons that are not well understood, children may have a problem with calcium levels that are too high. Irritability and colic are common in early development, especially in children with high calcium levels. Delays are typically seen in reaching developmental milestones, and children with Williams syndrome generally exhibit learning disabilities and may be easily distractible with some form of attention deficit disorder. Cognitive, verbal and motor deficits are universal, and about three quarters of children will be determined to have **mental retardation** in the course of their care. Young children with Williams syndrome often have extremely sensitive hearing, although this tends to become less significant as children get older.

Demographics

Williams syndrome is estimated to occur in one of every 20,000 births. In most families, only one child will be affected and there is no significant family history of Williams syndrome in other relatives.

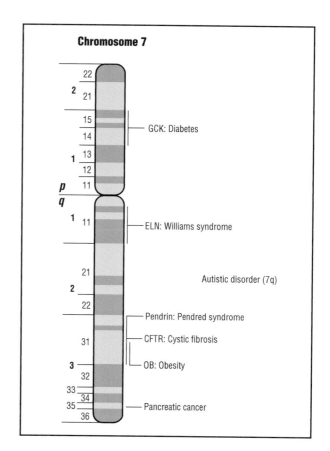

Williams syndrome, on chromosome 7. *(Gale Group.)*

Causes and symptoms

Williams syndrome is most often caused by a chromosome deletion involving loss of a gene called elastin on chromosome number 7, and may involve the loss of other neighboring genes as well.

Diagnosis

Because of the variability in the way that Williams syndrome affects different people, it often goes undiagnosed for many years. Although there is a chromosome deletion in over 98% of children born with Williams syndrome, the deletions are so small that they are usually not detectable under the microscope using standard methods. Diagnosis requires the use of a special test called fluorescence in situ hybridization (FISH) in which a DNA probe for the elastin gene is labeled with a brightly colored fluorescent dye.

Treatment team

Medical care for children with Williams syndrome should be provided by a physician with specific knowledge or experience with Williams syndrome, and growth charts specific to children with Williams syndrome are

Key Terms

Autosomal dominant   A pattern of inheritance in which only one of the two copies of an autosomal gene must be abnormal for a genetic condition or disease to occur. An autosomal gene is a gene that is located on one of the autosomes or non-sex chromosomes. A person with an autosomal dominant disorder has a 50% chance of passing it to each of their offspring.

Elastin   A protein that gives skin the ability to stretch and then return to normal.

available. The services of a medical geneticist should be available to the treating physician.

Treatment

Treatment is supportive and varies according to the symptoms displayed. Special attention is given to monitoring for heart and blood vessel disease, along with blood calcium levels. Multivitamin supplementation should generally be avoided unless directed by a physician because of the potential for problems caused by vitamin D.

Recovery and rehabilitation

Teens and adults with Williams syndrome face a variety of challenges that come with aging. Involvement of the family in support groups with other families that have direct experience with Williams syndrome can be helpful in anticipating and avoiding the common pitfalls. Most adults with Williams syndrome continue to live at home with parents or in special group home situations, with rare individuals living and functioning independently.

Prognosis

There is no cure for Williams syndrome as it is a genetically determined disease. Research is underway to determine the roles of approximately 20 genes in the area of chromosome 7 that are critical to the development of Williams syndrome.

Special concerns

Individuals who have Williams syndrome have a 50% chance of passing it on to their offspring if they have children because one of their two copies of chromosome 7 is missing some vital information, and each sperm or egg will receive one copy of chromosome 7 at random. This inheritance pattern is called autosomal pseudodominant because it so closely resembles the pattern of transmission seen for autosomal dominant single gene traits.

Resources

BOOKS

Semel, Eleanor, and Sue R. Rosner. *Understanding Williams Syndrome: Behavioral Patterns and Interventions.* Mahwah, NJ: Lawrence Erlbaum Assoc, 2003.

PERIODICALS

Committee on Genetics American Academy of Pediatrics. "Health care supervision for children with Williams syndrome." *Pediatrics* 107 (2001): 1192–1204.

OTHER

"NINDS Williams Syndrome Information Page." *National Institute of Neurological Disorders and Stroke.* (February 11, 2004). <http://www.ninds.nih.gov/health_and_medical/disorders/williams.htm#Is_there_any_treatment>.

ORGANIZATIONS

Williams Syndrome Association. P.O. Box 297, Clawson, MI 48017-0297. (248) 244-2229 or (800) 806-1871; Fax: (248) 244-2230. info@williams-syndrome.org. <http://www.williams-syndrome.org>.

National Organization for Rare Disorders (NORD), P.O. Box 1968 (55 Kenosia Avenue), Danbury, CT 06813-1968. (203) 744-0100 or (800) 999-NORD (6673); Fax: (203) 798-2291. orphan@rarediseases.org, <http://www.rarediseases.org>.

Robert G. Best, PhD

Wilson disease

Definition

Wilson disease (WD) is an inherited disorder of copper metabolism, transmitted as an autosomal recessive trait. This type of inheritance means unaffected parents who each carry the WD gene have a 25% risk in each pregnancy of having an affected child. The disorder is caused by a defective copper-binding protein found primarily in the liver, which leads to excess copper circulating through the bloodstream. Over time, the copper is deposited and increased to toxic levels in various body tissues, especially the liver, brain, kidney, and cornea of the eye. Left untreated, WD is invariably fatal.

Description

In 1912, Dr. Samuel Kinnear Wilson described a disorder he called "progressive lenticular degeneration." He noted the familial nature of the condition, and also that it was likely to be caused by a toxin affecting the liver. The toxin was later discovered to be excess copper. Another,

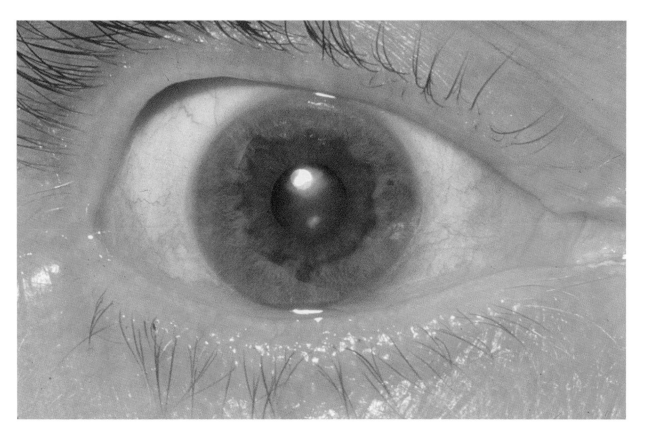

Eye afflicted with a Kayser-Fleischer ring, a brownish ring overlying the outer rim of the iris of the eye; it is caused by Wilson's disease. *(Photo Researchers, Inc. Reproduced by permission.)*

little-used name for the disorder is "hepatolenticular degeneration" (degeneration of the liver and lens), which omits the contribution of neurological symptoms.

The classic triad of signs for WD includes lenticular degeneration, cirrhosis of the liver, and neuropsychiatric symptoms. Errors in a specific gene produce a defective copper-binding protein in the liver, which results in an inability to excrete excess copper. While some copper is necessary for normal metabolic processes in the body, too much can be toxic. The disease is present at birth, but symptoms typically do not show until years later. WD is progressive because the underlying cause cannot be corrected. Effective treatments are available, but without treatment, people with WD will eventually die of liver failure.

Demographics

WD has an incidence of about one in 30,000, which means one in 90 individuals is a silent carrier of the WD gene. There seems to be no specific ethnic group or race that has a higher frequency of the disease. Only a man and woman who are both silent carriers of the WD gene can have a child with the condition. Unlike a disease with dominant inheritance, which usually implies a definite

family history, WD only rarely has occurred in a previous family member.

Causes and symptoms

WD is caused by errors in a gene located on chromosome 13, which produces a protein named ATP7B. Errors in the ATP7B gene produce a protein with decreased ability to bind copper. Unused copper is then absorbed back into the bloodstream where it is transported to other organs. A person who is a carrier of WD has one normally functioning copy of the ATP7B gene, and this produces enough functional protein to rid the body of excess copper.

A little more than half of all patients with WD first show symptoms of hepatitis. In addition, those who have liver-related symptoms first, do so at a younger age than do those who first present with neuropsychiatric symptoms—15 years and 25 years on average, respectively. However, the symptoms and their severity are quite variable, and the diagnosis of WD has been made in children as young as three years old, and in adults in their 60s.

Neurological symptoms are primarily the result of copper's toxic effects in the basal ganglia, a portion of the brain that controls some of the subconscious aspects of

Key Terms

Ceruloplasmin A protein circulating in the bloodstream that binds with copper and transports it.

Cirrhosis A chronic degenerative disease of the liver, in which normal cells are replaced by fibrous tissue and normal liver function is disrupted. The most common symptoms are mild jaundice, fluid collection in the tissues, mental confusion, and vomiting of blood. Cirrhosis is associated with portal hypertension and is a major risk factor for the later development of liver cancer. If left untreated, cirrhosis leads to liver failure.

Chelation The process by which a molecule encircles and binds to a metal and removes it from tissue.

Hepatitis An inflammation of the liver, with accompanying liver cell damage or cell death, caused most frequently by viral infection, but also by certain drugs, chemicals, or poisons. May be either acute (of limited duration) or chronic (continuing). Symptoms include jaundice, nausea, vomiting, loss of appetite, tenderness in the right upper abdomen, aching muscles, and joint pain. In severe cases, liver failure may result.

Penicillamine A drug used to bind to and remove heavy metals (such as copper or lead) from the blood, to prevent kidney stones, and to treat rheumatoid arthritis. Brand names include Cuprimine and Depen.

voluntary movement such as accessory movements and inhibiting tremor. These symptoms include:

- Dystonia. Prolonged muscular contractions that may cause twisting (torsion) of body parts, repetitive movements, and increased muscular tone.

- Dysarthria. Difficulty in articulating words, sometimes accompanied by drooling.

- Dysphagia. Difficulty swallowing.

- Pseudosclerosis. Symptoms similar to multiple sclerosis.

Diagnosis

While the diagnosis of WD may be suspected on clinical grounds, it can only be confirmed using laboratory tests. An easily detectable physical sign is the presence of Kayser-Fleisher rings in the eye, which are bluish rings around the iris, caused by copper deposition in the cornea.

The easiest biochemical test is measurement of ceruloplasmin, a blood protein that is nearly always decreased in patients with WD. While low levels of ceruloplasmin are highly suggestive, a liver **biopsy** to detect excess copper levels is much more accurate. Testing for mutations in the ATP7B gene is nearly definitive, but the large number of mutations catalogued in the gene means that only certain individuals may benefit from testing. A consultation with a genetics professional is always recommended.

Treatment team

A gastroenterologist will treat and monitor liver disease, while a **neurologist** and psychiatrist (or neuropsychiatrist) should evaluate and treat neuropsychiatric symptoms. Since many individuals achieve remission of their neurologic symptoms once treatment is started, neuropsychiatric consultations may only be short term. If necessary, periodic consultations with a geneticist can provide updated information on genetic testing.

Treatment

Treatment of WD revolves around the process of copper chelation. A chelating agent binds to excess copper in the bloodstream so that it can be excreted from the body. Penicillamine is the most effective and commonly used medication, but about 20% of all patients suffer serious side effects, which may include joint **pain**, blood disorders, fever, an increase in neurologic symptoms, and systemic **lupus** erythematosus.

Trientine and zinc salts given orally are somewhat less effective, but have fewer side effects than penicillamine. In addition, zinc salts may take several months to have any noticeable effect. A diet low in copper will also have some preventive effect. Finally, for those patients in advanced stages of liver disease, liver transplantation may be the only method of averting liver failure and death.

Recovery and rehabilitation

The earlier in the course of the disorder that treatment is started, the more beneficial the effects will be. For some individuals, liver function may return to near normal, and often dramatic improvements in the neuropsychiatric symptoms can be seen shortly after beginning treatment. For others who have gone untreated for longer periods, or who have a more severe form of the disease, only modest improvements may be seen. Treatment must be lifelong.

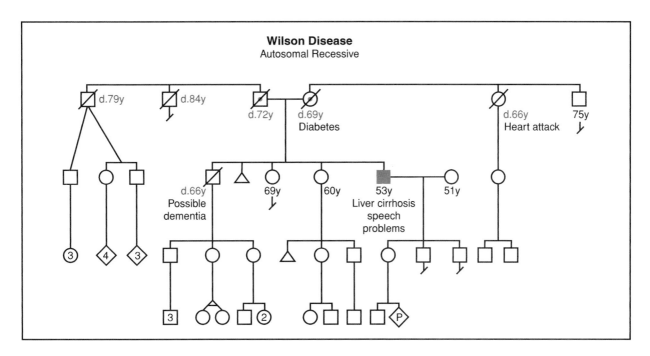

Wilson Disease
Autosomal Recessive

See Symbol Guide for Pedigree Charts. *(Gale Group.)*

Clinical trials

A newer copper chelating agent currently being investigated is tetrathiomolybdate. The hope is that it will prove to have fewer side effects than penicillamine, yet be more effective than Trientine. Possible suppression of bone marrow function may yet be a risk for some patients.

Prognosis

For those who begin treatment early in the progression of the disorder, or even before symptoms are noted, the prognosis is excellent, as long as the patients comply with the treatment regimen. For others, the prognosis may be more difficult to predict, but nearly every patient with WD sees at least some improvement once treatment is begun. For those who go untreated, the prognosis is very poor.

Special concerns

The rarity of WD, combined with its diverse and varied symptoms that can mimic other conditions, makes it difficult to diagnose. This is of special concern because it is a progressive fatal condition; yet it can be easily and effectively treated if caught early. The autosomal recessive nature of the condition means that there is almost never a previous family history (other than a diagnosed sibling) to alert anyone to the risk. Because the diagnosis is easily established by measuring serum ceruloplasmin levels, with subsequent liver biopsy for copper levels, anyone contracting hepatitis or cirrhosis with no obvious cause, with or without neuropsychiatric symptoms, should be tested for WD.

Resources

BOOKS

Gilroy, John. *Basic Neurology*, 3rd ed. New York: The McGraw-Hill Companies, Inc., 2000.

Weiner, William J., and Christopher G. Goetz, eds. *Neurology for the Non-Neurologist*, 4th ed. Philadelphia: Lippincott Williams & Wilkins, 1999.

PERIODICALS

El-Youssef, Mounif. "Wilson Disease." *Mayo Clinic Proceedings* 78 (September 2003): 1126–1136.

Gow, P. J., et al. "Diagnosis of Wilson's Disease: An Experience over Three Decades." *Gut* 46 (2000): 415–19.

Sellner, H. Ascher. "Wilson's Disease." *Exceptional Parent Magazine* (March 2001): 34–35.

Vechina, Joe, and Marlene Vechina. "Never Give Up Hope." *Exceptional Parent Magazine* (March 2001): 30–32.

OTHER

"NINDS Wilson's Disease Information Page." *The National Institute of Neurological Disorders and Stroke.* December 27, 2001 (April 4, 2004). <http://www.ninds.nih.gov/health_and_medical/disorders/wilsons_doc.htm>.

ORGANIZATIONS

Wilson's Disease Association. 4 Navaho Drive, Brookfield, CT 06804-3124. (800) 399-0266; Fax: (203) 775-9666. <http://www.wilsondisease.org>.

National Center for the Study of Wilson's Disease. 432 West 58th Street, Suite 614, New York, NY 10019. (212) 523-8717; Fax: (212) 523-8708.

Scott J. Polzin, MS, CGC

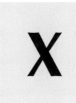

X

X-linked spinal and bulbar muscular
atrophy *see* **Kennedy disease**

Z

Zellweger syndrome

Definition

Zellweger syndrome is a severe and fatal genetic disorder affecting the brain, liver, and kidneys. It can be inherited by children of individuals that carry mutations for a specific gene.

Description

Zellweger syndrome is a fatal disorder that damages the brain, liver, and kidneys. There are related syndromes that have Zellweger-like symptoms and involve defects in the distinct cytoplasm organelles of cells called the peroxisomes; these include neonatal **adrenoleukodystrophy**, infantile **Refsum disease**, and hyperpipecolic acidemia. Zellweger syndrome is the most severe of these related syndromes.

Demographics

The incidence of Zellweger syndrome worldwide is roughly one in 100,000 births.

Causes and symptoms

Mutations in one of the many genes that cause Zellweger syndrome lead to a dysfunctional protein that is important for the cells' ability to import newly synthesized proteins into small cytoplasmic organelles called peroxisomes. Zellweger syndrome is characterized by the reduction or absence of these peroxisomes. Key enzymes that are critical for various chemical reactions, in particular oxidation, are contained within the peroxisomes.

Functional and structural abnormalities of the peroxisomes can lead to the disease development observed in Zellweger syndrome. Because peroxisomes are abundant in the liver and the kidney, these organs are affected in Zellweger syndrome. Toxic molecules that enter the bloodstream are detoxified by the peroxisomes, although there are additional mechanisms for detoxification. For example, when consuming large amounts of ethanol from alcoholic beverages, roughly 5–25% of the ethanol can be oxidized by the peroxisomes. Peroxisomes can also function in the organic creation of key compounds and play important roles in the various chemical reactions.

Zellweger syndrome is caused by mutations in any one of several different genes involved in the function of the peroxisome. These include peroxin-1 (PEX1), peroxin-2 (PEX2) peroxin-3 (PEX3), peroxin-5 (PEX5), peroxin-6 (PEX6), and peroxin-12 (PEX12). Each of these gene locations are biochemically and genetically distinct and are found on different chromosomes.

The observable clinical features of Zellweger syndrome can include facial, developmental, and ocular (eye) defects. Characteristic features commonly include a high forehead, upslanting eyes, and skin folds, called epicanthal folds, along the medial (nasal) borders of the palpebral fissures (space between upper and lower eyelids) of the eyes. Typically, babies with Zellweger syndrome have severe weakness, hyptonia (loss of muscle tone), and often have neonatal **seizures**. There are also several ocular abnormalities that can affect eyesight.

Diagnosis

Absent peroxisomes in the liver and kidney was initially demonstrated by American pathologist S. L. Goldfischer in 1985. The absence of these organelles in the liver is currently thought to be the hallmark of this disorder. Patients with Zellweger syndrome have been found to have remarkably fewer peroxisomes in both the brain and cultured skin fibroblasts. Fibroblasts are a type of skin cell and, in Zellweger syndrome, these cells appear to have ghost-like peroxisomes, which are caused by an absence of specific proteins inside the organelles that are recruited into the membranes.

Peroxisomes play an important role in organ development. Brain abnormalities can be explained by the disrupted migration of nerve cells called neurons (or

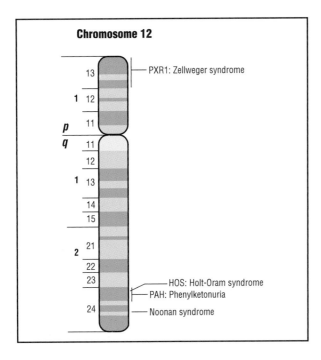

Chromosome 12

p

13 — PXR1: Zellweger syndrome
1 12
11

q 11
12
1 13
14
15

21
2 22
23 — HOS: Holt-Oram syndrome
— PAH: Phenylketonuria
24 — Noonan syndrome

Zellweger syndrome, on chromosome 12. *(Gale Group.)*

neuroblasts at this stage of development) around the third month of gestation. This defect occurs in a specific area of the brain called the cerebrum and leads to small or thick convolutions in brain tissue. This brain abnormality allows Zellweger syndrome to be distinguished from other diseases that involve brain abnormalities. Other tissues involved in the disease development include the liver, kidney, cartilage, heart, and muscle. Most patients have cysts on their kidneys.

Zellweger syndrome is diagnosed by measuring metabolic compounds in blood samples from patients. Various fatty acids, plasmalogens, pipecolic acid, and bile acid intermediates are usually studied. Aside from plasmalogen levels, which are diminished, these compounds are typically increased in affected individuals. It is also possible to detect fatty acid levels and plasmalogen synthesis before birth by obtaining cells in the fluid of the amnion, a process called amniocentesis. Thus, pregnant mothers who have previously had an affected baby can opt to have prenatal diagnosis to determine if the fetus is affected.

Treatment team

Physicians, nurses, and therapists provide the basis of the treatment team for a person with Zellweger's syndrome. Geneticists also provide diagnostic and genetic counseling services. Support services are available for families.

Treatment

There is no cure for Zellweger syndrome and treatment is based solely on lessening the symptoms and supporting the involved organs.

Recovery and rehabilitation

Physical, occupational, respiratory, and speech therapists can provide supportive strategies and devices to maintain posture, independent breathing, speech, eating, and other daily activities according to the infant or child's developmental stage for as long as practically possible.

Clinical trials

As of 2004, there is one clinical trial sponsored by the FDA Office of Orphan Products Development for the treatment of Zellweger syndrome (which is under review by the National Institutes of Health). It involves determining the effectiveness of giving oral bile acids (cholic acid, chenodeoxycholic acid, and ursodeoxycholic acid) as therapy for affected individuals.

Prognosis

Persons with Zellweger syndrome rarely live more than one year after diagnosis, with death due mostly to severe feeding difficulties, liver complications, respiratory distress, and cardiac defects.

Special concerns

Because Zellweger syndrome is usually fatal within the first year of life, genetic counseling and prenatal diagnosis are usually assigned a high priority for parents identified or concerned that they may be at risk for having a baby with the syndrome.

Resources
PERIODICALS
Collins, C. S., and S. J. Gould. "Identification of a Common PEX1 Mutation in Zellweger Syndrome." *Hum Mutat* (1999) 14: 45–53.
Depreter, M., M. Espeel, and F. Roels. "Human Peroxisomal Disorders." *Microsc Res Tech* (2003) 61: 203–23.
Gootjes, J., et al. "Biochemical Markers Predicting Survival in Peroxisome Diogenesis Disorders." *Neurology* (2002) 59: 1746–9.
Gould, S. J., G. V. Raymond, and D. Valle. "The Peroxisome Biogenesis Disorders." In *The Metabolic and Molecular Bases of Inherited Disease*, C. R. Scriver, A. L. Beaudet, W. S. Sly, and D. Valle, editors, 8th ed. New York: McGraw-Hill, 3181–218.

OTHER
Johns Hopkins University School of Medicine. *The Peroxisome.* January 3, 2004 (March 2, 2004). <http://www.peroxisome.org/Layperson/layperson.html>.

Key Terms

Cytoplasm The substance within a cell including the organelles and the fluid surrounding the nucleus.

Peroxisome A cellular organelle containing different enzymes responsible for the breakdown of waste or other products.

National Institute of Neurological Disorders and Stroke. *NINDS Zellweger Syndrome Information Page* January 3, 2004 (March 2, 2004). <http://www.ninds.nih.gov/health_and_medical/disorders/zellwege_doc.htm>.

ORGANIZATIONS

National Organization for Rare Disorders. P.O. Box 1968, Danbury, CT 06813-1968. (203) 744-0100. orphan@rarediseases.org. <http://www.rarediseases.org>.

United Leukodystrophy Foundation, Inc. 2304 Highland Drive, Sycamore, IL 60178. (800) 728-5483; Fax: (815) 895-2432. ulf@tbcnet.com. <http://www.ulf.org>.

Bryan Richard Cobb, PhD

Zonisamide

Definition

Zonisamide is an anti-convulsant used to control **seizures** in the treatment of **epilepsy**, a neurological dysfunction in which excessive surges of electrical energy are emitted in the brain.

Purpose

Zonisamide decreases abnormal activity and excitement within the brain that may trigger seizures. While zonisamide controls the partial seizures (focal seizures) associated with epilepsy, there is no known cure for the disease.

Some physicians have also used zonisamide in the treatment of mood disorders. As of 2004, zonisamide is additionally under study for the treatment of migraine **headaches** and neuropathic (nerve) **pain**.

Description

In the United States, zonisamide is sold under the brand name Zonegran. Zonisamide is classified as a sulfonamide anticonvulsant. The precise mechanisms by which it works are unknown.

Recommended dosage

Zonisamide is taken by mouth in tablet form. It is prescribed by physicians in varying dosages, usually from 100 mg to 400 mg daily.

Beginning a course of treatment which includes zonisamide requires a gradual dose-increasing regimen. Adults and teenagers 16 years or older typical take 100 mg per day for the first two weeks. Daily dosages of zonisamide may then be increased 100 mg once every two weeks until reaching the full daily dose (usually not more than 400 mg.) It may take several weeks to realize the full benefits of zonisamide.

Persons should not take a double dose of anticonvulsant medications. If a daily dose is missed, it should be taken as soon as possible. However, if it is almost time for the next dose, the missed dose should be skipped.

When discontinuing treatment with zonisamide, physicians typically direct patients to gradually reduce their daily dosages. Stopping the medicine suddenly may cause seizures to occur or become more frequent.

Precautions

Persons taking zonisamide should avoid alcohol and **central nervous system** depressants (medications including antihistimines, sleep medications, and some pain medications). Combining these substances with zonisamide can exacerbate (heighten) the side effects of alcohol and other medications.

A physician should be consulted before taking zonisamide with certain non-perscription medications, such as medicines for asthma, appetite control, coughs, colds, sinus problems, allergies, and hay fever.

Zonisamide may inhibit perspiration, causing body temperature to increase during physical activity. Persons taking zonisamide are at a greater risk for heat **stroke**. Caution should be used during strenuous **exercise**, prolonged exposure during hot weather, and while using saunas or hot tubs.

Zonisamide may not be suitable for persons with a history of liver or kidney disease, mental illness, high blood presure, angina (chest pain), irregular heartbeats, or other heart problems.

Before beginning treatment with zonisamide, patients should notify their physician if they consume a large amount of alcohol, have a history of drug use, are pregnant, or plan to become pregnant. Most physicians recommend using effective birth control while taking zonisamide, as it may cause defects to a developing fetus. Patients who become pregnant while taking zonisamide should contact their physician.

Side effects

Research indicates that zonisamide is generally well tolerated. However, it may case a variety of usually mild side effects. Headache, nausea and **fatigue**, and weakness are the most frequently reported side effects of zonisamide. Other possible side effects include:

- difficulty sleeping
- nervousness
- anxiety
- abdominal pain
- difficulty with memory
- double vision
- loss of appetite
- restlessness
- drowsiness
- diarrhea or constipation
- indigestion
- aching joints and muscles
- unpleasant taste in mouth or dry mouth
- tingling or prickly feeling on the skin

Many of these side effects disappear or occur less frequently during treatment as the body adjusts to the medication. However, if any symptoms persist or become too uncomfortable, the prescribing physician should be consulted.

Other, uncommon side effects of zonisamide can be serious. A patient taking zonisamide who experiences any of the following symptoms should contact their physician:

- rash or bluish patches on the skin
- discouragement, feeling sad or empty
- mood or mental changes
- shakiness or unsteady walking
- lack of appetite
- kidney stones
- difficulty breathing
- chest pain
- slow or irregular heartbeat
- faintness
- confusion or loss of consciousness
- persistent, severe headaches
- persistent fever or pain

Interactions

Zonisamide may have negative interactions with some antifungal medications, antihistimines, antidepressants, antibiotics, and monoamine oxidase inhibitors (MAOIs).

Key Terms

Epilepsy A disorder associated with disturbed electrical discharges in the central nervous system that cause seizures.

Seizure A convulsion, or uncontrolled discharge of nerve cells that may spread to other cells throughout the brain.

Sulfonamides A group of antibiotics used to treat a wide range of bacterial infections.

Other medications such as **diazepam** (Valium), fluoxetine (Prozac, Sarafem), fluvoxamine (Luvox), HIV protease inhibitors (indinavir), ritonavir (Norvir), ipratropium (Atrovent), isoniazid, **phenobarbital** (Luminal, Solfoton), nefazodone, metronidazole, **acetazolamide** (Diamox), phenytoin (Dilantin), **primidone**, propranolol (Inderal); and rifampin (Rifadin, Rimactane) may also adversely react with zonisamide.

Zonisamide is sometimes prescribed as part of a combination of drugs to prevent seizures. The physician will carefully monitor the combination drug therapy, as sometimes zonisamide will potentite (enhance) the effects of other anticonvulsant medications.

Zonisamide may decrease the effectiveness of some forms of oral contraceptives (birth control pills).

Zonisamide should not be taken by those allergic to sulfa drugs.

Resources

BOOKS

Weaver, Donald F. *Epilepsy and Seizures: Everything You Need to Know.* Richmond Hill, Ontario: Firefly Books, 2001.

OTHER

"Zonisamide." *Medline Plus.* National Library of Medicine. (March 20, 2004). <http://www.nlm.nih.gov/medlineplus/druginfo/uspdi/500137.html>.

ORGANIZATIONS

Epilepsy Foundation. 4351 Garden City Drive, Landover, MD 20785-7223. (800) 332-1000. <http://www.epilepsyfoundation.org>.

American Epilepsy Society. 342 North Main Street, West Hartford, CT 06117-2507. (860)586-7505. <http://www.aesnet.org>.

Adrienne Wilmoth Lerner

GLOSSARY

A

ABSCESS. A localized collection of pus or infection that is walled off from the rest of the body.

ABSENCE SEIZURE. A type of generalized seizure in which the person may temporarily appear to be staring into space and/or have jerking or twitching muscles. Previously called a petit mal seizure.

ABSTRACTION. Ability to think about concepts or ideas separate from specific examples.

ACALCULIA. The inability to perform basic calculation (addition, subtraction, multiplication, division).

ACETYLCHOLINE. A chemical called a neurotransmitter that functions primarily to mediate activity of the nervous system and skeletal muscles.

ACHALASIA. An esophageal disease of unknown cause in which the lower sphincter muscle is unable to relax normally, resulting in obstruction, either partial or complete.

ACOUSTIC. A term that refers to hearing.

ACOUSTIC NERVE. The cranial nerve VIII, involved in both hearing and balance.

ACROPARESTHESIAS. Painful burning sensation in hands and feet.

ACTION POTENTIAL. The wave-like change in the electrical properties of a cell membrane, resulting from the difference in electrical charge between the inside and outside of the membrane.

ACUITY. Sharpness.

ADJUVANT. A medication or other substance given to aid another drug, such as a tranquilizer given to ease the anxiety of a cancer patient in addition to an analgesic for pain relief.

ADRENAL INSUFFICIENCY. Problems with the adrenal glands that can be life-threatening if not treated. Symptoms include sluggishness, weakness, weight loss, vomiting, darkening of the skin, and mental changes.

ADVANCED BONE AGE. The bones, on x ray, appear to be those of an older individual.

AFFECTIVE PSYCHOSIS. Abnormalities in mood, emotions, feelings, sensibility, or mental state.

AFLATOXIN. A toxin produced by a fungus that infests grains, peanuts, soybeans, and corn that have been stored in warm, moist conditions.

AGNOSIA. Inability to notice or process sensory stimuli.

AGRAPHIA. The inability to write.

AIDS. Acquired Immune Deficiency Syndrome is a sexually transmitted disease caused by the Human Immunodeficiency Virus (HIV). It weakens the immune system and makes a person susceptible to many infections and malignancies.

ALEXANDER TECHNIQUE. A form of movement therapy that emphasizes correct posture and the proper positioning of the head with regard to the spine.

ALGORITHMS. A sequence of steps designed to calculate or determine a task.

ALLERGEN. Any substance that irritates only those who are sensitive (allergic) to it.

ALZHEIMER DISEASE. A neurological disorder characterized by slow, progressive memory loss due to a gradual loss of brain cells.

AMAUROSIS FUGAX. A type of transient ischemic attack (TIA) caused by decreased blood flow through the carotid artery, characterized by blindness or decreased vision in one eye.

AMENORRHEA. The absence or abnormal stoppage of menstrual periods.

AMINO ACID. An organic compound composed of both an amino group and an acidic carboxyl group. Amino acids are the basic building blocks of proteins. There are 20 types of amino acids (eight are "essential amino acids" that the body cannot make and must therefore be obtained from food).

AMNESIA. A general medical term for loss of memory that is not due to ordinary forgetfulness. Amnesia can be caused by head injuries, brain disease, or epilepsy, as well as by dissociation. Includes: 1) Anterograde amnesia: inability to retain the memory of events occurring after the time of the injury or disease that brought about the amnesic state. 2) Retrograde amnesia: inability to recall the memory of events that occurred prior to the time of the injury or disease that brought about the amnesic state.

AMNIOCENTESIS. A procedure performed at 16-18 weeks of pregnancy in which a needle is inserted through a woman's abdomen into her uterus to draw out a small sample of the amniotic fluid from around the baby. Either the fluid itself or cells from the fluid can be used for a variety of tests to obtain information about genetic disorders and other medical conditions in the fetus.

AMNIOTIC FLUID. The fluid that surrounds a developing baby during pregnancy.

AMNIOTIC SAC. Contains the fetus, which is surrounded by amniotic fluid.

AMYGDALA. An almond-shaped brain structure in the limbic system that is activated in stressful situations to trigger the emotion of fear. Hallucinations related to post-traumatic stress are thought to be caused by the activation of memory traces in the amygdala that have not been integrated and modified by other parts of the brain.

AMYLOID PLAQUE. A waxy, translucent, starch-like protein that is deposited in tissues during the course of certain chronic diseases such as rheumatoid arthritis and Alzheimer disease.

AMYLOIDOSIS. The accumulation of amyloid deposits in various organs and tissues in the body so that normal functioning is compromised. Primary amyloidosis usually occurs as a complication of multiple myeloma. Secondary amyloidosis occurs in patients suffering from chronic infections or inflammatory diseases such as tuberculosis, rheumatoid arthritis, and Crohn's disease.

AMYOTROPHIC LATERAL SCLEROSIS. ALS, also called Lou Gehrig's disease is a progressive neuromuscular condition due to degeneration of the motor nerve cells and fiber tracts in the spinal cord. The cause is not yet well defined. It is characterized by progressive weakening of the limb muscles and those involved in swallowing and breathing. It is fatal within a couple of years of onset.

AMYOTROPHY. A type of neuropathy resulting in pain, weakness, and/or wasting in the muscles.

ANAEROBIC. Describes an organism that grows and thrives in an oxygen-free environment.

ANALGESICS. A class of pain-relieving medicines, including aspirin and Tylenol.

ANEMIA. A condition in which there is an abnormally low number of red blood cells in the bloodstream. It may be due to loss of blood, an increase in red blood cell destruction, or a decrease in red blood cell production. Major symptoms are paleness, shortness of breath, unusually fast or strong heart beats, and tiredness.

ANEURYSM. A weakened area in the wall of a blood vessel that causes an outpouching or bulge. Aneurysms may be fatal if these weak areas burst, resulting in uncontrollable bleeding.

ANGINA PECTORIS. Chest pain caused by an insufficient supply of oxygen and decreased blood flow to the heart muscle. Angina is frequently the first sign of coronary artery disease.

ANGIOFIBROMA. Non-cancerous growth of the skin, which are often reddish in color and filled with blood vessels.

ANGIOGRAPHY. A mapping of the brain's blood vessels, using x-ray imaging.

ANGIOKERATOMA. Skin rash comprised of red bumps. Rash most commonly occurs between the navel and the knees.

ANGIOMYOLIPOMA. Non-cancerous growth in the kidney, most often found in tuberous sclerosis.

ANGULAR GYRUS. A ridge (outfolding) in the parietal lobe of the brain.

ANNULUS FIBROSUS. A fibrous and cartilage ring that forms the circumference of a vertebrae.

ANOREXIA. Loss of appetite.

ANOXIA. Lack of oxygen.

ANTERIOR CIRCULATION. The blood supply to most of the front part of the brain known as the cerebrum, including the frontal, parietal, and temporal lobes.

ANTERIOR VITREITIS. Inflammation of the corpus vitreum, which surrounds and fills the inner portion of the eyeball between the lens and the retina.

ANTEROGRADE AMNESIA. Amnesia for events that occurred after a physical injury or emotional trauma but before the present moment.

ANTIBODY. A special protein made by the body's immune system as a defense against foreign material (bacteria, viruses, etc.) that enters the body. It is uniquely designed to attack and neutralize the specific antigen that triggered the immune response.

ANTICHOLINERGIC DRUGS. Drugs that block the action of the neurotransmitter acetylcholine. They are used to lessen muscle spasms in the intestines, lungs, bladder, and eye muscles.

ANTICIPATION. Genetic phenomenon in which a triple repeat DNA mutation expands in a future generation, causing symptoms to develop earlier.

ANTICONVULSANT DRUGS. Drugs used to prevent convulsions or seizures. They often are prescribed in the treatment of epilepsy.

ANTIEMETIC. A type of drug given to stop vomiting.

ANTIEPILEPTIC. A drug that prevents or limits the spread of epileptic seizures.

ANTIGEN. A substance (usually a protein) identified as foreign by the body's immune system, triggering the release of antibodies as part of the body's immune response.

ANTIOXIDANT. Any substance that reduces the damage caused by oxidation, such as the harm caused by free radicals.

ANTIPLATELET AGENTS. Drugs that reduce the tendency of platelets to clump together, used to reduce the risk of transient ischemic attack (TIA) or stroke.

ANTIVIRAL. A drug that prevents viruses from replicating and therefore spreading infection.

ANXIETY. Worry or tension in response to real or imagined stress, danger, or dreaded situations. Physical reactions such as fast pulse, sweating, trembling, fatigue, and weakness may accompany anxiety.

ANXIETY DISORDER. A psychiatric disorder involving the presence of anxiety that is so intense or so frequently present that it causes difficulty or distress for the individual.

AORTA. The major artery that carries oxygenated blood from the heart to be delivered by arteries throughout the body.

APHASIA. Loss of the ability to speak or to understand written or spoken language. A person who cannot speak or understand language is said to be aphasic.

APHERESIS. A procedure in which the blood is removed and filtered in order to rid it of particular cells, then returned to the patient.

APNEA. An irregular breathing pattern characterized by abnormally long periods of the complete cessation of breathing.

APRAXIA. Inability to carry out ordinary purposeful movements in the absence of paralysis.

ARACHNOID MEMBRANE. One of the three membranes that sheath the spinal cord and brain; the arachnoid is the middle membrane. Also called the arachnoid mater.

ARBOVIRUSES. Viruses harbored by arthropods (mosquitoes and ticks) and transferred to humans by their bite. An arbovirus is the cause of West Nile infection, and arboviruses are one cause of encephalitis.

AREFLEXIA. Absence of a reflex; a sign of possible nerve damage.

ARTERIOGRAM. An x-ray study of an artery that has been injected with a contrast dye.

ARTERIOSCLEROSIS. A chronic condition characterized by thickening and hardening of the arteries and the build-up of plaque on the arterial walls. Arteriosclerosis can slow or impair blood circulation.

ARTERIOVENOUS MALFORMATION. Abnormal, direct connection between the arteries and veins. Arteriovenous malformations can range from very small to large.

ASPERGER SYNDROME. A developmental disorder of childhood characterized by autistic behavior but without the same difficulties acquiring language that children with autism have.

ASPIRATION. Inhalation of food or liquids into the lungs.

ASPIRATION PNEUMONIA. Infection of the lungs, caused by the presence of foreign material such as food.

ASTHENIA. Muscle weakness.

ASTHMA. A disease in which the air passages of the lungs become inflamed and narrowed.

ASTROCYTES. Types of neuroglial cells in the central nervous system that help support other nerve cells.

ATAXIA. A condition marked by impaired muscular coordination, most frequently resulting from disorders in the brain or spinal cord.

ATHEROSCLEROTIC PLAQUE. A deposit of fatty and calcium substances that accumulate in the lining of the artery wall, restricting blood flow. The disease is called atherosclerosis.

ATHETOSIS. A condition marked by slow, writhing, involuntary muscle movements.

ATONIC SEIZURE. A seizure characterized by a sudden loss of muscle tone, causing the individual to fall to the floor.

ATRIAL FIBRILLATION. A type of heart arrhythmia in which the upper chamber of the heart quivers instead of pumping in an organized way. In this condition, the upper chambers (atria) of the heart do not completely empty when the heart beats, which can allow blood clots to form.

ATROPHY. The progressive wasting and loss of function of any part of the body.

AUDIOLOGIST. A healthcare professional who specializes in diagnostic testing of hearing impairments and rehabilitation of patients with hearing problems.

AUDITORY. Pertaining to the sense of hearing.

AUDITORY NERVE. A bundle of nerve fibers that carries hearing information between the cochlea and the brain.

AURA. A group of visual or other sensations that precedes the onset of a migraine attack.

AUTISM. A developmental disability that appears early in life, in which normal brain development is disrupted and social and communication skills are retarded, sometimes severely.

AUTISTIC PSYCHOPATHY. Hans Asperger's original name for the condition now known as Asperger's disorder. It is still used occasionally as a synonym for the disorder.

AUTOANTIBODIES. Antibodies that attack the body's own cells or tissues.

AUTOIMMUNE. Pertaining to an immune response by the body against its own tissues or types of cells.

AUTOIMMUNE DISEASE. One of a group of diseases, like rheumatoid arthritis and systemic lupus erythematosus, in which the immune system is overactive and has lost the ability to distinguish between self and non-self. The body's immune cells turn on the body, attacking various tissues and organs.

AUTOMATISMS. Movements during a seizure that are semi-purposeful but involuntary.

AUTONOMIC FAILURE. Refers to failure in the autonomic nervous system, which comprises two divisions called the parasympathetic nervous system, which slows heart rate, increases intestinal and gland activity, and relaxes sphincter muscles; and the sympathetic nervous system, which accelerates heart rate, raises blood pressure, and constricts blood vessels.

AUTONOMIC NERVOUS SYSTEM. The part of the nervous system that controls so-called involuntary functions, such as heart rate, salivary gland secretion, respiratory function, and pupil dilation.

AUTOSOMAL. Relating to any chromosome besides the X and Y sex chromosomes. Human cells contain 22 pairs of autosomes and one pair of sex chromosomes.

AUTOSOMAL DOMINANT. A pattern of inheritance in which only one of the two copies of an autosomal gene must be abnormal for a genetic condition or disease to occur. An autosomal gene is a gene that is located on one of the autosomes or non-sex chromosomes. A person with an autosomal dominant disorder has a 50% chance of passing it to each of their offspring.

AUTOSOMAL RECESSIVE. A pattern of inheritance in which both copies of an autosomal gene must be abnormal for a genetic condition or disease to occur. An autosomal gene is a gene that is located on one of the autosomes or non-sex chromosomes. When both parents have one abnormal copy of the same gene, they have a 25% chance with each pregnancy that their offspring will have the disorder.

AXILLARY. Referring to the armpit.

AXON. The long, hairlike extension of a nerve cell that carries a message to a nearby nerve cell.

AXONTOMESIS. Loss of the protective sheet of tissue that covers the axon (the part of the nerve cell that carries a transmission).

B

BABESIOSIS. A disease caused by protozoa of the genus *Babesia* characterized by a malaria-like fever, anemia, vomiting, muscle pain, and enlargement of the spleen. Babesiosis, like Lyme disease, is carried by a tick.

BACILLUS. A rod-shaped bacterium, such as the diphtheria bacterium.

BALANCED CHROMOSOME TRANSLOCATION. A rearrangement of the chromosomes in which two chromosomes have broken and exchanged pieces without the loss of genetic material.

BALLISMUS. Involuntary violent flinging movements that may take the form of uncontrollable flailing. It is also called ballism. Ballismus that occurs with chorea is known as choreoballismus or choreoballism.

BARBITURATE. A class of drugs including phenobarbital that have sedative properties and depress respiratory rate, blood pressure, and nervous system activity.

BASAL GANGLIA. Brain structure at the base of the cerebral hemispheres involved in controlling movement.

BASILAR MIGRAINE. A type of migraine with aura that involves the basilar artery at the base of the brain. It occurs most commonly in young women, and may include vision problems, confusion, and loss of consciousness as well as headache.

BATTERY. A number of separate items (such as tests) used together. In psychology, a group or series of tests given with a common purpose, such as personality assessment or measurement of intelligence.

BEHAVIOR DISORDERS. Disorders characterized by disruptive behaviors such as conduct disorder, oppositional defiant disorder, and attention-deficit/hyperactivity disorder.

BENIGN. In medical usage, benign is the opposite of malignant. It describes an abnormal growth that is stable, treatable, and generally not life-threatening.

BENZODIAZEPINES. A class of drugs with hypnotic, antianxiety, anticonvulsive, and muscle-relaxant properties. They are used in the treatment of anxiety and sleeping disorders, to relax muscles, and to control seizures. Diazepam (Valium), alprazolam (Xanax), and chlordiazepoxide (Librium) are all benzodiazepines.

BILATERAL. Occurring on both sides of the body.

BIOCHEMICAL TESTING. Measuring the amount or activity of a particular enzyme or protein in a sample of blood or urine or other tissue from the body.

BIOFEEDBACK. A training technique that enables an individual to gain some element of control over involuntary or automatic body functions.

BIOLOGICAL MARKER. An indicator or characteristic trait of a disease that facilitates differential diagnosis (the process of distinguishing one disorder from other, similar disorders).

BIOPSY. The surgical removal and microscopic examination of living tissue for diagnostic purposes or to follow the course of a disease. Most commonly the term refers to the collection and analysis of tissue from a suspected tumor to establish malignancy.

BIOTRANSFORMATION. The conversion of a compound from one form to another by the action of enzymes in the body of an organism.

BIPOLAR DISORDER. A psychiatric disorder marked by alternating episodes of mania and depression. Also called bipolar illness, manic-depressive illness.

BLOOD VESSELS. General term for arteries, veins, and capillaries that transport blood throughout the body.

BODYWORK. Any technique involving hands-on massage or manipulation of the body.

BOLUS. A mass of a substance to be swallowed.

BOTULINUM TOXIN. A potent bacterial toxin or poison made by *Clostridium botulinum*; causes paralysis in high doses, but is used medically in small, localized doses to treat disorders associated with involuntary muscle contraction and spasms, in addition to strabismus. Commonly known as Botox.

BRACHIAL PLEXUS. A group of lower-neck and upper-back spinal nerves supplying the arm, forearm, and hand.

BRADYKINESIA. Extremely slow movement.

BRAIN STEM. The part of the brain that is continuous with the spinal cord and controls most basic life functions. It is the last part of the brain that is destroyed by Alzheimer's disease.

BREECH PRESENTATION. Buttocks presentation during delivery.

BRONCHITIS. Inflammation of the air passages of the lungs.

BRUIT. An abnormal sound heard with the stethoscope placed over the carotid artery in the neck, suggesting decreased blood flow through the vessel.

BRUXISM. Habitual clenching and grinding of the teeth, especially during sleep.

BULBAR MUSCLES. Muscles of the mouth and throat responsible for speech and swallowing.

C

CALCIFICATION. A process in which tissue becomes hardened due to calcium deposits.

CAPILLARY BED. A dense network of tiny blood vessels that enables blood to fill a tissue or organ.

CAPSAICIN. An alkaloid derived from hot peppers that can be used as a topical anesthetic.

CARBIDOPA. A drug combined with levodopa to slow the breakdown of the levodopa, used to treat the symptoms of Parkinson's disease.

CARBONIC ANHYDRASE. An enzyme that shifts the rate of reaction to favor the conversion of carbon dioxide and water into carbonic acid, bicarbonate ions, and free protons.

CARCINOGEN. A substance known to cause cancer.

CARDIAC TAMPONADE. A condition in which blood leaking into the membrane surrounding the heart puts pressure on the heart muscle, preventing complete filling of the heart's chambers and normal heartbeat.

CARDIOMYOPATHY. A disease of the heart muscle that leads to generalized deterioration of the muscle and its pumping ability.

CARDITIS. Inflammation of the heart tissue.

CAROTID ARTERY. One of the major arteries supplying blood to the head and neck.

CAROTID ENDARTERECTOMY. Surgical procedure designed to reduce the accumulation of plaque in the carotid artery and thus, prevent stroke.

CAROTID ULTRASONOGRAPHY. A painless and harmless test using high-frequency sound waves to determine if there is narrowing or plaque formation in the carotid arteries.

CARPAL TUNNEL SYNDROME. A condition caused by compression of the median nerve in the carpal tunnel of the hand, characterized by pain.

CARRIER. A person who possesses a gene for an abnormal trait without showing signs of the disorder. The person may pass the abnormal gene on to offspring.

CATAPLEXY. A symptom of narcolepsy marked by a sudden episode of muscle weakness triggered by strong emotions. The muscle weakness may cause the person's knees to buckle or the head to drop. In severe cases the patient may become paralyzed for a few seconds to minutes.

CATARACTS. Abnormal clouding or opacities within the lens of the eye.

CATATONIA. A fixed, motionless stupor.

CATECHOLAMINES. Chemicals such as epinephrine, dopa, and norepinephrine; often at high levels in the urine if a pheochromocytoma is present.

CATHETER. A long, thin, flexible tube used in angiography to inject contrast material into the arteries.

CAUDATE. A region of gray matter near the lateral ventricle of the brain; also called caudate nucleus.

CENTRAL APNEA. Abnormal breathing as a result of the medulla being pushed down, such as from an Arnold-Chiari, Type II malformation.

CENTRAL NERVOUS SYSTEM. The brain, spinal cord and the nerves throughout the body.

CENTRAL SLEEP APNEA. A less-common form of sleep apnea in which the brain does not properly signal respiratory muscles to begin breathing.

CEPHALALGIA. The medical term for headache.

CEREBELLAR ATAXIA. Unsteadiness and lack of coordination caused by a progressive degeneration of the part of the brain known as the cerebellum.

CEREBELLUM. The part of the brain involved in the co-ordination of movement, walking, and balance.

CEREBRAL ANEURYSM. An abnormal, localized bulge in a blood vessel that is usually caused by a congenital weakness in the wall of the vessel.

CEREBRAL COLLATERAL BLOOD FLOW. Anatomical and physiological mechanisms that allow blood destined for one hemisphere of the brain to crossover and nourish tissue on the other side of the brain when the supply to the other side of the brain is impaired.

CEREBRAL CORTEX. The thin, convoluted surface of the brain consisting mainly of nerve cell bodies. This brain region is responsible for reasoning, mood, and perception.

CEREBRAL DOMINANCE. The preeminence of one cerebral hemisphere over the other in the control of cerebral functions.

CEREBRAL EMBOLISM. A blockage of blood flow through a vessel in the brain by a blood clot that formed elsewhere in the body and traveled to the brain.

CEREBRAL HERNIATION. Movement of the brain against the skull.

CEREBRAL INFARCTION. Brain-tissue damage caused by interrupted flow of oxygen to the brain.

CEREBRAL ISCHEMIA. Lack of oxygen to the brain, which may result in tissue death.

CEREBRAL OXIDATIVE METABOLISM. Using oxygen to generate energy by complex chemical reactions that occur in brain cells.

CEREBRAL PALSY. A nonprogressive movement disability caused by abnormal development of or damage to motor control centers of the brain.

CEREBRAL THROMBOSIS. A blockage of blood flow through a vessel in the brain by a blood clot that formed in the brain itself.

CEREBRAL VASCULAR ACCIDENT. Damage to brain cells caused by lack of blood flow in the brain from emboli (clots) plaque, or hemorrhage.

CEREBROSPINAL FLUID. The clear, normally colorless fluid that fills the brain cavities (ventricles), the subarachnoid space around the brain, and the spinal cord and acts as a shock absorber.

CEREBRUM. The main portion of the brain (and the largest part of the central nervous system), occupying the upper portion of the cranial cavity. It is responsible for higher functions such as speech, thought, vision, and memory.

CERULOPLASMIN. A protein circulating in the bloodstream that binds with and transports copper.

CERVICAL. Referring to the neck. Cervical vertebrae are the first 7 bones of the spine.

CHELATION. The process by which a molecule encircles and binds to a metal and removes it from tissue.

CHEMOTHERAPY. Chemical medical treatment often used for cancer.

CHOREA. A term that refers to rapid, jerky, involuntary movements of the limbs or face that characterize several different disorders of the nervous system, including chorea of pregnancy, Huntington's chorea, and Sydenham's chorea.

CHOREA GRAVIDARUM. Chorea occurring in the early months of pregnancy.

CHORIONIC VILLUS SAMPLING. A medical procedure done during weeks 10-12 of a pregnancy. A needle is inserted into the placenta and a small amount of fetal tissue is withdrawn for analysis.

CHOROID. A vascular membrane that covers the back of the eye between the retina and the sclera and serves to nourish the retina and absorb scattered light.

CHOROID PLEXUS. Specialized cells located in the ventricles of the brain that produce cerebrospinal fluid.

CHROMATIN. The readily stainable portion of a cell nucleus, consisting of DNA, RNA, and various proteins. It coils and folds itself to form chromosomes during the process of cell division. Rett syndrome (RS) is sometimes described as a chromatin disease.

CHROMOSOME. A microscopic thread-like structure found within each cell of the human body and consisting of a complex of proteins and DNA. Humans have 46 chromosomes arranged into 23 pairs. Chromosomes contain the genetic information necessary to direct the development and functioning of all cells and systems in the body. They pass on hereditary traits from parents to child (like eye color) and determine whether the child will be male or female. Changes in either the total number of chromosomes or their shape and size (structure) may lead to physical or mental abnormalities.

CHRONIC. Refers to a disease or condition that progresses slowly but persists or recurs over time.

CIRCLE OF WILLIS. Also known as the circulus arteriosus; formed by branches of the internal carotid arteries and the vertebral arteries.

CIRRHOSIS. A chronic degenerative disease of the liver, in which normal cells are replaced by fibrous tissue and normal liver function is disrupted. The most common symptoms are mild jaundice, fluid collection in the tissues, mental confusion, and vomiting of blood. Cirrhosis is associated with portal hypertension and is a major risk factor for the later development of liver cancer. If left untreated, cirrhosis leads to liver failure.

CLAUDICATION. Cramping or pain in a leg caused by poor blood circulation. This condition is frequently caused by hardening of the arteries (atherosclerosis). Intermittent claudication occurs only at certain times, usually after exercise, and is relieved by rest.

CLAVICLE. Also called the collarbone. Bone that articulates with the shoulder and the breast bone.

CLEFT PALATE. A birth defect in which the roof of the mouth (palate) has an abnormal opening (cleft).

CLONIC. A type of seizure characterized by rhythmic jerking of the arms and legs.

CLOSED HEAD INJURY. Traumatic brain injury (TBI) in which the head strikes or is struck by an object without breaking the skull.

CLUBFOOT. Abnormal positioning of the feet and legs, when they are turned inward towards each other.

CLUSTER HEADACHE. A painful recurring headache associated with the release of histamine from cells.

CLUTTER. A fluency disorder where speech delivery is either abnormally fast, irregular, or both.

COCHLEA. A spiral-shaped tubular structure resembling a snail's shell that forms part of the inner ear.

COCHLEAR IMPLANT. A device used for treating deafness that consists of one or more electrodes surgically implanted inside or outside the cochlea, an organ in the inner ear that transforms sound vibrations in the inner ear into nerve impulses for transmission to the brain.

COGNITIVE DELAY. Impairment or slowing of the mental processes of thinking and acquiring knowledge.

COLLAGEN. The main supportive protein of cartilage, connective tissue, tendon, skin, and bone.

COMA. A decreased level of consciousness with deep unresponsiveness.

COMMAND HALLUCINATION. A type of auditory hallucination in which the person hears voices ordering him or her to perform a specific act.

COMMUNITY MENTAL HEALTH CENTERS. Organizations that manage and deliver a comprehensive range of mental health services, education, and outreach to residents of a given community.

COMORBID. A term used to refer to a disease or disorder that is not directly caused by another disorder but occurs at the same time.

COMPULSION. A repetitive or stereotyped act or ritual.

CONCUSSION. Injury to the brain causing a sudden, temporary impairment of brain function.

CONDUCTIVE HEARING LOSS. A type of medically treatable hearing loss in which the inner ear is usually normal, but there are specific problems in the middle or outer ears that prevent sound from getting to the inner ear in a normal way.

CONGENITAL. Present at birth.

CONGENITAL MYOPATHY. Any abnormal condition or disease of muscle tissue that is present at birth; it is characterized by muscle weakness and wasting.

CONNECTIVE TISSUE. Supportive tissue in the body that joins structures together, lending strength and elasticity.

CONSTRUCTIONAL APRAXIA. Difficulty or inability to copy a drawing.

CONTRACTURE. A tightening or shortening of muscles that prevents normal movement of the associated limb or other body part.

CONTRECOUP. An injury to the brain opposite the point of direct impact.

CONTUSION. A focal area of swollen and bleeding brain tissue.

CORDOTOMY. Surgery to relieve pain by destroying bundles of nerve fibers on one or both sides of the spinal cord.

CORNEA. The clear, dome-shaped outer covering of the eye that lies in front of the iris and pupil. The cornea lets light into the eye.

COROLLARY DISCHARGE. A mechanism in the brain that allows one to distinguish between self-generated and external stimuli or perceptions.

CORPUS CALLOSUM. A thick bundle of nerve fibers deep in the center of the forebrain that provides communications between the right and left cerebral hemispheres.

CORPUS STRIATUM. Region of the brain that contains the caudate nucleus and putamen.

CORTICAL ATROPHY. A wasting away and decrease in size of the outer portion of the brain, or cerebral cortex.

CORTICOSPINAL TRACT. A tract of nerve cells that carries motor commands for voluntary body movements from the brain to the spinal cord.

CORTICOSTEROIDS. A group of hormones produced naturally by the adrenal gland or manufactured synthetically. They are often used to treat inflammation. Examples include cortisone and prednisone.

CORTISOL. A steroid hormone secreted by the adrenal cortex that is important for maintenance of body fluids, electrolytes, and blood sugar levels. Also called hydrocortisone.

CRANIAL NERVES. The set of twelve nerves found on each side of the head and neck that control the sensory and muscle functions of the eyes, nose, tongue, face, and throat.

CRANIAL SUTURES. The fibrous joints (sutures) that hold together the five bones comprising the skull of a newborn.

CRANIOSYNOSTOSIS. A birth defect of the brain characterized by the premature closure of one or more of the cranial sutures, the fibrous joints between the bones of the skull

CRANIOTOMY. A surgical procedure in which part of the skull is removed (then replaced) to allow access to the brain.

CRANIUM. Skull; the bony framework that holds the brain.

CREATININE PHOSPHOKINASE. A chemical normally found in the muscle fibers that is released into the bloodstream when the muscles undergo damage and breakdown. Testing for it can prove the occurrence of a heart attack or other muscle damage. It used to be called creatine kinase.

CRYOABLATION. Using very cold temperatures to remove a foreign substance or body.

CRYOTHERAPY. Using very cold temperatures to treat a disease.

CUTANEOUS. Relating to the skin.

CYST. An abnormal sac or enclosed cavity in the body that is filled with liquid or partially solid material. Also refers to a protective, walled-off capsule in which an organism lies dormant.

CYSTADENOMA. Non-cancerous growth, in which fluid-filled, gas, or semi-solid areas may be present.

CYTOGENETICS. The branch of biology that combines the study of genetic inheritance with the study of cell structure.

CYTOMEGALOVIRUS (CMV). A common human virus causing mild or no symptoms in healthy people, but permanent damage or death to an infected fetus, a transplant patient, or a person with HIV.

CYTOPLASM. The substance within a cell including the organelles and the fluid surrounding the nucleus.

CYTOSKELETON. A network of filaments that give structure and shape to the cell.

CYTOTOXIC T-CELLS. A type of white blood cells, T-lymphocytes, that can kill body cells infected by viruses or transformed by cancer.

D

DANDY WALKER MALFORMATION. A complex structural abnormality of the brain frequently associated with hydrocephalus, or accumulation of excess fluid in the brain. Abnormalities in other areas of the body may also be present. Individuals with Dandy-Walker malformation have varying degrees of mental handicap or none at all.

DECEREBRATE POSTURE. Stiff, rigid posture indicative of severe damage to brain stem.

DECONDITIONING. Loss of physical strength or stamina resulting from bed rest or lack of exercise.

DECORTICATE POSTURE. A stiff, rigid posture indicative of damage to nerve tracts that run between spinal cord and brain.

DEINSTITUTIONALIZATION. The process of moving people out of mental hospitals into treatment programs or halfway houses in local communities. With this movement, the responsibility for care shifted from large (often governmental) agencies to families and community organizations.

DELIRIUM. A condition characterized by waxing-and-waning episodes of confusion and agitation.

DELTOID MUSCLE. A muscle near the clavicle bone that is responsible for arm movement.

DELUSION. A false belief that a person maintains in spite of obvious proof or evidence to the contrary.

DEMENTIA. Loss of memory and other higher functions, such as thinking or speech, lasting six months or more.

DEMENTIA PUGILISTICA. Syndrome of brain damage caused by repeated head trauma. People with this kind of damage are sometimes described as "punch drunk."

DEMYELINATING DISEASES. A group of diseases characterized by the breakdown of myelin, the fatty sheath surrounding and insulating nerve fibers. This breakdown interferes with nerve function and can result in paralysis. Multiple sclerosis is a demyelinating disorder.

DEMYELINATION. Disruption or destruction of the myelin sheath, leaving a bare nerve. It results in a slowing or stopping of the impulses that travel along that nerve.

DEPOLARIZATION. Occurs when a neuron exchanges ions, causing an influx of sodium and calcium inside the cell and an efflux of potassium out of the cell.

DEPOT. A type of drug preparation and administration that involves the slow, gradual release from an area of the body where the drug has been injected.

DEPRESSED SKULL FRACTURE. A fracture in which fragments of broken skull press into brain tissue.

DEPRESSION. A psychiatric disorder in which the mood is low for a prolonged period of time, and feelings of hopelessness and inadequacy interfere with normal functioning.

DEPRESSIVE DISORDER. A psychiatric disorder of varying degrees characterized by feelings of hopelessness, physical responses such as insomnia, and withdrawal from normal activities.

DERMATOME. An area of skin that receives sensations through a single nerve root.

DESMIN. A protein that provides part of the structure to heart, skeletal, and smooth muscle cells.

DEVELOPMENTAL DELAY. The failure to meet certain developmental milestones such as sitting, walking, and talking at the average age. Developmental delay may indicate a problem in development of the central nervous system.

DEVELOPMENTAL DISABILITIES. Disabilities that are present from birth and delay or prevent normal development, such as mental retardation or autism.

DIABETES MELLITUS. The clinical name for common diabetes. It is a chronic disease characterized by the inability of the body to produce or respond properly to insulin, a hormone required by the body to convert glucose to energy.

DIABETIC NEUROPATHY. A complication of diabetes mellitus in which the peripheral nerves are affected. Diabetic neuropathy is primarily due to metabolic imbalance and secondarily to nerve compression.

DIALYSIS. Process by which special equipment purifies the blood of a patient whose kidneys have failed.

DIENCEPHALON. A part of the brain that binds the mesencephalon to the cerebral hemispheres, it includes the thalamus and the hypothalmus. It acts as a relay station for impulses concerning sensation and movement.

DIFFUSE. Widespread.

DILATATION. Increasing in caliber.

DIPLOPIA. Also known as double vision, it is a visual disorder resulting from unequal action of the eye muscles, which causes two images of a single object to be seen.

DISCECTOMY. Surgery to relieve pressure on a nerve root caused by a bulging disc or bone spur.

DISCOGRAPHY. A test in which dye is injected into a disc space thought to be causing back pain, allowing the surgeon to confirm that an operation on that disc will be likely to relieve pain.

DISEASE ERADICATION. A status whereby no further cases of a diseases occur anywhere, and continued control measures are unnecessary.

DISSECTION. Tear in the wall of an artery that causes blood from inside the artery to leak into the wall and thereby narrows the lumen of the blood vessel.

DISSEMINATED. Scattered or distributed throughout the body. Lyme disease that has progressed beyond the stage of localized erythema migrans (EM) is said to be disseminated.

DISTAL. Situated away from the center of the body.

DISTAL MUSCLES. Muscles farthest away from the center of the body, such as muscles in the fingers and toes.

DIURETIC DRUGS. A group of medications that increase the amount of urine produced and relieve excess fluid buildup in body tissues. Diuretics may be used in treating high blood pressure, lung disease, premenstrual syndrome, and other conditions.

DIZYGOTIC TWINS. Twins that share the same environment during development in the uterus.

DNA. Deoxyribonucleic acid; the genetic material in cells that holds the inherited instructions for growth, development, and cellular functioning.

DNA TESTING. Analysis of DNA (the genetic component of cells) in order to determine changes in genes that may indicate a specific disorder.

DOMINANT DISORDER. A disorder resulting from an inheritance pattern where one parent has a single, faulty dominant gene, and has a 50% chance of passing on that faulty gene to offspring with each pregnancy.

DOPAMINE. A neurotransmitter made in the brain that is involved in many brain activities, including movement and emotion.

DORSAL. Pertaining in direction to the back or upper surface of an organ.

DORSAL COLUMNS. This refers to nerve fiber tracts that run in the portion of the spinal cord that is closest to the back. They carry sensory information like position sense and deep pain from the legs and arms to the brain.

DORSAL HORN. The part of the spinal cord that receives and processes pain messages from the peripheral nervous system.

DOUBLE BLIND STUDY. A study or clinical trial designed to minimize any bias, in that neither participant or study director knows who is assigned to the control group and who is assigned to the test group until the end of the study.

DOWN SYNDROME. A genetic disorder characterized by an extra chromosome 21 (trisomy 21), mental retardation, and susceptibility to early-onset Alzheimer's disease.

DUPLICATION. Extra genetic material due to a duplicate copy.

DURA MATTER. The strongest and outermost of three membranes that protect the brain, spinal cord, and nerves of the cauda equina.

DYNATOME. An area in which pain is felt when a given spinal nerve is irritated.

DYSARTHRIA. Imperfect articulation of speech (slurred speech) due to muscular weakness resulting from damage to the central or peripheral nervous system.

DYSAUTONOMIA. A disorder or dysfunction of the autonomic nervous system.

DYSCALCULIA. Difficulty with basic arithmetic and calculations.

DYSESTHESIA. A painful feeling of numbness, tingling, or heat.

DYSGRAPHIA. Difficulty writing.

DYSKINESIA. Impaired ability to make voluntary movements.

DYSLEXIA. A type of reading disorder often characterized by reversal of letters or words.

DYSPHAGIA. Difficulty in swallowing.

DYSPHONIA. Disordered phonation or voice production.

DYSPLASIA. The abnormal growth or development of a tissue or organ.

DYSTHYMIA. A chronic mood disorder characterized by mild depression.

DYSTONIA. Painful involuntary muscle cramps or spasms.

DYSTROPHIN. A large protein that stabilizes the plasma membrane of a muscle cell during muscle contractions. Dystrophin is absent or reduced in the most common forms of muscular dystrophy.

E

ECHOCARDIOGRAM. Ultrasound of the heart, which shows heart structure in detail.

ECHOLALIA. Involuntary echoing of the last word, phrase, or sentence spoken by someone else.

EDEMA. An accumulation of watery fluid that causes swelling of the affected tissue.

ELASTIN. A protein that gives skin the ability to stretch and then return to normal.

ELBOW EXTENSION. Movement away from the body at a jointed point.

ELECTROACUPUNCTURE. A variation of acupuncture in which the practitioner stimulates the traditional acupuncture points electronically.

ELECTROCARDIOGRAM. Test that shows a heart's rhythm by studying its electrical current patterns.

ELECTROENCEPHALOGRAM (EEG). A record of the tiny electrical impulses produced by the brain's activity picked up by electrodes placed on the scalp. By measuring characteristic wave patterns, the EEG can help diagnose certain conditions of the brain.

ELECTROLYTES. Salts and minerals that produce electrically charged particles (ions) in body fluids. Common human electrolytes are sodium chloride, potassium, calcium, and sodium bicarbonate. Electrolytes control the fluid balance of the body and are important in muscle contraction, energy generation, and almost all major biochemical reactions in the body.

ELECTROMYOGRAPHY (EMG). A diagnostic test that records the electrical activity of muscles. Small electrodes are placed on or in the skin and the patterns of electrical activity are projected on a screen or over a loudspeaker. This procedure is used to test for muscle disorders, including muscular dystrophy.

ELECTRON. One of the small particles that make up an atom. An electron has the same mass and amount of charge as a positron, but the electron has a negative charge.

ELISA PROTOCOLS. ELISA is an acronym for "enzyme-linked immunosorbent assay"; it is a highly sensitive technique for detecting and measuring antigens or antibodies in a solution.

EMBOLISM. A blood clot, air bubble, or clot of foreign material that travels and blocks the flow of blood in an artery. When blood supply blocks a tissue or organ with an embolism, infarction (death of the tissue the artery feeds) occurs. Without immediate and appropriate treatment, an embolism can be fatal.

EMBOLIZATION. A technique to stop or prevent hemorrhage by introducing a foreign mass, such as an air-filled membrane (balloon), into a blood vessel to block the flow of blood. This term also refers to an alternative to splenectomy that involves injecting silicone or a similar substances into the splenic artery to shrink the size of the spleen.

EMBOLUS. A fragment of plaque or thrombus that breaks off from its original location and travels downstream to progressively narrower arteries, where it may block the vessel.

EMPHYSEMA. An irreversible lung disease in which breathing becomes increasingly difficult.

ENCEPHALITIS. Inflammation of the brain, usually caused by a virus. The inflammation may interfere with normal brain function and may cause seizures, sleepiness, confusion, personality changes, weakness in one or more parts of the body, and even coma.

ENCEPHALOGRAM. Machine that detects brain activity by measuring its electrical impulses.

ENCEPHALOPATHIC. Widespread brain disease or dysfunction.

ENCEPHALOPATHY. Any abnormality in the structure or function of brain tissues.

ENDODONTIST. A dentist who specializes in the treatment of diseases and injuries that affect the tooth root, dental pulp, and the tissues surrounding the tooth root.

ENDOLYMPH. The fluid contained inside the membranous labyrinth of the inner ear.

ENDOLYMPHATIC HYDROPS. Another term for Ménière's disease. It defines the disorder in terms of increased fluid pressure in the inner ear.

ENDOLYMPHATIC SAC TUMOR. Growths that develop within inner ear structures called endolymph sacs.

ENDORPHINS. A group of chemicals resembling opiates that are released in the body in response to trauma or stress. Endorphins react with opiate receptors in the brain to reduce pain sensations.

ENDOSCOPY. A clinical technique using an instrument called an endoscope, used for visualization of structures within the body.

ENDOTHELIUM. A layer of cells called endothelial cells that lines the inside surfaces of body cavities, blood vessels, and lymph vessels.

ENKEPHALINS. Polypeptides that serve as neurotransmitters and short-acting pain relievers. Enkephalins also influence a person's perception of painful sensations.

ENTRAPMENT NEUROPATHY. A disorder of the peripheral nervous system in which a nerve is damaged by compression as it passes through a bony or fibrous passage or canal. Many repetitive motion disorders are associated with entrapment neuropathies.

ENZYME. A protein that catalyzes a biochemical reaction or change without changing its own structure or function.

EPIDIDYMIS. Male genital structure usually connected to the testis; an area where sperm collect.

EPIDURAL HEMATOMA. Bleeding into the area between the skull and the dura, the tough, outermost brain covering.

EPIDURAL SPACE. The space immediately surrounding the outermost membrane (dura mater) of the spinal cord.

EPILEPSY. A neurological disorder characterized by recurrent seizures with or without a loss of consciousness.

EQUINUS. Excess contraction of the calf, causing toe walking.

ERB POINT. A point 2-3 centimeters above the clavicle.

ERGONOMICS. The branch of science that deals with human work and the efficient use of energy, including anatomical, physiological, biomechanical, and psychosocial factors.

ERGOT. A compound produced by a fungus that grows on rye plants. It is used in the production of some abortive antimigraine drugs.

ERYTHEMA. Redness of the skin due to congestion of the capillaries, usually due to injury, infection, or inflammation.

ERYTHROCYTE SEDIMENTATION RATE. A test that measures the rate at which red blood cells settle out in a tube of anticoagulated blood, expressed in millimeters per hour; elevated sedimentation rates indicate the presence of inflammation.

ESOPHAGUS. The tube leading from the back of the mouth, down the throat, and into the stomach.

ESSENTIAL TREMOR. An uncontrollable (involuntary) shaking of the hands, head, and face. Also called familial tremor because it is sometimes inherited, it can begin in the teens or in middle age. The exact cause is not known.

ETIOLOGY. The cause or origin of disease.

EUDYNIA. The medical term for acute pain, or pain that is a symptom of an underlying disease or disorder.

EUPHORIA. An exaggerated state of psychological and physical well being.

EUTHYROID. State of normal function of the thyroid gland.

EXCISIONAL BIOPSY. Removal of an entire lesion for microscopic examination.

EXCLUSION CRITERIA. A predetermined set of factors that make a potential participant not eligible for inclusion in a clinical trial or study.

EXECUTIVE FUNCTIONS. A set of cognitive abilities that control and regulate other abilities and behaviors. Necessary for goal-directed behavior, they include the ability to initiate and stop actions, to monitor and change behavior as needed, and to plan future behavior when faced with novel tasks and situations.

EXTENSIVE SUPPORT. Ongoing daily support required to assist an individual in a specific adaptive area, such as daily help with preparing meals.

EXTRAPYRAMIDAL SYSTEM. A functional rather than anatomical unit, it is comprised of nuclei and nerve fibers that are chiefly involved with subconscious, automatic aspects of motor coordination, but which also assist in the regulation of postural and locomotor movements.

F

FACIAL NERVE. A cranial nerve that controls the muscles in the face.

FAILURE TO THRIVE. Significantly reduced or delayed physical growth.

FASCICULATIONS. Small involuntary muscle contractions visible under the skin.

FAST FOURIER TRANSFER. A digital processing of the recorded signal resulting in a decomposition of its frequency components.

FATAL FAMILIAL INSOMNIA . A rare, progressive neurological disease that is believed to be transmitted via an abnormal protein called a prion.

FEBRILE CONVULSION. Seizures occurring mainly in children between three months and five years of age that are triggered by fever.

FEMORAL ARTERY. An artery located in the groin area that is the most frequently accessed site for arterial puncture in angiography.

FETAL. Refers to the fetus. In humans, the fetal period extends from the end of the eighth week of pregnancy to birth.

FETAL TISSUE TRANSPLANTATION. A method of treating Parkinson's and other neurological diseases by grafting brain cells from human fetuses onto the affected area of the human brain. Human adults cannot grow new brain cells but developing fetuses can. Grafting fetal tissue stimulates the growth of new brain cells in affected adult brains.

FIBROMYALGIA. A condition characterized by aching and stiffness, fatigue, and sleep disturbance, as well as pain at various sites on the body.

FILUM TERMINALE. The strand of elastic, fibrous tissue that secures the lower end of the spinal cord.

FINGER AGNOSIA. Inability to identify a particular finger.

FLACCID PARALYSIS. Loss of muscle tone resulting from injury or disease of the nerves that innervate the muscles.

FLAIL. To swing freely.

FLASHBACK. A vivid sensory or emotional experience that happens independently of the initial event or experience. Flashbacks resulting from the use of LSD are sometimes referred to as hallucinogen persisting perception disorder, or HPPD.

FLUORESCEIN DYE. An orange dye used to illuminate the blood vessels of the retina in fluorescein angiography.

FLUOROSCOPE. An imaging device that displays x rays of the body. Fluoroscopy allows the radiologist to visualize the guide wire and catheter moving through the patient's artery.

FOCAL. Limited to a defined area.

FORAMEN MAGNUM. Large opening in the back of the skull, where the spinal cord connects with the brain.

FORAMINOTOMY. Surgery to enlarge the bony hole, or foramen, where a nerve root enters or exits the spinal canal.

FRAGILE X SYNDROME. A genetic condition related to the X chromosome that affects mental, physical, and sensory development. It is the most common form of inherited mental retardation.

FREE RADICAL. An unstable molecule that causes oxidative damage by stealing electrons from surrounding molecules, thereby disrupting activity in the body's cells.

FRONTAL CORTEX. The part of the human brain associated with aggressiveness and impulse control. Abnormalities in the frontal cortex are associated with an increased risk of suicide.

FRONTAL LOBE. The area of the brain responsible for higher thinking.

G

GAIT. The way in which one walks.

GAMMA RAY. A high-energy photon emitted by radioactive substances.

GANGLION. A mass of nerve cells usually found outside the central nervous system, from which axons arrive from the periphery and proceed to the spinal cord or brain; plural form: ganglia .

GANGLIOSIDE. A fatty (lipid) substance found within the brain and nerve cells.

GANGRENE. The death of tissue caused by loss of blood supply. Gangrene is a serious potential side effect of taking ergot alkaloids.

GASTROPARESIS. Nerve damage of the stomach that delays or stops stomach emptying, resulting in nausea, vomiting, bloating, discomfort, and weight loss.

GELASTIC SEIZURES. Seizures manifesting with brief involuntary laughter

GENE. A building block of inheritance, it contains the instructions for the production of a particular protein and is made up of a molecular sequence found on a section of DNA. Each gene is found at a precise location on a chromosome.

GENERALIZED ANXIETY DISORDER. An anxiety disorder characterized by excessive worry or fear about a number of activities or events.

GENOME. The entire collection of genes of an individual.

GENOTYPE. The genetic makeup of an organism or a set of organisms.

GINGIVAL FIBROMA. Small non-cancerous growth on the toe or finger nail beds.

GLASGOW COMA SCALE. A measure of level of consciousness and neurological functioning after traumatic brain injury (TBI).

GLAUCOMA. A common eye disease characterized by increased fluid pressure in the eye that damages the optic nerve, which carries visual impulses to the brain. Glaucoma can be caused by another eye disorder, such as a tumor or congenital malformation, or it can appear without obvious cause. If untreated it generally leads to blindness.

GLIAL CELL. Nerve tissue of the central nervous system other than the signal-transmitting neurons. Glial cells are interspersed between neurons, providing support and insulation.

GLIOMA. A tumor that originates in the cells supporting and nourishing brain neural tissue (glial cells).

GLOBOID CELLS. Large cells containing excess toxic metabolic "waste" of galactosylceramide and psychosine.

GLUCOCORTICOID MEDICATIONS. A group of medications that produces effects of the body's own cortisone and cortisol. Glucocorticoids are commonly called steroids and, among other functions, work to reduce inflammation,

GLUCOSYLCERAMIDE. A chemical substance composed of glucose (sugar) and lipid (fat).

GLYCOGEN. The principle form of carbohydrate energy (glucose) stored within the muscles and liver.

GOITER. A swelling or enlargement of the thyroid gland.

GRAY MATTER. Areas of the brain and spinal cord that are comprised mostly of unmyelinated nerves.

GUIDE WIRE. A wire that is inserted into an artery to guide a catheter to a certain location in the body.

GUSTATORY. Pertaining to the sense of taste.

H

HALLUCINATION. A false or distorted perception of objects, sounds, or events that seems real. Hallucinations usually result from drugs or mental disorders.

HALLUCINOGEN. A drug or other substance that induces hallucinations.

HAMARTOMA. Abnormal growth that may resemble cancer, but is not cancerous.

HANDEDNESS. The preference of either the right or left hand as the dominant hand for the performance of tasks such as writing.

HAPTIC. Pertaining to the sense of touch.

HEMANGIOBLASTOMA. Tumor often found in the brain, as in von Hippel-Lindau disease.

HEMATOMA. A localized collection of blood, often clotted, in body tissue or an organ, usually due to a break or tear in the wall of blood vessel.

HEMICHOREA. Chorea that affects only one side of the body.

HEMIPARESIS. Muscle weakness of one side of the body.

HEMIPLEGIA. Paralysis on one side of the body.

HEMIPLEGIC MIGRAINE. Migraine accompanied by temporary paralysis on one side of the body.

HEMISPHERE. One side of the brain, right or left.

HEMOPHILIAC. A person with the blood disorder hemophilia, an inherited deficiency in blood-clotting ability. Hemophiliacs require regular administration of blood products, and were especially at risk of acquiring AIDS from HIV-contaminated blood during the early years of the evolving AIDS epidemic, before tests were developed to identify the HIV virus in donated blood.

HEMORRHAGE. Severe, massive bleeding that is difficult to control. The bleeding may be internal or external.

HEPATIC ENCEPHALOPATHY. A change in mental state due to toxic substance buildup in the blood that is caused by liver failure.

HEPATITIS. An inflammation of the liver, with accompanying liver cell damage or cell death, caused most frequently by viral infection, but also by certain drugs, chemicals, or poisons. May be either acute (of limited duration) or chronic (continuing). Symptoms include jaundice, nausea, vomiting, loss of appetite, tenderness in the right upper abdomen, aching muscles, and joint pain. In severe cases, liver failure may result.

HEPATOSPLENOMEGALY. Enlargement of the liver and spleen.

HEPATOTOXICITY. Damaging or destructive to the liver.

HEREDITARY ATAXIA. One of a group of hereditary degenerative diseases of the spinal cord or cerebellum. These diseases cause tremor, spasm, and wasting of muscle.

HERNIATED DISC. A blisterlike bulging or protrusion of the contents of the disk out through the fibers that normally hold them in place. It is also called a ruptured disk, slipped disk, or displaced disk.

HERPES. A virus that causes cold sores, sexually transmitted diseases, shingles, or chicken pox.

HERPES SIMPLEX VIRUS. A virus that can cause fever and blistering on the skin and mucous membranes. Herpes simplex 1 infections usually occur on the face (cold sores) and herpes simplex 2 infections usually occur in the genital region.

HERPES VARICELLA ZOSTER VIRUS. The virus that typically causes chicken pox in children; then may reactivate later in life to cause shingles.

HIB DISEASE. An infection caused by *Haemophilus influenza*, type b (Hib). This disease mainly affects children under the age of five. In that age group, it is the leading cause of bacterial meningitis, pneumonia, joint and bone infections, and throat inflammations.

HIPPOCAMPUS. A part of the brain that is involved in memory formation and learning. The hippocampus is shaped like a curved ridge and belongs to an organ system called the limbic system.

HISTAMINE. A substance released by immune system cells in response to the presence of an allergen. It stimulates widening of blood vessels and increased porousness of blood vessel walls so that fluid and protein leak out from the blood into the surrounding tissue, causing localised inflammation of the tissue.

HISTOLOGIC. Pertaining to histology, the study of cells and tissues at the microscopic level.

HISTOLOGY. The study of tissue structure.

HOLOPROSENCEPHALY. Brain, cranial, and facial malformations present at birth that are caused by incomplete cleavage of the brain during embryologic development.

HOMEOSTASIS. The balanced internal environment of the body and the automatic tendency of the body to maintain this internal "steady state." Also refers to the tendency of a family system to maintain internal stability and to resist change.

HORMONE. Chemical substance produced by certain endocrine glands that is released into the bloodstream where it controls and regulates functioning of several other tissues.

HUMAN IMMUNODEFICIENCY VIRUS (HIV). A transmissible retrovirus that causes AIDS in humans. Two forms of HIV are now recognized: HIV-1, which causes most cases of AIDS in Europe, North and South America, and most parts of Africa; and HIV-2, which is chiefly found in West African patients. HIV-2, discovered in 1986, appears to be less virulent than HIV-1 and may also have a longer latency period.

HYDROCEPHALUS. An abnormal accumulation of cerebrospinal fluid within the brain. This accumulation can be harmful by pressing on brain structures and thereby damaging them.

HYPERCAPNIA. Excess carbon dioxide in the blood.

HYPEREMESIS GRAVIDARUM. Uncontrollable nausea and vomiting associated with pregnancy. Acupuncture appears to be an effective treatment for women with this condition.

HYPEREXTENSION. Extension of a limb or body part beyond the normal limit.

HYPERFUNCTION. Term used to describe excess effort or strain involved in producing an action.

HYPERHIDROSIS. Excessive sweating. Hyperhidrosis can be caused by heat, overactive thyroid glands, strong emotion, menopause, or infection.

HYPERLIPIDEMIA. A condition characterized by abnormally high levels of lipids in blood plasma.

HYPERPIGMENTATION. An excess of melanin, leading to abnormal areas of increased dark skin color.

HYPERREFLEXIA. An increased reaction to reflexes.

HYPERTENSION. Abnormally high arterial blood pressure, which if left untreated can lead to heart disease and stroke.

HYPERTHERMIA. Elevated body temperature.

HYPERTHYROID. State of excess thyroid hormone in the body.

HYPERTHYROIDISM. Abnormally high levels of thyroid hormone. About 2% of patients with this condition develop chorea.

HYPERTONUS. Increased tension of a muscle or muscle spasm.

HYPERVENTILATION. A pattern of rapid but shallow breathing that is frequently found in patients with Rett syndrome.

HYPNOGOGIC. Pertaining to drowsiness. It is usually used to describe hallucinations that occur as a person falls asleep.

HYPNOGOGIC HALLUCINATION. A vivid, dream-like hallucination, such as the sensation of falling, that occurs at the onset of sleep.

HYPNOPOMPIC. Persisting after sleep. It is usually used to describe hallucinations that occur as a person awakens.

HYPNOTICS. A class of drugs that are used as sedatives and sleep aids.

HYPOCALCEMIA. A condition characterized by an abnormally low level of calcium in the blood.

HYPOMELANOTIC MACULE. Skin patch that is lighter in color than the area around it.

HYPOPIGMENTATION. A deficiency of melanin, leading to abnormal areas of lighter skin color.

HYPOPITUITARISM. A condition characterized by underactivity of the pituitary gland.

HYPOTHALAMUS. The lowermost part of the diencephalon, containing several nuclei, nerve tracts, and the pituitary gland; it is the regulatory seat of the autonomic nervous system, controlling heartbeat, body temperature, thirst, hunger, blood pressure, blood sugar levels, and other functions.

HYPOTHYROIDISM. A disorder in which the thyroid gland produces too little thyroid hormone causing a decrease in the rate of metabolism with associated effects on the reproductive system. Symptoms include fatigue, difficulty swallowing, mood swings, hoarse voice, sensitivity to cold, forgetfulness, and dry/coarse skin and hair.

HYPOTONIA. Having reduced or diminished muscle tone or strength.

HYPOTONUS. Decreased tension of a muscle, or abnormally low muscle tone.

HYPOXEMIA. Abnormally low blood oxygen.

HYPOXIA. A condition characterized by insufficient oxygen in the cells of the body

HYPOXIC. Oxygen deficient.

HYPSARRHYTHMIA. Typical brain wave activity found in infantile spasms.

I

ICHTHYOSIS. Dry, thickened, rough, coarse skin, sometimes with evident scaling.

ICTAL EEG. An electroencephalogram (EEG) done to determine the type of seizure characteristic of a person's disorder. During this EEG, seizure medicine may be discontinued in an attempt to induce as seizure during the testing period.

IDIOPATHIC. Of unknown cause or spontaneous origin. Ménière's disease and some headaches are considered idiopathic disorders.

ILLUSION. A false visual perception of an object that others perceive correctly. A common example is the number of sightings of UFOs that turn out to be airplanes or weather balloons.

IMMUNOADSORPTION. A procedure that can remove harmful antibodies from the blood.

IMMUNOCOMPROMISED. A state in which the immune system is suppressed or not functioning properly.

IMMUNOGLOBULIN. A protein molecule formed by mature B-cells in response to foreign proteins in the body; the building blocks for antibodies.

IMMUNOHISTOCHEMISTRY. A method of detecting the presence of specific proteins in cells or tissues.

IMMUNOSUPPRESSANTS. Drugs that reduce or eliminate the body's ability to make an immune response.

INBORN ERROR OF METABOLISM. One of a group of rare conditions characterized by an inherited defect in an enzyme or other protein. Inborn errors of metabolism can cause brain damage and mental retardation if left untreated. Phenylketonuria, Tay-Sachs disease, and galactosemia are inborn errors of metabolism.

INCISIONAL BIOPSY. Removal of a small part of a sample tissue area for microscopic examination.

INCLUSION BODY. A small intracellular body found within the cytoplasm or nucleus of another cell, characteristic of disease.

INCLUSION CRITERIA. A predetermined set of factors that make a potential participant eligible for inclusion in a clinical trial or study.

INCONTINENCE. Inability to control excretory functions such as defecation and urination.

INCOORDINATION. Loss of voluntary muscle control resulting in irregular movements.

INCREASED INTRACRANIAL PRESSURE. Increased overall pressure inside the skull.

INFARCT. An area of dead tissue caused by inadequate blood supply; in the brain, this condition is called a stroke.

INFLAMMATION. The body's response to injury, resulting in swelling, warmth, redness, pain.

INGUINAL. Referring to the groin area.

INNERVATION. Distribution or supply of nerves to a structure.

INSIDIOUS. Developing in a stealthy or gradual manner.

INSULIN. A hormone or chemical produced by the pancreas that is needed by cells of the body in order to use glucose (sugar), a major source of energy for the human body.

INTENTION TREMOR. A rhythmic purposeless shaking of the muscles that begins with purposeful (voluntary) movement. This tremor does not affect muscles that are resting.

INTERFERON ALFA. A potent immune-defense protein that is used as an anti-cancer drug.

INTERLEUKINS. Chemicals released in the body as a result of stress.

INTERMEDIATE CARE FACILITY. An inpatient facility that provides periodic nursing care.

INTERVERTEBRAL DISCS. Gelatinous structures separating the spinal vertebrae and acting as shock absorbers.

INTRACEREBRAL HEMATOMA. Bleeding within the brain caused by trauma to a blood vessel.

INTRACEREBRAL HEMORRHAGE. A cause of some strokes in which vessels within the brain begin bleeding.

INTRACRANIAL HYPERTENSION. Increase in pressure in the brain.

INTRACRANIAL PRESSURE. The overall pressure within the skull.

INTRAOCULAR. Inside the eye.

INTRAVENTRICULAR HEMORRHAGE. Bleeding into the brain, specifically into the ventricles.

IONIZING RADIATION. High-energy radiation such as that produced by x rays.

IRIS. The circular membrane that forms the colored portion of the eye and expands or contracts around the pupil.

IRITIS. Inflammation of the iris, the membrane in the pupil, the colored portion of the eye. It is characterized by photophobia, pain, and inflammatory congestion.

IRRITATIVE HALLUCINATIONS. Hallucinations caused by abnormal electrical activity in the brain.

ISCHEMIA. A decrease in the blood supply to an area of the body caused by obstruction or constriction of blood vessels.

J

JAUNDICE. Yellowing of the skin or eyes due to excess of bilirubin in the blood.

K

KARYOTYPE. A standard arrangement of photographic or computer-generated images of chromosome pairs from a cell in ascending numerical order, from largest to smallest.

KETOACIDOSIS. Usually caused by uncontrolled type I diabetes, when the body isn't able to use glucose for energy. As an alternate source of energy, fat cells are broken down, producing ketones, toxic compounds that make the blood acidic. Symptoms of ketoacidosis include excessive thirst and urination, abdominal pain, vomiting, rapid breathing, extreme tiredness, and drowsiness.

KI. The Japanese spelling of qi, the traditional Chinese term for vital energy or the life force.

KINETIC. Word taken from the Greek (kinesis): motion.

KYPHOSIS. An abnormal convex (outward) curvature of the upper portion of the spinal column, sometimes called a humpback or hunchback.

L

LABYRINTH. The inner ear. It consists of the membranous labyrinth, which is a system of sacs and ducts made of soft tissue; and the osseous or bony labyrinth, which surrounds and contains the membranous labyrinth.

LABYRINTHECTOMY. Surgical removal of the labyrinth of the ear. It is done to treat Ménière's disease only when the patient has already suffered severe hearing loss.

LACINATING PAIN. Piercing, stabbing, or darting pain.

LAMINA. Flat plates of bone that form part of a vertebrae.

LARYNGEAL STRIDOR. Constriction of the voice box, causing vocal hoarseness.

LARYNX. The "voice box," located between the pharynx (upper area of the throat) and the trachea (windpipe).

LATERAL FLEXION. To flex toward a side.

LATERAL GENICULATE NUCLEI. A structure that receives and processes impulses from the optic nerve; it sends these impulses farther into the brain for more processing.

LEFT VENTRICULAR ENLARGEMENT. Abnormal enlargement of the left lower chamber of the heart.

LEPTOMENINGEAL ANGIOMA. A swelling of the tissue or membrane surrounding the brain and spinal cord, which can enlarge with time.

LESION. A disruption of the normal structure and function of a tissue by an injury or disease process. Wounds, sores, rashes, and boils are all lesions.

LEUKEMIA. A cancer of the blood-forming organs (bone marrow and lymph system) characterized by an abnormal increase in the number of white blood cells in the tissues. There are many types of leukemias and they are classified according to the type of white blood cell involved.

LEUKOCYTOSIS. An elevated white blood cell count.

LEUKODYSTROPHY. A disease that affects the white matter called myelin in the central nervous system (CNS).

LEUKOMALACIA. Softening of the brain's white matter.

LEVODOPA. A substance used in the treatment of Parkinson's disease. Levodopa can cross the blood-brain barrier that protects the brain. Once in the brain, it is converted to dopamine and thus can replace the dopamine lost in Parkinson's disease.

LEWY BODIES. Spheres, found in the bodies of dying cells, that are considered to be a marker for Parkinson's disease.

LIGAMENT. A type of tough, fibrous tissue that connects bones or cartilage and provides support and strength to joints.

LIMBIC SYSTEM. A group of structures in the brain that includes the hypothalamus, amygdala, olfactory bulbs, and hippocampus. The limbic system plays an important part in the regulation of human moods and emotions. Many psychiatric disorders are related to malfunctioning of the limbic system.

LIMITED SUPPORT. A predetermined period of assistance required to deal with a specific event, such as training for a new job.

LIPIDS. Organic compounds not soluble in water but soluble in fat solvents such as alcohol. Lipids are stored in the body as energy reserves and are important components of cell membranes. Commonly known as fats.

LIPOPIGMENTS. Substances made up of fats and proteins found in the body's tissues.

LIPOPROTEINS. Compounds of protein that carry fats and fat-like substances such as cholesterol in the blood.

LISCH NODULE. A benign growth within the iris of the eye.

LIVER ENCEPHALOPATHY. A condition in which the brain is affected by a buildup of toxic substances that would normally be removed by the liver. The condition occurs when the liver is too severely damaged to cleanse the blood effectively.

LOCOMOTOR. Means of or pertaining to movement or locomotion.

LORDOSIS. Anterior curvature of the spine, creating a swayback appearance.

LUMBAR. Referring to the lower back. There are five lumbar vertebrae.

LUMBAR PUNCTURE. A diagnostic procedure in which a needle is inserted into the lower spine to withdraw a small amount of cerebrospinal fluid.

LYME BORRELIOSIS. Another name for Lyme disease.

LYMPHADENOPATHY. Swelling of the lymph glands.

LYMPHANGIOLEIMYOMA. Non-cancerous growth in the lung, typical of tuberous sclerosis.

LYMPHOCYTE. A type of white blood cell that participates in the immune response. The two main groups are the B-cells that have antibody molecules on their surface and T-cells that destroy antigens.

LYMPHOCYTIC MENINGITIS. Benign infection of brain coverings that protect the brain

LYMPHOMA. A malignant tumor of the lymph nodes.

LYSOSOME. Membrane-enclosed compartment in cells, containing many hydrolytic enzymes; where large molecules and cellular components are broken down.

M

MACROPHAGE. A large, versatile immune cell that acts as a scavenger, engulfing dead cells, foreign substances, and other debris.

MACULE. A small, flat area of abnormal color on the skin.

MAGNETIC RESONANCE IMAGING (MRI). An imaging technique used in evaluation and diagnoses of the brain and other parts of the body.

MAJOR DEPRESSIVE DISORDER. A mood disorder characterized by overwhelming and persistent feelings of hopelessness, often accompanied by sleep disturbances, withdrawal from normal social and personal care activities, and an inability to concentrate.

MALABSORPTION. The inability to adequately or efficiently absorb nutrients from the intestinal tract.

MALDYNIA. The medical term for chronic pain, or pain that has become a disease in and of itself as a result of changes in the patient's nervous system.

MALINGERING. Knowingly pretending to be physically or mentally ill in order to get out of some unpleasant duty or responsibility, or for economic benefit.

MANIC. A period of excess mental activity, often accompanied by elevated mood and disorganized behavior.

MASTOID BONE. The bony areas behind and below the ears. Also called the mastoid process.

MEDIAN NERVE. A nerve that runs through the wrist and into the hand. It provides sensation and some movement to the hand, the thumb, the index finger, the middle finger, and half of the ring finger.

MEDICAID. A program jointly funded by state and federal governments that reimburses hospitals and physicians for the care of individuals who cannot pay for their own medical expenses. These individuals may be in low-income households or may have chronic disabilities.

MEDULLA. The lowermost portion of the brain stem (it borders the spinal cord) that controls vital functions like respiration, blood pressure, swallowing, and heart rate. Also called the medulla oblongata.

MENINGES. The three-layered membranous covering of the brain and spinal cord.

MENINGIOMA. A tumor made up of cells of the lining of the brain and spinal cord (meninges).

MENINGITIS. An infection or inflammation of the membranes that cover the brain and spinal cord (the meninges). It is usually caused by bacteria or a virus.

MERIDIANS. In traditional Chinese medicine, the channels that run beneath the skin through which the body's energy, chi (sometimes spelled "qi" or "ki") flows.

METABOLIC. Refers to the chemical reactions in living organisms.

METABOLIC ACIDOSIS. Overly acidic condition of the blood.

METABOLISM. The group of biochemical processes within the body that release energy in support of life.

METANEPHRINE. A byproduct of epinephrine, found elevated in urine if a pheochromocytoma is present.

METASTASIS. The spread of cancer from one part of the body to another. Cells in the metastatic (secondary) tumor are like those in the original (primary) tumor.

MICROCEPHALY. An abnormally small head and underdeveloped brain.

MICROTUBULES. Slender, elongated, anatomical channels.

MIGRAINE. Recurrent severe headaches generally accompanied by an aura (classic migraine), nausea, vomiting, and dizziness.

MILLIGRAM. One thousandth of a gram; the metric measure that equals 0.035 ounces.

MINERALOCORTICOID. A steroid hormone, like aldosterone, that regulates the excretion of salt, potassium, and water.

MITOCHONDRIA. Spherical or rod-shaped structures of the cell. Mitochondria contain genetic material (DNA and RNA) and are responsible for converting food to energy.

MITOCHONDRIAL DNA. The genetic material found in mitochondria, the organelles that generate energy for the cell. Because reproduction is by cloning, mitochondrial DNA is usually passed along female lines.

MITRAL VALVE PROLAPSE. A heart defect in which one of the valves of the heart (which normally controls blood flow) becomes floppy. Mitral valve prolapse may be detected as a heart murmur, but there are usually no symptoms.

MONOAMINE OXIDASE INHIBITORS. A class of antidepressants used to treat certain types of mental depression. MAO inhibitors are especially useful in treating people whose depression is combined with other problems such as anxiety, panic attacks, phobias, or the desire to sleep too much.

MONONEUROPATHY. Disorder involving a single nerve.

MONOZYGOTIC TWINS. Twins that are genetically identical and are always of the same gender.

MOTOR. Of or pertaining to motion, the body structures involved in movement, or the brain functions that direct such deliberate movement.

MOTOR FUNCTION. The ability to produce body movement by complex interaction of the brain, nerves and muscles.

MOTOR NERVES. Motor or efferent nerve cells, they carry impulses from the brain to muscle or organ tissue.

MOTOR NEURON. A nerve cell that specifically controls and stimulates voluntary muscles.

MOTOR NEURON DISEASE. A neuromuscular disease, usually progressive, that causes degeneration of motor neuron cells and loss or diminishment of voluntary muscle control.

MOTOR UNIT ACTION POTENTIALS. Spikes of electrical activity recorded during an electromyogram (EMG) that reflect the number of motor units (motor neurons and the muscle fibers they transmit signals to) activated when the patient voluntarily contracts a muscle.

MOVEMENT EDUCATION. A term that refers to the active phase of bodywork, in which clients learn to move with greater freedom and to maintain the proper alignment of their bodies.

MOXIBUSTION. A technique in traditional Chinese medicine that involves burning a "Moxa," or cone of dried wormwood leaves, close to the skin to relieve pain. When used with acupuncture, the cone is placed on top of the needle at an acupuncture point and burned

MUCOPOLYSACCHARIDE. A complex molecule made of smaller sugar molecules strung together to form a chain. It is found in mucous secretions and intercellular spaces.

MULTIPLE MONONEUROPATHY. Neuropathy affecting several individual nerve trunks.

MULTIPLE SCLEROSIS. A progressive, autoimmune disease of the central nervous system characterized by damage to the myelin sheath that covers nerves. The disease, which causes progressive paralysis, is marked by periods of exacerbation and remission.

MUSCLE TONE. Also termed tonus; the normal state of balanced tension in the tissues of the body, especially the muscles.

MUTATION. A permanent change in the genetic material that may alter a trait or characteristic of an individual, or manifest as disease. It can be transmitted to offspring.

MYASTHENIA. Muscular weakness or a group of chronic muscular diseases characterized by muscle weakness.

MYASTHENIA GRAVIS. A chronic, autoimmune, neuromuscular disease with symptoms that include muscle weakness and sometimes paralysis.

MYELIN. A fatty sheath surrounding nerves throughout the body that helps them conduct impulses more quickly.

MYELOGRAM. An x-ray exam of the spinal cord, nerves, and other tissues within the spinal cord that are highlighted by injected contrast dye.

MYELOGRAPHY. A test in which dye is injected into the spinal canal and the patient is then tilted in different directions on a special table, allowing dye to outline the spinal cord and nerve roots and to show areas of compression.

MYELOMENINGOCELE. A sac that protrudes through an abnormal opening in the spinal column.

MYELOPATHY. A disorder in which the tissue of the spinal cord is diseased or damaged.

MYOCARDIAL INFARCTION. Commonly known as a heart attack, a myocardial infarction is an episode in which some of the heart's blood supply is severely cut off or restricted, causing the heart muscle to suffer and die from lack of oxygen.

MYOCLONUS. Involuntary contractions of a muscle or an interrelated group of muscles. Also known as myoclonic seizures.

MYOFILAMENT. Ultrastructural microscopic unit of a muscle that is made up of proteins that contract.

MYOPATHY. Any abnormal condition or disease of muscle tissue, characterized by muscle weakness and wasting.

MYOSITIS. Inflammation of a muscle.

MYOTONIA. The inability to normally relax a muscle after contracting or tightening it.

N

NARCOLEPSY. A life-long sleep disorder marked by four symptoms: sudden brief sleep attacks, cataplexy (a sudden loss of muscle tone usually lasting up to 30 minutes), temporary paralysis, and hallucinations. The hallucinations are associated with falling asleep or the transition from sleeping to waking.

NARCOTIC. Another term for opioid drugs that refers to their ability to produce drowsiness as well as relieve pain.

NASAL POLYPS. Drop-shaped overgrowths of the nasal membranes.

NECROSIS. Cellular or tissue death; skin necrosis may be caused by multiple, consecutive doses of radiation from fluoroscopic or x-ray procedures.

NEOPLASM. An abnormal growth of tissue or cells (a tumor) that may be either malignant (cancerous) or benign.

NERVE. Fibers that carry sensory information, movement stimuli, or both from the brain and spinal cord to other parts of the body and back again. Some nerves, including the vagus nerve, innervate distantly separated parts of the body.

NERVE CONDUCTION. The speed and strength of a signal being transmitted by nerve cells. Testing these factors can reveal the nature of nerve injury, such as damage to nerve cells or to the protective myelin sheath.

NERVE CONDUCTION STUDY. Testing that shows electrical impulse activity along nerves.

NERVE CONDUCTION VELOCITY. A recording of how well a nerve conducts electrical impulses.

NERVE IMPULSE. The electrochemical signal carried by an axon from one neuron to another neuron.

NERVE ROOT. Two groups of nerves that run from the spinal cord to join and form the spinal nerves.

NEURAL TUBE. A hollow column of ectodermal tissue that forms in early embryonic development and goes on to become the spinal cord and spinal column.

NEURAL TUBE DEFECT. A birth defect caused by abnormal closure or development of the neural tube, the embryonic structure that gives rise to the central nervous system.

NEURALGIA. Pain along the pathway of a nerve.

NEUROBLASTOMA. A malignant tumor of nerve cells that strikes children.

NEUROCUTANEOUS. Conditions involving unique manifestations of the skin, hair, teeth, and nervous system, usually with familial tendencies.

NEURODEGENERATIVE. Relating to the deterioration of nerve tissues.

NEURODEGENERATIVE DISEASE. A disease in which the nervous system progressively and irreversibly deteriorates.

NEUROFIBRILLARY TANGLES. Abnormal structures composed of twisted masses of protein fibers within nerve cells. They are found in the brains of persons with Alzheimer's disease.

NEUROFIBROMAS. Soft, rubbery, flesh-colored tumors made up of the fibrous substance that covers peripheral nerves.

NEUROFIBROMATOSIS. Also called von Reclinghausen's disease; a disease in which tumors grow on nerve cells throughout the body.

NEUROGENIC. Caused by or originating in the nerves.

NEUROGENIC PAIN. Pain originating in the nerves or nervous tissue and following the pathway of a nerve.

NEUROLEPTIC. Another name for the older type of antipsychotic medications, such as haloperidol and chlorpromazine, prescribed to treat psychotic conditions.

NEUROMUSCULAR. Involving both the muscles and the nerves that control them.

NEUROMUSCULAR DISEASE. Disease involving both the muscles and the nerves that control them.

NEUROMUSCULAR JUNCTION. The site at which nerve impulses are transmitted to muscles.

NEURON. A cell specialized to conduct and generate electrical impulses and to carry information from one part of the brain to another.

NEURONAL CEROID LIPOFUSCINOSES. A family of four progressive neurological disorders.

NEURONAL MIGRATION. A step of early brain development in which nerve cells travel over large distances to different parts of the brain.

NEUROPATHIC BLADDER. Improper or lack of bladder function, due to a nerve problem.

NEUROPATHY. A disease or abnormality of the peripheral nerves (the nerves outside the brain and spinal cord). Major symptoms include weakness, numbness, paralysis, or pain in the affected area.

NEUROSYPHILIS. This is the slowly progressive destruction of the brain and spinal cord due to untreated tertiary (late-stage) syphilis. It can be asymptomatic or cause different disorders like tabes dorsalis, general paresis, and meningovascular syphilis.

NEUROTOXIN. A poison that acts directly on the central nervous system.

NEUROTRANSMISSION. The process in which a neurotransmitter travels across the synapse to act on the target cell to either inhibit or excite it.

NEUROTRANSMITTER. A chemical messenger that transmits an impulse from one nerve cell to the next.

NOCICEPTOR. A specialized type of nerve cell that senses pain.

NOREPINEPHRINE. A hormone that controls blood pressure and heart rate. It is also a chemical found in the brain that is thought to play a role in attention deficit hyperactivity disorder (ADHD).

NUCLEUS PULPOSUS. Central core of a vertebrae.

NYSTAGMUS. An involuntary, rhythmic movement of the eyes.

O

OBSESSION. A persistent or recurrent thought, image, or impulse that is unwanted and distressing.

OBSTRUCTIVE SLEEP APNEA. The most common form of sleep apnea characterized by repeated episodes of upper airway obstruction during sleep.

OCCIPITAL LOBE. The back part of the brain that functions as a visual interpretation center.

OCCIPITAL NERVES. Two pairs of nerves that originate in the area of the second and third vertebrae of the neck. They are part of a network that innervate the neck, upper back, and head.

OCCLUSION. Blockage.

OLFACTORY. Pertaining to the sense of smell.

OPHTHALMIC ARTERY. The artery supplying the eye and adjacent structures with blood.

OPHTHALMOPARESIS. Paralysis of one or more of the muscles of the eye.

OPHTHALMOPLEGIA. Paralysis of the motor nerves of the eye, resulting in wandering or floating eye movements or drooping eyelids.

OPIOID. Any natural or synthetic substance that produces the same effects as an opiate, such as pain relief, sedation, constipation, and respiratory depression. Some opioids are produced by the human body (e.g., endorphins), while others are produced in the laboratory (e.g., methadone).

OPPORTUNISTIC INFECTION. An infection in a person with an impaired immune system caused by an organism that does not usually cause disease in people with healthy immune systems.

OPSOCLONUS. Often called "dancing eyes," this symptom involves involuntary, quick darting movements of the eyes in all directions.

OPTIC NERVE. The bundle of nerve fibers that carry visual messages from the retina to the brain.

OPTIC NEURITIS. Inflammation of the optic nerve, often accompanied by vision loss.

OREXIN. Another name for hypocretin, a chemical secreted in the hypothalmus that regulates the sleep/wake cycle. Narcolepsy is sometimes described as an orexin deficiency syndrome.

ORGANELLE. A specialized structure within a cell, which is separated from the rest of the cell by a membrane composed of lipids and proteins, where chemical and metabolic functions take place.

ORGANIC BRAIN SYNDROME. A brain disorder that is caused by defective structure or abnormal functioning of the brain.

ORTHOSTATIC HYPOTENSION. A drop in blood pressure that causes faintness or dizziness and occurs when an individual rises to a standing position. Also known as postural hypotension.

ORTHOTIC DEVICE. An external device, such as a splint or a brace, that prevents or assists movement. Also called an orthosis.

OSSICLES. Tiny bones in the middle ear—the incus, malleus, and stapes—that convey sound impulses from the eardrum to the inner ear.

OSTEOPOROSIS. Literally meaning "porous bones," this condition occurs when bones lose an excessive amount of their protein and mineral content, particularly calcium. Over time, bone mass and strength are reduced leading to increased risk of fractures.

OTITIS MEDIA. Inflammation, usually with infection, of the middle ear.

OTOLARYNGOLOGIST. A physician who specializes in medical and surgical treatment of disorders of the ear, nose, throat, and larynx.

OTOLARYNGOLOGY. The branch of medicine that treats disorders of the ear, nose, and throat.

OTOLITH ORGANS. Organs in the vestibular apparatus that sense horizontal and vertical movements of the head.

OTOLOGY. The branch of medicine that specializes in medical or surgical treatment of ear disorders.

OTOSCLEROSIS. Abnormal bone development in the middle ear, resulting in progressive hearing loss.

P

PAIN MEDICINE. The medical specialty that deals with the study and prevention of pain, and with the evaluation, treatment, and rehabilitation of patients with acute or chronic pain.

PALLIDOTOMY. A surgical procedure that destroys a small part of a tiny structure within the brain called the globus pallidus internus. This structure is part of the basal ganglia, a part of the brain involved in the control of willed (voluntary) movement of the muscles.

PALPITATION. A heartbeat that is more pronounced, often felt physically.

PALSY. Uncontrollable tremors.

PANDEMIC. Widespread epidemic.

PANIC DISORDER. An anxiety disorder in which people have sudden and intense attacks of fear in certain situations. Symptoms such as shortness of breath, sweating, dizziness, chest pain, and extreme fear often accompany the attacks.

PAPILLEDEMA. Swelling of the optic disk inside the eye (the portion of the optic nerve that collects nerves from the light sensitive layer of the eye, the retina); often caused by increased pressure inside the head.

PARALYSIS. Loss of the ability to move one or more parts of the body voluntarily due to muscle or nerve damage.

PARANEOPLASTIC SYNDROME. A set of symptoms associated with cancer but not directly caused by the cancer.

PARAPARESIS. Weakness of the legs.

PARAPLEGIA. Loss of voluntary movement and sensation of both lower extremities.

PARASITE. An organism that lives and feeds in or on another organism (the host) and does nothing to benefit the host.

PARASYMPATHETIC NERVOUS SYSTEM. A branch of the autonomic nervous system that tends to induce secretion, increase the tone and contraction of smooth muscle, and cause dilation of blood vessels.

PARESIS. Partial or total loss of movement or sensation.

PARESTHESIA. An abnormal sensation often described as burning, tickling, tingling, or "pins and needles."

PARIETAL LOBE. One of two brain hemispheres responsible for associative processes.

PARKINSONIAN. Related to symptoms associated with Parkinson's disease, a nervous system disorder characterized by abnormal muscle movement of the tongue, face, and neck; inability to walk or move quickly; walking in a shuffling manner; restlessness; or tremors.

PARKINSONISM. A set of symptoms originally associated with Parkinson's disease that can occur as side effects of neuroleptic medications. The symptoms include trembling of the fingers or hands, a shuffling gait, and tight or rigid muscles.

PARTIAL SEIZURE. An episode of abnormal activity in a specific part of the brain that causes changes in attention, movement, or behavior.

PATHOGEN. A disease-causing organism.

PATHOPHYSIOLOGY. The changes in body functions associated with a disorder or disease.

PENETRANCE. The degree to which individuals possessing a particular genetic mutation express the trait that this mutation causes. One hundred percent penetrance is expected to be observed in truly dominant traits.

PENETRATING HEAD INJURY. Traumatic brain injury (TBI) in which an object pierces the skull and enters brain tissue.

PENICILLAMINE. A drug used to bind to and remove heavy metals (such as copper or lead) from the blood, to prevent kidney stones, and to treat rheumatoid arthritis. Brand names include Cuprimine and Depen.

PERCUTANEOUS ABLATION. Attempting to remove a foreign body by a method just above the skin, like using an ointment.

PERILYMPH. The fluid that lies between the membranous labyrinth of the inner ear and the bony labyrinth.

PERIPHERAL NERVES. Nerves outside the brain and spinal cord that provide the link between the body and the central nervous system.

PERIPHERAL NERVOUS SYSTEM. The part of the nervous system that is outside the brain and spinal cord. Sensory, motor, and autonomic nerves are included. PNS nerves link the central nervous system with sensory organs, muscles, blood vessels, and glands.

PERISTALSIS. Waves of involuntary muscle contraction and relaxation.

PERIUNGUAL FIBROMA. Small non-cancerous growth on the toe- or fingernail beds.

PERIVENTRICULAR. Located around the brain's ventricles.

PERONEAL. Related to the legs.

PEROXISOME. A cellular organelle containing enzymes responsible for the breakdown of waste or other products.

PES CAVUS. A highly arched foot.

PHARYNGITIS. Inflammation of the throat, accompanied by dryness and pain. Pharyngitis caused by a streptococcal infection is the usual trigger of Sydenham's chorea.

PHARYNX. The part of the airway that is located at the back of the throat.

PHENOTYPE. The physical expression of an individual's genes.

PHENYLKETONURIA (PKU). A rare, inherited metabolic disorder in which the enzyme necessary to break down and use phenylalanine, an amino acid necessary for normal growth and development, is lacking. As a result, phenylalanine builds up in the body causing mental retardation and other neurological problems.

PHEOCHROMOCYTOMA. A tumor that originates from the adrenal gland's chromaffin cells, causing overproduction of catecholamines, powerful hormones that induce high blood pressure and other symptoms.

PHOBIA. An intense and irrational fear of a specific object, activity, or situation that leads to avoidance.

PHONEME. A discrete unit of a language that corresponds to a similar discrete unit of speech sound. It is the smallest meaningful segment of language; for example, the word "cat" has three phonemes, "kuh," "aah," and "tuh."

PHONICS. A system to teach reading by teaching the speech sounds associated with single letters, letter combinations, and syllables.

PHOTON. A light particle.

PIA MATER. The innermost of the three meninges covering the brain.

PICKWICKIAN SYNDROME. A distinctive form of obstructive sleep apnea associated with being overweight, having a large neck, fat buildup around the soft tissues of the neck, and loss of muscle tone with aging.

PITCH. The property of sound that is determined by the frequency of sound wave vibrations reaching the ear.

PITUITARY GLAND. The most important of the endocrine glands (glands that release hormones directly into the bloodstream), the pituitary is located at the base of the brain. Sometimes referred to as the "master gland," it regulates and controls the activities of other endocrine glands and many body processes including growth and reproductive function. Also called the hypophysis.

PLACEBO. A drug containing no active ingredients, such as a sugar pill, that may be used in clinical trials to compare the effects of a given treatment against no treatment.

PLAQUE. A deposit, usually of fatty material, on the inside wall of a blood vessel. Also refers to a small, round demyelinated area that develops in the brain and spinal cord of an individual with multiple sclerosis.

PLASMA CELL. A type of white blood cell that produces antibodies; derived from an antigen-specific B-cell.

PLASMAPHERESIS. A procedure in which harmful cells are removed from the blood plasma.

PNEUMOTHORAX. A condition in which air or gas is present in the chest cavity.

POLIO. A disease caused by the poliovirus that can result in muscle weakness and/or paralysis.

POLIOVIRUS. The virus responsible for the disease called polio.

POLYARTHRITIS. Inflammation of several joints at the same time.

POLYDACTYLY. The presence of extra fingers or toes.

POLYDIPSIA. Excessive thirst.

POLYMORPHISM. A difference in DNA sequence among individuals; genetic variation.

POLYNEUROPATHY. Peripheral neuropathy affecting multiple nerves.

POLYP. Piece of skin that pouches outward.

POLYSOMNOGRAM. A machine that is used to diagnose sleep disorders by measuring and recording a variety of body functions related to sleep, including heart rate, eye movements, brain waves, muscle activity, breathing, changes in blood oxygen concentration, and body position.

POLYURIA. Excessive production and excretion of urine.

POOR MUSCLE TONE. Muscles that are weak and floppy.

PORPHYRIA. A disorder in which porphyrins build up in the blood and urine.

PORPHYRIN. A type of pigment found in living things.

PORTAL HYPERTENSION. A condition caused by cirrhosis of the liver, characterized by impaired or reversed blood flow from the portal vein to the liver, an enlarged spleen, and dilated veins in the esophagus and stomach.

PORTAL VEIN THROMBOSIS. The development of a blood clot in the vein that brings blood into the liver. Untreated portal vein thrombosis causes portal hypertension.

POSITRON. One of the small particles that make up an atom. A positron has the same mass and amount of charge as an electron, but the positron has a positive charge.

POSTERIOR CIRCULATION. The blood supply to the back part of the brain, including the occipital lobe, cerebellum, and brain stem.

POSTERIOR FOSSA. Area at the base of the skull attached to the spinal cord.

POSTERIOR SUBCAPSULAR LENTICULAR OPACITY. A type of cataract in the eye.

POSTICTAL. The time period immediately following a seizure.

POSTURAL DRAINAGE. The use of positioning to drain secretions from the bronchial tubes and lungs into the trachea or windpipe.

POSTURAL HYPOTENSION. A drop in blood pressure that causes faintness or dizziness and occurs when an individual rises to a standing position. Also known as orthostatic hypotension.

PREGNANCY CATEGORY. A system of classifying drugs according to their established risks for use during pregnancy. Category A: Controlled human studies have demonstrated no fetal risk. Category B: Animal studies indicate no fetal risk, but no human studies have been conducted, or, adverse effects have been shown in animal studies, but not in well-controlled human studies. Category C: No adequate human or animal studies, or adverse fetal effects in animal studies, but no available human data. Category D: Evidence of fetal risk, but benefits outweigh risks. Category X: Evidence of fetal risk. Risks outweigh any benefits.

PREMUTATION CARRIERS. Individuals who have the genetic protein repeats associated with a particular disorder, but not in sufficient numbers to cause the disorder.

The repeats may expand in these carriers' offspring, causing the disorder to occur.

PRENATAL TESTING. Testing for a disease such as a genetic condition in an unborn baby.

PRESBYCUSIS. Loss of hearing that gradually occurs because of age-related changes in the inner or middle ear.

PRESYNAPTIC. Before the synapse.

PRIMARY HEADACHE. A headache that is not caused by another disease or medical condition. Migraine headaches are one type of primary headache.

PRIMARY TUMOR. Abnormal growths that originated in the location where they were diagnosed.

PRION. A protein particle lacking nucleic acid and thought to be the cause of certain infectious diseases of the central nervous system, such as Creutzfeldt-Jakob disease.

PRODROMAL. Symptomatic of the approaching onset of an attack or a disease.

PRODROME. A symptom or group of symptoms that appears shortly before an acute attack of illness. The term comes from a Greek word that means "running ahead of."

PROGRESSIVE SUPRANUCLEAR PALSY. A rare disease that gradually destroys nerve cells in the parts of the brain that control eye movements, breathing, and muscle coordination. The loss of nerve cells causes palsy, or paralysis, that slowly gets worse as the disease progresses. The palsy affects ability to move the eyes, relax the muscles, and control balance.

PROJECTILE VOMITING. Forceful vomiting that is not preceded by nausea. It is usually associated with increased pressure inside the head.

PRONATION. The motion of the forearm to turn the palm downwards.

PROPHYLACTIC. Treatment given to protect against or ward off disease. Many doctors give antibiotics to patients who have been bitten by ticks as a prophylactic measure against Lyme disease.

PROPHYLAXIS. A measure taken to prevent disease or an acute attack of a chronic disorder. Migraine prophylaxis refers to medications taken to reduce the frequency of migraine attacks.

PROPRIOCEPTION. The ability to sense the location, position, orientation, and movement of the body and its parts.

PROSENCEPHALON. The part of the brain that develops from the front portion of the neural tube.

PROSTAGLANDINS. A group of hormone-like molecules that exert local effects on a variety of processes including fluid balance, blood flow, and gastrointestinal function. They may be responsible for the production of some types of pain and inflammation.

PROTEIN. Important building blocks of the body, composed of amino acids, involved in the formation of body structures and controlling the basic functions of the human body.

PROTEINURIA. Excess protein in the urine.

PROXIMAL MUSCLES. Muscles closest to the center of the body, such as muscles used in breathing and sitting upright.

PSYCHOMETRIC. The development, administration, and interpretation of tests to measure mental or psychological abilities. Psychometric tests convert an individual's psychological traits and attributes into a numerical estimation or evaluation.

PSYCHOMOTOR. Movement produced by action of the mind or will.

PSYCHOMOTOR RETARDATION. Slowing of movement and speech.

PSYCHOSIS. A severe mental disorder characterized by loss of contact with reality. Hallucinations are associated with such psychotic disorders as schizophrenia and brief psychotic disorder.

PSYCHOTHERAPY. Psychological counseling that seeks to determine the underlying causes of a patient's depression. The form of this counseling may be cognitive/behavioral, interpersonal, or psychodynamic.

PTOSIS. Drooping of the upper eyelid.

PUTAMEN. Structure in the brain that is connected to the caudate nucleus and a component of the corpus striatum.

Q

QI. The Chinese term for energy, life force, or vital force.

QUADRIPARESIS. Partial or incomplete paralysis of all four limbs.

QUADRIPLEGIA. Permanent paralysis of the trunk, lower and upper limbs. It is caused by injury or disease affecting the spinal cord at the neck level.

R

RADICULONEURITIS. Inflammation of a spinal nerve.

RADICULONEUROPATHY. Disease of the nerve roots and nerves.

RADIOISOTOPE. One of two or more atoms with the same number of protons but a different number of neutrons with a nuclear composition. In nuclear scanning, radioactive isotopes are used as a diagnostic agent.

RADIOLOGIST. A physician who specializes in imaging techniques such as x rays, CT scans, MRI scans, and certain scans using radioactive isotopes.

RADIOTHERAPY. The use of x rays or other radioactive substances to treat disease.

REBOUND HEADACHE. A type of primary headache caused by overuse of migraine medications or pain relievers. It is also known as analgesic abuse headache.

RECEPTOR. A structure located on the outside of a cell's membrane that causes the cell to attach to specific molecules; the molecules are then internalized, taken inside the cell, and they either activate or inhibit certain cellular functions.

RECESSIVE GENE. A type of gene that is not expressed as a trait unless inherited by both parents.

RECOMBINANT DNA. DNA that has been altered by joining genetic material from two different sources. It usually involves putting a gene from one organism into the genome of a different organism.

RECOMBINANT HUMAN GROWTH HORMONE. A synthetic form of growth hormone that can be given to a patient to help skeletal growth.

RELEASE HALLUCINATIONS. Hallucinations that develop after partial loss of sight or hearing, and represent images or sounds formed from memory traces rather than present sensory input. They are called "release" hallucinations because they would ordinarily be blocked by incoming sensory data.

RENAL CELL CARCINOMA. A type of kidney cancer.

RESONATOR. As used in regard to the human speech mechanism, it is the cavity extending from the vocal folds to the lips, which selectively amplifies and modifies the energies produced during speech and voice production. It is synonymous with the term vocal tract.

RESTLESS LEGS SYNDROME. A condition that causes an annoying feeling of tiredness, uneasiness, and itching deep within the muscle of the leg. It is accompanied by twitching and sometimes pain. The only relief is in walking or moving the legs.

RETICULAR ACTIVATING SYSTEM. A network of structures, including the brain stem, medulla, and thalamus, and nerve pathways, which function together to produce and maintain arousal.

RETINA. The inner, light-sensitive layer of the eye containing rods and cones. The retina transforms the image it receives into electrical signals that are sent to the brain via the optic nerve.

RETINAL ACHROMIC PATCH. Small area of the retina that is lighter than the area around it.

RETINITIS PIGMENTOSA. A family of genetically linked retinal diseases that causes progressive deterioration of peripheral vision and eventually blindness.

RETROCOLLIS. Muscular spasms that affect the neck muscles located in the back.

RETROGRADE AMNESIA. A form of amnesia, or memory loss, in which the memories lost are those that occurred before a traumatic injury.

RETROVIRUS. A family of ribonucleic acid (RNA) viruses containing a reverse transcriptase enzyme that allows the viruses' genetic information to become part of the genetic information of the host cell upon replication. Human immunodeficiency virus (HIV) is a retrovirus.

REYE SYNDROME. A serious, life-threatening illness in children, usually developing after a bout of flu or chicken pox, and often associated with the use of aspirin. Symptoms include uncontrollable vomiting, often with lethargy, memory loss, disorientation, or delirium. Swelling of the brain may cause seizures, coma, and in severe cases, death.

RHABDOMYOLYSIS. Breakdown of muscle fibers resulting in release of muscle contents into the blood.

RHABDOMYOMA. Non-cancerous growth in the heart muscle.

RHABDOMYOSARCOMA. A tumor of the tendons, muscles, or connective tissue.

RHEUMATIC FEVER. Fever following a throat infection with group A Streptococcus, typically affecting children and young adults.

RHINITIS. Inflammation and swelling of the nasal membranes.

RHIZOTOMY. Surgery to relieve pain by cutting the nerve root near its point of entry to the spinal cord.

RNA. Ribonucleic acid, a nucleic acid that transmits messages in the DNA to other elements in the cell.

RODENTICIDES. Chemical that kills rodents

ROTE LEARNING. Learning by means of repetition and memorization, usually without significant understanding of the concepts involved.

S

SACCULAR ANEURYSM. A type of aneurysm that resembles a small sack of blood attached to the outer surface of a blood vessel by a thin neck.

SACROILIAC JOINT. The joint between the triangular bone below the spine (sacrum) and the hip bone (ilium).

SACRUM. An area in the lower back, below the lumbar region.

SCAPULA. The bone also known as the shoulder blade.

SCHIZOPHRENIA. A severe mental illness in which a person has difficulty distinguishing what is real from what is not real. It is often characterized by hallucinations, delusions, and withdrawal from people and social activities.

SCHWANN CELL. A type of supportive cell in the nervous system that makes up the myelin sheath around nerve fibers, providing both insulation and increasing the speed of nerve conduction.

SCIATIC NERVE. The nerve controlling the muscles of the back of the knee and lower leg, and providing sensation to the back of the thigh, part of the lower leg, and the sole of the foot.

SCIATICA. A common form of nerve pain related to compression of fibers from one or more of the lower spinal nerve roots, characterized by burning low back pain radiating to the buttock and back of the leg to below the knee or even to the foot.

SCLERA. The tough white membrane that forms the outer layer of the eyeball.

SCOLIOSIS. An asymmetric curvature of the spine to one side.

SECONDARY HEADACHE. A headache that is caused by another disease or disorder.

SEDATIVE. A medication that has a calming effect and may be used to treat nervousness or restlessness. Sometimes used as a synonym for hypnotic.

SEIZURE. A sudden attack, spasm, or convulsion produced by an abnormal electrical discharge of neurons in the brain.

SEMICIRCULAR CANALS. A set of three fluid-filled loops in the inner ear that are important for balance.

SENSORIUM. The place in the brain where external expressions are localized and processed before being perceived.

SENSORY. Related to the senses, or the ability to feel.

SENSORY NERVES. Sensory or afferent nerves carry impulses of sensation from the periphery or outward parts of the body to the brain. Sensations include feelings, impressions, and awareness of the state of the body.

SEPSIS. A severe systemic infection in which bacteria have entered the bloodstream or body tissues.

SEPTUM PELLUCIDUM. Two-layered thin wall separating the right and the left anterior horn of lateral ventricle.

SEQUENCING. Genetic testing in which the entire sequence of deoxyribonucleic acid (DNA) bases that make up a gene is studied, in an effort to find a mutation.

SEROTONIN. A widely distributed neurotransmitter that is found in blood platelets, the lining of the digestive tract, and the brain, and that works in combination with norepinephrine. It causes very powerful contractions of smooth muscle and is associated with mood, attention, emotions, and sleep. Low levels of serotonin are associated with depression.

SEROTONIN SYNDROME. A potentially fatal drug interaction caused by combining drugs that raise the level of serotonin in the patient's nervous system to dangerously high levels. The symptoms of serotonin syndrome include shivering, overreactive reflexes, nausea, low-grade fever, sweating, delirium, mental confusion, and coma.

SERUM. The fluid part of the blood that remains after blood cells, platelets, and fibrogen have been removed. Also called blood serum.

SHAGREEN PATCHES. Patches of skin with the consistency of an orange peel.

SHAKEN BABY SYNDROME. A severe form of traumatic brain injury (TBI) resulting from shaking an infant or small child forcibly enough to cause the brain to jar against the skull.

SHINGLES. A disease caused by an infection with the herpes zoster virus, the same virus that causes chicken pox. Symptoms of shingles include pain and blisters along one nerve, usually on the face, chest, stomach, or back.

SKILLED NURSING FACILITY. An inpatient facility that provides 24-hour nursing services to individuals in need of extended care.

SKIN TAG. Abnormal outward pouching of skin, with a varying size.

SKULL. All of the bones of the head.

SLEEP APNEA. A condition in which a person temporarily stops breathing during sleep.

SLEEP PARALYSIS. An abnormal episode of sleep in which the patient cannot move for a few minutes, usually occurring while falling asleep or waking up. Sleep paralysis is often found in patients with narcolepsy.

SOMATIC EDUCATION. A term used in both Hellerwork and the Feldenkrais method to describe the integration of bodywork with self-awareness, intelligence, and imagination.

SOMATOFORM DISORDERS. A group of psychiatric disorders in the *Diagnostic and Statistical Manual of Mental Disorders,* Fourth Edition (DSM-IV) classification that are characterized by external physical symptoms or complaints related to psychological problems rather than organic illness.

SOUND WAVES. Changes in air pressure that produce an oscillating wave that transmits sound.

SPASM. Sudden involuntary muscle movement or contraction.

SPASTIC. Refers to a condition in which the muscles are rigid, posture may be abnormal, and fine motor control is impaired.

SPASTIC QUADRIPLEGIA. Inability to use and control movements of the arms and legs.

SPASTICITY. Increased muscle tone, or stiffness, which leads to uncontrolled, awkward movements.

SPEECH SYNTHESIZER. A computerized device that accepts input, interprets data, and produces audible language.

SPHENOID. A bone of the skull.

SPHENOIDAL ELECTRODES. Fine wire electrodes that are implanted under the cheek bones, used to measure temporal seizures.

SPHINCTER. A band of muscle that encircles an opening in the body, allowing the opening to open and close (anal sphincter, esophageal sphincter).

SPIKE WAVE DISCHARGE. Characteristic abnormal wave pattern in the electroencephalogram that is a hallmark of an area that has the potential of generating a seizure.

SPINA BIFIDA. A birth defect (a congenital malformation) in which part of the vertebrae fail to develop completely so that a portion of the spinal cord, which is normally protected within the vertebral column, is exposed. People with spina bifida can suffer from bladder and bowel incontinence, cognitive (learning) problems, and limited mobility.

SPINA BIFIDA OCCULTA. A relatively mild form of spina bifida in which the defect is not visible from the surface. This condition is most often asymptomatic.

SPINAL CORD. The part of the central nervous system that extends from the base of the skull and runs through the vertebral column in the back. It acts as a relay to convey information between the brain and the periphery.

SPINAL DEGENERATION. Wear and tear on the intervertebral discs, which can narrow the spinal canal and cause back stiffness and pain.

SPINAL FUSION. A surgical procedure that stabilizes the spine and prevents painful movements, but with resulting loss of flexibility.

SPINAL STENOSIS. A congenital narrowing of the spinal canal.

SPIROCHETE. A bacterium shaped like a loosely coiled spiral. The organism that causes Lyme disease is a spirochete.

SPONDYLITIS. Inflammation of the spinal joints, characterized by chronic back pain and stiffness.

SPONDYLOLISTHESIS. A more extreme form of spondylosis, with slippage of one vertebra relative to its neighbor.

SPONDYLOSIS. A condition in which one or more of the vertebral joints in the spine becomes stiff or fixed in one position.

SPORE. A dormant form assumed by some bacteria, such as anthrax, that enable the bacterium to survive high temperatures, dryness, and lack of nourishment for long periods of time. Under proper conditions, the spore may revert to the actively multiplying form of the bacteria. Also refers to the small, thick-walled reproductive structure of a fungus.

STATUS EPILEPTICUS. A serious condition involving continuous seizures with no conscious intervals.

STATUS MIGRAINOSUS. The medical term for an acute migraine headache that lasts 72 hours or longer.

STENOSIS. A condition in which an opening or passageway in the body is narrowed or constricted.

STERNOCLEIDOMASTOID MUSCLE. A muscle located in front of the neck that functions to turn the head from side to side.

STEROID. A class of drugs resembling normal body substances that often help control inflammation in the body tissues.

STIMULANT. Any chemical or drug that has excitatory actions in the central nervous system.

STORAGE DISEASES. Diseases in which too much of a substance (usually fats, glycogen, or certain enzymes) builds up in specific cells of the body and causes metabolic or tissue disorders.

STRABISMUS. Deviation of one eye from parallelism with the other.

STRESS. A physical and psychological response that results from being exposed to a demand or pressure.

STRIATUM. Area located deep within the brain.

STRIDOR. A high-pitched sound made when breathing, caused by the narrowing of the airway.

STROKE. Interruption of blood flow to a part of the brain with consequent brain damage. A stroke may be caused by a blood clot or by hemorrhage due to a burst blood vessel. Also known as a cerebrovascular accident.

STRUCTURAL INTEGRATION. The term used to describe the method and philosophy of life associated with Rolfing. Its fundamental concept is the vertical line.

STUTTERING. A disorder characterized by speech that has more dysfluencies (involuntary hesitations and repetitions) than is considered average.

SUBARACHNOID. The space underneath the layer of meningeal membrane called the arachnoid.

SUBARACHNOID HEMORRHAGE. A cause of some strokes in which arteries on the surface of the brain begin bleeding.

SUBARACHNOID SPACE. The space between two membranes surrounding the spinal cord and brain, the arachnoid and pia mater.

SUBCORTICAL. The neural centers located below (inferior to) the cerebral cortex.

SUBDURAL ELECTRODES. Strip electrodes that are placed under dura mater (the outermost, toughest, and most fibrous of the three membranes [meninges] covering the brain and spinal cord). They are used to locate foci of epileptic seizures prior to epilepsy surgery.

SUBDURAL HEMATOMA. A localized accumulation of blood, sometimes mixed with spinal fluid, in the space between the middle (arachnoid) and outer (dura mater) membranes covering the brain. It is caused by an injury to the head that tears blood vessels.

SUBEPENDYMAL GIANT CELL ASTROCYTOMA. Specific type of cancerous brain tumor found in tuberous sclerosis.

SUBSTANTIA NIGRA. One of the movement control centers of the brain. It can become depleted of a specific neurotransmitter, dopamine, and cause symptoms of Parkinson's disease.

SULFONAMIDES. A group of antibiotics used to treat a wide range of bacterial infections.

SUPERIOR OBLIQUE MUSCLE. One of six extraocular muscles concerned with eye movement. The superior oblique muscle pushes the eye down, turns it inward and rotates it outward.

SYLVIAN FISSURE. The lateral fold separating the brain hemisphere into the frontal and temporal lobes.

SYMPATHETIC NERVOUS SYSTEM. A branch of the autonomic nervous system that regulates involuntary reactions to stress such as increased heart and breathing rates, blood vessel contraction, and reduction in digestive secretions.

SYMPATHETIC SKIN RESPONSE. Minute change of palmar and plantar electrical potential.

SYNAPSE. A junction between two neurons. At a synapse the neurons are separated by a tiny gap called the synaptic cleft.

SYNCOPE. A loss of consciousness over a short period of time, caused by a temporary lack of oxygen in the brain.

SYNDROME. A group of symptoms that together characterize a disease or disorder.

SYPHILIS. Sexually transmitted disease caused by a corkscrew shaped bacterium called *Treponema pallidum*. It is characterized by three clinical stages, namely primary, secondary, and tertiary or late syphilis.

SYRINGOMYELIA. Excessive fluid in the spinal cord.

SYRINX. Abnormal fluid-filled cavities within the spinal cord.

T

TACHYCARDIA. Elevated heart rate.

TACHYPNEA. Elevated breathing rate.

TELANGIECTASIS. Very small arteriovenous malformations, or connections between the arteries and veins. The result is small red spots on the skin known as "spider veins."

TEMPORAL LOBE. A large lobe of each hemisphere of the brain that is located on the side of the head, nearest the ears. It contains a sensory area associated with hearing.

TENDON REFLEX. This is a simple circuit that consists of a stimulus, like a sharp tap delivered to a tendon, and the response, muscle contraction. It is used to test the integrity of the nervous system.

TERATOGEN. A substance that has been demonstrated to cause physical defects in the developing human embryo.

TERATOGENIC. Able to cause birth defects.

TETANUS. Denotes continuous, involuntary contraction of voluntary muscles due to repetitive stimuli from nerve endings. It can occur due to infection with a bacterium called *Clostridium tetani*.

THALAMOTOMY. A surgical procedure that destroys part of a large oval area of gray matter within the brain that acts as a relay center for nerve impulses. The thalamus is an essential part of the nerve pathway that controls intentional movement. By destroying tissue at a particular spot on the thalamus, the surgeon can interrupt the nerve signals that cause tremor.

THALAMUS. A pair of oval masses of gray matter within the brain that relay sensory impulses from the spinal cord to the cerebrum.

THALIDOMIDE. A mild sedative that is teratogenic, causing limb, neurologic, and other birth defects in infants exposed during pregnancy. Women used thalidomide (early in pregnancy) in Europe and in other countries between 1957 and 1961. It is still available in many places, including the United States, for specific medical uses (leprosy, AIDS, cancer).

THERMOGRAPHY. A test using infrared sensing devices to measure differences in temperature in body regions thought to be the source of pain.

THORACIC. Referring to the area of the torso commonly called the chest. There are 12 thoracic vertebrae.

THROMBOSIS. The formation of a blood clot in a vein or artery that may obstruct local blood flow or may dislodge, travel downstream, and obstruct blood flow at a remote location. The clot or thrombus may lead to infarction, or death of tissue, due to a blocked blood supply.

THROMBUS. A blood clot, which may form at the site of an atherosclerotic plaque and block the artery.

THYMOMA. A tumor that originates in the thymus, a small gland located in the upper chest just below the neck, that produces hormones necessary for the development of certain components of the immune system.

THYROTOXICOSIS. The most common form of hyperthyroidism, characterized by bulging eyes, rapid heart rate, and other symptoms. Also called Graves' disease.

THYROXINE. Hormone produced by the thyroid gland.

TIC. A brief and intermittent involuntary movement or sound.

TINNITUS. A noise, ranging from faint ringing or thumping to roaring, that originates in the ear not in the environment.

TONIC. A type of seizure characterized by episodes of stiffening in all the limbs for up to one or two minutes.

TOPICAL. For application to the surface of the skin.

TORTICOLLIS. Twisting of the neck to one side that results in abnormal carriage of the head and is usually caused by muscle spasms. Also called wryneck.

TOURETTE SYNDROME. An abnormal condition that causes uncontrollable facial grimaces and tics and arm and shoulder movements. Tourette syndrome is perhaps best known for uncontrollable vocal tics that include grunts, shouts, and use of obscene language (coprolalia).

TRACHEOSTOMY. A surgical procedure that makes an opening in the windpipe to bypass the obstructed airway.

TRACTION. Spinal stretching using weights applied to the spine, once thought to decrease pressure on the nerve roots but now seldom used.

TRANSCRIPTION FACTOR. A protein that acts to regulate the expression of genes.

TRANSIENT ISCHEMIC ATTACK (TIA). A brief interruption of the blood supply to part of the brain, it causes a temporary impairment of vision, speech, or movement. Usually the episode lasts for just a few moments, but it may be a warning sign for a full-scale stroke.

TRANSMISSIBLE SPONGIFORM ENCEPHALOPATHY. A term that refers to a group of diseases, including kuru, Creutzfeldt-Jakob disease, Gerstmann-Straussler-Scheinker syndrome, fatal familial insomnia, and new variant Creutzfeldt-Jakob disease. These diseases share a common origin as prion diseases, caused by abnormal proteins that accumulate within the brain and destroy brain tissue, leaving spongy holes.

TRANSVERSE MYELITIS. A neurologic syndrome caused by inflammation of the spinal cord.

TRAPEZIUS. Muscle of the upper back that rotates the shoulder blade, raises the shoulder, and flexes the arm.

TREMOR. Involuntary shakiness or trembling.

TREMOR CONTROL THERAPY. A method for controlling tremor by self-administered shocks to the part of the brain that controls intentional movement (thalamus). An electrode attached to an insulated lead wire is implanted in the brain; the battery power source is implanted under the skin of the chest, and an extension wire is tunneled under the skin to connect the battery to the lead. The patient turns on the power source to deliver the electrical impulse and interrupt the tremor.

TRICEPS. Muscle of the back of the upper arm, primarily responsible for extending the elbow.

TRIGEMINAL NERVE. The main sensory nerve of the face and motor nerve for chewing muscles.

TRIGEMINAL NEURALGIA. Brief episodes of severe shooting pain on one side of the face caused by inflammation of the root of the trigeminal nerve. Also referred to as tic douloureux.

TRIGGER FINGER. An overuse disorder of the hand in which one or more fingers tend to lock or "trigger" when the patient tries to extend the finger.

TRINUCLEOTIDE. A sequence of three nucleotides.

TRINUCLEOTIDE REPEAT EXPANSION. A sequence of three nucleotides that is repeated too many times in a section of a gene.

TRIPTANS. Also known as serotonin agonists or 5-hydroxytryptamine receptor agonists, triptans are a class of drugs that are used in the treatment of migraine headaches.

TRISOMY. An abnormality in chromosomal development. In a trisomy syndrome, an extra chromosome is present so that the individual has three of a particular chromosome instead of the normal pair. An extra chromosome 18 (trisomy 18) causes mental retardation.

TSUBO. In shiatsu, a center of high energy located along one of the body's meridians. Stimulation of the tsubos during a shiatsu treatment is thought to rebalance the flow of vital energy in the body.

TUBEROUS SCLEROSIS. A genetic condition that affects many organ systems including the brain, skin, heart, eyes, and lungs. Benign (non-cancerous) growths or tumors called hamartomas form in various parts of the body, disrupting their normal function.

TUBERS. Firm growths in the brain, named for their resemblance in shape to potato stems.

TUMOR. An abnormal growth of cells. Tumors may be benign (noncancerous) or malignant (cancerous).

TUMORIGENESIS. Formation of tumors.

U

ULNAR NERVE. The nerve that supplies some of the forearm muscles, the elbow joint, and many of the short muscles of the hand.

ULTRASONOGRAPHY. A medical test in which sound waves are directed against internal structures in the body. As sound waves bounce off the internal structure, they create an image on a video screen. Ultrasonography is often used to diagnose fetal abnormalities, gallstones, heart defects, and tumors. Also called ultrasound imaging.

UNILATERAL. Refers to one side of the body or only one organ in a pair.

URINARY INCONTINENCE. Lacking the ability to control urinary excretion.

UVEITIS. Inflammation of all or part the uvea. The uvea is a continuous layer of tissue that consists of the iris, the ciliary body, and the choroid. The uvea lies between the retina and sclera.

V

VAGINISMUS. An involuntary spasm of the muscles surrounding the vagina, making penetration painful or impossible.

VAGUS NERVE. Tenth cranial nerve and an important part of the autonomic nervous system, influencing motor functions in the larynx, diaphragm, stomach, and heart, and sensory functions in the ears and tongue.

VALSALVA MANEUVER. A strain against a closed airway combined with muscle tightening, such as happens when a person holds his or her breath and tries to move a heavy object. Most people perform this maneuver several times a day without adverse consequences, but it can be dangerous for anyone with cardiovascular disease. Pilots perform this maneuver to prevent black-outs during high-performance flying.

VASCULAR. Related to the blood vessels.

VASCULITIS. Inflammation of the walls of the blood vessels.

VASOCONSTRICTIVE. Causing a blood vessel to become narrower, thus decreasing blood flow.

VASODILATOR. Any drug that relaxes blood vessel walls.

VASOMOTOR. Referring to the regulation of the diameter of blood vessels.

VECTOR. A carrier organism (such as a fly or mosquito) that serves to deliver a virus (or other agent of infection) to a host. Also refers to a retrovirus that had been modified and is used to introduce specific genes into the genome of an organism.

VENTRAL. Pertaining in direction to the front or lower surface of an organ.

VENTRICLES. In neurology, the four fluid-filled chambers, or cavities, found in the two cerebral hemispheres of the brain, at the center of the brain, and between the brain stem and cerebellum. They are linked by channels, or ducts, allowing cerebral fluid to circulate through them.

VENTRICULOPERITONEAL SHUNT. A tube equipped with a low-pressure valve, one end of which is inserted into a cerebral ventricle, the other end of which is routed into the peritoneum, or abdominal cavity.

VENTRICULOSTOMY. Surgery that drains cerebrospinal fluid from the brain to treat hydrocephalus or increased intracranial pressure.

VERMIS. The central portion of the cerebellum, which divides the two hemispheres. It functions to monitor and control movement of the limbs, trunk, head, and eyes.

VERTEBRAE. Singular, vertebra. The individual bones of the spinal column that are stacked on top of each other. There is a hole in the center of each bone through which the spinal cord passes.

VERTEX PRESENTATION. Head presentation during delivery.

VERTIGO. A feeling of dizziness together with a sensation of movement and a feeling of rotating in space.

VESICLE. A small, raised lesion filled with clear fluid.

VESTIBULAR. A term that refers to the organs of balance.

VESTIBULAR SYSTEM. The sensory system located in the inner ear that allows the body to maintain balance.

VIRUS. A small infectious agent consisting of a core of genetic material (DNA or RNA) surrounded by a shell of protein. A virus needs a living cell to reproduce.

VISCERAL. Generally related to the digestive, respiratory, urogenital, or endocrine organs.

VISUAL FIELD. A field of vision that is visible without eye movement.

VITAMINS. Small compounds required for metabolism that must be supplied by diet, microorganisms in the gut (vitamin K), or sunlight (UV light converts pre-vitamin D to vitamin D).

VOLUNTARY MUSCLE. A muscle under conscious control; contrasted with smooth muscle and heart muscle which are not under voluntary control.

W

WESTERN BLOT. A sensitive laboratory blood test for specific antibodies; useful in confirming the diagnosis of AIDS.

WHITE MATTER. A substance, composed primarily of myelin fibers, found in the brain and nervous system that protects nerves and allows messages to be sent to and from the brain and various parts of the body. Also called white substance.

WHITE MATTER RADIAL MIGRATION LINE. White lines seen on a brain scan, signifying abnormal movement of neurons (brain cells) at that area.

WITHDRAWAL SYMPTOMS. A group of physical or mental symptoms that may occur when a person suddenly stops using a drug upon which he or she has become dependent.

WOODS LAMP. Lamp that uses ultraviolet light, making subtle skin changes more obvious.

WRAPAROUND. A relatively new form of mental health service delivery that strives to accommodate all family members based on self-defined needs, flexibly incorporating both formal and informal community services.

X

X INACTIVATION. The process in which each cell in a girl's body selects at random and turns off one of its two X chromosomes. X inactivation is one reason why some patients with Rett syndrome (RS) have more severe symptoms than others.

X RAY. Electromagnetic radiation of very short wavelength and very high energy.

Y

YIN AND YANG. In traditional Chinese medicine and philosophy, a pair of opposing forces whose harmonious balance in the body is necessary for good health.

INDEX

Numbers before a colon indicate volume. Numbers after a colon indicate page references. **Boldface** page numbers indicate the main essay for a topic. *Italicized* page numbers indicate photographs or illustrations.

A

AAMR (American Association on Mental Retardation), 2:526

AAN (American Academy of Neurology), 2:602

AB42 protein, 1:37

ABCN (American Board of Clinical Neuropsychology), 2:610

Abducens nerve, 2:906

Abetalipoproteinemia. *See* Bassen-Kornzweig syndrome

Ablative lesions, 2:650

ABPP (American Board of Professional Psychology), 2:610

Absence seizures, 2:755, 756, 798, 816

Abulia, 1:**1–2**

Abuse. *See* Child neglect or abuse; Drug abuse

Abusive head trauma. *See* Shaken baby syndrome

Acanthocytosis. *See* Bassen-Kornzweig syndrome

ACC (Agenesis of the corpus callosum), 1:**16–20**, *498*

Accidental ingestion of medication, 1:112

Acetaminophen, 1:**280–282**, 446–447

Acetazolamide, 1:**2–3**, 2:708

Acetyl-CoA-alpha-glucosaminide acetyltransferase, 2:554

Acetylcholine (ACh)
  anticholinergics effects, 1:62, 263
  cholinergic stimulants effects, 1:228, 229
  congenital myasthenia, 1:237
  history, 2:615
  Lambert-Eaton myasthenic syndrome, 1:471
  motor neuron diseases, 2:543
  myasthenia, congenital, 2:573
  myasthenia gravis, 2:574–576
  neuromuscular blockers effects, 2:602

in sympathetic preganglionic synapses, 2:660

Acid alpha-glucosidase, 2:685

Acid sphingomyelinase (ASM), 2:617

ACPA (American Chronic Pain Association), 2:639

Acquired brain injuries. *See* Traumatic brain injuries

Acquired Creutzfeldt-Jakob disease, 1:250

Acquired immunodeficiency syndrome. *See* AIDS

Acrodermatitus chronica atrophicans, 1:507

ACT (Assertive community treatment) programs, 2:749

ACTH. *See* Adrenocorticotropin

Acupuncture, 1:**3–7**, *5, 6*
  for back pain, 1:136
  for headaches, 1:408
  for Mèniére's disease, 2:522
  for pain, 2:639
  for repetitive motion disorders, 2:725, 726

Acute confusional state. *See* Delirium

Acute disseminated encephalomyelitis (ADE), 1:**8–9**, 274

Acute flaccid paralysis. *See* Guillain-Barré syndrome

Acute idiopathic polyneuritis. *See* Guillain-Barré syndrome

Acute inflammatory demyelinating polyneuropathy (AIDP). *See* Guillain-Barré syndrome

Acute thyrotoxic myopathy, 2:843

Acyclovir, 1:83, 336

Addams, Jane, 2:773

Addiction. *See* Alcohol abuse; Drug abuse

Addison disease, 1:10

ADE (Acute disseminated encephalomyelitis), 1:**8–9**, 274

Adenine deaminase deficiency, 1:383

Adenosine triphosphate (ATP), 2:536, 842

ADHD. *See* Attention deficit hyperactivity disorder

ADLP gene, 1:489

ADM (Amyopathic dermatomyositis). *See* Dermatomyositis

Adolescents, ADHD treatment, 1:122

Adrenal glands
  adrenoleukodystrophy, 1:9–12
  Cushing syndrome, 1:254, 255–256
  glucocorticoid manufacture, 1:390
  von Hippel-Lindau disease, 2:914, 915

Adrenocorticotropin (ACTH)
  Cushing syndrome, 1:254–255
  infantile spasms, 1:453
  opsoclonus myoclonus, 2:624–625

Adrenoleukodystrophy (ALD), 1:**9–13**, 114, 489, 491

Adrenomyeloneuropathy, 1:10

Adult day care, 2:727

Affective disorders, 1:**13–16**

AFP (Alpha-fetoprotein), 2:792

Africa (encephalitis lethargica cases), 1:338
  See also World health issues

African trypansomiasis. *See* Encephalitis lethargica

Agenesis of the corpus callosum (ACC), 1:**16–20**, *498*

Ageusia, 1:60–61

Aggrenox, 2:861

Aging
  exercise and, 1:355
  hearing disorders, 1:410
  nerve impulse speed, 2:596
  shingles, 2:761
  transient global amnesia, 2:856
  visual disturbances, 2:907

Agnosia, 1:**20–22**

AIDP (Acute inflammatory demyelinating polyneuropathy). *See* Guillain-Barré syndrome

E

H

M

N

O

P

T

U